CW01590185

Atlas of

Neurosurgery

Basic Approaches to Cranial and Vascular Procedures

Fredric B. Meyer, M.D.
Consultant
Department of Neurologic Surgery
Mayo Clinic and Mayo Foundation
Professor of Neurosurgery
Mayo Medical School
Rochester, Minnesota

Illustrations by
Gillian Duncan, M.S.

CHURCHILL LIVINGSTONE
A Division of Harcourt Brace & Company
Edinburgh London Philadelphia San Francisco

CHURCHILL LIVINGSTONE
A Division of Harcourt Brace & Company

The Curtis Center
Independence Square West
Philadelphia, Pennsylvania 19106

Library of Congress Cataloging-in-Publication Data

Meyer, Fredric B.
Atlas of neurosurgery/Fredric B. Meyer.—1st ed.

p. cm.

ISBN 0–443–08951–5

1. Brain—Surgery—Atlases. 2. Nervous system—Surgery—Atlases.
I. Title.
[DNLM: 1. Neurosurgical Procedures atlases. 2. Brain—surgery atlases. WL 17 M612a 1999]

RD594.M49 1999 617.4′8—dc21

DNLM/DLC 98–18407

ATLAS OF NEUROSURGERY ISBN 0–443–08951–5

Copyright © 1999 by Mayo Foundation.

All rights reserved. No part of this publication may be reproduced or transmitted in any form or by any means, electronic or mechanical, including photocopy, recording, or any information storage and retrieval system, without permission in writing from the publisher.

Printed in the United States of America.

Last digit is the print number: 9 8 7 6 5 4 3 2 1

Atlas of

Neurosurgery

Basic Approaches to
Cranial and Vascular Procedures

Preface

The purpose of this *Atlas* is to provide neurosurgeons an educational tool useful when preparing to perform common intracranial and vascular procedures. Originally, this *Atlas* was intended to be a manual of practical information for my neurosurgical residents. Over the years, the conception has developed from a pen and ink spiral-bound manual into the present full-color book. The operations chosen for review in this *Atlas* were based on a list created by determining the frequency of each procedure performed on my service, excluding those required to treat traumatic lesions.

The discussions on anatomy are purposely brief to focus on information that should be immediately helpful when performing an operation. In fact, the *Atlas* is organized from the perspective of a surgical approach. Each of the operations considered deserves a special monograph of its own (and many such detailed monographs are available); nonetheless, the simplified text of the *Atlas* is intended to provide a framework for the surgeon to review ways of accessing a region and performing a particular surgical procedure.

The operative approaches described here reflect my synthesis of the techniques and surgical skills I have learned from my teachers and colleagues. I am indebted to my neurosurgical colleagues—past and present—at the Mayo Clinic: the late Dr. Thoralf M. Sundt, Jr., vascular and brain tumor surgery; Dr. Burton M. Onofrio, skull base and spine approaches; Dr. David G. Piepgras, vascular, brain tumor, and skull base surgery; Dr. Edward R. Laws, brain tumor, epilepsy, and pituitary surgery; Dr. Patrick J. Kelly, brain tumor and stereotactic surgery; Dr. Michael J. Ebersold, brain tumor and skull base surgery; Dr. W. Richard Marsh, brain tumor and epilepsy surgery; Dr. Dudley H. Davis, brain tumor surgery and general neurosurgical approaches; Dr. Robert J. Coffey, stereotactic and functional surgery; Dr. William E. Krauss, spine and skull base surgery; Dr. John L. D. Atkinson, vascular and brain tumor surgery; Dr. Corey Raffel, pediatric neurosurgery; and Dr. Bruce E. Pollock, stereotactic and functional surgery. Dr. Pollock, with the assistance of Dr. Atkinson, wrote the chapter on percutaneous procedures for the treatment of facial pain.

The following general rules of conduct and practice are ones I attempt to follow and encourage neurosurgical residents to adopt:

1. Always remember the patient who suffered a complication and learn from that event to avoid making the same mistake in the future.
2. Be humble, especially with a great result.
3. Only recommend an operation that you would choose for yourself if you had the same condition as the patient. Too often, the choice to proceed with surgery is based primarily on emotion. When making a surgical decision, your intellect should control your emotions.
4. Be realistic about your technical skills.
5. Take a minimalist approach. When treating any lesion surgically, consider the simplest solution. Avoid grandiose, involved options.
6. Use the professional resources available to you, including neuroradiology and neurology. Be willing to get and to listen to advice.
7. Know the anatomy of the area being operated on.
8. Do not "pick" (e.g., glioma resection margin, endarterectomy bed, ventricular ependymal surface after resection of a trigone meningioma). A corollary of this rule is do not finick or repeatedly reposition an aneurysm clip if the overall placement is acceptable.
9. Know a few instruments well. Most of the cranial operations on my surgical service are performed with interchangeable #5 or #7 suction tips, 0.7- and 1.0-mm tip bipolar cautery, micro ball tip dissector, small black dissecting spatula, straight or angled Gimmick dissector, Penfield #1 and #3 dissectors, Gerald forceps, straight and curved microscissors, knot-tying forceps, Castroviejo microneedle holder, and ring curets.
10. Use one retractor blade. It is exceedingly rare that a second retractor is ever required. In fact, many operations can be performed without a retraction blade.
11. Always use magnification with illumination. The operating microscope is essential for most neurosurgical procedures.
12. Be courteous and thankful to the paramedical staff who assist you.

It is a pleasure to acknowledge the great help I received from the following persons. First, Ms. Gillian Duncan, MS, an expert medical illustrator. Each drawing was meticulously created and then recreated after she spent many hours in the operating room and anatomy laboratory. In addition to her great artistic talent, I appreciate the patience she showed in working with me. Mr. Robert Benassi, Emeritus Head of the Section of Visual Information, assisted with the initial stages of several drawings. Thanks also to Mr. Steven D. Orwoll, Ms. Sue Mundy, Mr. James J. Tidwell, Mr. Thomas E. Bibby, and Mr. Fred Graszer, in the Section of Computer Graphics, for their superb computer colorization of the drawings and to Dr. O. E. Millhouse, Mrs. Roberta J. Schwartz, Mrs. Sharon L. Wadleigh, and Mrs. Dorothy L. Tienter, in the Section of Publications, for help in editing and preparing the manuscript for publication. I am also indebted to Mr. Robert E. Anderson for expertly supervising our Thoralf M. Sundt, Jr. Research Laboratory, Mrs. Wanda L. Windschitl for her outstanding patient care, and to my long-time dedicated operating room technicians, Mrs. Helen Morrison and Ms. Eileen M. Zirbel. Special thanks to my secretaries, Ms. Mary M. Soper, for sifting through tedious writing, dictation, and redictation to produce readable drafts of each chapter, and Ms. Marylin J. Witts, for her remarkable kindness in helping me take care of neurosurgical patients and for her patience with me. I am also indebted to our neurosurgical residents whose enthusiasm and intellectual drive continue to teach and inspire me.

Most importantly, I thank my lovely wife Irene, who is not only a devoted mother of five children but also a clinical neurologist at the Mayo Clinic. To my children Jenna, Ilana, Benjamin, Jacob, and Robert, you continue to teach me that in the end the only thing that truly matters is coming home.

FREDRIC B. MEYER, M.D.

NOTICE

Medicine is an ever-changing field. Standard safety precautions must be followed, but as new research and clinical experience broaden our knowledge, changes in treatment and drug therapy become necessary or appropriate. Readers are advised to check the product information currently provided by the manufacturer of each drug to be administered to verify the recommended dose, the method and duration of administration, and the contraindications. It is the responsibility of the treating physician relying on experience and knowledge of the patient to determine dosages and the best treatment for the patient. Neither the Publisher nor the editor assumes any responsibility for any injury and or damage to persons or property.

THE PUBLISHER

Contents

1

Pterional Approach

Copyright © 1999 Mayo Foundation.

PROCEDURE

Although Dandy noted the importance of the keyhole bur hole to approach the optic chiasm and neurosurgeons have long used the subfrontal approach, Yasargil deserves credit for developing the pterional approach. He emphasized that combining the frontotemporal approach with resection of the outer sphenoid wing provides access to the circle of Willis, with minimal retraction of the brain.

In the classic pterional approach, the temporalis muscle and its investing fascia are cut off the bone at the junction between the posterior orbital rim and the zygomatic arch, and through an incision in the temporal line, the muscle can be dissected posteriorly without injury to its nerve or blood supply, thereby minimizing muscle atrophy. However, with this intrafascial approach, there is risk of injury to the frontalis branch of the facial nerve from retraction or dissection. With the muscle-splitting flap described below (and advocated by many surgeons), approximately the front half of the temporalis muscle is dissected anteriorly in conjunction with the skin flap. In this way, there is minimal risk of injury to the facial nerve. One disadvantage of this is that the angle of the approach is altered ever so slightly, and this sometimes requires more retraction of the brain to achieve exposure.

Head Position

For the muscle-splitting flap, the head is extended slightly; this allows the frontal lobe to fall away from the skull base, thus decreasing the need for brain retraction. The head is also rotated approximately 25 to 30 degrees opposite to the side of the craniotomy. Occasionally, it is necessary to put a towel under the patient's shoulder on the side of the craniotomy. Minimal shaving of the head is required. The incision is made 1.0 to 1.5 cm behind the hairline, so that the scar is not visible.

Skin Flap

The incision is started in front of the ear and carried to the midline, avoiding the anterior limb of the superficial temporal artery. The incision is made through both the skin and the temporalis muscle, and together, they are swept forward. The muscle fibers can be dissected off the cranium with a periosteal elevator and with bipolar coagulation of arterial feeders. This reduces the degree of atrophy of the temporalis muscle (atrophy can occur when a monopolar cutting current is used to separate the muscle from the skull). The skin flap and temporalis muscle are retracted with 3 to 4 fishhooks placed under tension.

Bone Flap

With current craniotomes, it is not necessary to place multiple bur holes. Still, it is helpful to mark on the skull surface the four bur holes that would be required if Gigli saws were used. When a craniotome is used, there is a tendency to limit the craniotomy, thereby compromising exposure. The critical keyhole bur hole is placed just behind the orbital rim, immediately superior to the frontal zygomatic suture. This keyhole provides access to both the anterior and middle cranial fossae. The second bur hole is placed just above the orbital rim, between the inner canthus and the mid-pupillary line. By placing this bur hole medial to the mid-pupillary line, the surgeon can use a more subfrontal approach, if required. The lower this bur hole, the less brain retraction required. Although it is preferable to stay out of the frontal sinus, exposure should never be sacrificed only to preserve the integrity of the sinus. If the frontal sinus is entered and the mucosa has not been violated, a piece of temporalis muscle should be placed in the opening to obliterate the communication. Alternatively, if the mucosa has been violated, it should be removed. A piece of temporalis muscle is used to plug the deep ostium. A third bur hole is placed in the parietal bone 4 cm posterior to the second bur hole in the linea temporalis near the coronal suture. A fourth bur hole is placed low in the squamous temporal bone behind the sphenoid temporal suture. When making the cut between this fourth bur hole and the keyhole bur hole, it is important that the incision swing low and anterior along the floor of the middle cranial fossa. A diamond bur can be used instead of a craniotome to create this fourth cut. This has the advantage of ensuring that the cut is low and anterior, to better expose the temporal lobe. A low and anterior bone cut becomes important when a lateral approach or line of site along the sphenoid wing is desirable for approaching difficult posterior communicating artery aneurysms.

After elevation of the bone flap, it is helpful to remove the outer one-third to one-half of the sphenoid wing down close to the superior orbital fissure. First, the dura mater is stripped off the sphenoid wing with a Penfield dissector or periosteal elevator. Next, a diamond bur is used to drill off the outer sphenoid wing for a depth of approximately 3 cm. Approximately a 1.0- to 1.5-cm width of outer sphenoid wing can be removed to improve exposure and to decrease the need for brain retraction. Occasionally, part of the orbital roof is removed inadvertently, but this is of little concern. If the patient has a thick frontal bone, it may be helpful to remove the inner one-half table of bone between the sphenoid wing and orbital bur hole to increase exposure and to minimize brain retraction.

Opening of the Dura Mater

If the dura mater is going to be closed with a graft, it is best to open the dura mater and to tack it to the bone and muscle margins. If this is done, there is no risk that the underlying cerebral cortex will be injured inadvertently by a tack suture. However, if the dura mater is going to be closed primarily, it is necessary to tack the dura before it is opened by placing the tack sutures in the outer layer of the dura mater. The dura mater is opened in a way that allows it to be reflected over the sphenoid wing and tacked to the temporalis muscle. This will decrease the amount of blood running into the wound. A small "t" is extended over the temporal lobe and tacked to the edge of the bone to facilitate exposure of the Sylvian fissure. The remaining dura mater is tacked to the bone margins but left intact to protect the brain.

Division of the Sylvian Fissure

The Sylvian fissure can be divided with either a medial to lateral or a lateral to medial approach. In most circumstances, the latter method is better. However, in young patients or in some patients with a severe subarachnoid hemorrhage, the Sylvian fissure is obliterated or not present. In this case, the surgeon must temporarily retract the frontal lobe to initially identify the carotid artery adjacent to the clinoid process and then work from medial to lateral to divide the fissure. It is for this reason—that is, to minimize the degree of brain retraction in case an initial subfrontal approach is required—that it is important to ensure that the frontal cut made during the craniotomy is low and just above the orbital ridge.

In the more standard dissection of the Sylvian fissure, the frontal lobe first is protected with hemostatic fabric (Surgicel) covered by a large cottonoid (Americot). By placing the hemostatic fabric first, it will be easier to remove the cottonoid from the brain at the end of the operation and there will be less risk of subpial hemorrhage. Gently, the frontal lobe is retracted medially and upward, which places tension on the arachnoid between the frontal and temporal lobes. Under the operating microscope, a small incision is made in the arachnoid with a #11 blade knife. Any large Sylvian veins should be kept lateral with the temporal lobe. After the initial incision is made in the arachnoid, it is enlarged with either a straight microscissors or bipolar forceps. Occasionally, small veins that bridge the Sylvian fissure must be cauterized and divided. There is wide variation in vascular anatomy among patients, and in some, the middle cerebral artery is quite superficial and prone to injury. After the outer, or superficial, Sylvian fissure has been divided, the frontal retractor is repositioned to provide new tension on the deep arachnoid. The dissection of the arachnoid along the Sylvian fissure is extended down to the carotid bifurcation.

At this point, it is best to incise the arachnoid on both sides of the carotid artery to achieve vascular control, especially in cases of cerebral aneurysm. After the carotid bifurcation has been dissected free of arachnoid, the lesion dictates the approach to dissecting the arachnoid off the anterior cerebral artery. Specifically, if the operation is for a craniopharyngioma, the arachnoid between the anterior cerebral artery and the optic chiasm should be incised. This will allow the anterior cerebral artery to be retracted, with the frontal lobe still protected by arachnoid. Alternatively, if the lesion is an anterior communicating artery aneurysm, the arachnoid on both sides of the proximal anterior cerebral artery needs to be incised for control of proximal blood vessels.

NEUROSURGICAL ANATOMY

Because the optic nerve is the anatomic landmark and serves as a reference to all other structures in this region, it should be identified early in the exposure. There is significant variation among patients regarding the diameter and length of the internal carotid artery, the location of the carotid bifurcation, the size and extent of the anterior clinoid process, and whether the optic chiasm is prefixed or postfixed. The anatomic publications of Yasargil and Rhoton and their colleagues are required reading.

Ophthalmic Artery

The ophthalmic artery originates medially from the internal carotid artery as it emerges from the cavernous sinus underneath the anterior clinoid process. The ophthalmic artery arises from the subdural portion of the internal carotid artery in 90 percent of patients and at the carotid-dural ring in 2 percent. In the other 8 percent of patients, its origin is extradural, from the cavernous carotid artery. As the ophthalmic artery leaves the internal carotid artery, it runs along the inferior surface of the optic nerve, delicately attached by loose connective tissue. The artery enters the optic canal inferiorly to the optic nerve by piercing the dural sheath of the optic nerve. As the artery runs through the optic canal, it is inferior to the optic nerve. The artery penetrates the orbit and curves medially, either above or below the optic nerve.

Superior Hypophysial Artery

Several small arteries, named the superior hypophysial arteries, usually exit from the inferior medial portion of the internal carotid artery underneath the optic nerve and supply the pituitary stalk, anterior lobe of the pituitary, and the inferior surface of the optic nerve and chiasm. These small arteries anastomose with their counterparts from the opposite internal carotid artery and with the inferior hypophysial arteries form a vascular plexus around the pituitary stalk.

Posterior Communicating Artery

The next major branch of the internal carotid artery is the posterior communicating artery. It originates from the inferior lateral wall of the supraclinoid internal carotid artery, 2 to 7 mm distal to the anterior clinoid process, and exits from the carotid cistern by penetrating the arachnoid posteriorly and inferiorly to enter the interpeduncular cistern. This portion of the posterior communicating artery is covered by arachnoid. As the artery runs posteriorly, it is adjacent to the posterior clinoid process, to which it is occasionally adherent. In approximately 60 percent of patients, the posterior communicating artery is 2 mm or less in diameter. Its diameter is larger in children than in adults. In approximately 10 percent of patients, the posterior communicating artery is hypoplastic or absent. Rarely, it can have a duplication or fenestration. After it leaves the internal carotid artery, the posterior communicating artery runs medially and, thus, is hidden from view if the surgeon uses a subfrontal approach to this region. If a more lateral or temporal approach along the axis of the sphenoid wing is used, the artery can be followed further into the interpeduncular cistern. Approximately 3 mm from its origin, the posterior communicating artery gives rise to 2 to 10 branches that run posteriorly, inferiorly, and medially into the interpeduncular cistern to supply the optic chiasm and tract, tuber cinereum, mammillary bodies, hypothalamus, and inferior thalamus. These branches are long and variable in caliber.

Anterior Choroidal Artery

The anterior choroidal artery arises 2 to 5 mm distal to the origin of the posterior communicating artery and runs laterally to this artery, following the optic tract posteriorly. The anterior choroidal artery varies greatly in diameter (0.5 to 1.5 mm) and may arise as more than one vessel (it is duplicated in 30 percent of patients). If it originates as a single trunk that divides into two vessels, one of them, the "uncal artery," ramifies almost immediately to supply the uncus, part of the amygdala, and the anterior hippocampus. The main trunk of the anterior choroidal artery continues posteriorly inferior to the optic tract to the choroidal fissure, where its supplies the choroid plexus of the temporal horn and anastomoses distally with branches of the posterior lateral choroidal artery. In its course through the carotid cistern, the anterior choroidal artery gives off branches that supply the inferior surface of the optic chiasm, the posterior two-thirds of the optic tract, the medial globus pallidus, the genu of the internal capsule, the middle third of the cerebral peduncle, part of the red nucleus, the subthalamus, and thalamic nuclei. As the anterior choroidal artery enters the choroidal fissure to supply the choroid plexus of the temporal horn, it gives off branches that supply the anterior lateral half of the lateral geniculate body, the anterior half of the posterior internal capsule, the retrolenticular part of the internal capsule, and the optic radiations. Considering the territory that is irrigated by the anterior choroidal artery, it is clear that loss of this vessel has devastating neurologic consequences for the patient.

Middle Cerebral Artery

The middle cerebral artery is 2.5 to 4.6 mm in diameter at its origin. The part of this artery that extends from its origin to its bifurcation—approximately 15 mm in length—is referred to as the "M_1," "sphenoidal," or "pterional segment." The M_1 segment gives off two sets of branches: the superior lateral (or temporal) and the inferior medial (or deep) perforating branches. Typically, 1 to 3 branches form the superior lateral group and are labeled the "uncal," "polar temporal," and "anterior temporal arteries." Occasionally, the uncal branch originates from the posterior internal carotid artery just distal to the anterior choroidal artery. Often, the polar temporal artery is small or absent. In this case, the remaining anterior temporal artery is large. Occasionally, the polar temporal and anterior temporal arteries are both absent and are replaced by a large branch from the anterior trunk of the M_2 segment of the middle cerebral artery.

The inferior medial branches of the M_1 segment are the lenticulostriate arteries. There usually are 3 to 5 of these arteries, although up to 15 perforating vessels have been reported. They enter the lateral two-thirds of the anterior perforated substance and supply the anterior commissure, the putamen, the lateral globus pallidus, the superior half of the internal capsule, and the head and body of the caudate nucleus. Sometimes, there is only one large lenticulostriate artery that divides into many smaller branches that perfuse the above territory. This larger lenticulostriate artery usually originates just proximal to the bifurcation of the middle cerebral artery and runs medially. This vessel can be injured if the clip is placed too deep during repair of a middle cerebral artery aneurysm.

The part of the middle cerebral artery that is distal to its bifurcation is called the "M_2 segment." It usually consists of a superior branch and inferior branch, but in approximately 20 percent of patients, there are three branches—a trifurcation instead of a bifurcation. The proximal branches of the M_2 segment include the lateral orbitofrontal, prefrontal, frontal auricular, precentral, central sulcus, angular, and posterior temporal arteries. The branches originating from the superior trunk typically supply inferior frontal cortex, frontal auricular cortex, and parietal and central sulcus regions. Branches from the inferior trunk usually supply the temporal, temporooccipital, angular, and posterior parietal gyri. Rarely, an accessory middle cerebral artery has been reported to originate from the anterior cerebral artery complex.

Anterior Cerebral Artery

The size and configuration of the anterior cerebral artery complex and its branches vary significantly. The A_1 segment of the anterior cerebral artery extends from the bifurcation of the internal carotid artery to the anterior communicating artery. Typically, one A_1 segment is dominant, with the opposite A_1 segment being either quite small in caliber or absent. The average diameter of the A_1 segment is 2.5 mm. Perforating arteries arise from the inferior posterior portion of the proximal anterior cerebral artery and supply the optic chiasm and penetrate the anterior perforated substance to supply part of the fornix, the anterior limb of the internal capsule, the anterior inferior part of the striatum, and the anterior hypothalamus. These branches of the A_1 segment may originate from one larger vessel, the medial proximal striate artery, which may have a reciprocal relationship with the lenticulostriate arteries that originate from the M_1 segment of the middle cerebral artery.

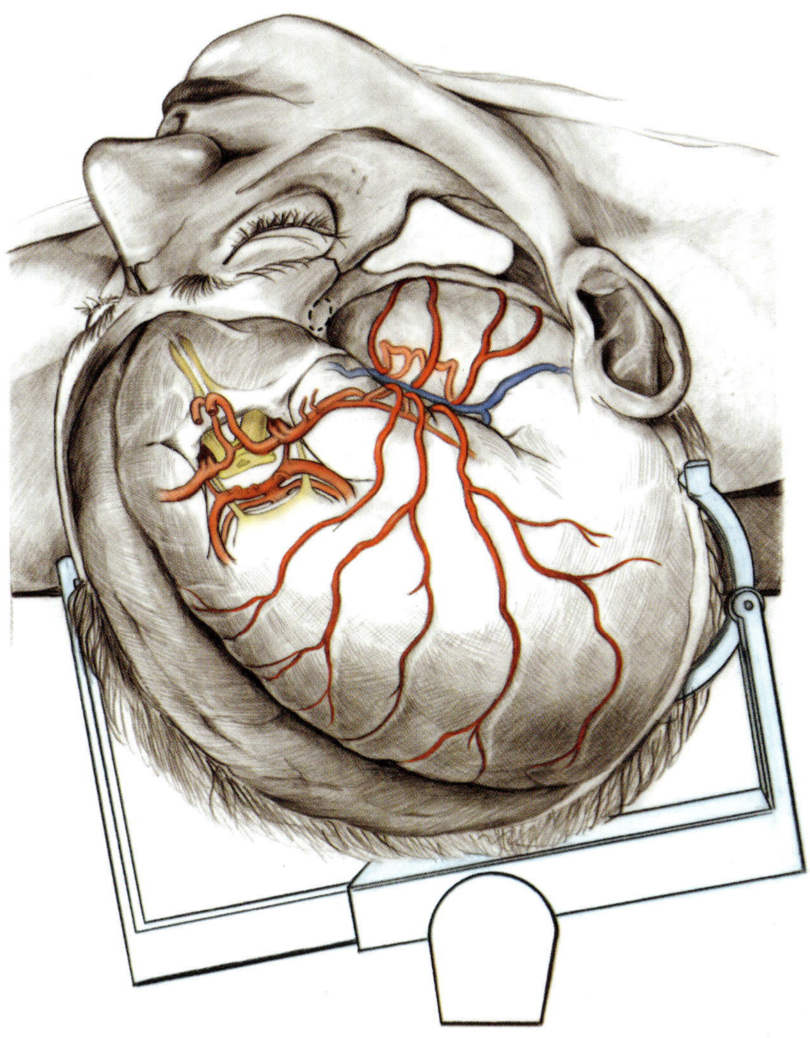

Figure 1–1.

The optic nerve and the supraclinoid part of the internal carotid artery serve as the landmarks or reference points for all the structures exposed during a standard pterional craniotomy. The approach to these structures is along the long axis of the sphenoid wing. The two routes of access are the trans-Sylvian and the subfrontal. Which of these two routes is used is determined primarily by whether the patient has a Sylvian fissure that can be divided easily. In young patients or those who are obese or have a subarachnoid hemorrhage, the Sylvian fissure is often obscured. In this case, a subfrontal approach can be used, and the medial aspect of Sylvian fissure can be identified and incised from medial to lateral.

The anterior communicating artery is 0.1 to 3.0 mm long. Typically, a large A_1 branch divides into two distal A_2 segments, and the anterior communicating artery is the apparent attachment or entry point of the hypoplastic contralateral A_1 segment. In 75 percent of patients, the anterior communicating artery is a single vessel, and in the other 25 percent, it has various anomalies, including fenestrations or duplications. Perforating arteries, which vary in number and diameter, arise from the posterior inferior aspect of the anterior communicating artery and the distal A_1 segment, at its junction with the anterior communicating artery. They supply the infundibulum, optic chiasm, and preoptic area of the hypothalamus. Yasargil reported that if the A_1 segments are equal in size, the perforating vessels arise from the midportion of the anterior communicating artery. However, if the A_1 segments are unequal, the perforating branches arise from the anterior communicating artery on the side of the larger A_1 segment. Because this relationship is similar to that observed for aneurysms in this location, these vessels typically are found on the anterior inferior side of the neck of the aneurysm.

Recurrent Artery of Heubner

A recurrent artery of Heubner is almost always present and usually originates from the A_1 or A_2 segment, adjacent to the origin of the anterior communicating artery. It originates from the A_2 segment in approximately 80 percent of patients and is bilateral in 95 percent. The reported diameters for the recurrent artery of Heubner range from 0.2 to 2.9 mm. It runs parallel to the anterior cerebral artery before entering the anterior perforated substance to supply the anterior part of the caudate nucleus, the anterior putamen, part of the globus pallidus, and the anterior limb of the internal capsule. During exposure of the anterior communicating artery complex, any vessel that runs laterally along the inferior frontal lobe must be presumed to be the recurrent artery of Heubner and, therefore, protected. This is particularly true if partial resection of the gyrus rectus is necessary. Of note is that the recurrent artery of Heubner occasionally originates from the frontal polar branch of the anterior cerebral artery.

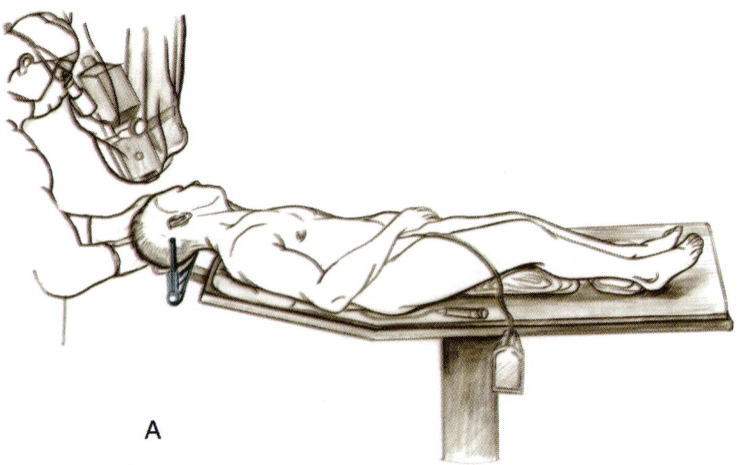

A

Figure 1–2.

Step 1. *A*, The patient's head is fixed in a pinion, extended slightly, and rotated approximately 25 to 30 degrees opposite the side of the craniotomy. With extension of the head, the frontal lobe falls away from the floor of the frontal cranial fossa, thereby lessening the degree of brain retraction.

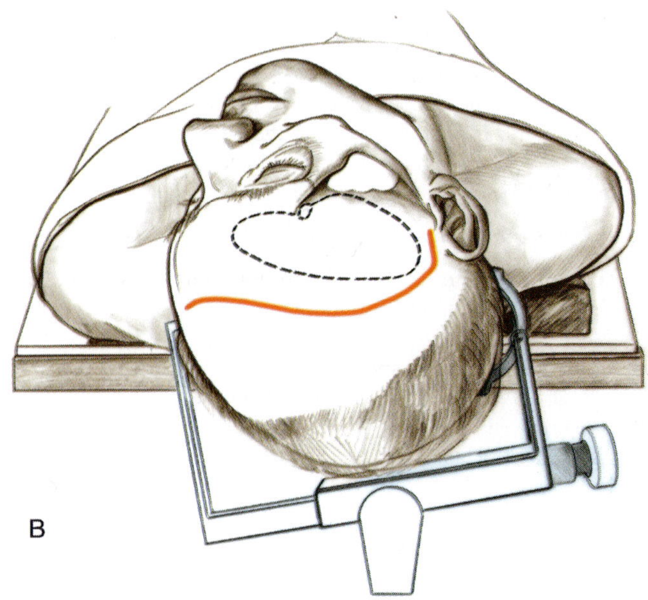

B

B, The keyhole bur hole allows access to both the frontal and middle cranial fossae. It is important to extend the bone flap just medial to the mid-pupillary line to increase exposure in case a subfrontal approach is required.

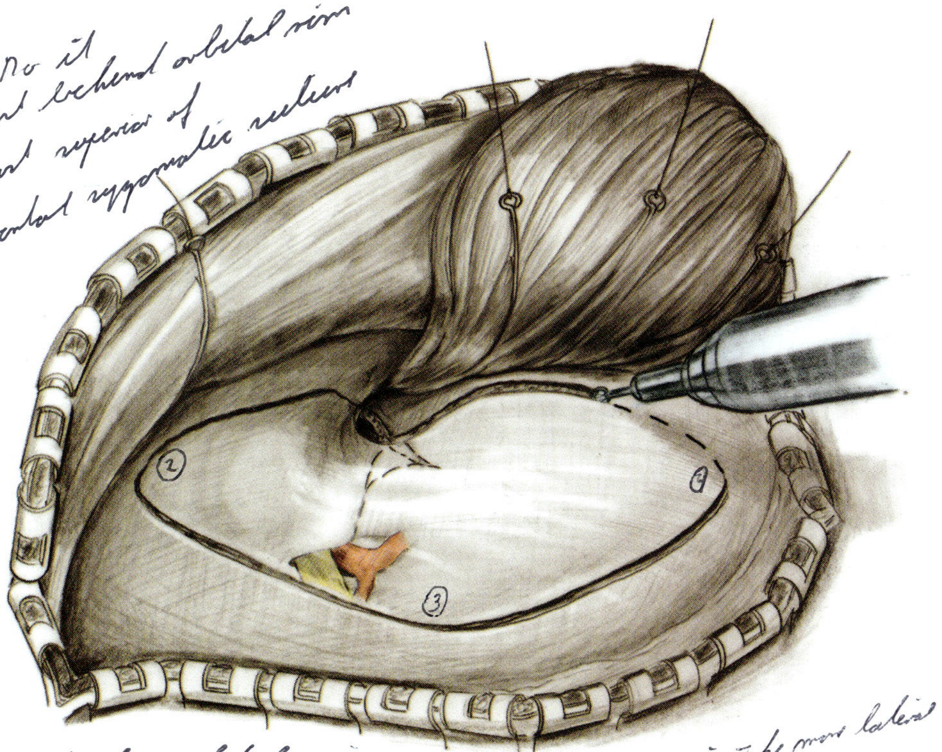

Figure 1–3.

Step 2. Several techniques can be used to cut the bone flap, including standard bur holes and Gigli saws or newer craniotomes. It is helpful to mark the extent of the bone flap when using a craniotome to prevent minimizing the size of the craniotomy. It is important to extend the bone flap down toward the base of the middle cranial fossa. Sometimes, the optimal method is to perform two-thirds of the craniotomy with a craniotome and then use a high-speed air drill with a diamond bur to make the last one-third of the cut along the floor of the middle cranial fossa over the outer sphenoid wing up to the keyhole bur hole. With this method, the bone flap is not minimized.

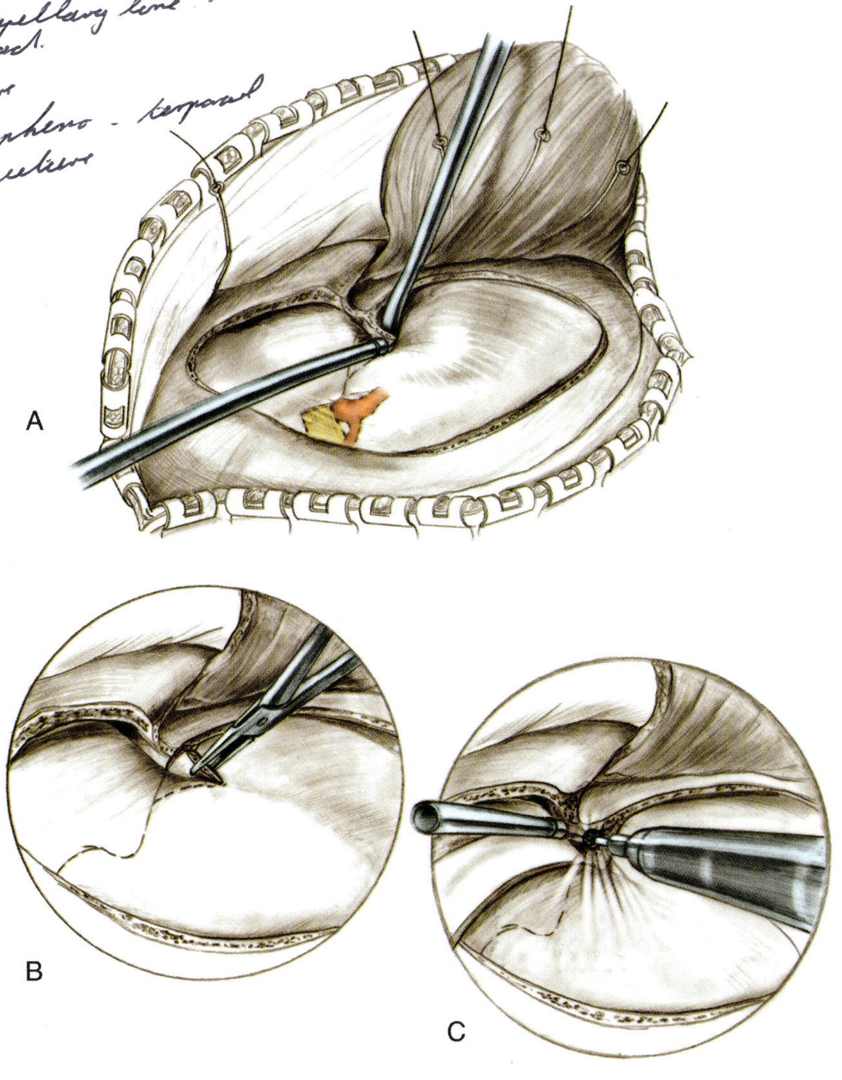

Figure 1–4.

Step 3. *A*, After removing the bone flap, the outer sphenoid wing is removed down to the superior orbital fissure. This increases the exposure by approximately 1.5 cm. The dura mater along the sphenoid wing is sharply dissected free with a periosteal elevator.

B, The outer sphenoid wing is removed with a small orbital rongeur.

C, A Yasargil retractor is used to displace the dura mater, and, under the microscope, a high-speed air drill with a diamond bur is used to remove the deeper portion of the sphenoid wing. In fact, removal of the sphenoid wing can be extended deep to include the clinoid process, which allows the anterior clinoid process to be removed without incising the dura mater. This is described later in the chapter. In some patients, the frontal bone is thick and the diamond bur can be used to remove the inner one-half of the frontal bone, which also increases exposure, especially if a subfrontal approach to the internal carotid artery is being used.

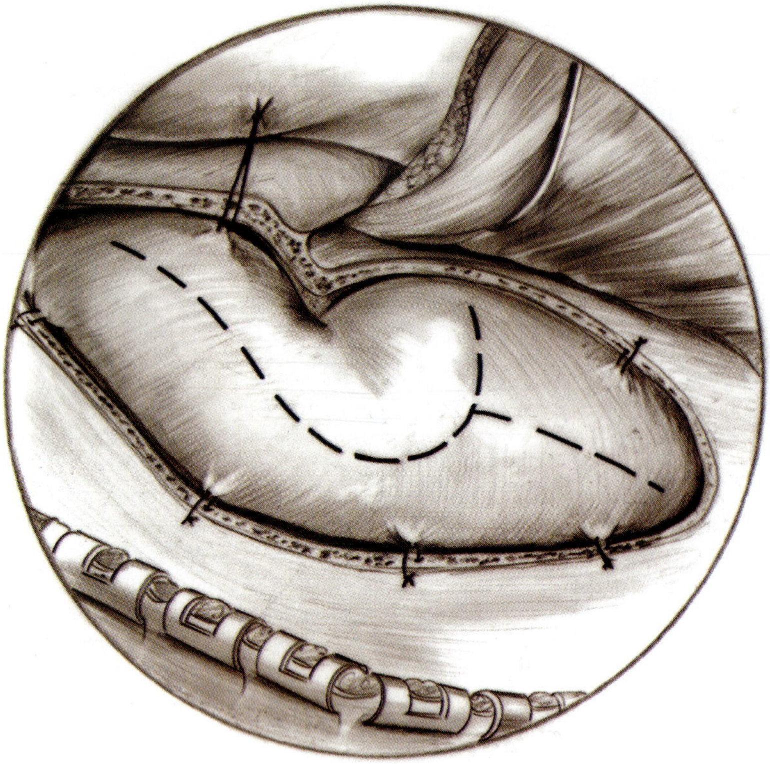

Figure 1–5.

Step 4. The dura mater is tacked to the bone margins. If a dural graft is going to be used, the dura mater can be opened and then tacked. In this way, there is no risk of inadvertently injuring the underlying cerebral cortex. However, if the dura mater is going to be closed primarily, it is best to tack it to the bone before opening it. In patients with a large frontal sinus, the frontal tack stitch should be sewn to the muscle to avoid a tack hole going into the frontal sinus, which can lead to rhinorrhea postoperatively.

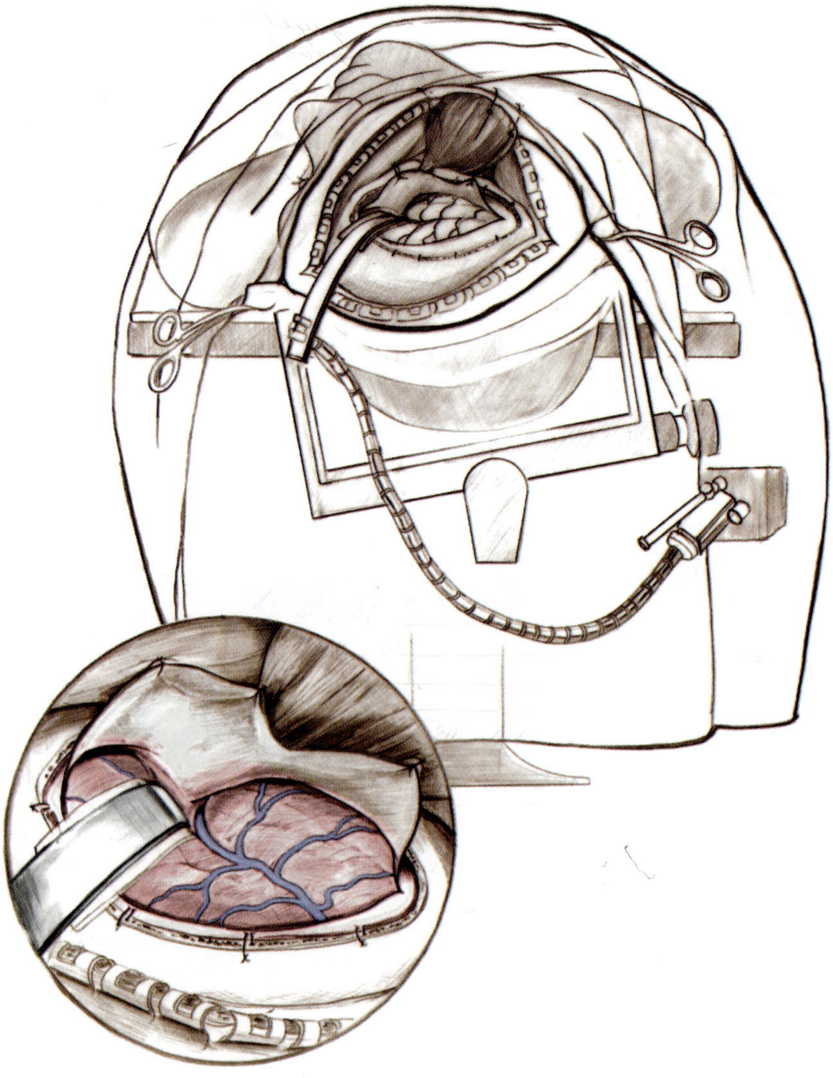

Figure 1–6.

Step 5. The dura mater is opened and reflected over the sphenoid wing and temporalis muscle to prevent blood from running into the operative field. The frontal lobe is lined with hemostatic fabric and cottonoids and then gently retracted to place the Sylvian fissure under tension. Correct orientation of the Yasargil bar, head, and arm will increase the effectiveness of this retractor. As described by Sundt, the Yasargil arm should hang straight down and touch the drapes approximately 5 cm from the blade, forming a gentle "S" shape. With this arrangement, gravity assists the retraction and the distal arm has a fulcrum. To achieve this straight up-and-down orientation, the Yasargil head off the bar needs to be in the correct position. The surgeon can determine this by attaching the arm to the unsecured Yasargil head on the bar. The arm is held in the correct orientation, and the head is rotated around the bar until there is no torque. Next, the head is secured to the bar. A common mistake is not to insert the Yasargil bar far enough into the clamp along the side of the operating room table to prevent excessive outward looping of the arm.

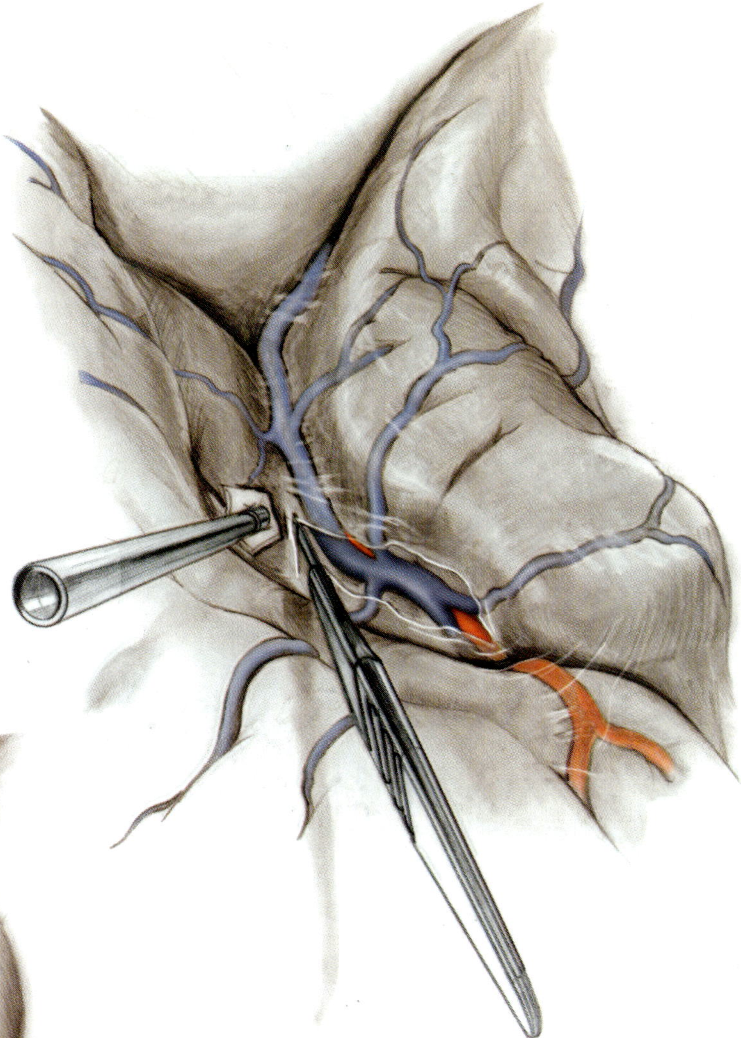

Figure 1–7.

Step 6. With a #5 or #7 straight suction tip and small cottonoid, the frontal lobe adjacent to the lateral Sylvian fissure is retracted gently to place the arachnoid under tension. In the process of dividing the Sylvian fissure, both the suction tip and cottonoid are "walked down" the fissure, placing under tension the next part of the arachnoid to be cut. Under the operating microscope, an incision is made in the arachnoid with a #11 blade knife.

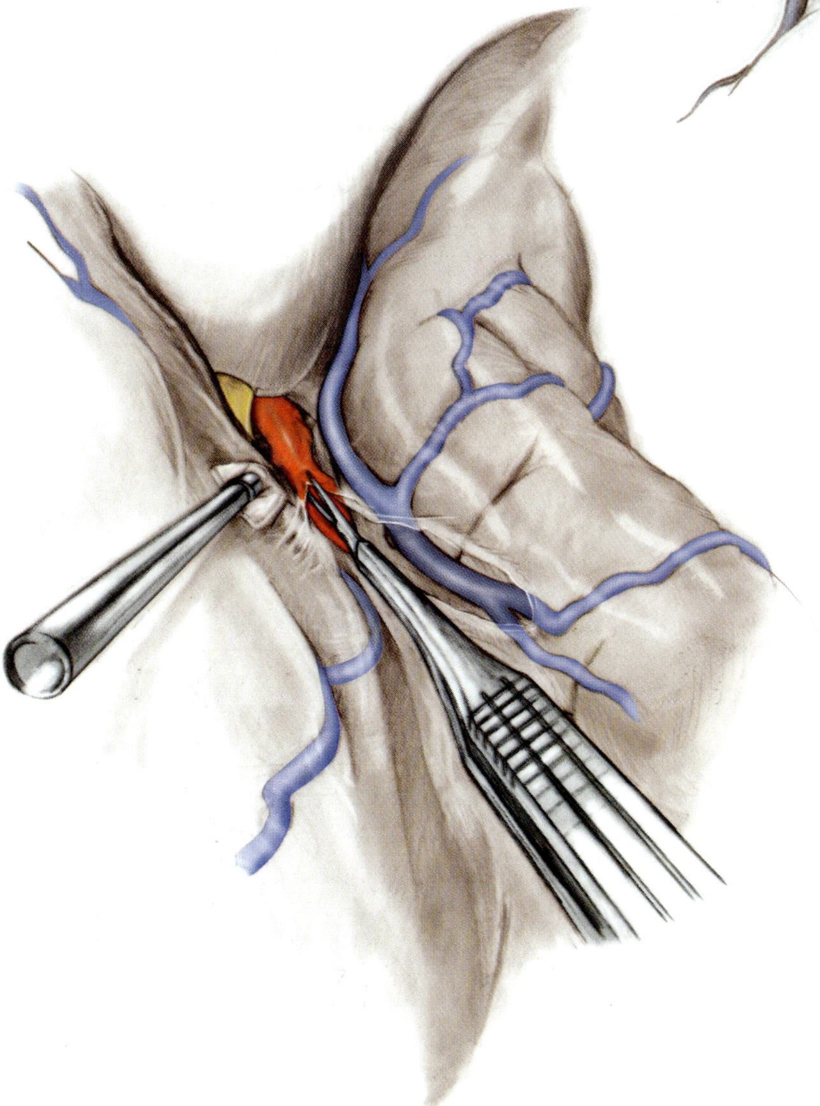

Figure 1–8.

This incision in the arachnoid is extended downward or medially along the Sylvian fissure by separating the arachnoid with bipolar forceps. Alternatively, the arachnoid can be lifted and cut with a straight microscissors. Large Sylvian veins should be left intact and displaced laterally with the temporal lobe. Small bridging veins across the Sylvian fissure can be safely cauterized and divided.

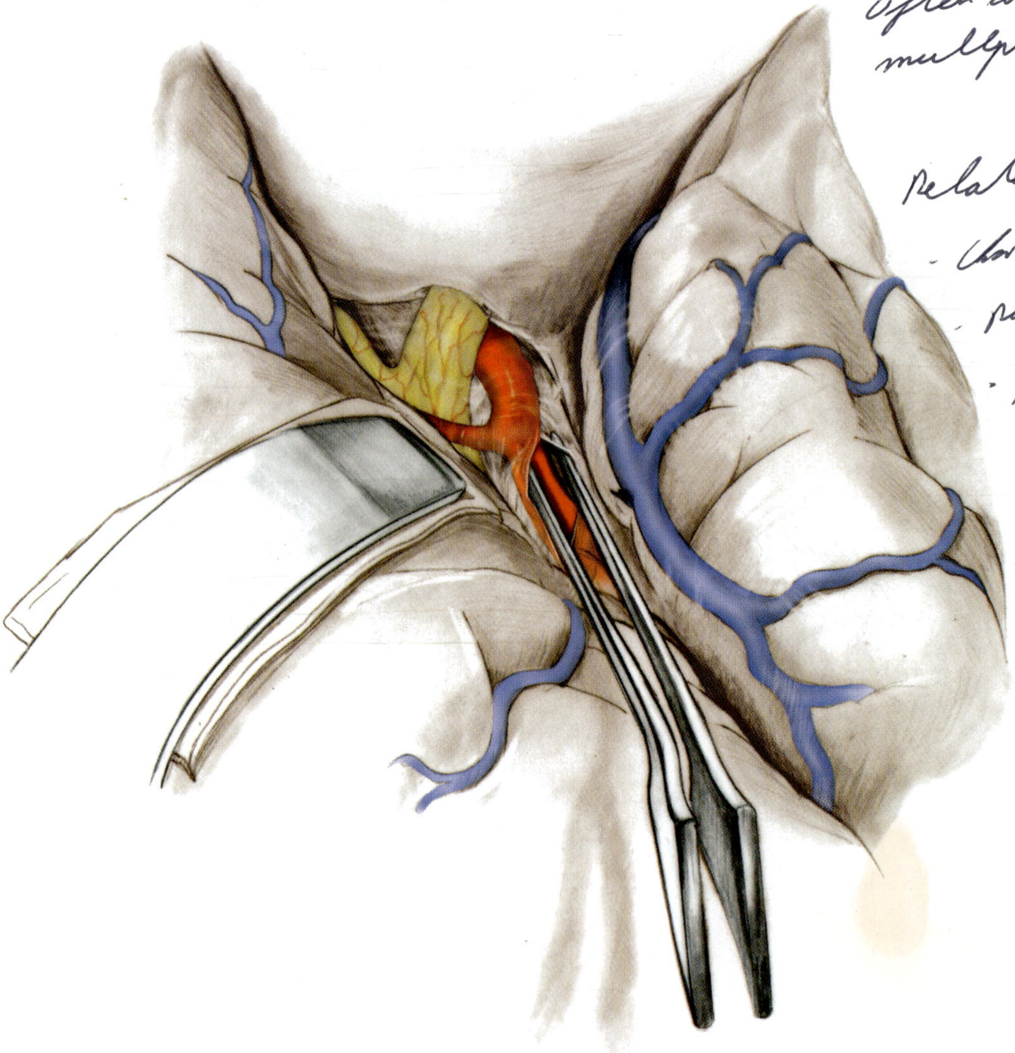

Figure 1–9.

As the Sylvian fissure becomes more broadly split, the frontal lobe is increasingly retracted upward to place the deep arachnoid under tension. If a lumbar drain has been placed, it is best not to remove cerebrospinal fluid until the Sylvian fissure has been divided. Removal of cerebrospinal fluid through the drain will decompress the Sylvian fissure and, thus, make it more difficult to dissect the arachnoid. The arachnoid incision is carried down on top of the internal carotid artery.

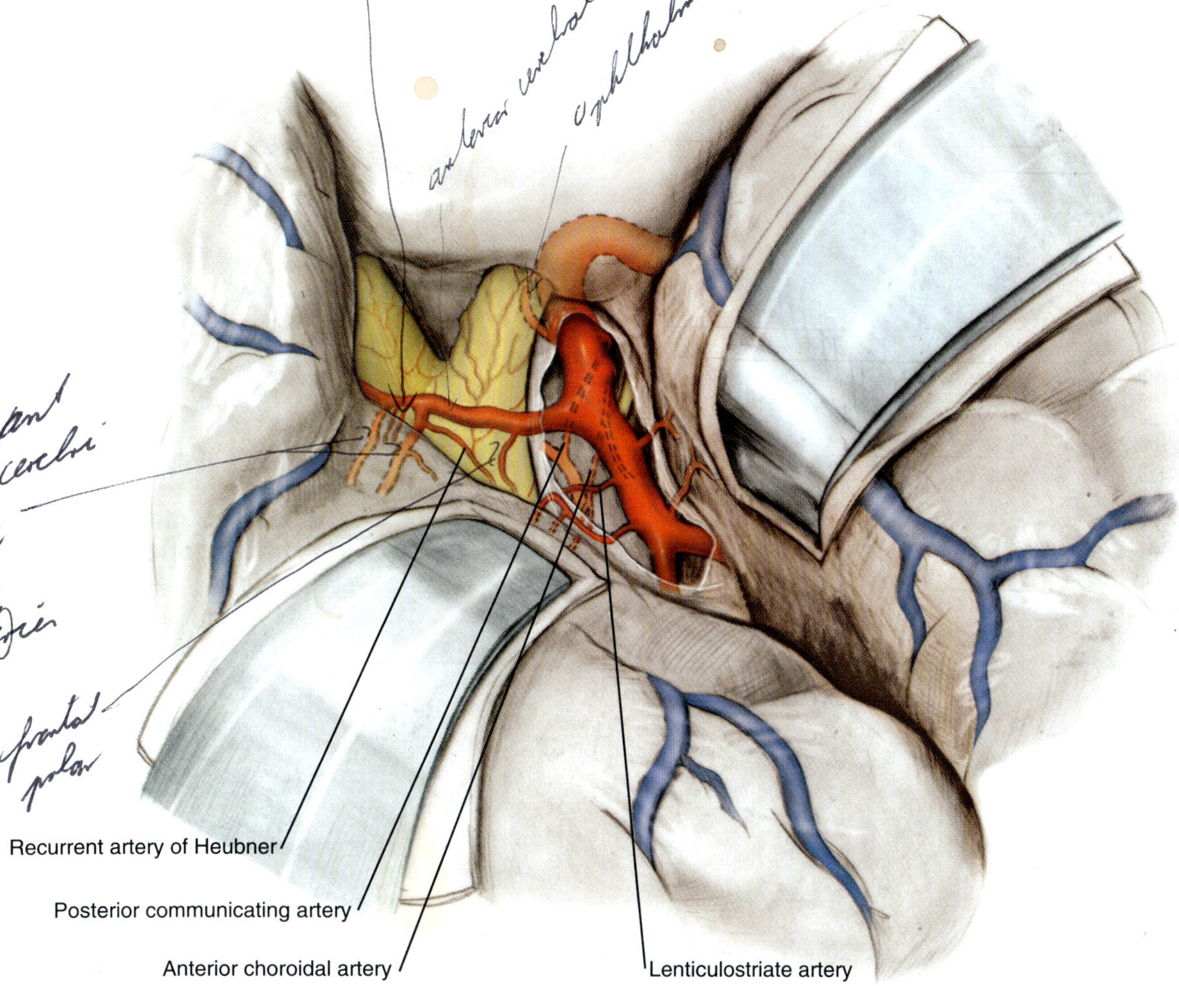

Figure 1–10.

With a straight or angled dissector, the arachnoid is teased off the internal carotid artery both medially and laterally, especially in cases of aneurysm. Accordingly, immediate proximal control has been obtained. Next, the arachnoid is incised medially between the anterior cerebral artery and the optic chiasm. This incision is carried over to the opposite optic nerve. By cutting the arachnoid between the anterior cerebral artery and the optic chiasm, the A_1 segment and its perforating vessels are lifted with the frontal lobe and, therefore, moved out of harm's way. If an anterior cerebral artery–anterior communicating artery aneurysm is being treated, both sides of the proximal A_1 segment need to be dissected to provide proximal arterial control. After the Sylvian fissure is divided, the temporal lobe can be retracted laterally if necessary. There often are bridging veins off the tip of the temporal lobe that are under tension. These can be supported and protected with a piece of absorbable gelatin sponge (Gelfoam). If required, these bridging veins can safely be cauterized and divided.

POSTERIOR COMMUNICATING ARTERY ANEURYSM

Aneurysms in this location are best exposed by first identifying the medial surface of the internal carotid artery adjacent to the optic nerve. This is called the "optic-carotid triangle." In most instances, these aneurysms project laterally toward the tentorium cerebelli and the oculomotor nerve. Not unexpectedly, they often are associated with hemorrhage into the temporal lobe. Occasionally, these aneurysms are located proximally, necessitating resection of the anterior clinoid process.

After the medial surface of the internal carotid artery is identified, a dissector is used to incise the arachnoid over the lateral aspect of the artery. This allows proximal arterial control to be achieved and, if necessary, a temporary clip to be placed. Typically, the aneurysms arise from the axilla of the posterior communicating artery, at its origin from the internal carotid artery. The base of the aneurysm usually projects at a 45-degree angle away from the origin of the posterior communicating artery. It is important to dissect the origin of the posterior communicating artery from the anterior wall of the aneurysm so that the artery can be preserved when a clip is placed across the base. After the posterior communicating artery is identified and the arachnoid that tethers the aneurysm to the artery is incised, a piece of absorbable gelatin sponge (Gelfoam) can be placed to displace this artery. A dissector is then used to identify the origins of the anterior choroidal artery. A piece of absorbable gelatin sponge is also placed between this artery and the neck of the aneurysm. Placement of small bits of absorbable gelatin sponge keep the important arteries out of harm's way when an aneurysm clip is placed. In rare instances, the posterior communicating artery originates from the neck of the aneurysm in such a way that the posterior communicating artery has to be occluded at its origin from the internal carotid artery before the aneurysm can be obliterated. Before concluding that this is indeed the case, it is mandatory that the surgeon ensure that there is no plane between the artery and neck of the aneurysm and that the posterior communicating artery has a small diameter. Furthermore, the preoperative angiogram should show retrograde filling of the posterior communicating artery on the vertebral study. In this rare case, it is acceptable to place the aneurysm clip in a way that both the neck of the aneurysm and the origin of the posterior communicating artery are occluded. This will be tolerated by the patient because the posterior communicating artery fills retrogradely.

For all aneurysms, it is necessary to ensure that after the clip has been placed, the aneurysm has been obliterated completely and no vessels are trapped by the jaws of the clip. It is useful to aspirate the aneurysm, especially large lesions, to collapse the structure. After this is done, the dome of the aneurysm can be manipulated with a #5 or #7 straight suction tip, and the underside of the neck of the aneurysm and the clip can be inspected. After a posterior communicating artery aneurysm is clipped, the anterior choroidal artery is viewed from a lateral perspective to make sure that it has not been compromised. The same is true for the posterior communicating artery. Depending on the location of the aneurysm clip, it may be difficult to visualize the posterior communicating artery. If this is so, the artery and its branches can be viewed from a medial perspective between the optic nerve and the internal carotid artery by gently displacing the medial wall of the internal carotid artery laterally. After these vessels have been inspected, papaverine can be applied topically with a cottonoid to relieve mechanically induced vasospasms.

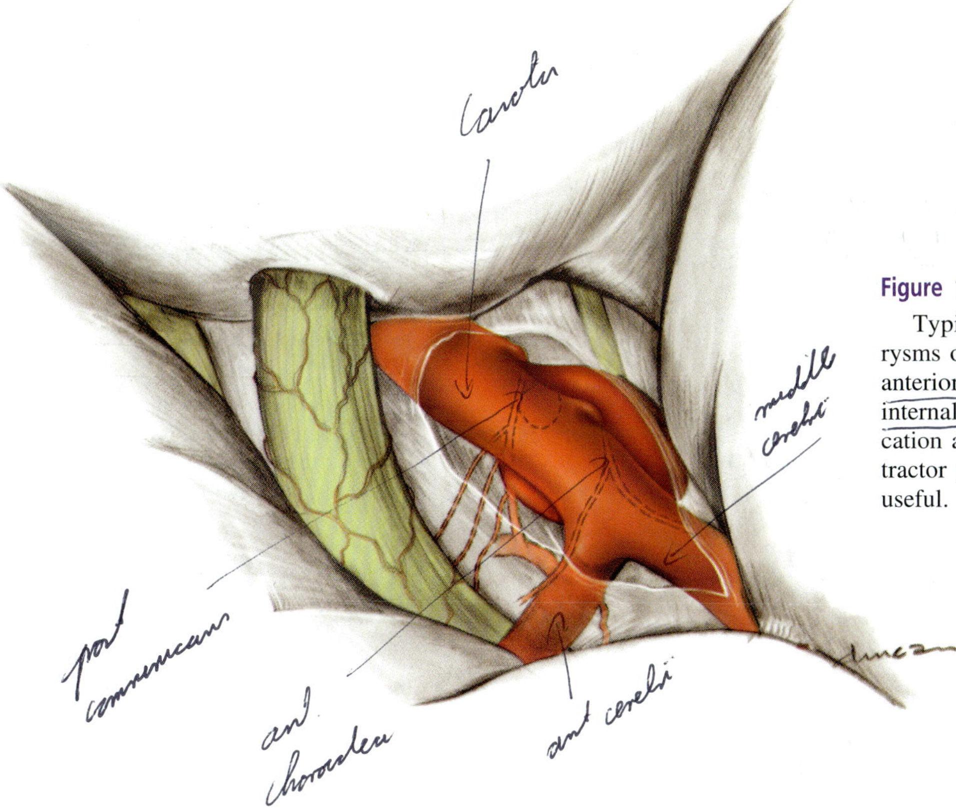

Figure 1–11.

Typical operative exposure used for aneurysms of the posterior communicating artery, anterior choroidal artery, or bifurcation of the internal carotid artery. Depending on the location and projection of the aneurysm, a retractor placed on the temporal lobe can be useful.

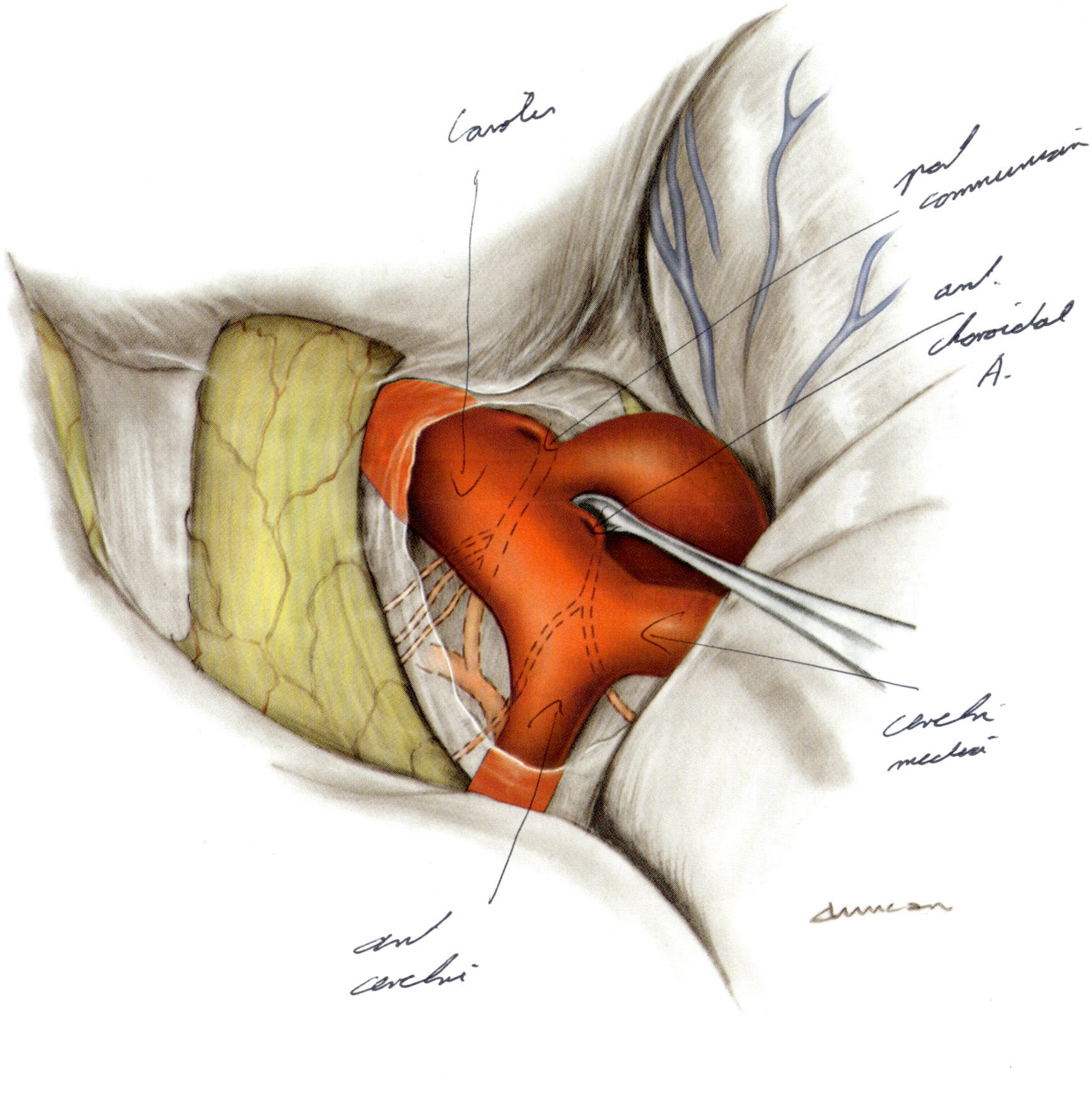

Figure 1–12.

Step 1. Under the operating microscope, it is mandatory to dissect the neck of the aneurysm of the posterior communicating artery off both the anterior choroidal artery and the posterior communicating artery.

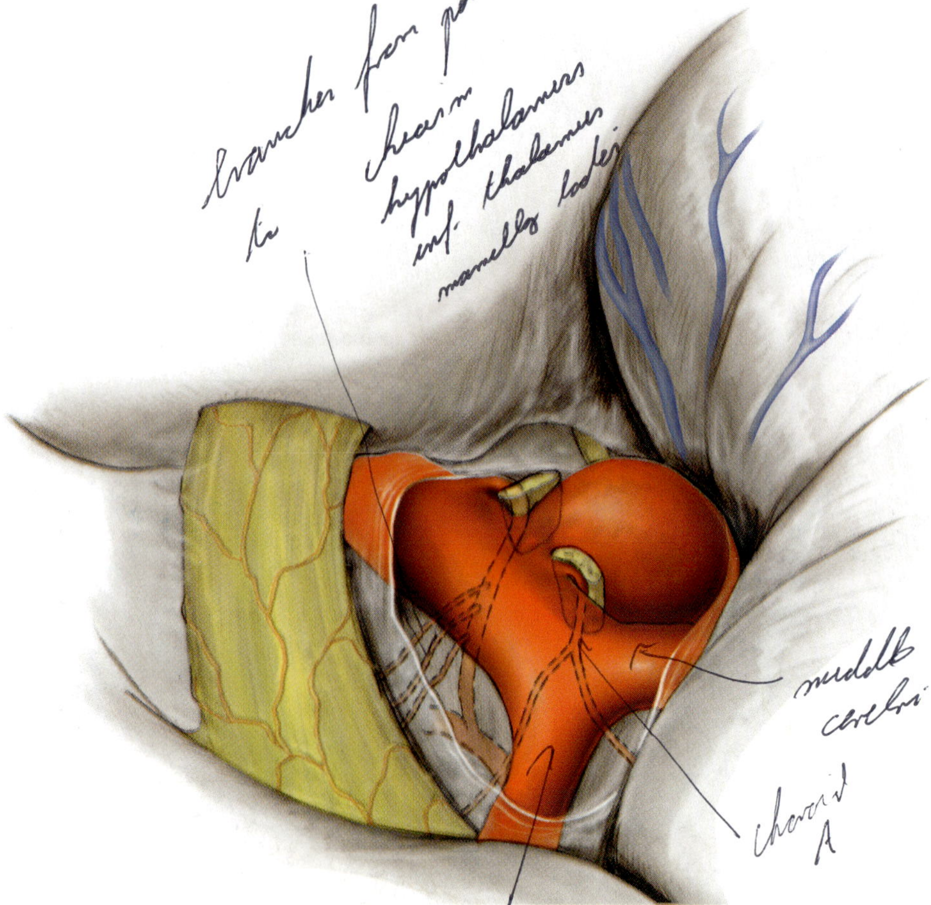

Figure 1–13.

Step 2. A useful step in all aneurysm surgery is to displace dissected vessels from the neck of the aneurysm by using small pieces of absorbable gelatin sponge (Gelfoam).

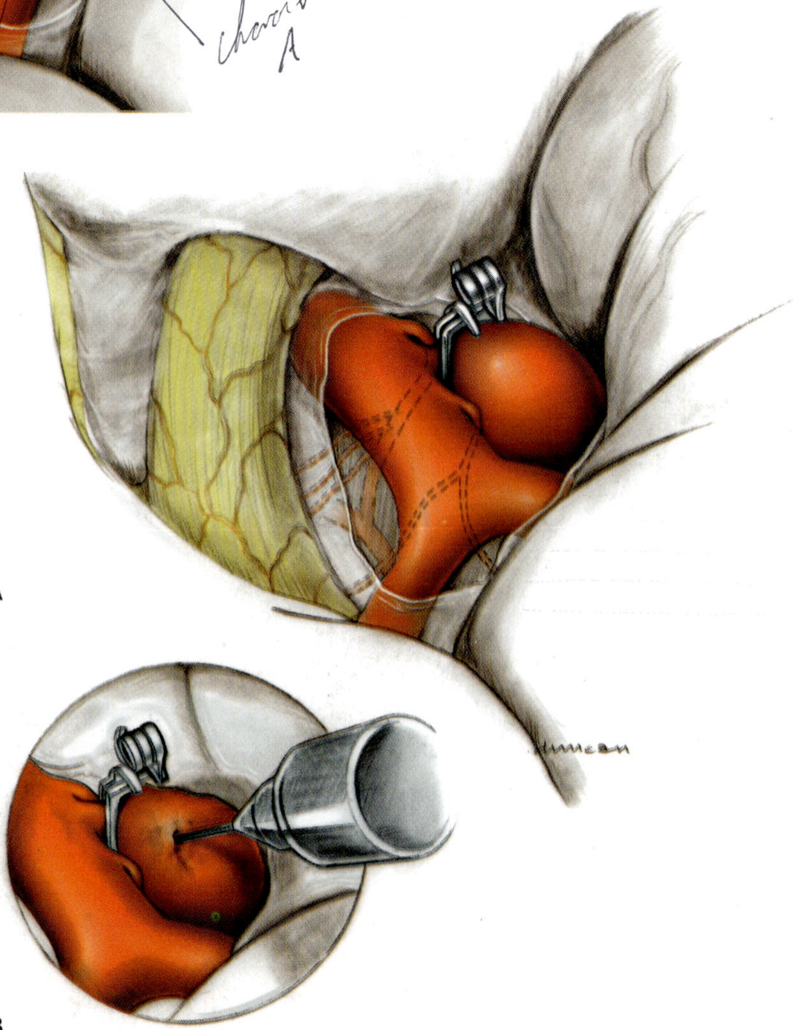

A

B

Figure 1–14.

Step 3. *A*, Usually a straight, bayonet, or 45-degree-angled aneurysm clip is best for aneurysms of the posterior communicating artery or anterior choroidal artery. When placing the clip, it is important to ensure that neither the perforating vessels nor the internal carotid artery is compromised or constricted.

B, After the aneurysm is clipped, its dome is aspirated if the surgeon believes that the neck has been occluded completely with the clip. Aspirating the dome of the aneurysm enhances the exposure, thus allowing better inspection of the underlying perforating vessels.

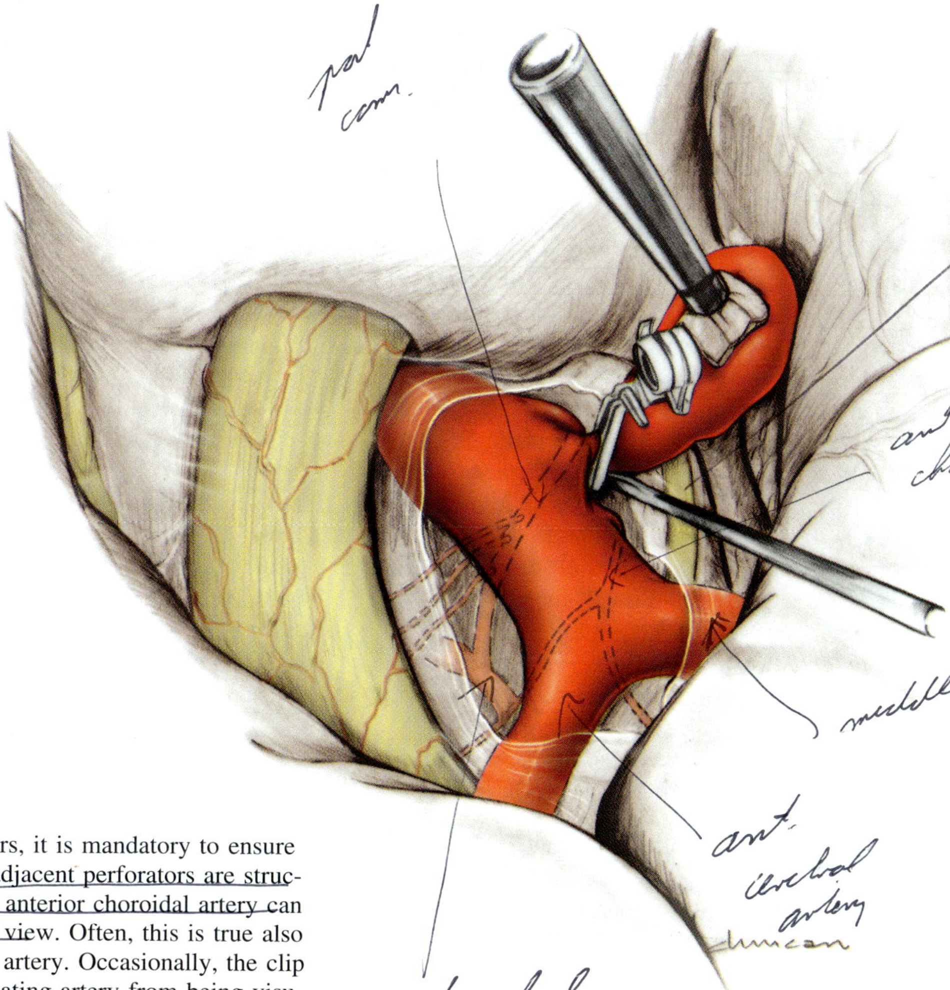

Figure 1–15.

Step 4. In all aneurysm repairs, it is mandatory to ensure that both the parent vessel and adjacent perforators are structurally intact. The takeoff of the anterior choroidal artery can be visualized best from a lateral view. Often, this is true also for the posterior communicating artery. Occasionally, the clip prevents the posterior communicating artery from being visualized. In that case, it can be viewed from a medial to lateral perspective, looking between the optic nerve and internal carotid artery through the optic-carotid triangle.

ANTERIOR COMMUNICATING ARTERY ANEURYSM

It is easiest to expose an aneurysm of the anterior communicating artery from a more subfrontal than sphenoidal approach through a pterional craniotomy. Therefore, the head should not be rotated more than 30 degrees opposite the side of the craniotomy. It usually is best to approach the aneurysm from the side of the dominant feeding artery, unless there has been severe hemorrhage into the opposite gyrus rectus. Because it occasionally is necessary to remove part of the gyrus rectus to expose the aneurysm, it is preferable to remove tissue that has already been damaged by a hemorrhage.

After the Sylvian fissure is divided, the carotid bifurcation is identified. A hemostatic fabric and cottonoids are placed over the frontal lobe, which is then retracted upward and posteriorly. This increases tension on the arachnoid over the anterior cerebral artery. The arachnoid between the anterior cerebral artery and the chiasmatic cistern is opened and the proximal A_1 segment is identified in case a temporary clip has to be placed should the aneurysm rupture. The arachnoid is dissected free between the anterior cerebral artery and the optic chiasm. It is not necessary to separate the arachnoid completely between the frontal lobe and the anterior cerebral artery, because this might increase the risk of injury to the perforating arteries that originate from the A_1 segment. To prevent inadvertent rupture during exposure, the surgeon must bear in mind the direction of the dome of the aneurysm.

The incision in the arachnoid is extended medially over the optic chiasm so that the opposite A_1 segment can be visualized. With a #11 blade knife, the cistern of the lamina terminalis in the interhemispheric fissure is incised between the two gyri recti. If the lamina terminalis can be identified clearly, it may be useful to incise it to drain cerebrospinal fluid from the third ventricle to increase brain relaxation. If a lumbar spinal drain is being used, this maneuver is not required. If necessary, a small portion of the gyrus rectus can be removed with a bipolar cautery and suction. It is important not to coagulate or to divide any perforating vessels in this area. Furthermore, the frontal polar artery must not be mistaken for the recurrent artery of Huebner. After the gyrus rectus is removed, the ipsilateral A_2 segment is identified. Therefore, at this point in the operation, three of the four major trunks have been visualized except for the opposite A_2 segment. With a typical posteriorly pointing aneurysm, it is best to start dissecting the aneurysm at the junction between the ipsilateral A_2 segment and the anterior communicating artery. This dissection usually starts posteriorly behind the aneurysm, with the aneurysm being elevated with a #5 or #7 straight suction tip and small cottonoid. Typically, perforating vessels are ensheathed in their own arachnoid and can be dissected off the back wall of the aneurysm as a single sheet or layer. As the aneurysm is gently rotated anteriorly, the opposite A_2 segment usually can be identified and dissected free. Thereafter, a small piece of absorbable gelatin sponge is placed between the opposite A_2 segment, arachnoid and perforating vessels, and the ipsilateral A_2 segment and the neck of the aneurysm. After clipping, it is important to decompress the aneurysm to allow manipulation of the dome to verify that the anterior communicating artery complex and its perforating vessels are intact and not entrapped by the jaws of the clip.

In large aneurysms, it may be necessary to perform a thrombectomy in order to place a clip and to preserve the surrounding vasculature. In this case, the dominant feeding A_1 segment is temporarily occluded. If perforating vessels originate from the A_1 segment, it is preferable to place the temporary clip distal to their takeoff, without compromising exposure of the neck of the aneurysm. An incision is made in the dome far distal to the neck. If an incision is made too close to the neck, then subsequent placement of an aneurysm clip may be compromised. Thrombectomy is performed with curets. If back bleeding is significant, it may be necessary to occlude the contralateral A_1 segment.

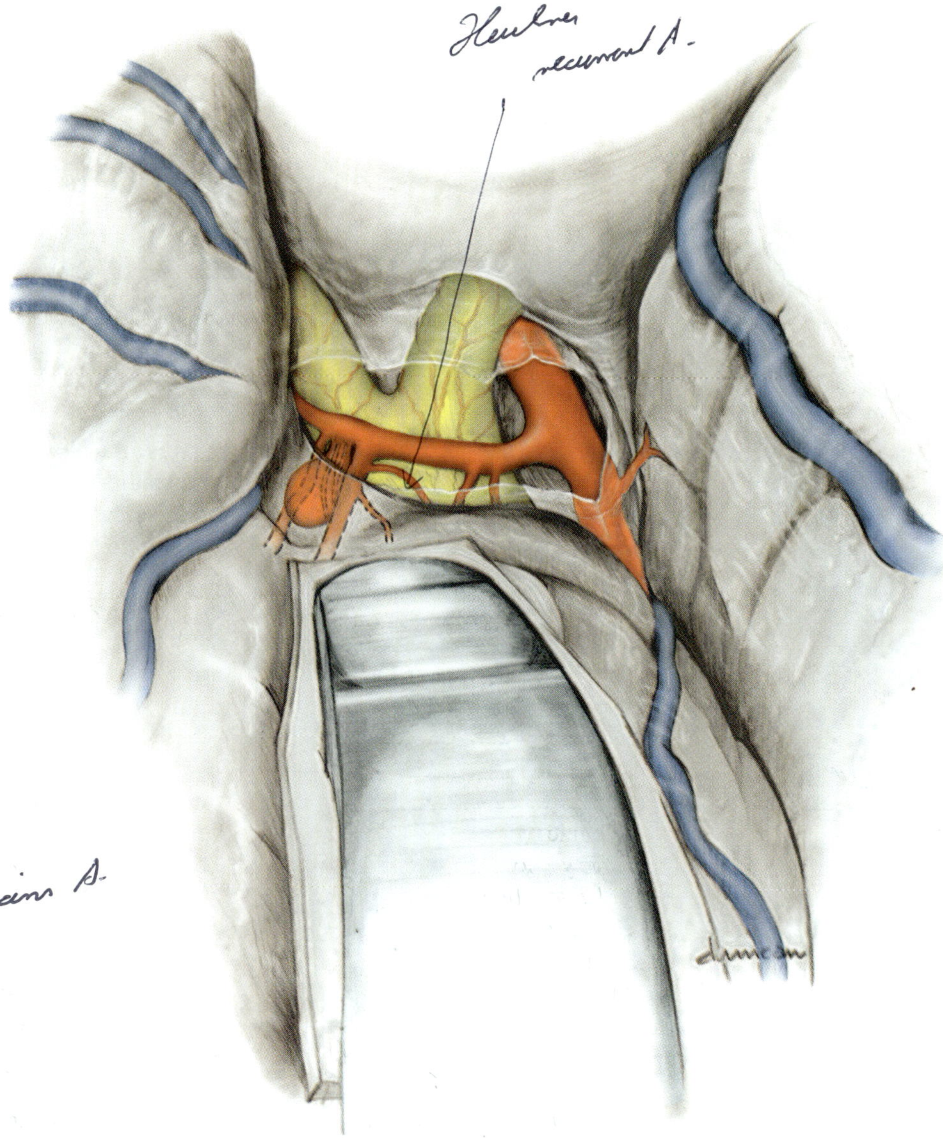

Figure 1–16.

Step 1. The approach to an anterior communicating artery aneurysm is more subfrontal than sphenoidal. After the Sylvian fissure is divided, the frontal lobe retractor is repositioned to lift the frontal lobe up and posteriorly to expose the carotid bifurcation. The arachnoid over the A_1 segment is incised to allow access in case a temporary clip has to be placed because of intraoperative rupture of the aneurysm. The arachnoid between the anterior cerebral artery and the optic chiasm is incised to identify the opposite A_1 segment.

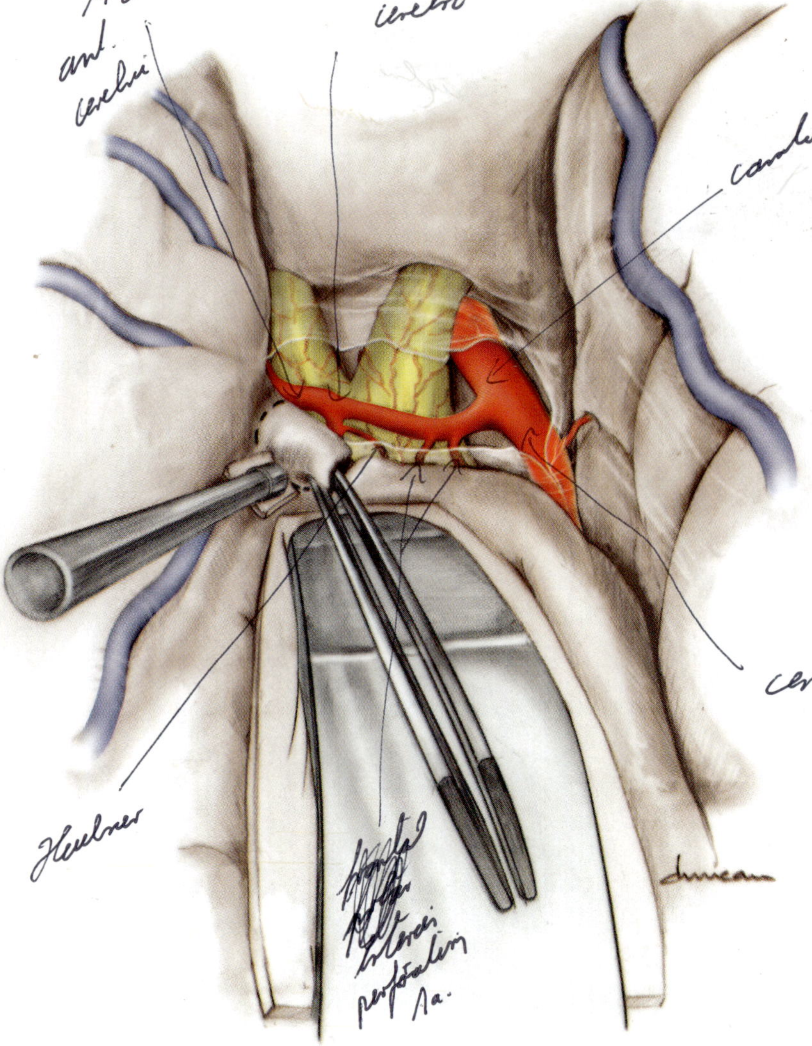

Figure 1–17.

Step 2. Despite the Sylvian fissure being divided and despite cerebrospinal fluid being aspirated from the suprachiasmatic cistern and drained through a lumbar drain or an incision in the lamina terminalis, exposure of the aneurysm can still be difficult. If exposure is a problem, part of the ipsilateral gyrus rectus may be removed with bipolar cautery and delicate suction. Any artery that runs lateral and horizontal to the A_1 segment should be protected and presumed to be the recurrent artery of Heubner.

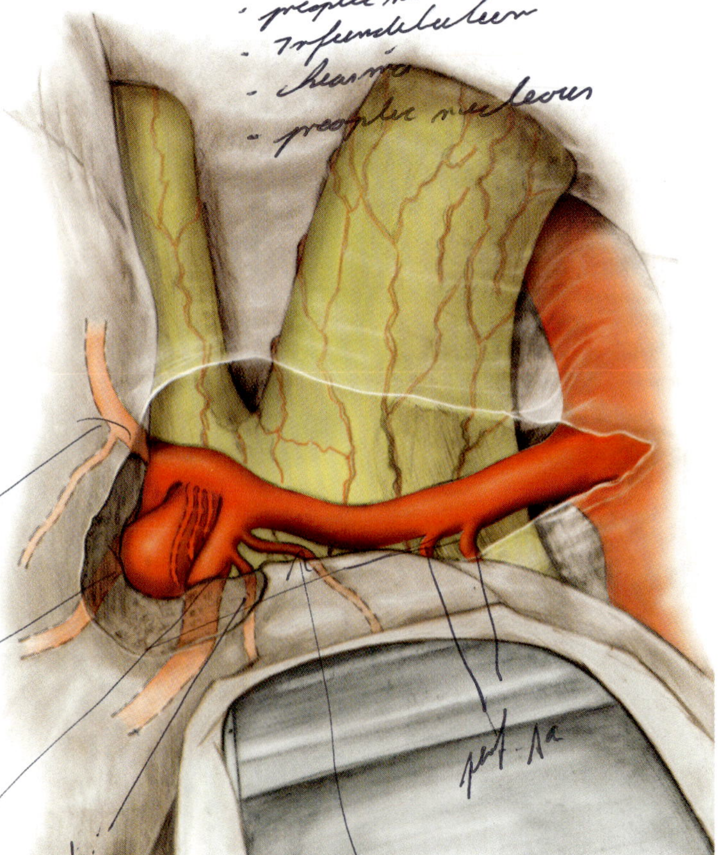

Figure 1–18.

Step 3. The frontal retractor is placed deeper to allow additional retraction of the frontal lobe and gyrus rectus. It is important to be sure that the interhemispheric arachnoid has been incised to decrease tension on the opposite frontal lobe. Before the aneurysm is dissected, it is mandatory to ensure good access to the dominant A_1 segment in case temporary clipping is necessary.

Figure 1–19.

Step 4. *A*, The neck of the aneurysm is carefully dissected free from the underlying perforating vessels and the adjacent A_1 and A_2 segments. It is best first to isolate the dominant A_1 segment and then the opposite A_1 for good proximal control. A spatula or dissector is used to dissect free the ipsilateral A_2 segment. The contralateral A_2 segment is the last structure identified. The perforating vessels originating from the anterior communicating artery usually are sheathed in arachnoid and can be separated in a plane en bloc. This is similar to dissecting perforating vessels off the basilar caput. The perforating vessels adjacent to the ipsilateral A_2 segment are identified first. The plane between these perforators and the neck of the aneurysm is developed and extended around the backside of the lesion.

B, A piece of absorbable gelatin sponge is used to displace these vessels before the aneurysm is clipped.

C, After placement of the clip, the dome is aspirated and manipulated to allow inspection of the clip and its relationship to all adjacent vascular structures.

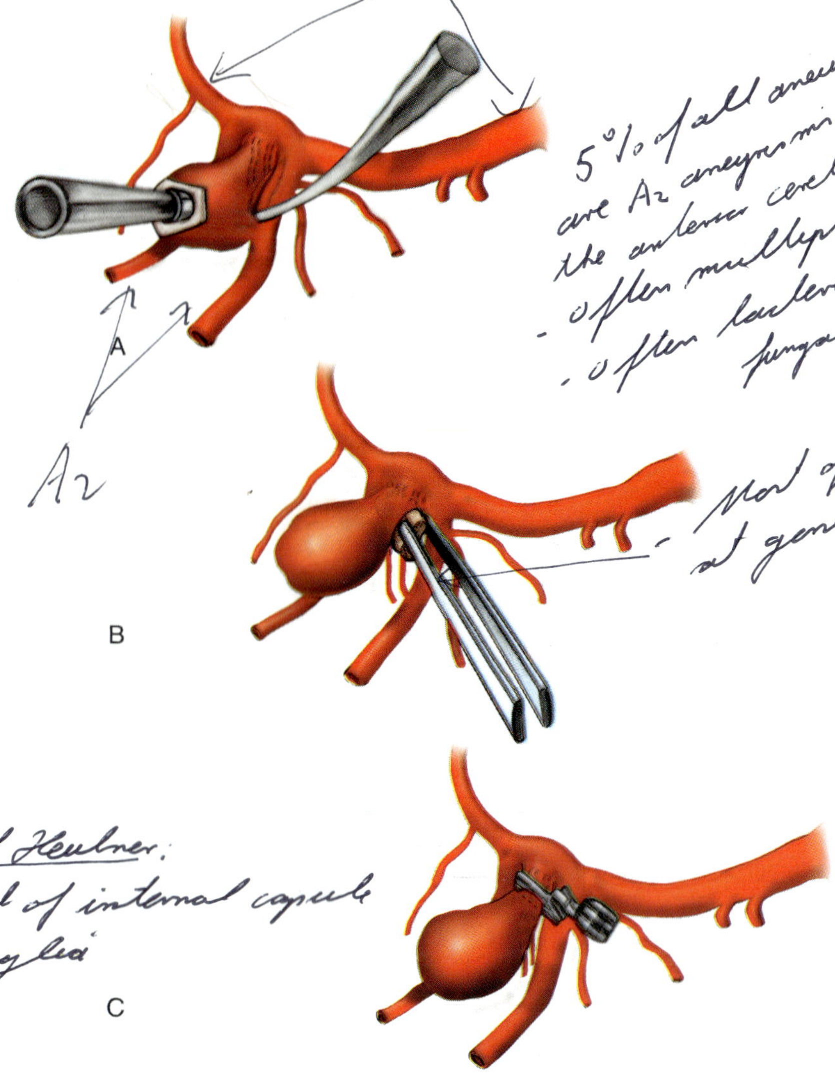

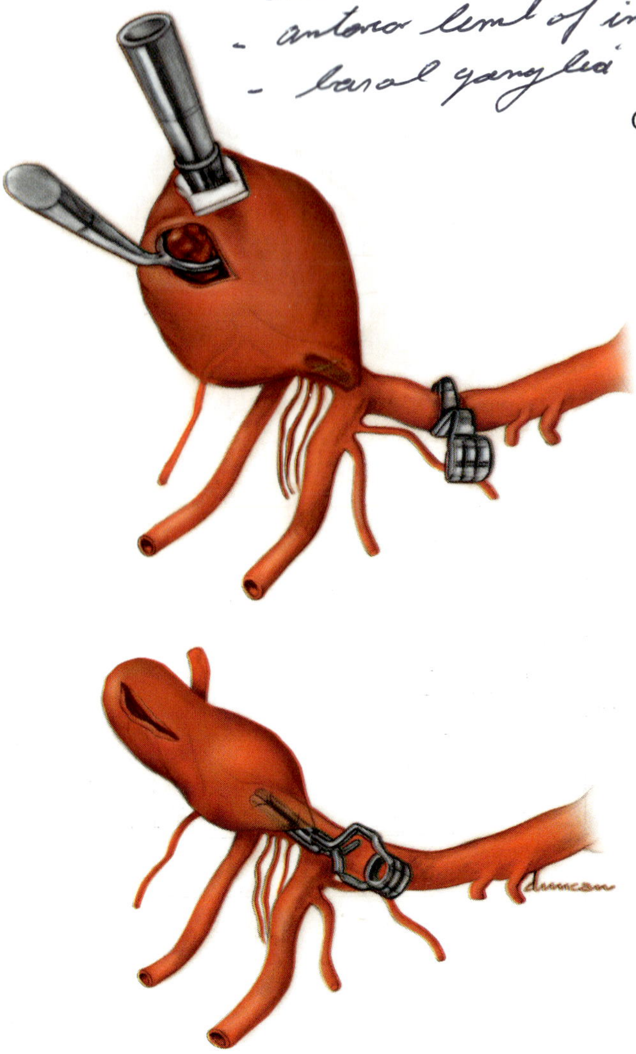

Figure 1–20.

Illustrated here is repair of a giant partially thrombosed aneurysm of the anterior communicating artery complex. With these lesions, thrombectomy must be performed. A temporary clip is placed on the dominant A_1 segment distal to any perforating vessels. The dome of the aneurysm is incised, and ring curets are used to remove the thrombus. It is important to make sure that the incision in the dome of the aneurysm is as far from the neck as possible. If there is significant back bleeding, it may be necessary to occlude temporarily the opposite anterior cerebral artery adjacent to the opposite optic nerve.

SUPRACLINOID INTERNAL CAROTID ARTERY ANEURYSM

As emphasized by Sundt, giant aneurysms of the supraclinoid internal carotid artery can be divided by the direction of their projection, including superior, posterior, medial, and lateral. In nearly all instances, it is necessary to resect the anterior clinoid process. This resection can be performed through either an intradural or an extradural approach. If the intradural approach is chosen, the dura mater overlying the anterior clinoid process is cauterized for a distance of 5 to 10 mm. The bone is then removed with a high-speed diamond air bit. When using the high-speed air drill, it is critical to remove all cottonoids from the wound, because the suction vacuum created by the drill can quickly wrap these cottonoids around the drill and create an "egg beater" in the wound. The extradural approach to removing the anterior clinoid process is described later in this chapter.

Posteriorly projecting aneurysms, as illustrated in this case, are typically the most treacherous because it often is difficult to reconstruct the parent internal carotid artery. Therefore, the surgeon must be prepared to perform a bypass graft either from the cervical carotid or petrous carotid artery, using a saphenous vein harvested from the leg. In this regard, it is useful to know preoperatively the potential for collateral blood flow by performing a trial balloon occlusion during the initial angiography, perhaps in combination with a xenon blood flow or a single photon emission computed tomographic (SPECT) blood flow study. Alternatively, the surgeon can expose the cervical carotid artery and perform a temporary occlusion in conjunction with intraoperative electroencephalographic or cerebral blood flow monitoring. If on inspection of the aneurysm it appears that it is not technically feasible to reconstruct the internal carotid artery and the patient does not tolerate the temporary occlusion, a reasonable option is to perform a saphenous vein bypass graft.

After the Sylvian fissure is divided, the internal carotid artery and optic nerve are first identified. The relationship between the internal carotid artery between the anterior clinoid process and the carotid bifurcation is inspected to determine whether primary clipping will be feasible technically. If the anterior clinoid process has not been removed through an extradural approach, it is removed through an intradural approach. This allows identification of the proximal neck of the aneurysm, which typically originates immediately under the anterior clinoid process.

After the proximal neck of the aneurysm is identified, attention is turned to the distal neck to establish the relationship between it and the anterior choroidal artery. The posterior communicating artery is often absent in posteriorly projecting aneurysms of the internal carotid artery. However, the anterior choroidal artery is often stretched just underneath the carotid bifurcation and must be dissected free. After the anterior choroidal artery is identified, a piece of absorbable gelatin sponge is placed between it and the neck of the aneurysm.

For most giant aneurysms in this location, temporary vessel occlusion and thrombectomy are necessary to facilitate clip placement. The internal carotid artery is occluded either in the neck just distal to the carotid bifurcation or intracranially as the carotid artery exits the cavernous sinus. In that regard, it is best to incise the distal carotid dural ring, which allows a temporary clip to be placed more proximally, thus increasing the amount of space along the proximal neck of the aneurysm. The second temporary clip is placed on the distal internal carotid artery if there is sufficient room. Otherwise, it may be necessary to occlude the proximal A_1 segment if back bleeding is sufficient after the aneurysm has been opened and decompressed. The patient's blood pressure is increased to a systolic pressure of 150 to 160 mm Hg to increase collateral blood flow. Intraoperative electroencephalography can be helpful in determining whether collateral cerebral blood flow is sufficient. If, during preoperative planning, the surgeon anticipates that occlusion of the internal carotid artery will be longer than 20 minutes because of the complexity of the aneurysm and trial balloon occlusion was not tolerated, serious consideration should be given to performing the operation under profound hypothermia or constructing a preocclusion bypass graft to the distal middle cerebral artery complex.

After the aneurysm is temporarily trapped, an incision is made in the dome as distal to the parent artery as possible. Thrombectomy is performed with ring curets. After the aneurysm is collapsed, a clip is placed across its neck in one of two directions. Placement of an angled clip underneath the internal carotid artery from lateral to medial is technically easier than using a cutout clip placed parallel to the internal carotid artery. Although it often is written that a cutout clip is less likely to stenose or to occlude the internal carotid artery, it is difficult to place the clip in a position in which the neck of the aneurysm is obliterated but the origin of the anterior choroidal artery is not compromised. For this reason, it is best to start out using an angled clip placed lateral to medial to determine whether the aneurysm can be obliterated without stenosing the carotid artery. After the clip is placed, blood flow through the carotid artery is confirmed with intraoperative Doppler, ultrasonography, or angiography. The anterior choroidal artery is inspected visually to make sure that it is patent.

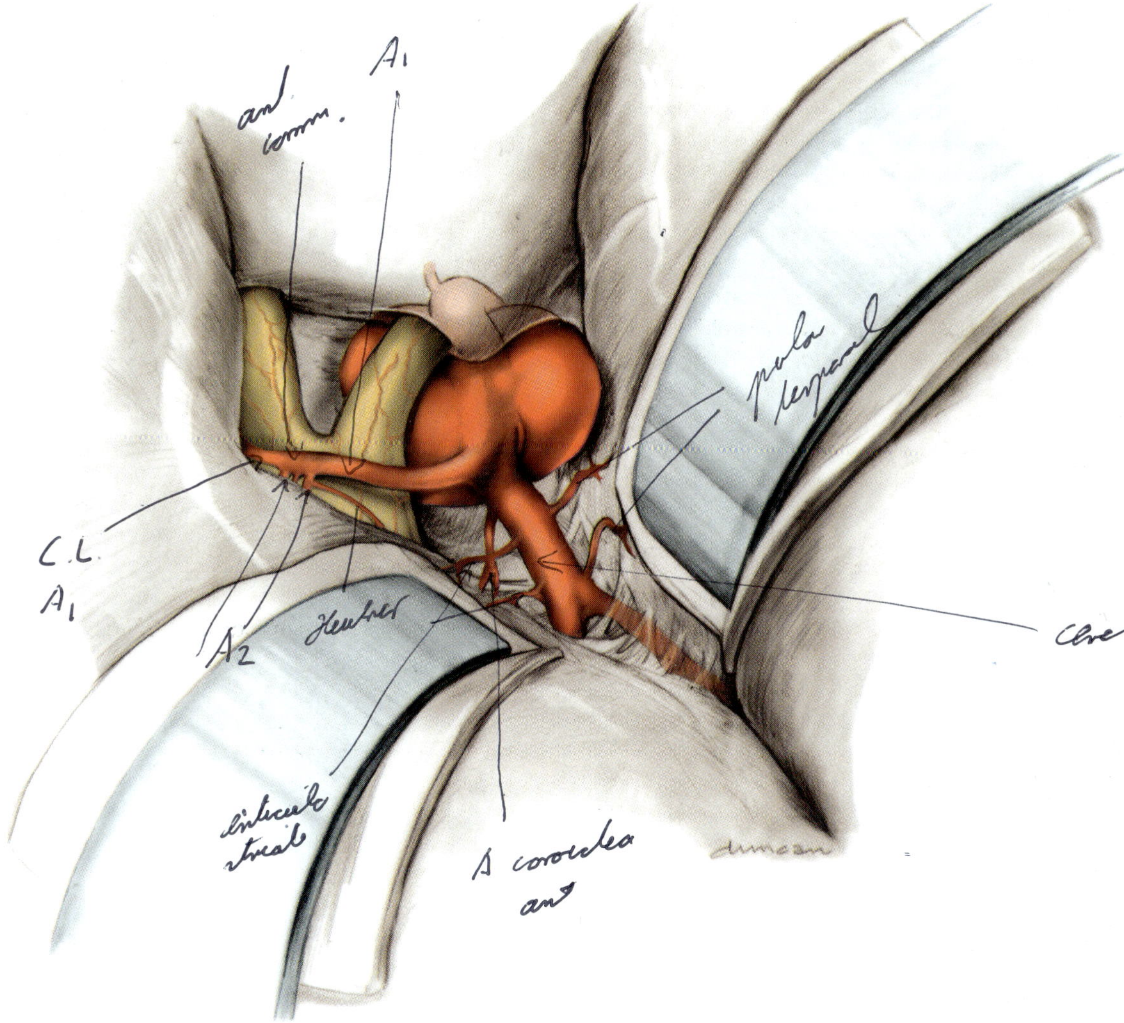

Figure 1–21.

Step 1. It is necessary to remove the anterior clinoid process and to expose the proximal internal carotid artery to obtain proximal control of the vessel and to identify the neck of the aneurysm. Some of these aneurysms can be transitional in that the neck originates from the clinoid segment and the dome of the aneurysm extends intradurally. Typically, the posterior communicating artery is not present. However, invariably, the anterior choroidal artery is intimately associated with the distal neck of the aneurysm and must be dissected free. It is necessary to separate widely the Sylvian fissure to identify the carotid bifurcation. It may be useful to place a retractor on the temporal lobe. However, depending on the angle of the clip to be placed, the temporal lobe retractor may be in the way and may need to be removed. With giant aneurysms in this location, exposure of the cervical carotid artery provides a safety net in case the aneurysm ruptures before proximal control of the carotid artery is achieved.

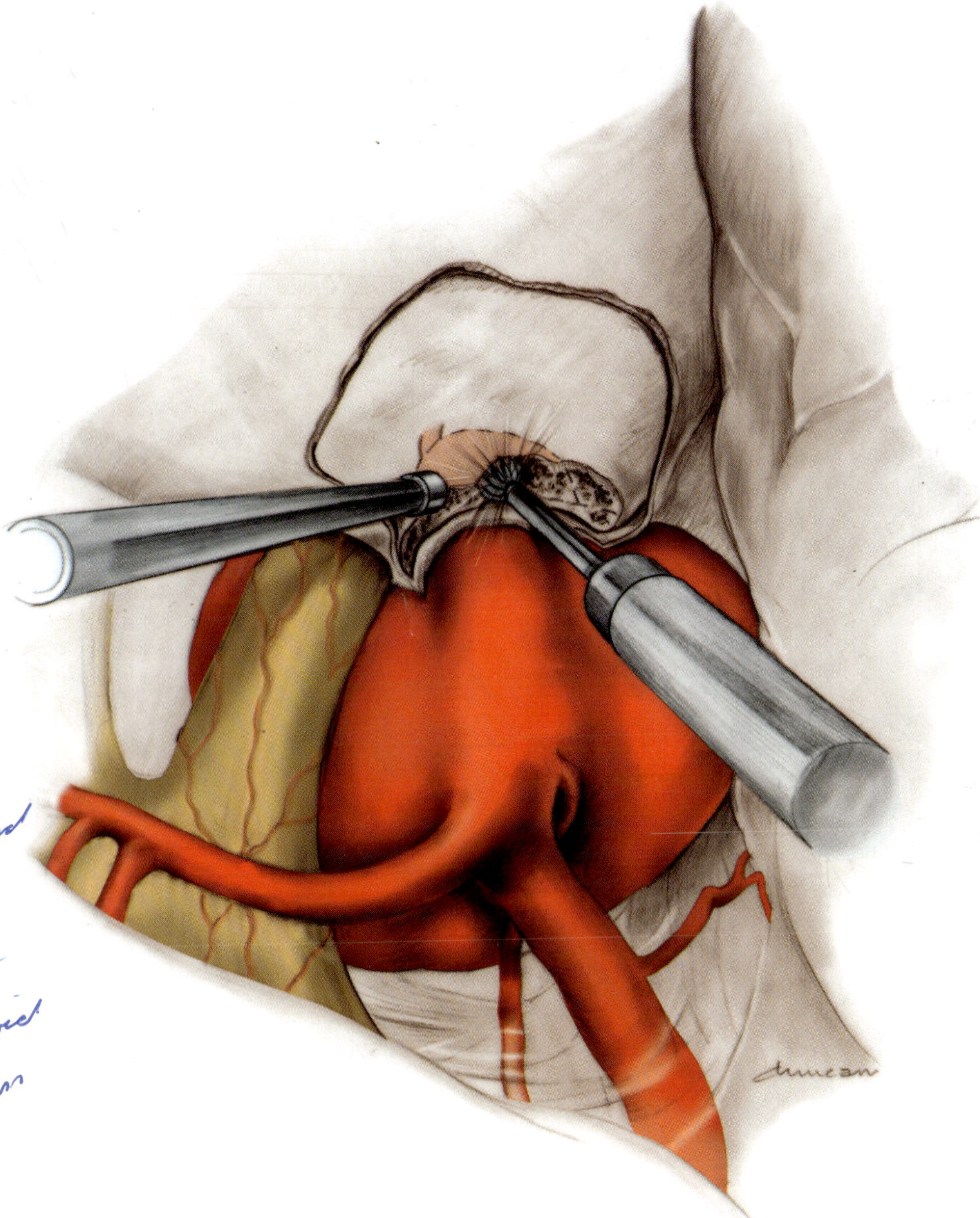

Figure 1–22.

Step 2. There are two ways to remove the anterior clinoid process. As illustrated here, it can be removed through an intradural approach. A small spatula is used to cauterize and to peel the dura mater off the anterior clinoid process. A small diamond bur is used to gently drill the clinoid process and expose the supraclinoid carotid artery. When the anterior clinoid process is thin, a small bone rongeur is used to bite off the rest of the bone. During removal of the anterior clinoid process, it is important to remove the bar of bone between the anterior clinoid process and the superior orbital fissure. Also, it is best to remove the optic strut bone just lateral to the optic nerve. This removal of bone medial and lateral to the anterior clinoid process creates more room, thereby increasing the options for placing and manipulating the clip. The other way to remove the anterior clinoid process is through an extradural approach, as pioneered by Dolenc. The advantage of the extradural approach is that there is dura mater between the bony removal and the aneurysm. Also, the surgeon can be more aggressive about the degree of bony removal of the medial sphenoid wing, which increases exposure of the intracavernous carotid artery. With the extradural approach, the outer sphenoid wing is removed with a small orbital rongeur. Under the operating microscope, the medial sphenoid wing is drilled off with a diamond bur, first identifying the superior orbital fissure. Next, the diamond bur is used to thin the bony bridge between the superior orbital fissure and the anterior clinoid process. The drill is also used to thin and to remove the orbital strut of bone between the optic canal and the anterior clinoid process. After these medial and lateral bony bridges have been thinned, small bone cups or forceps are used to bite bone and to wiggle the anterior clinoid process free. These same bony cups can be used to remove additional thin bone over the optic nerve medially and the superior orbital fissure laterally.

Figure 1–23.

Step 3. *A*, After the anterior clinoid process is removed, the internal carotid artery is mobilized by incising the distal dural ring. This distal dural ring is continuous with the dura mater that surrounds the optic nerve medially and the falciform ligament laterally.

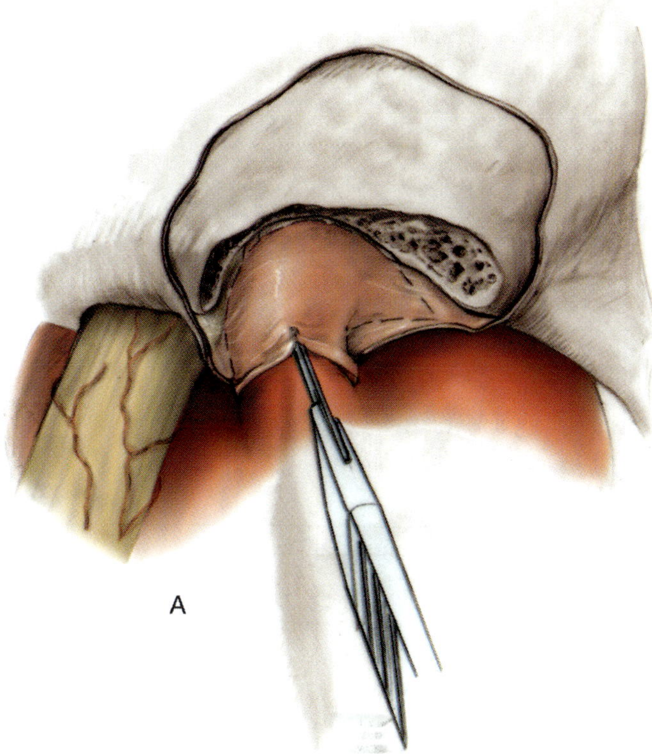

A

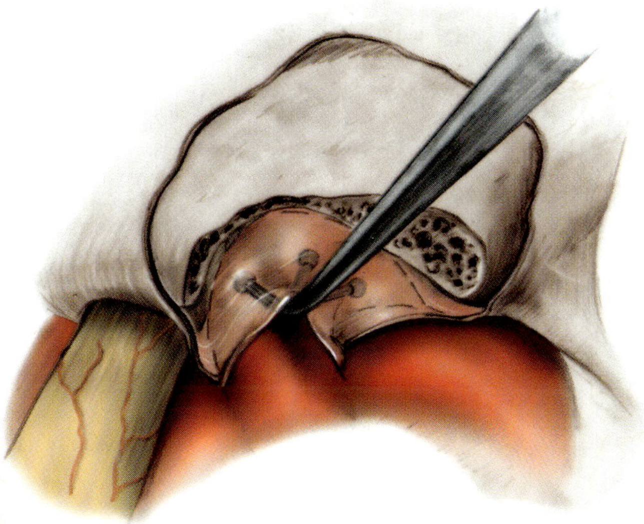

B

B, A ball-tip dissector can be used to dissect the plane between the internal carotid artery and the dural ring.

C, When this plane is established, a microscissors such as a micro Potts can be used to incise the dural ring. It is best to stay on top of the internal carotid artery during this incision. After the outer dural ring is cut, a small spatula can be used to sweep the dural reflections medially and laterally. In most transitional carotid aneurysms, the origin of the ophthalmic artery defines the medial extent of the neck of the aneurysm. Often, the ophthalmic artery originates from the extradural carotid artery. Therefore, it is necessary to carry the dissection proximal to the anterior genu of the internal carotid artery. Often, the very lateral and medial attachments of the carotid dural rings are adherent to the neck of the aneurysm and must be sharply dissected free with a spatula or, occasionally, a #11 blade knife.

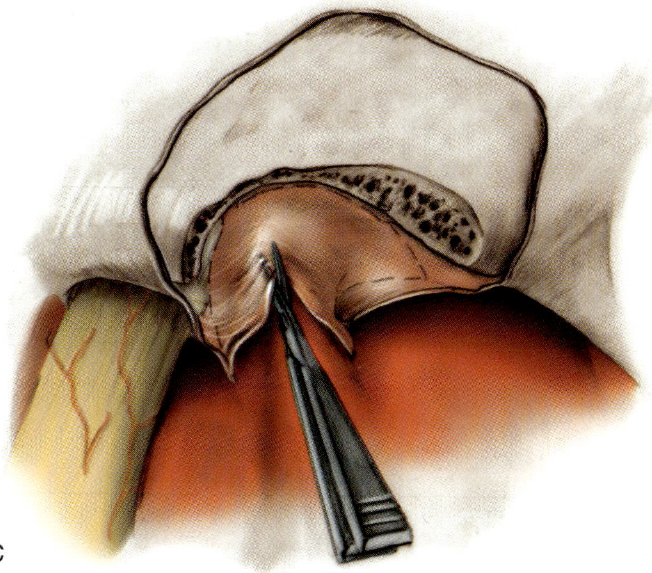

C

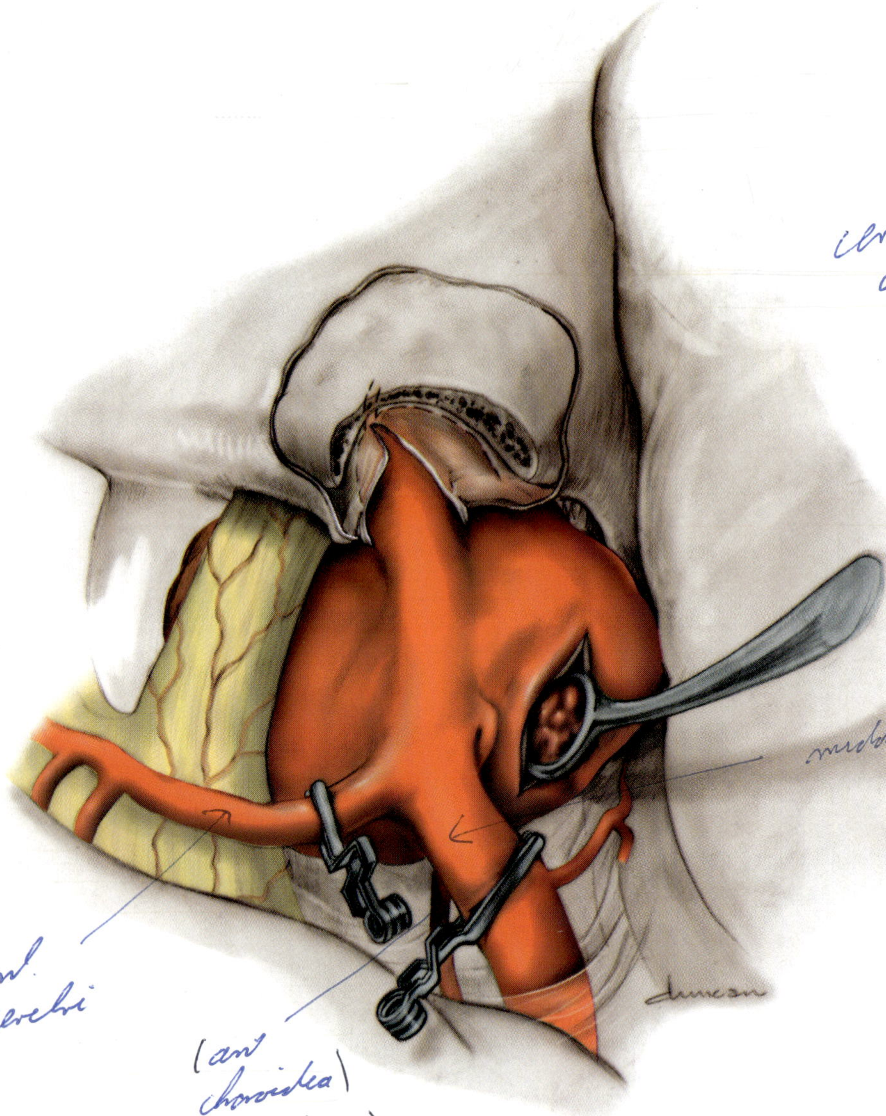

Figure 1–24.

Step 4. For most giant aneurysms, it is necessary to temporarily occlude some of the major arteries and to perform thrombectomy. In this example, removal of the anterior clinoid process is not sufficient to expose the proximal internal carotid artery to temporarily place a clip. Therefore, the cervical internal carotid artery is occluded. A temporary clip is also placed on the A_1 segment. Occasionally, it is possible to place a temporary clip proximal to the anterior choroidal artery, in which case there is continued perfusion of the anterior choroidal artery and the middle cerebral artery complex through the anterior communicating artery. More typically, as illustrated here, there is not enough room to place temporary clips proximal to the bifurcation. When incising the dome of the aneurysm, it is important to make the incision as distal to the neck as possible so that placement of the permanent clip will not be compromised.

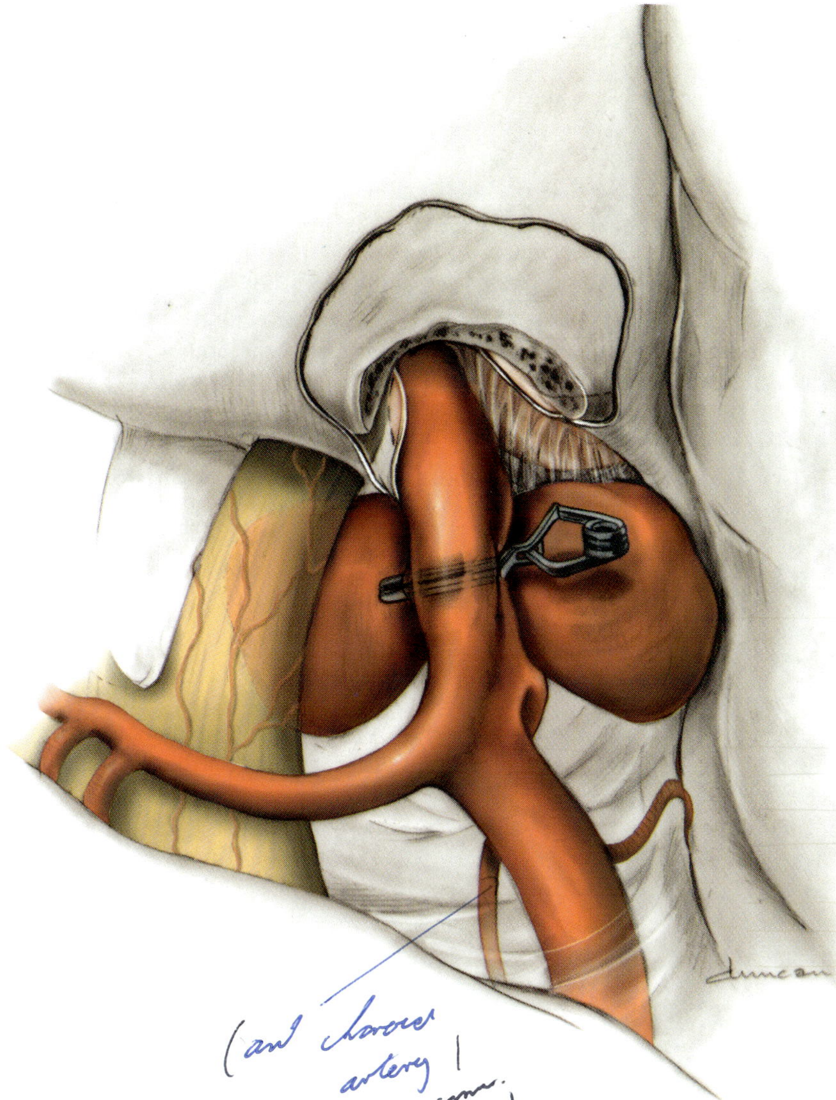

Figure 1–25.

Step 5. There are two ways to place the aneurysm clip—the one illustrated here and the one shown in Figure 1–26. Placing the clip perpendicular to the internal carotid artery is technically easier in terms of preserving the anterior choroidal artery. However, it may also cause kinking of the carotid artery and lead to stenosis or occlusion.

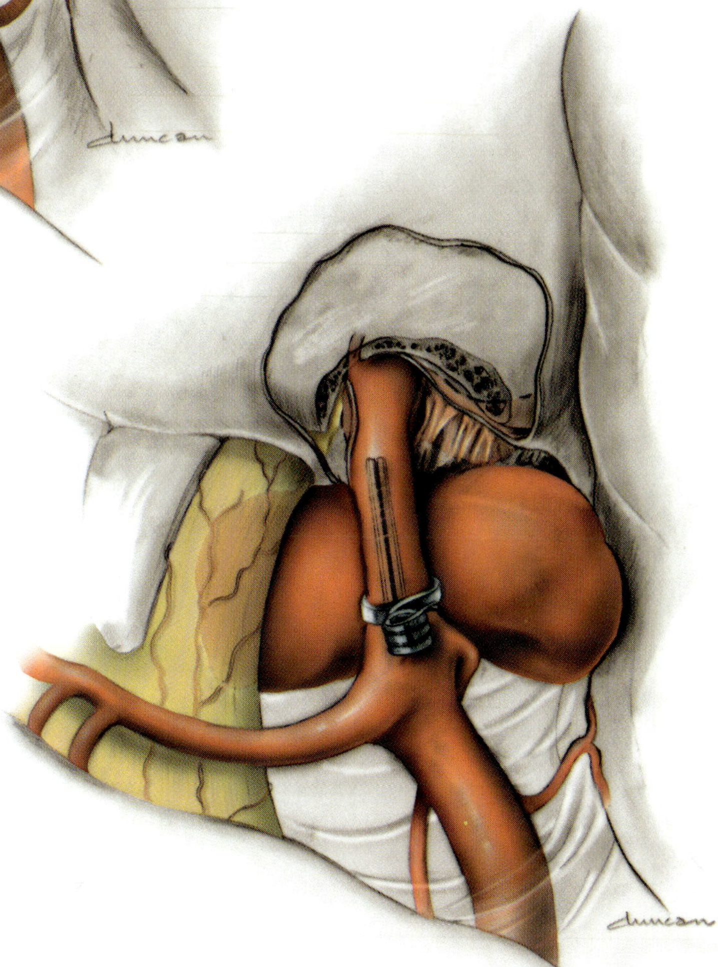

Figure 1–26.

An alternative clip placement is a cutout that runs parallel with the internal carotid artery. There is less risk of stenosis of the artery if the cutout has sufficient caliber. Regardless of the way the clip is placed, the more aggressive the thrombectomy, the easier the placement of the clip and the less risk of stenosis of the parent internal carotid artery. After the clip is placed in these complex cases, it is mandatory to determine that the internal carotid artery is patent. Although intraoperative micro Doppler or ultrasonography can be used to demonstrate patency, intraoperative angiography is superior because it reveals whether there is significant stenosis adjacent to the clip. If the ipsilateral cervical carotid artery has already been exposed, intraoperative angiography can be performed through a direct common carotid artery puncture.

CRANIOPHARYNGIOMA

There are several good exposures for removal of suprasellar craniopharyngiomas, including a frontotemporal orbital craniotomy and a standard pterional craniotomy. The true subfrontal approach, with removal of one orbital roof, can be advantageous when there is a large extension of the craniopharyngioma into the third ventricle (described in Chapter 3). However, a large extension into the third ventricle can also be removed through a standard pterional craniotomy by vigorous internal decompression of the tumor, often in combination with an incision in the lamina terminalis posterior to the optic chiasm. With a pterional craniotomy, the expanded optic-carotid triangle can be used to the surgeon's advantage. Sectioning the lamina terminalis during a pterional approach is often more difficult than expected, because the posterior margin of the optic chiasm may not be visible. In this case, it is best to perform an aggressive debulking of the tumor through the optic-carotid triangle and to collapse the third ventricular extension of the tumor into the subchiasmatic cistern. Occasionally, the infundibulum can be preserved, especially if the craniopharyngioma is largely cystic. However, if the tumor is more calcified and grumous, the infundibulum typically enters the tumor capsule and cannot be preserved.

After the Sylvian fissure is divided and the retractors are placed, the optic-carotid triangle is identified. Typically, the ipsilateral carotid artery is displaced laterally, the anterior cerebral artery and its perforating branches are pushed upward, and the optic chiasm is bowed medially and upward. The arachnoid is first incised between the tumor capsule and medial surface of the internal carotid artery. This incision is then carried distally between the anterior cerebral artery and the tumor capsule. Finally, the arachnoid between the optic nerve and chiasm and the tumor is incised. The arachnoid between the anterior cerebral artery and the frontal lobe is left intact. A Yasargil retractor is placed deeper along the inferior aspect of the frontal lobe, which helps to move the anterior cerebral artery out of harm's way.

The next step is to make a linear incision, 5 to 10 mm, in the tumor capsule. An internal decompression is then performed with ring curets. After the tumor has been partially decompressed, the lateral aspect of the tumor capsule is dissected off the medial aspect of the internal carotid artery. Typically, the posterior communicating artery and its branches are ensheathed in arachnoid, which facilitates dissection and separation from the lateral aspect of the tumor capsule. After this has been achieved, cottonoids are placed between the outer tumor capsule and the inner aspect of the internal carotid artery, the posterior communicating artery, and the anterior choroidal artery.

With a #5 or #7 straight suction tip and a cottonoid, the tumor is gently retracted medially and dissection is performed behind the tumor capsule, with preservation of the arachnoid overlying the basilar artery and its perforating vessels. The tumor is further decompressed internally to facilitate manipulation of the capsule wall. After the basilar artery, the basilar caput, and, possibly, the posterior cerebral arteries have been identified, cottonoids are placed deep to protect them.

Next, attention is directed to dissecting the tumor off the opposite anterior clinoid process and internal carotid artery. Typically, the arachnoid covers the internal carotid artery and posterior communicating artery, and if it is left intact, it will protect these structures. The tumor capsule is retracted toward the surgeon with a #5 or #7 straight suction tip, which stretches the adhesions between the capsule and the internal carotid artery, making it easier to divide the adhesions.

After the tumor has been dissected off the opposite internal carotid artery, the angle of the microscope is repositioned to allow a more direct view underneath the optic chiasm. It usually is necessary, once again, to debulk the tumor to facilitate retraction of the capsule. The tumor capsule is again retracted toward the ipsilateral internal carotid artery with the use of a #5 or #7 straight suction tip and cottonoid, which stretches the adhesions between the tumor capsule and the optic chiasm and the hypothalamus. They can be dissected free more easily, after which cottonoids are placed to protect the underside of the chiasm and the hypothalamic region.

It is important to emphasize that the residual tumor capsule should be removed through the optic-carotid triangle with gentle force. While the capsule is being removed, all aspects are inspected to make sure that no residual adhesions remain between the tumor capsule and the surrounding vascular and parenchymal structures. After the tumor is removed, the surgical bed is inspected. A malleable fiberoptic probe or mirrors are useful in inspecting the underside of the optic chiasm and the third ventricle for possible residual tumor.

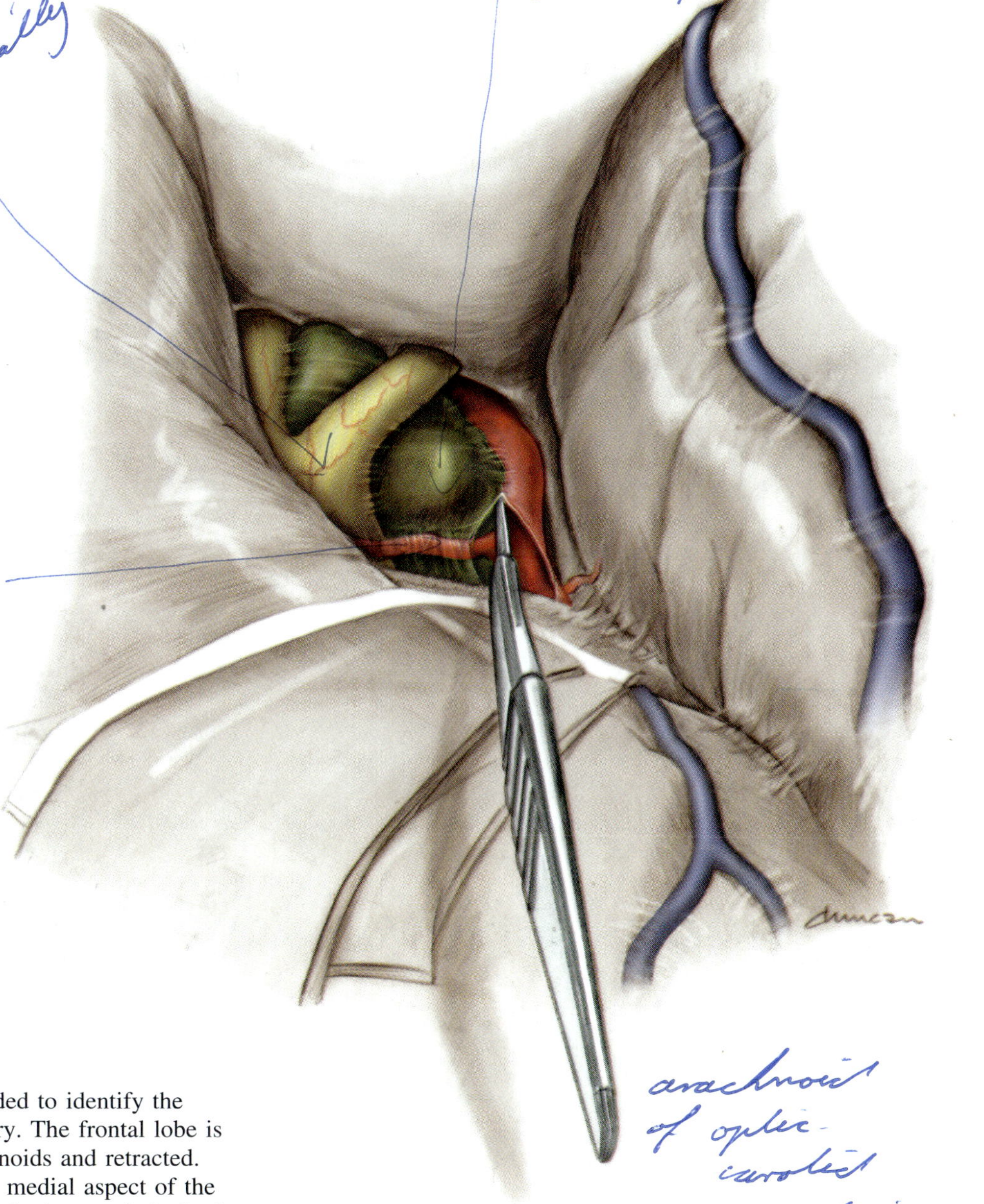

Figure 1–27.

Step 1. The Sylvian fissure is divided to identify the bifurcation of the internal carotid artery. The frontal lobe is lined with hemostatic fabric and cottonoids and retracted. The arachnoid between the tumor and medial aspect of the internal carotid artery and anterior cerebral artery is incised. The arachnoid between the anterior cerebral artery and the frontal lobe is left intact, so that when the frontal lobe is retracted the anterior cerebral artery is gently displaced. During the operation, most of the work is performed through the expanded optic-carotid triangle. Tumor debulking can also be performed between the two optic nerves if the chiasm is postfixed.

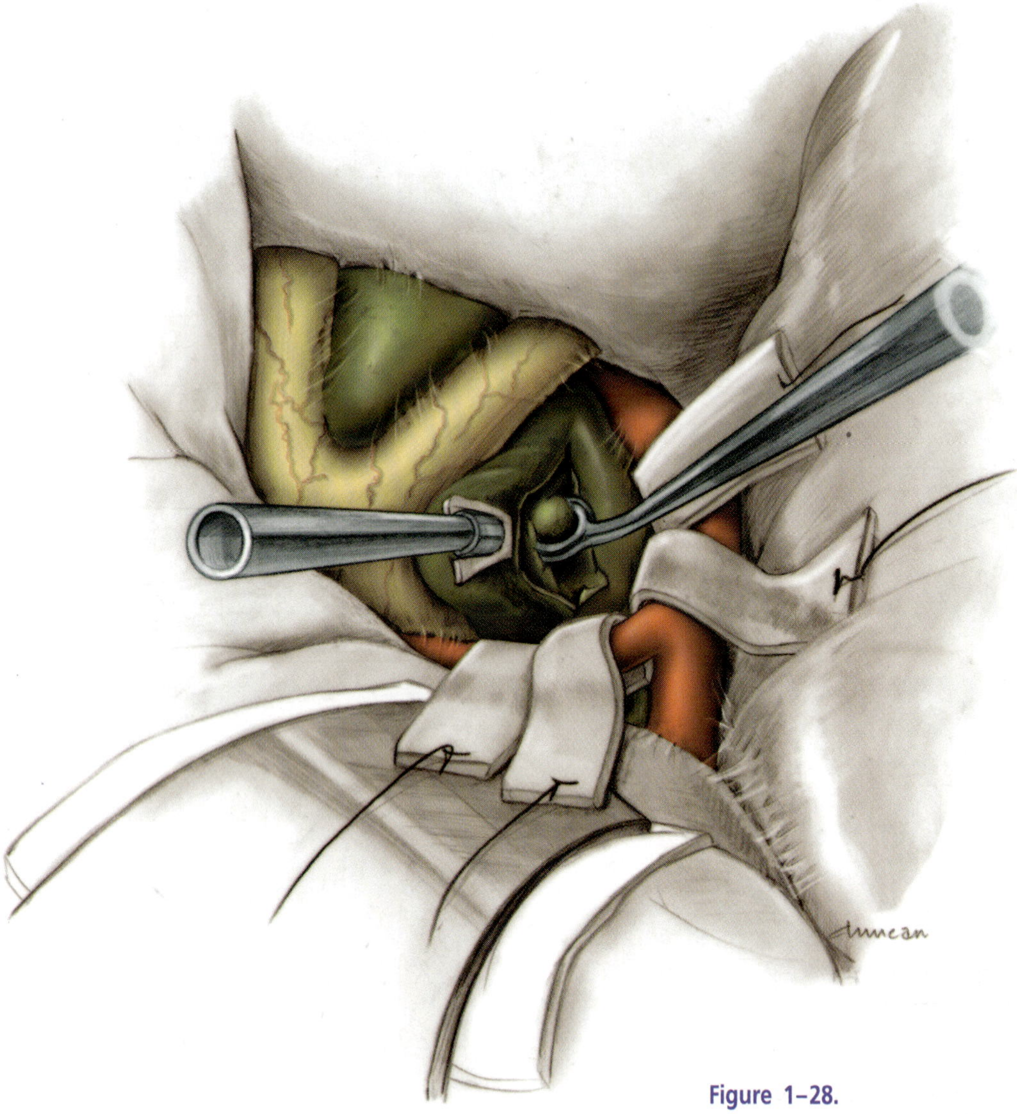

Figure 1–28.

Step 2. After the lateral aspect of the tumor capsule has been defined, a 5- to 10-mm incision is made in the tumor. Various ring curettes are used to begin debulking the tumor. During this process, it is important to make sure that traction is kept to a minimum on the optic apparatus.

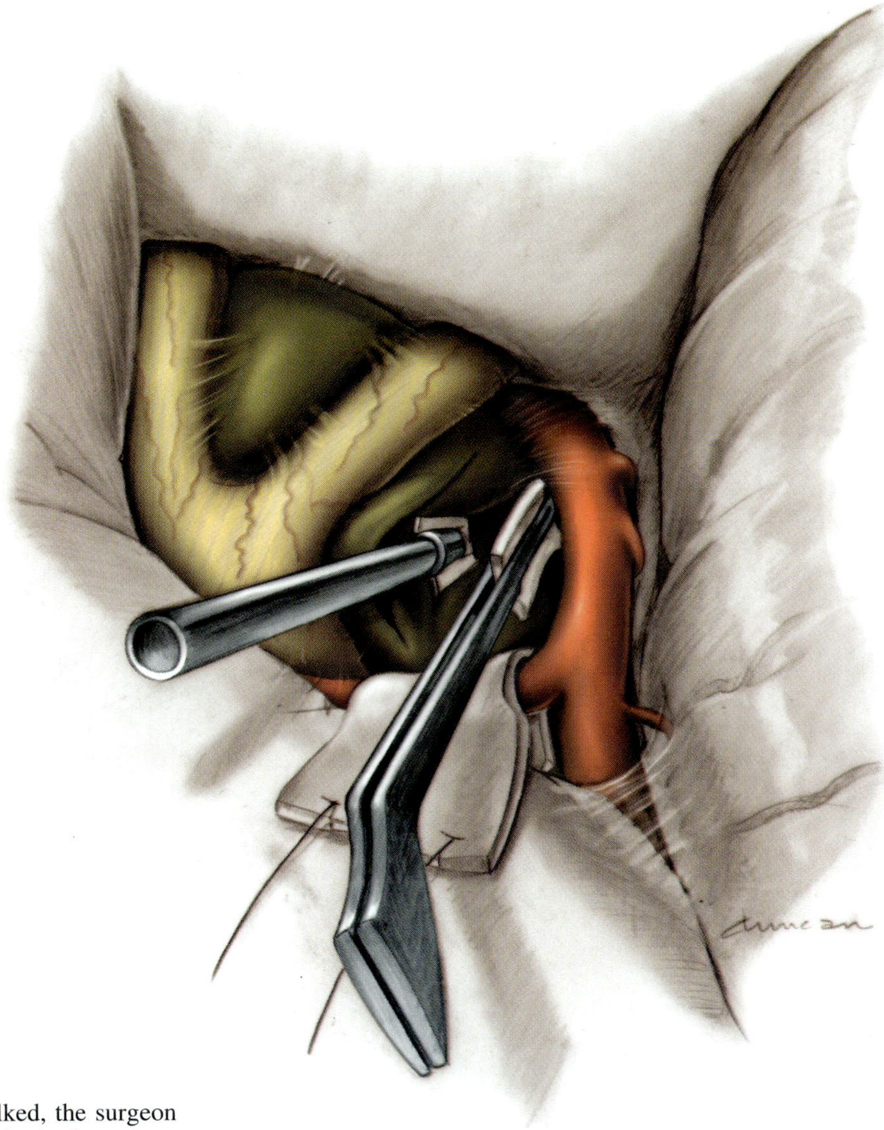

Figure 1–29.

Step 3. After the tumor is partially debulked, the surgeon dissects the lateral margin of the tumor off the ipsilateral internal carotid artery. There typically is a layer of arachnoid between the tumor capsule and the posterior communicating and anterior choroidal arteries and their perforating arteries. Respecting this arachnoid barrier will protect these vascular structures. The tumor capsule is gently displaced medially with a #5 or #7 straight suction tip and cottonoid. After the perforating arteries that come off the internal carotid artery are identified, they are protected with cottonoids.

Figure 1–30.

Step 4. The dissection is carried deeper to identify the basilar artery. The arachnoid that invests the posterior communicating artery extends deep between the tumor capsule and basilar artery. This arachnoid should not be violated. The tumor is retracted medially with a #5 or #7 straight suction tip and a cottonoid. After the posterior component of the tumor capsule has been identified, cottonoids are placed over the basilar artery.

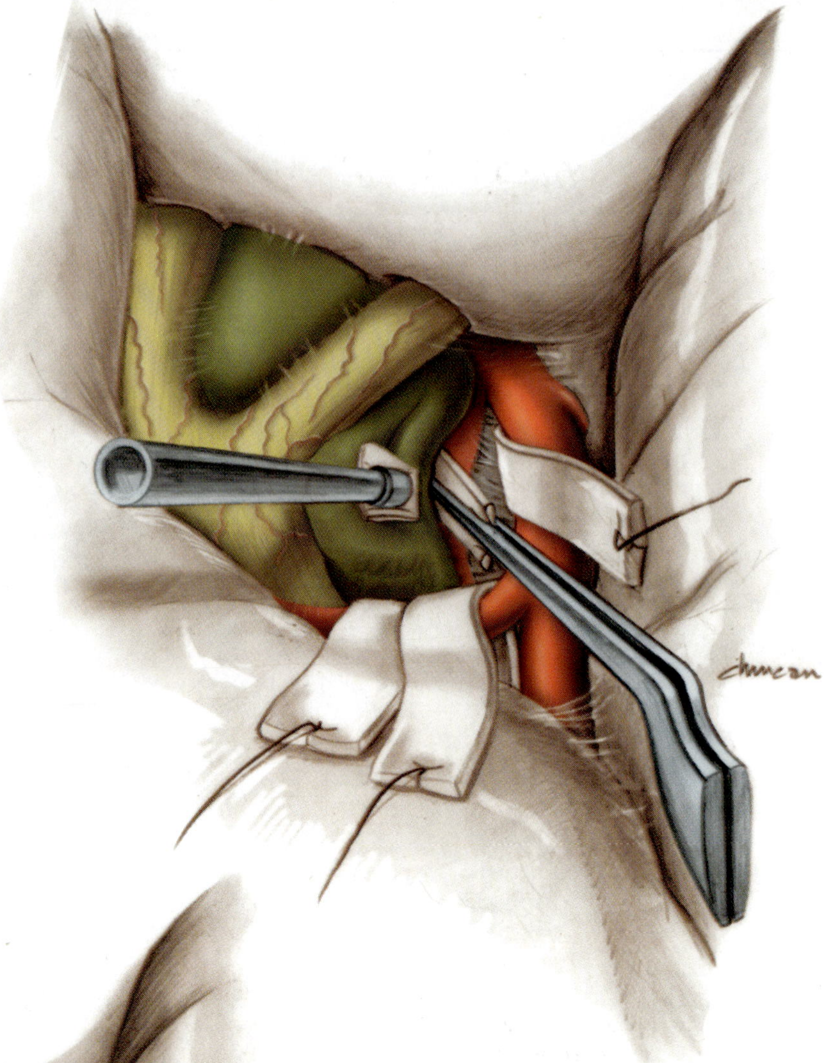

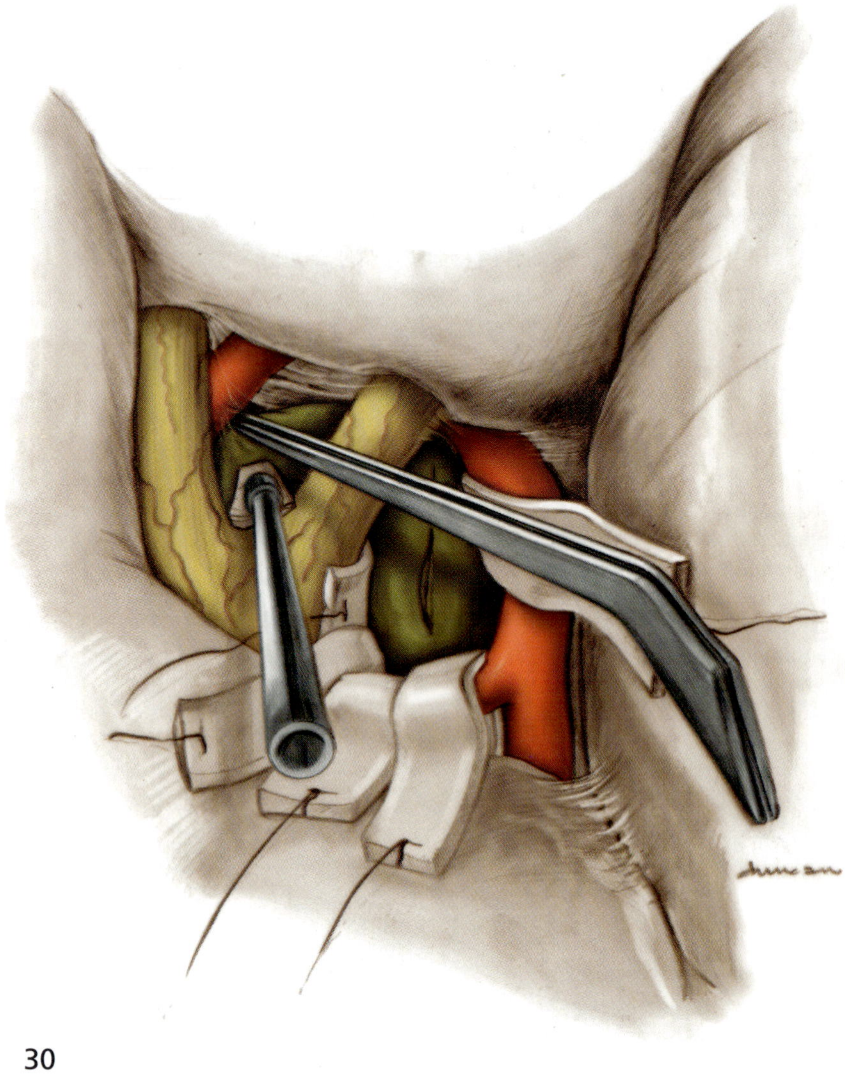

Figure 1–31.

Step 5. Next, the tumor capsule is dissected off the contralateral internal carotid artery and the anterior clinoid process. In this case, there is a postfixed chiasm; thus, the dissection is performed between the two optic nerves. The arachnoid plane between the carotid artery and its branches and the tumor capsule should be respected.

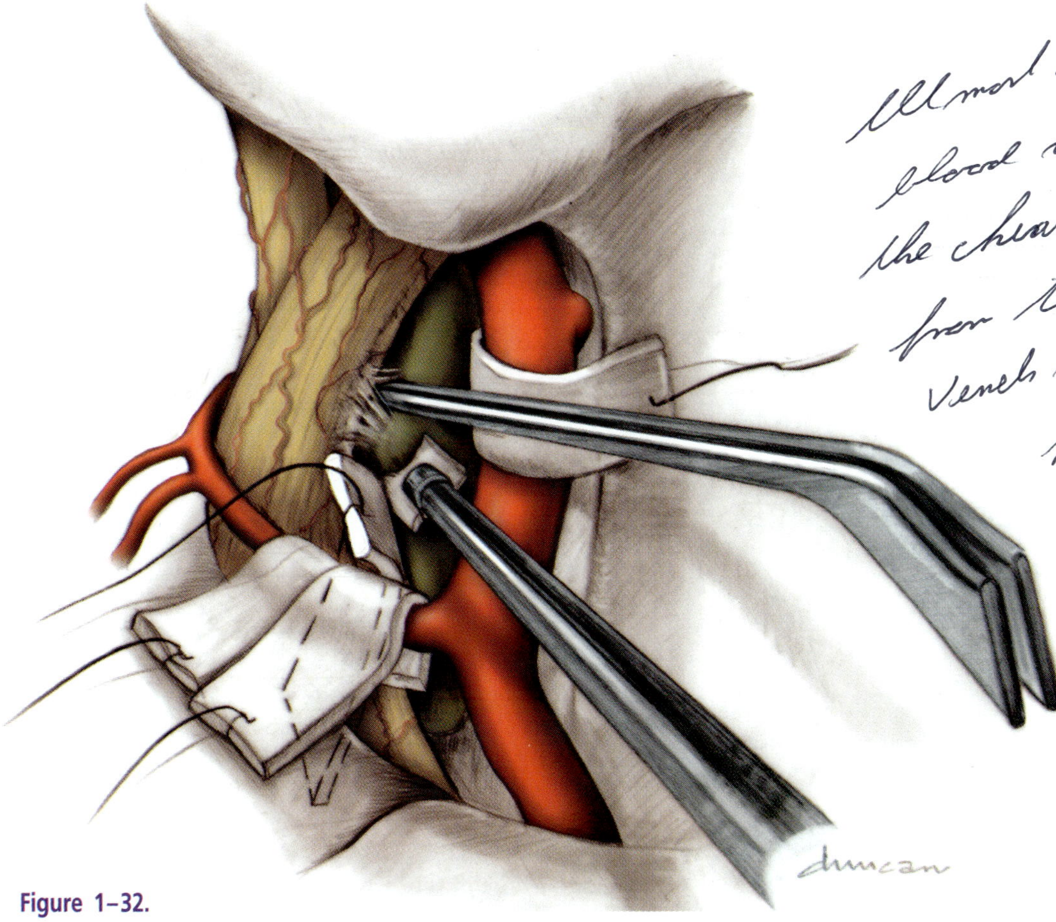

Figure 1–32.

Step 6. The tumor is further decompressed internally with ring curets. To work across the middle cranial fossa, the operating microscope is repositioned to provide a more lateral or horizontal view of the ipsilateral optic nerve. This permits dissection of the interface between the tumor and the optic nerve and chiasm. There is no arachnoid plane between these structures. The tumor capsule should be retracted downward; oftentimes, this retraction peels the tumor capsule off the underside of the chiasm. It is important to recognize that the primary blood supply to the chiasm is from the underside, and, therefore, all minute blood vessels must be preserved. In patients with a large extension of craniopharyngioma into the third ventricle or a prefixed optic chiasm, it is useful to remove this ventricular component through the lamina terminalis. This is described in Chapter 3.

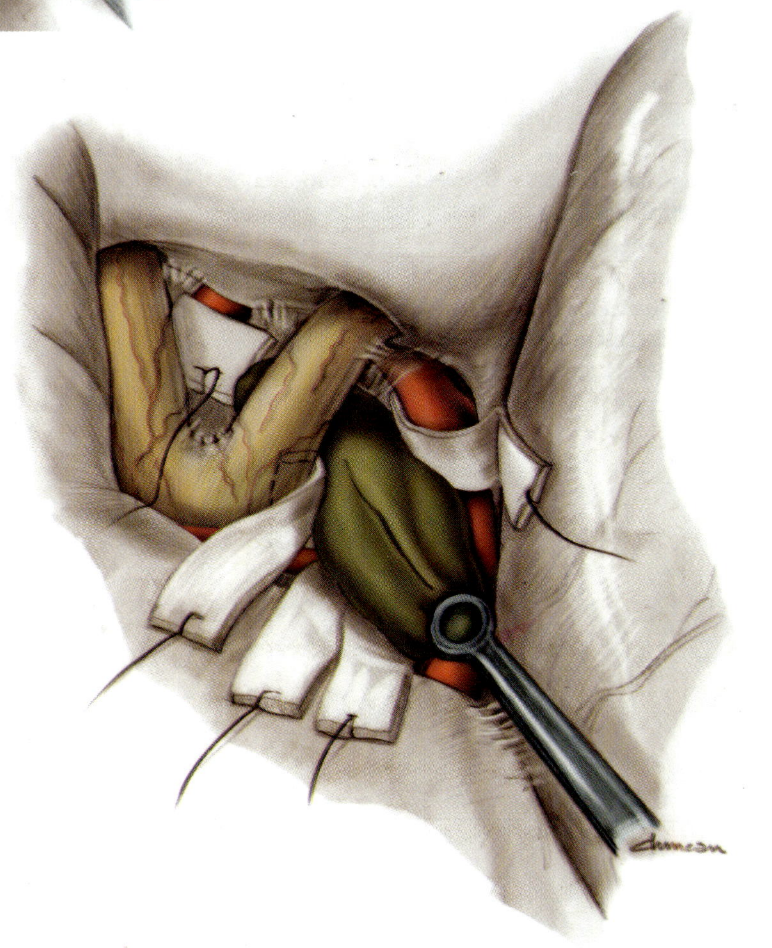

Figure 1–33.

Step 7. After the tumor has been dissected off the chiasm and extracted from the third ventricle, it is removed through the optic-carotid triangle with a forceps. After the tumor has been removed, the underside of the chiasm and the third ventricle are inspected with either mirrors or a malleable fiberoptic probe to make sure that the tumor has been resected completely.

SPHENOID WING MENINGIOMA

Meningiomas located along the medial two-thirds of the sphenoid wing are best approached through a standard pterional craniotomy, whereas those located on the lateral one-third should be approached through a larger frontotemporal craniotomy. It is important to recognize that often one or two perforating arteries off the middle cerebral artery enter the deep aspect of the tumor capsule. Thus, to prevent evulsing these branches, the tumor must not be pulled out before the underside or deep component of the tumor is dissected.

After the bone flap is removed, the outer sphenoid wing is removed with a high-speed air drill, under the operating microscope. This is useful in increasing exposure and devascularizing part of the tumor. The dura mater is opened widely, and any branches off the middle meningeal artery that were exposed when the outer sphenoid wing was removed are cauterized and divided because they typically feed the tumor. The brain is lined with hemostatic fabric and cottonoids, and the tumor capsule is separated from the overlying frontal and temporal lobes.

Separating the tumor from the overlying parenchyma is made easier by placing the brain under slight tension with a Yasargil retractor and providing countertraction on the tumor capsule with a #5 or #7 straight suction tip. This places tension on the adhesions between the tumor capsule and the arachnoid, easing separation. First, the lateral margin of the tumor is dissected free from the temporal lobe. Second, the distal Sylvian fissure is divided, identifying the interface between the tumor and the middle cerebral artery. After the middle cerebral artery is identified, cottonoids are placed over it for protection. The interface between the frontal lobe and the tumor is then identified and dissected free, and cottonoids are placed to protect the frontal and temporal lobes.

After an initial dissection has been performed between the tumor and the frontal and temporal lobes, the tumor capsule is cauterized and the tumor is decompressed internally with curets and an ultrasonic aspirator. The greater the internal decompression of the tumor, the easier it is to retract the tumor capsule from the neurovascular structures.

Typically, the blood supply of these tumors is from the dura mater of the sphenoid wing. Therefore, after debulking some of the tumor and clearly distinguishing the borders of the tumor from the frontal and temporal lobes, the tumor attachments to the sphenoid wing are cauterized. The tumor capsule is retracted with a #5 or #7 straight suction tip and cottonoids, thereby allowing better definition of the interface between the tumor and sphenoid wing. Bipolar cautery with irrigation is used to obtain hemostasis of the dura mater, which often is quite vascular.

The critical component in tumor resection is the deep aspect of the tumor and its relationship to the supraclinoid carotid artery, the middle cerebral artery, and the optic nerve. Occasionally, one can work from lateral to medial along the Sylvian fissure, identifying the middle cerebral artery and following it proximal to the carotid bifurcation. When this is achieved, much of the tumor can be removed. This leaves a small piece of tumor along the anterior clinoid process.

Underneath the anterior clinoid process, the internal carotid artery and optic nerve usually are separated from the tumor by overlying arachnoid. It is important to preserve this arachnoid (if possible) because it protects these structures. The residual bit of tumor is rolled outward along the sphenoid wing to identify the internal carotid artery and its bifurcation. Although the tumor may wrap itself around the internal carotid artery, the arachnoid plane between this artery and the tumor often allows removal of the tumor between the internal carotid artery and its branches laterally and the tentorial edge medially.

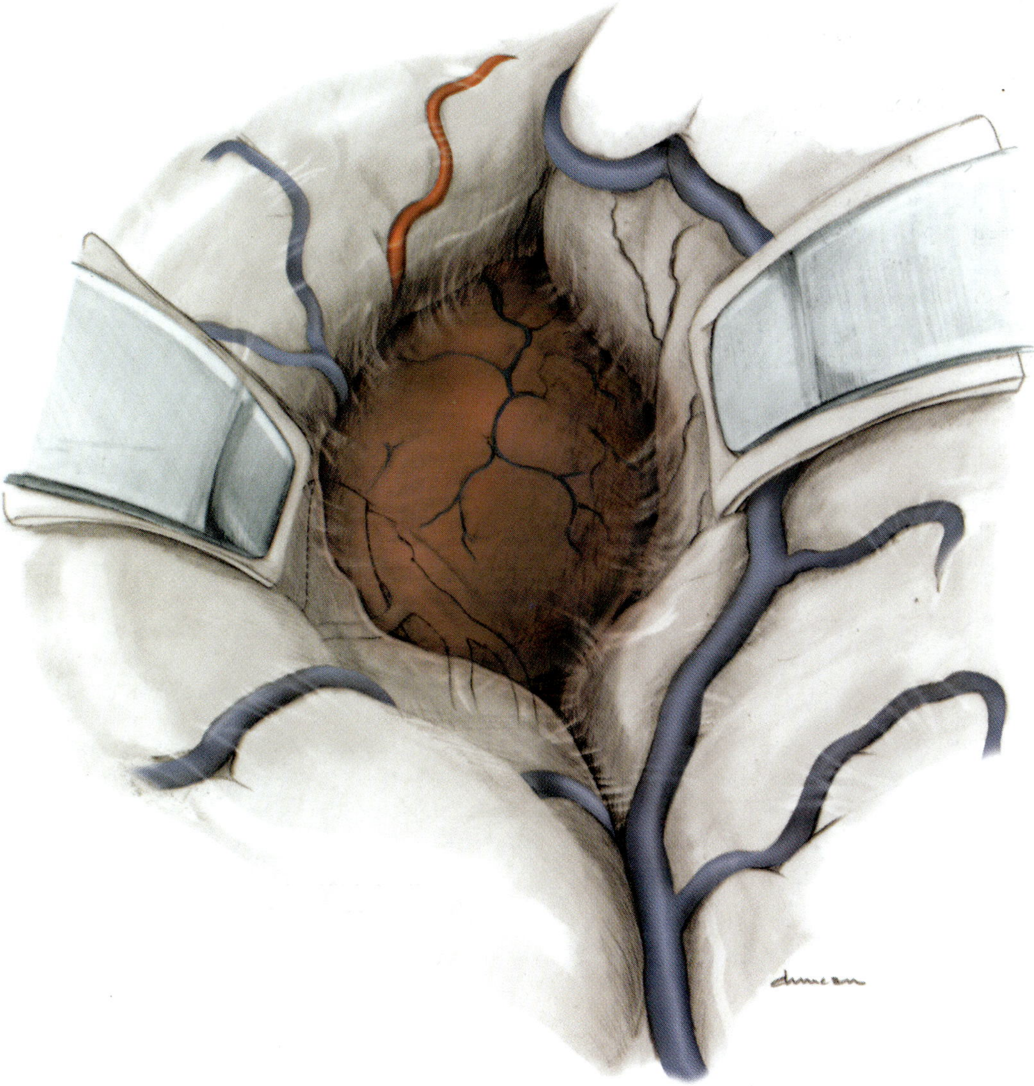

Figure 1–34.

The meningioma illustrated involves much of the sphenoid wing, both medially and laterally.

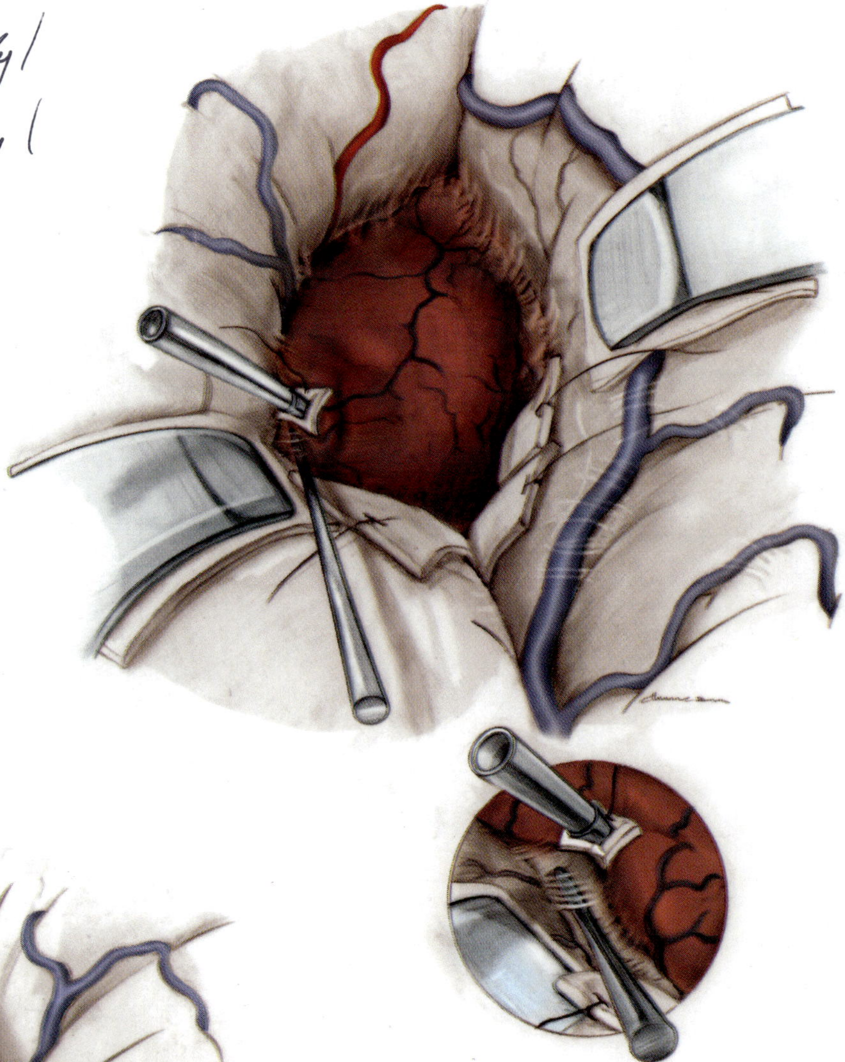

Figure 1–35.

Step 1. The interface between the tumor and the temporal lobe and, then, the frontal lobe is identified and separated. Typically, a Yasargil retractor is used to retract the brain and a #5 or #7 straight suction tip and cottonoid are used to place countertraction on the tumor capsule. This places the arachnoid adhesions under tension, allowing easier separation of the tumor from the brain.

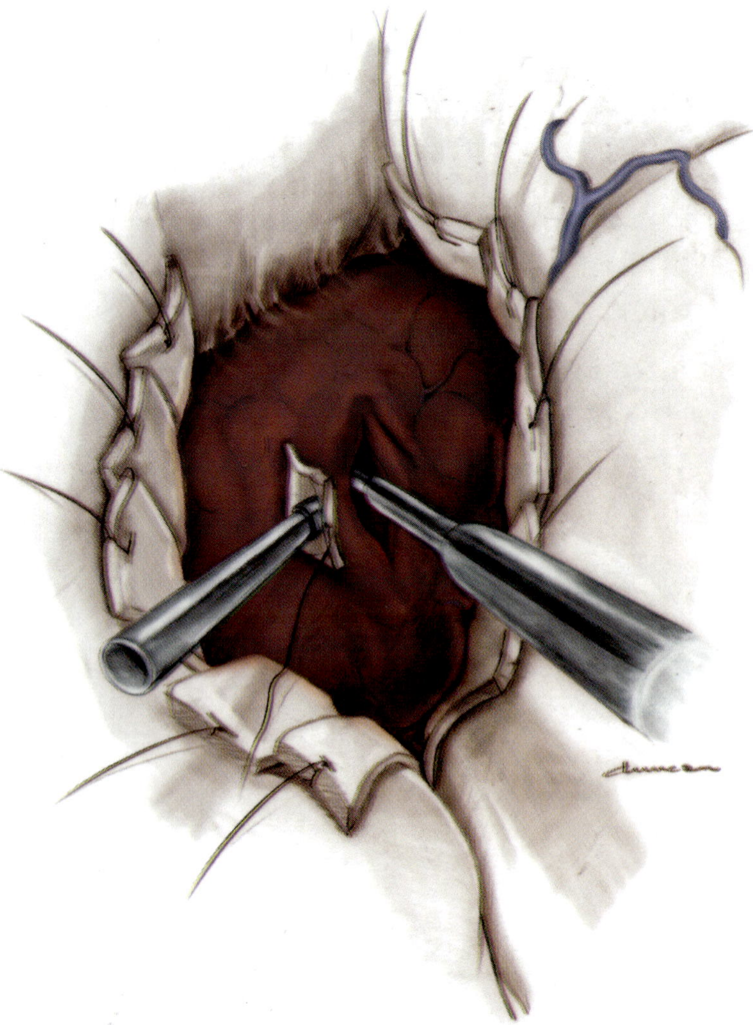

Figure 1–36.

Step 2. After the tumor is separated from the frontal and temporal lobes, it is decompressed with curets, laser, or an ultrasonic aspirator.

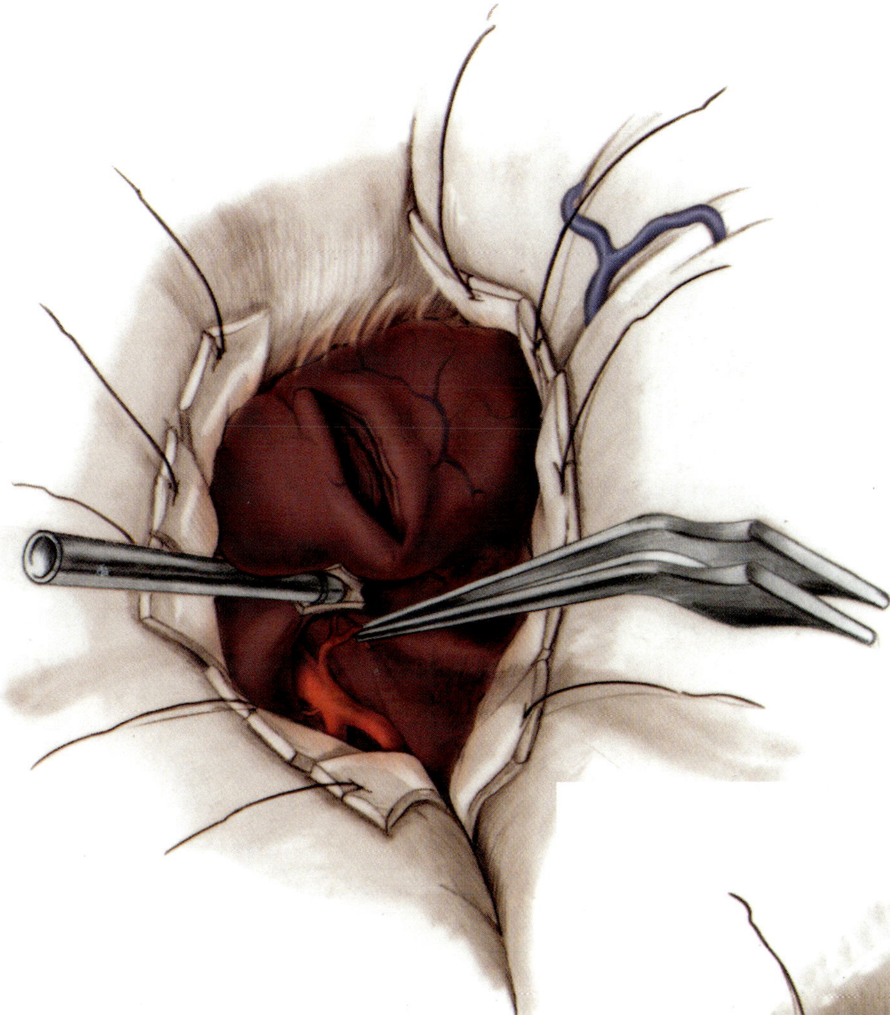

Figure 1–37.

Step 3. The outer or lateral Sylvian fissure is divided, and the relationship between the tumor and the middle cerebral artery is dissected free. Often, one or two branches off the middle cerebral artery are incorporated into the tumor capsule. Because of this, the underside of the tumor must be separated completely from the middle cerebral artery before the tumor is removed. Otherwise, some of the perforating branches of the middle cerebral artery may be evulsed. Also, the tumor may parasitize several of these vessels. Branches of the middle cerebral artery that clearly supply the tumor may be safely cauterized and divided.

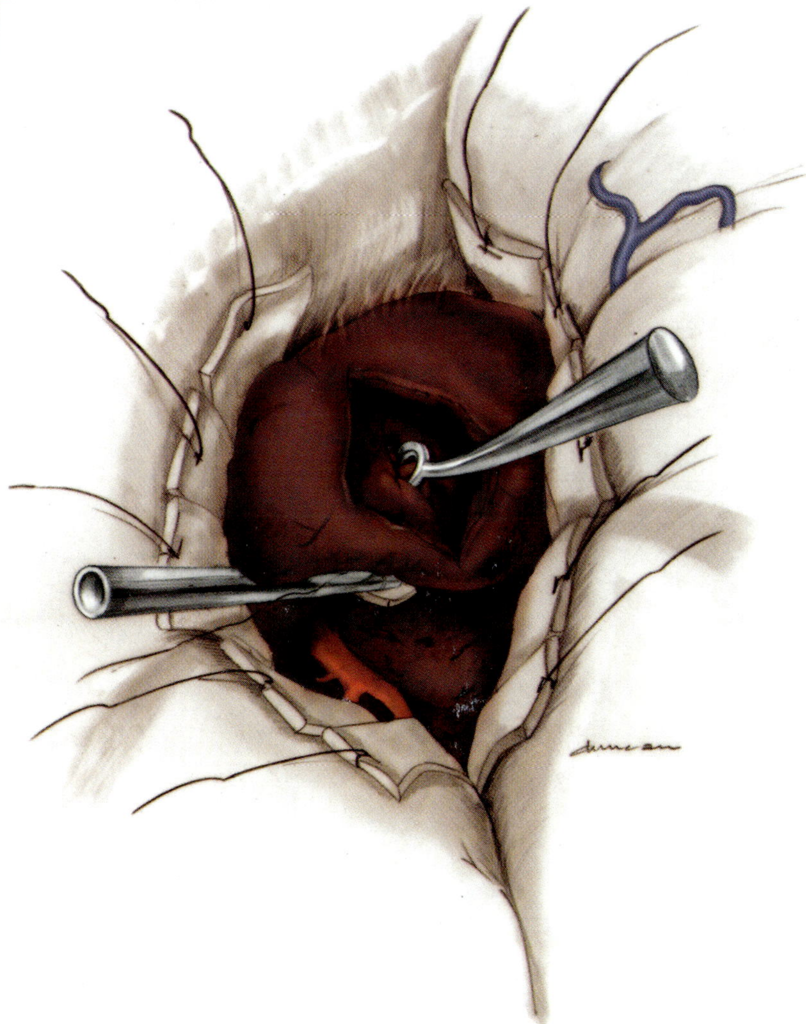

Figure 1–38.

Step 4. With increasing exposure, further internal decompression of large tumors is performed. This internal decompression facilitates the manipulation of the tumor capsule off the deeper neurovascular structures.

Figure 1–39.

Step 5. After extensive debulking of the tumor and dissection of its lateral and medial margins, the attachments of the tumor to the dura mater of the sphenoid wing are further cauterized and divided down to the anterior clinoid process.

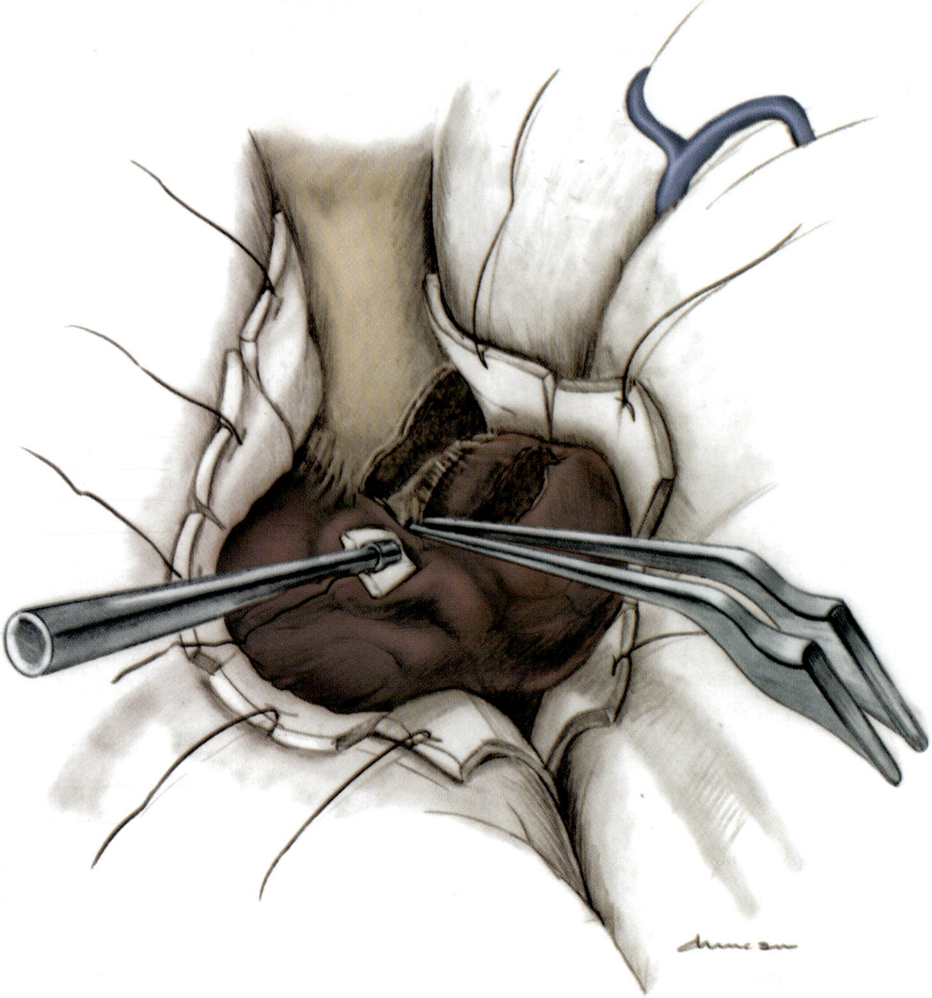

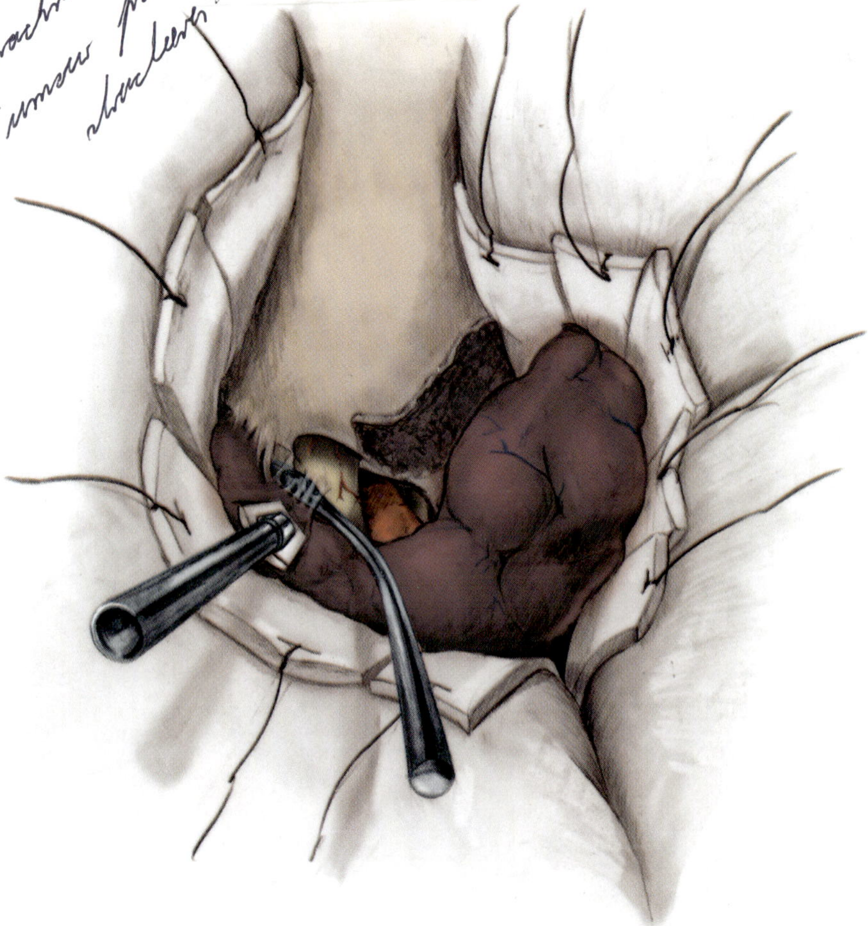

Figure 1–40.

Step 6. Typically, there is a layer of arachnoid between the deepest part of the tumor capsule and the underlying internal carotid artery and optic nerve. This arachnoid prevents injury to these structures during dissection of the tumor. The attachment of the tumor to the anterior clinoid process and the planum sphenoidal is cauterized and divided. Countertraction is provided by a #5 or #7 straight suction tip placed on the tumor capsule.

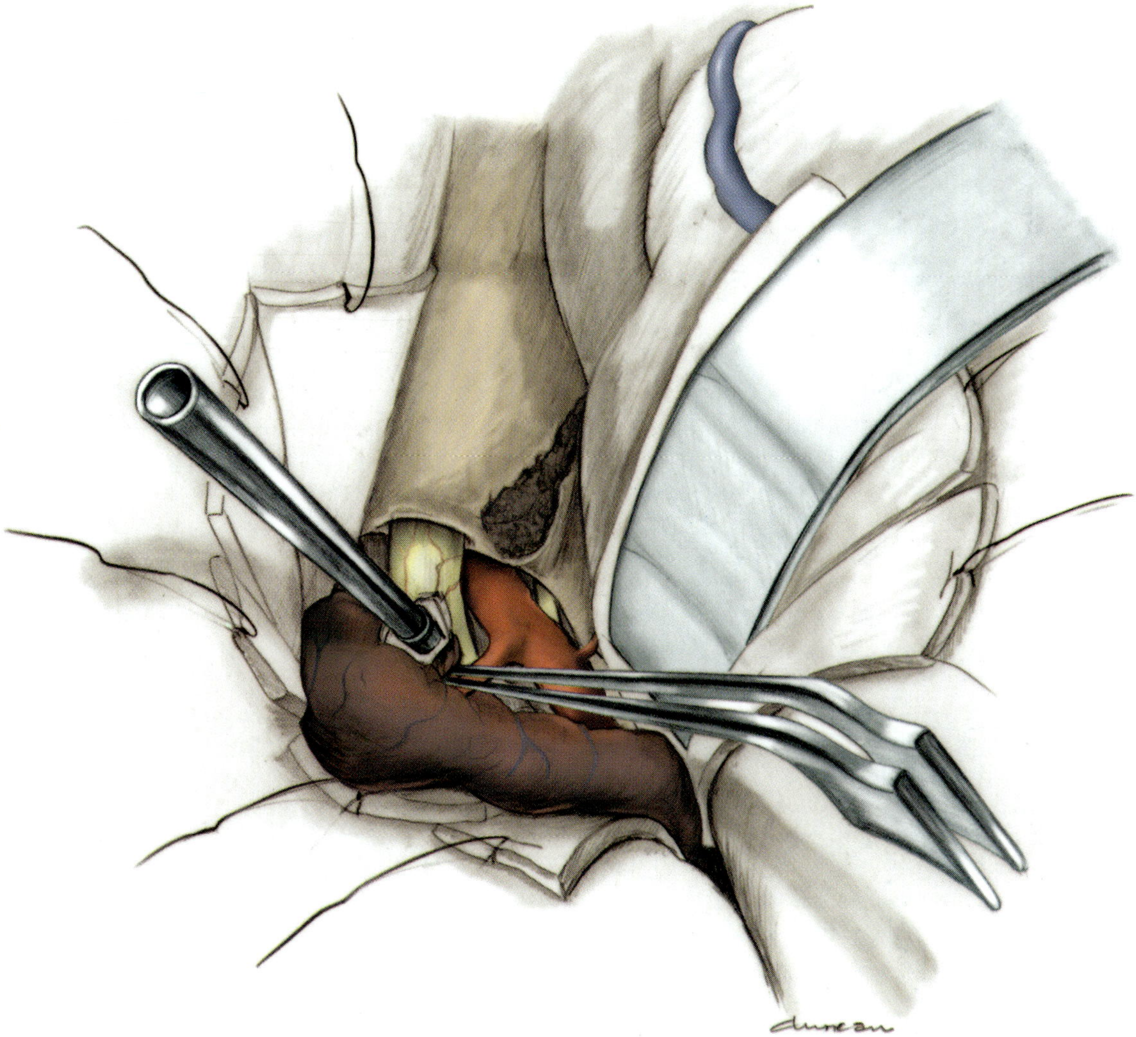

Figure 1–41.

Step 7. The residual piece of tumor is rotated medially and laterally as the tumor is dissected off the internal carotid artery and its branches. Often the tumor encircles part of the internal carotid artery, but it usually can be removed from the artery with gentle suction, fine spatulas, and bipolar cautery. Occasionally, one can visualize the tumor invading the adventitia of the internal carotid artery. Fine spatulas should be used to scrape the tumor off the artery. Any bleeding should be controlled with an absorbable gelatin sponge instead of bipolar cautery. Cauterizing small bleeders on the internal carotid artery can lead to arterial dissection and thrombosis.

TRANSITIONAL CAVERNOUS CAROTID ANEURYSM

Anatomy

It is mandatory for surgeons to understand exactly the three-dimensional anatomic relationships of the cavernous sinus before operating on a transitional cavernous carotid aneurysm. The important features are the course of the internal carotid artery through the cavernous sinus, the relationship of the cranial nerves to the internal carotid artery, and the enveloping and tethering reflections of the dura mater. When considering the anatomy and surgery of the cavernous sinus, neurosurgeons are indebted to the pioneering work of Parkinson and Dolenc. The following discussion of the anatomy of the cavernous sinus should be considered a bare minimum, or cursory, and relevant primarily to transitional cavernous carotid aneurysms.

The internal carotid artery enters the cavernous sinus through the foramen lacerum and runs superiorly and curves anteriorly toward the superior orbital fissure (Figure 1–42). The meningeal hypophysial trunk usually arises from the superior medial aspect of the internal carotid artery just distal to this curve. The three branches of the meningeal hypophysial trunk include the tentorial artery of Bernasconi and Cassinari, the dural meningeal artery, and the inferior hypophysial artery. There also may be an artery of the inferior cavernous sinus, which originates from the lateral side of the internal carotid artery and runs anteriorly to cross the abducens nerve and eventually anastomose with branches of the maxillary artery. Some of the anastomoses include the artery of the foramen rotundum, the recurrent meningeal artery along the superior orbital fissure, the accessory meningeal artery at the foramen ovale, and the middle meningeal artery at the foramen spinosum. Approximately 10 percent of patients have McConnell's capsular arteries, which originate from the medial side of the internal carotid artery and supply part of the pituitary gland.

Within the cavernous sinus, a dense venous plexus connects the ophthalmic vein, the superior and inferior petrosal sinuses, the pterygoid plexus, and the basilar venous plexus. This venous plexus surrounds the internal carotid artery. The oculomotor, trochlear, and trigeminal nerves run in the lateral wall of the cavernous sinus. The dura mater of the cavernous sinus is continuous with the connective tissue that tethers these cranial nerves to the wall of the sinus. The abducens nerve runs within the cavernous sinus and enters the superior orbital fissure under the ophthalmic division of the trigeminal nerve.

Several nomenclatures have been proposed for divisions of the internal carotid artery. The first was that of Fisher in 1938, subsequently modified by Fukushima in 1988. In this classic nomenclature, the C_1 segment begins at the carotid bifurcation and extends to the origin of the posterior communicating artery. The C_2 segment extends from the posterior communicating artery to the distal dural ring. This has also been described by Day as the "ophthalmic segment." The C_3 segment is the extradural extracavernous part of the artery and lies underneath the anterior clinoid process. The C_4 segment is the intracavernous segment, which extends to the origin of the meningeal hypophysial trunk. The C_5 segment extends from the meningeal hypophysial trunk to underneath the trigeminal nerve. The C_6 segment, the last segment, is the intrapetrous portion of the internal carotid artery, from where it crosses underneath the mandibular division of the trigeminal nerve to its entrance at the foramen lacerum. More recently, van Loveren and colleagues introduced a nomenclature that essentially reverses and modifies the numbering sequence to reflect the direction of blood flow. To avoid confusion, terms such as "horizontal segment" and "anterior genu" are used in this book.

There are two so-called carotid dural rings, and they are important anatomic landmarks (Figure 1–43). The proximal ring denotes where the internal carotid artery exits from the cavernous sinus to become the clinoid segment of the internal carotid artery. The distal ring is the point where the internal carotid artery becomes intradural. Accordingly, these two rings delineate the clinoid segment of the internal carotid artery. The distal dural ring surrounds the internal carotid artery and is continuous with the dura mater of the falciform ligament, the anterior clinoid process, and the cavernous sinus. It is attached to the adventitia of the internal carotid artery. The proximal dural ring, which incompletely surrounds the internal carotid artery, is made up of periosteum arising from the anterior clinoid process. The membrane between the internal carotid artery and the oculomotor nerve is sometimes called the "caroticooculomotor membrane."

The nine triangles of the cavernous sinus region need to be considered (Figure 1–44).

1. Anterior Medial Triangle

The anterior medial triangle is defined by the medial border of the optic nerve medially and the oculomotor nerve laterally. The base of the triangle is the dural edge

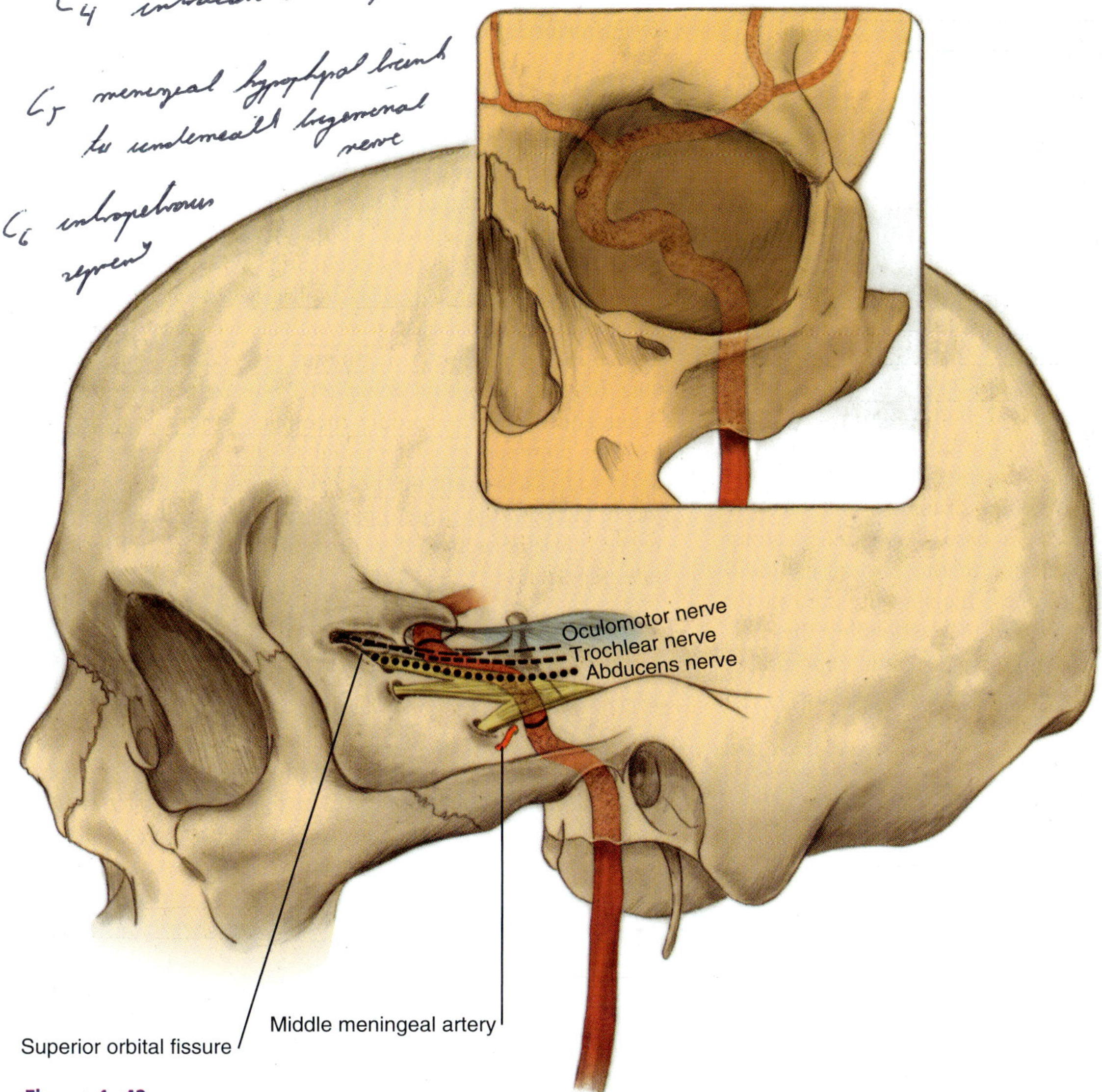
Oculomotor nerve
Trochlear nerve
Abducens nerve
Superior orbital fissure
Middle meningeal artery

Figure 1–42.

of the tentorium cerebelli. The anterior loop of the internal carotid artery lies in the floor of the triangle, along with trabeculated venous channels. This is called the "clinoid segment" of the internal carotid artery, and it is neither intradural nor intracavernous. Most transitional cavernous carotid aneurysms arise from this clinoid segment and penetrate through the distal dural ring to enter the subarachnoid space. Fibrous connective tissue in the apex of the triangle forms the proximal ring that ensheaths the internal carotid artery and delineates the anteromedial border of the cavernous sinus.

2. *Paramedial Triangle*

The two sides of the paramedial triangle are defined medially by the medial border of the oculomotor nerve and laterally by the lateral border of the trochlear nerve. The base of the triangle is the dural edge of the tentorium cerebelli. The anterior loop and part of the horizontal segment of the cavernous carotid artery can be visualized through this aperture. Some surgeons have extended the paramedial triangle to a "medial triangle" that has the above-mentioned margins but a base that extends along the dura mater from the anterior to the posterior clinoid process, "the oculomotor trigone." Incising the dura mater along this oculomotor trigone and then extending the incision into the paramedial triangle increases the exposure of the horizontal segment of the cavernous carotid artery.

3. *Parkinson's Triangle*

Parkinson's triangle is defined medially by the trochlear nerve and laterally by the first division of the trigeminal nerve. The base of this triangle is also the dural edge of the tentorium cerebelli. Access through this triangle provides visualization of the horizontal segment of the cavernous carotid artery.

4. *Anterior Lateral Triangle*

The anterior lateral triangle is defined medially by the ophthalmic division of the trigeminal nerve and laterally by the maxillary division of the trigeminal nerve. The base of the triangle is formed by a line running anteriorly between the superior orbital fissure and the foramen ovale. This triangle can be used to expose the superior orbital vein and to gain access to the anterior portion of the cavernous sinus.

5. *Lateral Triangle*

The lateral triangle is defined medially by the maxillary division of the trigeminal nerve and laterally by the mandibular division of the trigeminal nerve. The base is formed by a line extending from the foramen rotundum to the foramen ovale. The lateral triangle can be used when exposure of the anterior lateral part of the cavernous sinus is necessary for tumor excision.

6. *Posterior Lateral Triangle (Glasscock's Triangle)*

The posterior lateral triangle is defined by the posterior rim of the foramen ovale, the foramen spinosum, the posterior border of the mandibular division of the trigeminal nerve, and the cochlear apex (greater petrosal nerve). This triangle is important for obtaining proximal control of the horizontal segment of the intrapetrous internal carotid artery for temporary occlusion or bypass procedures. This space is approached extradurally. Often, the internal carotid artery can be seen or palpated because it is covered only by a fibrous membrane instead of bone. Exposure of this triangle is achieved by using a diamond bur. After control of the middle meningeal artery is achieved, drilling commences just medial to the foramen spinosum and progresses along the posterior border of the mandibular branch of the trigeminal nerve. The greater petrosal nerve must be sectioned to prevent traction on the geniculate ganglion.

7. *Posterior Medial Triangle (Kawase's Triangle)*

The posterior medial triangle is defined laterally by the greater superior petrosal nerve and medially by the petrosal sinus. The base is the trigeminal nerve. No pertinent neurovascular structures occur in this triangle. This ridge of petrous bone within Kawase's triangle may safely be removed to provide greater access to the posterior cranial fossa when performing a transtentorial approach. The posterior medial triangle also provides greater exposure of the trigeminal nerve.

8. *Inferior Medial Triangle*

The inferior medial triangle is defined medially by a line between the posterior clinoid process and the abducens nerve at Dorello's canal and laterally by a line running between Dorello's canal and the trochlear nerve at the edge of the tentorium. The base of the triangle is the petrous apex.

9. *Inferior Lateral Triangle*

The inferior lateral triangle is defined medially by a line running between Dorello's canal and the trochlear nerve at the edge of the tentorium cerebelli and laterally by a line between Dorello's canal and the petrosal vein at the petrosal sinus. The base is the tentorium cerebelli.

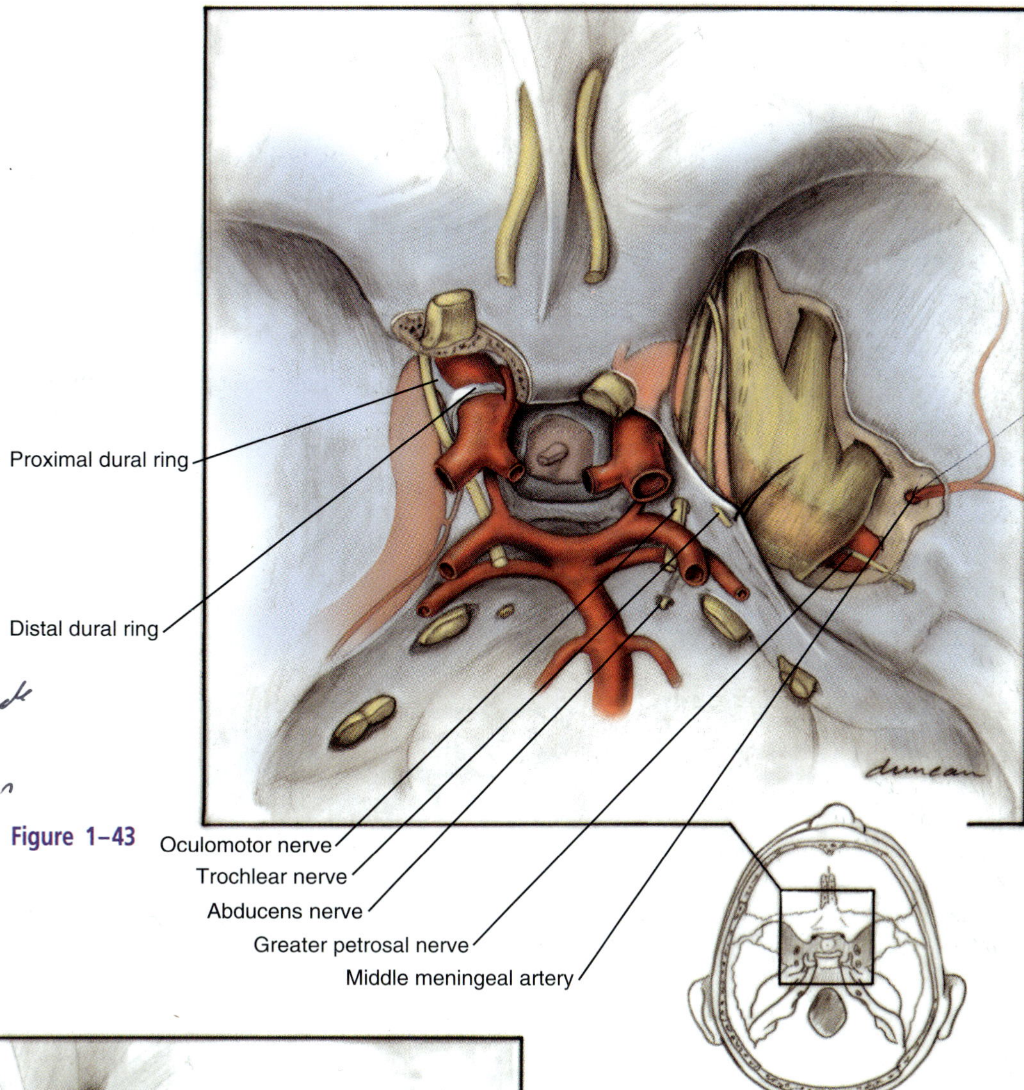

Figure 1–43

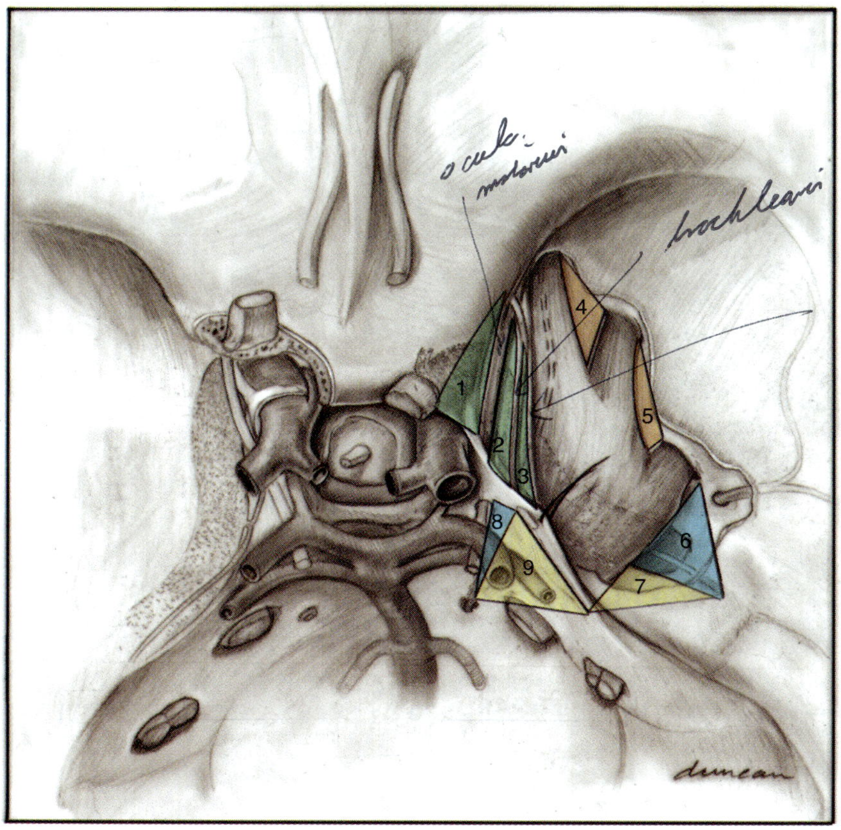

Figure 1–44.

Operation

Most transitional carotid cavernous aneurysms can be approached through a modified pterional craniotomy that requires more removal of temporal bone. Some surgeons prefer to approach these aneurysms through a frontotemporal zygomatic craniotomy. If the aneurysm extends proximally to the proximal carotid ring, removal of the zygoma will allow better exposure of the lateral cavernous sinus.

In most larger cavernous carotid aneurysms, proximal control of the internal carotid artery is desirable. This can be achieved through an extradural exposure of the petrous carotid artery. Alternatively, the cervical carotid artery can be exposed through a linear incision anterior to the sternocleidomastoid muscle. Exposure of the cervical carotid artery has the advantages of being easier technically and providing a route to perform intraoperative angiography if so needed. Exposure of either the cervical or petrous carotid offers the surgeon some degree of safety should the aneurysm inadvertently rupture intraoperatively.

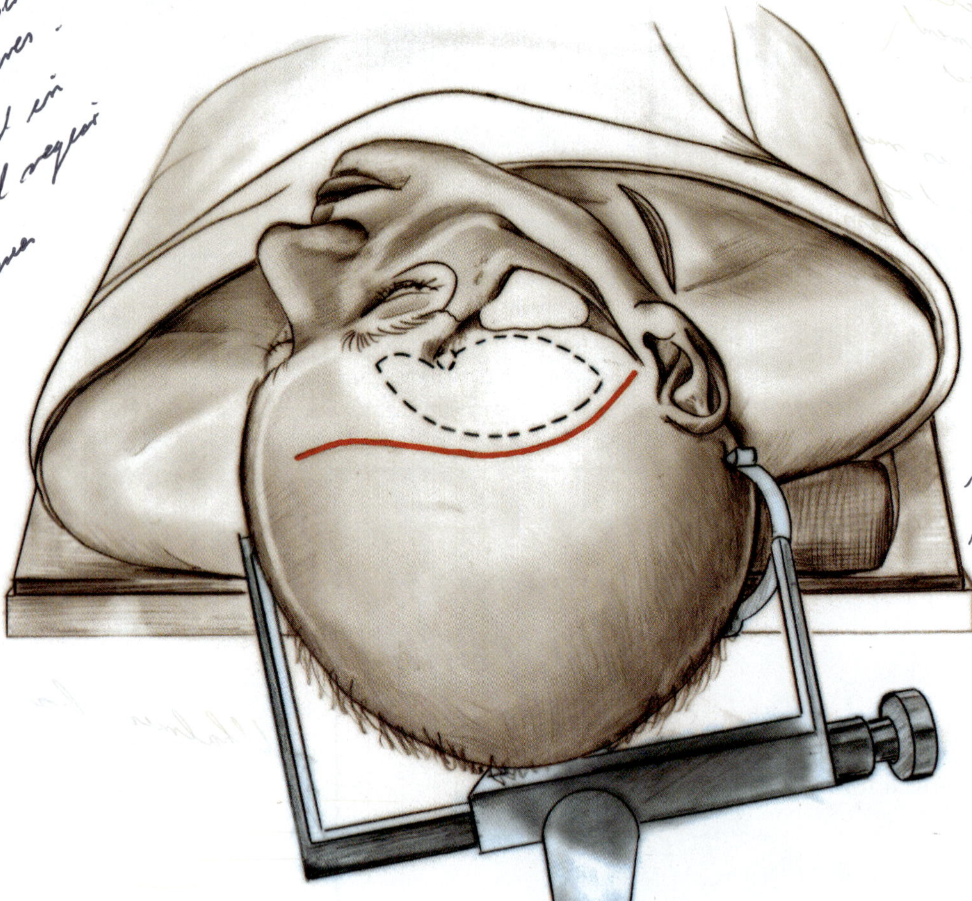

Figure 1–45.

Step 1. Most transitional cavernous carotid aneurysms can be explored through an enlarged pterional craniotomy that has some extension into the middle cranial fossa. As illustrated here, the cervical carotid artery is exposed to provide proximal blood vessel control should an inadvertent rupture occur intraoperatively. An alternative to this is a frontotemporal zygomatic craniotomy, with extradural exposure of the petrous carotid artery. Exposure of the cervical carotid artery is technically easier and quicker, and it provides an easier route for performing intraoperative angiography if needed. Note that the position of the patient's head is slightly more lateral than for a true pterional craniotomy to facilitate dissection of the cavernous sinus.

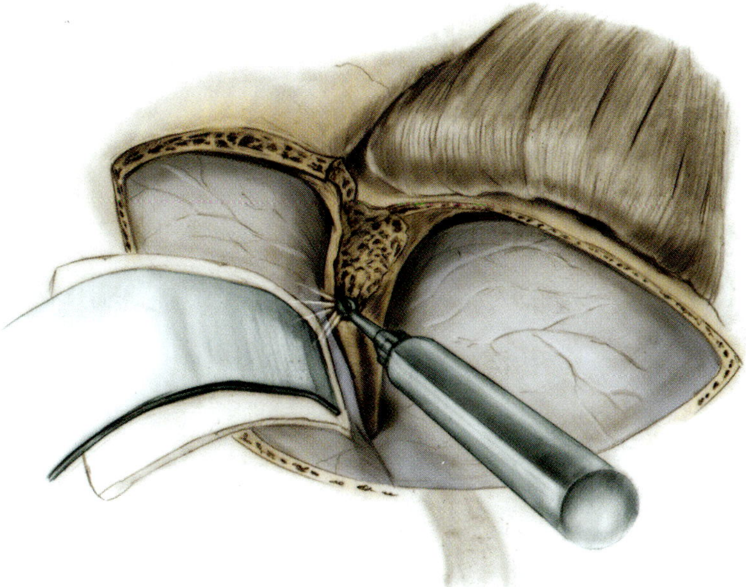

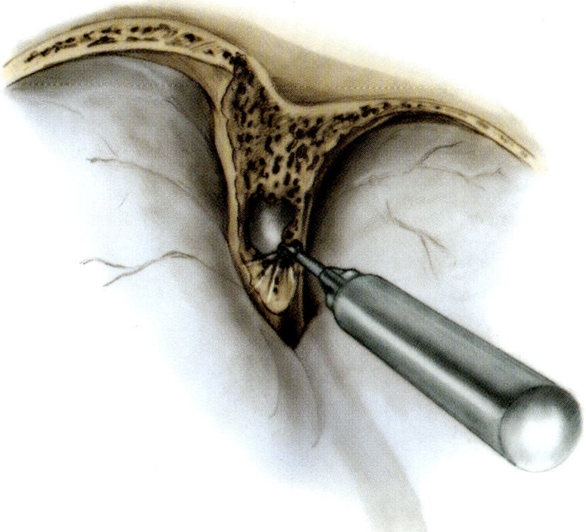

Figure 1–46.

Step 2. After the bone flap is elevated, the frontal and temporal dura mater are dissected off the sphenoid wing and protected with malleable retractors. The outer sphenoid wing is removed with a high-speed diamond air drill. Approximately 2 to 3 cm deep to the outer sphenoid wing, the drill is used to make a hole into the orbital roof.

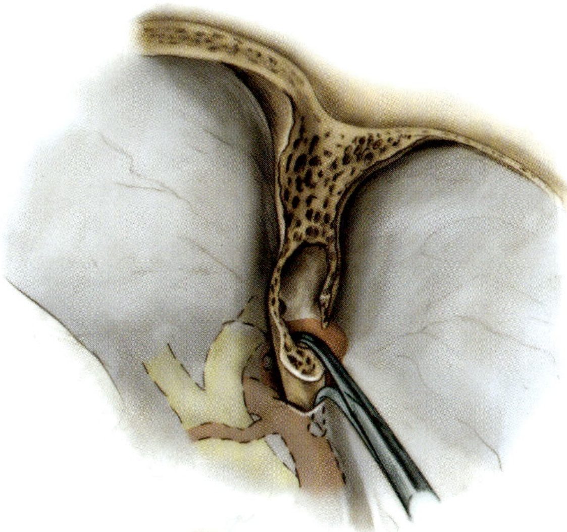

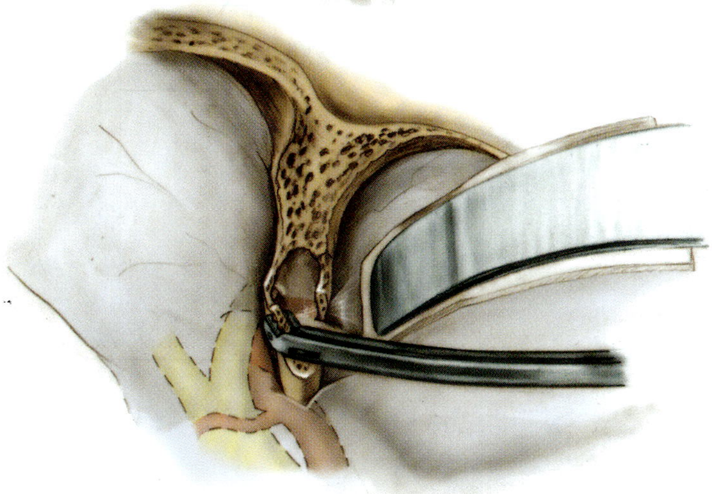

Figure 1–47.

Step 3. The hole created in the orbital roof is extended by using a small bone forceps or punch. Both small spatulas and ball-tip dissectors can be used to dissect the inner sphenoid wing and anterior clinoid process off both the orbital fascia and the frontal and temporal dura mater. As the dissection is extended deeper, two struts of bone tether the anterior clinoid process. Both of these struts, the optic strut and the lateral rim over the superior orbital fissure, can be removed with small bone forceps. After these two bony struts are removed, a fine spatula is used to dissect the anterior clinoid process off the dura mater. The dura mater is then grabbed with the bone forceps, gently rocked, and rotated medially and laterally until it is loose, and then it is pulled out of the junction between the frontal dura mater, temporal dura mater, and orbital fascia.

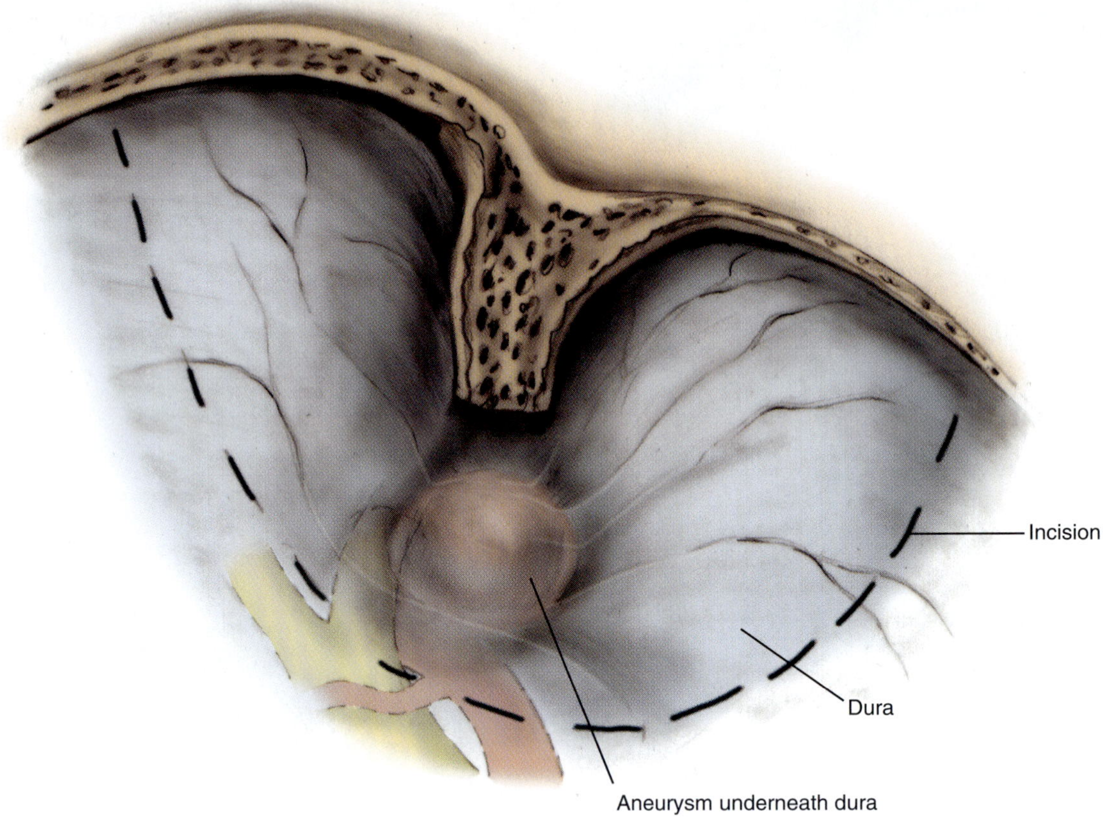

Figure 1–48.

Step 4. This figure illustrates the location of the aneurysm in relation to the removed part of the medial sphenoid wing and the anterior clinoid process. This extradural removal is advantageous because dura mater overlies the aneurysm, the internal carotid artery, and the optic nerve. The relationship of the optic nerve to the medial bony optic strut indicates why removal of this bone with bone forceps decreases the risk of thermal injury to the optic nerve, which might occur with a high-speed air drill.

The dura mater is opened in a curved fashion and tacked to the overlying temporalis muscle. This dural flap prevents blood from running into the wound. At the end of the operation, the dura mater can be closed either primarily or with a graft. In this way, the only dural defect that remains is the one in the cavernous sinus region, and the risk of postoperative leakage of cerebrospinal fluid and wound complications is minimized.

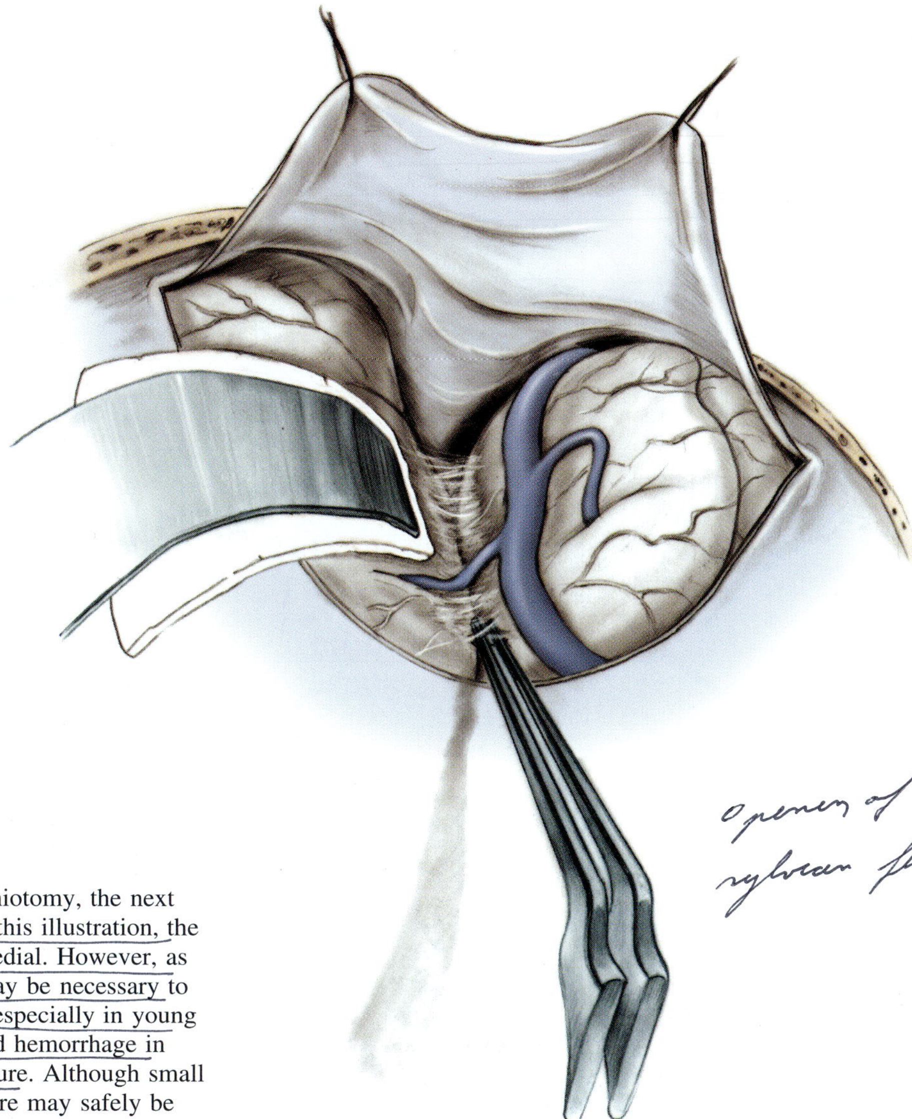

Figure 1–49.

Step 5. As in a standard pterional craniotomy, the next step is to separate the Sylvian fissure. In this illustration, the fissure is being divided from lateral to medial. However, as mentioned above, in some situations it may be necessary to divide the fissure from medial to lateral, especially in young patients or after a significant subarachnoid hemorrhage in which blood is packed in the Sylvian fissure. Although small bridging veins overlying the Sylvian fissure may safely be cauterized and divided, it is best to preserve the temporal veins by displacing them laterally with the temporal lobe. This will help decrease the risk of postoperative seizures and contusions of the temporal lobe.

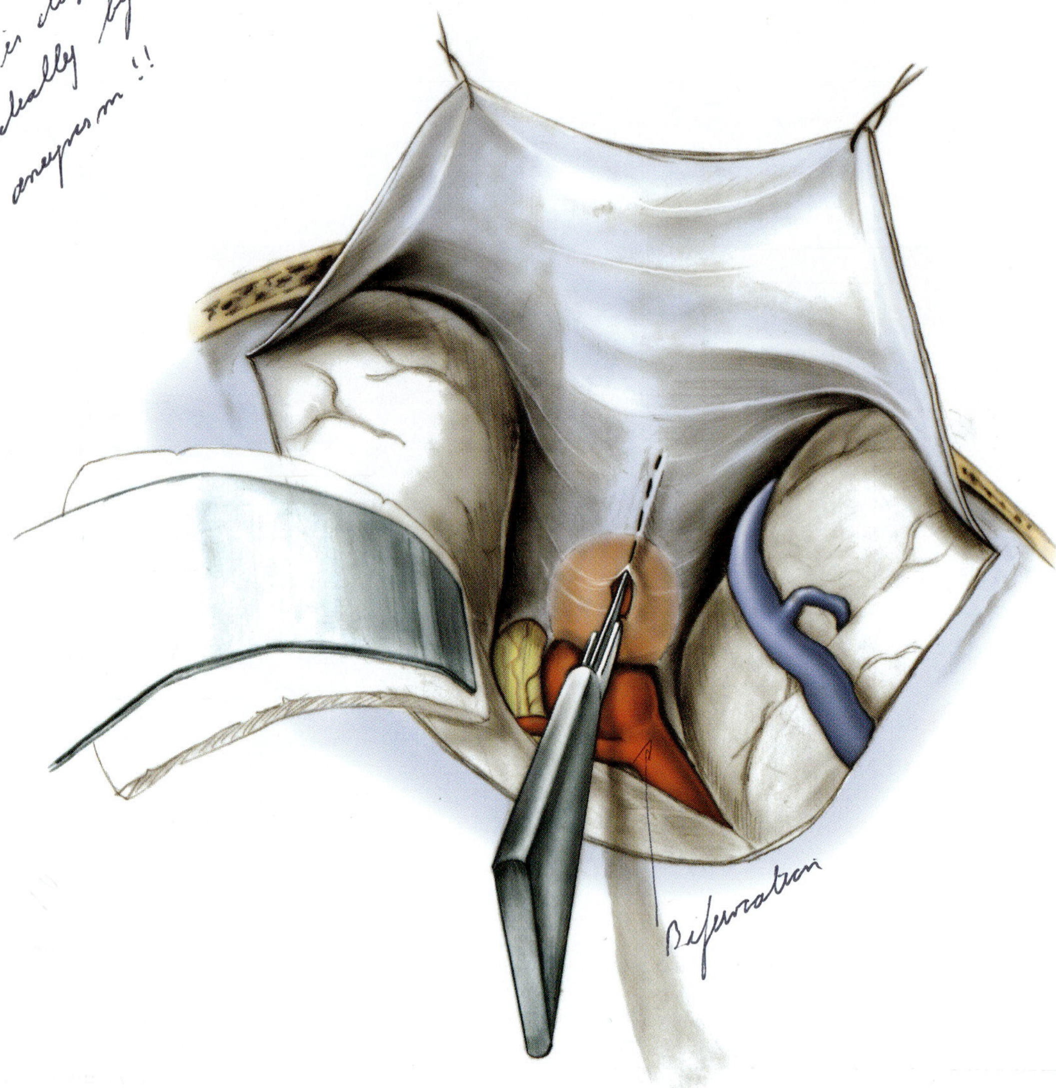

Figure 1–50.

Step 6. The Sylvian fissure is divided, and after the brain is protected with hemostatic fabric and cottonoids, the frontal lobe retractor is again repositioned deeper. The arachnoid over the supraclinoid carotid artery is divided to identify the bifurcation of the internal carotid artery. Typically, the rostral portion of the aneurysm is immediately apparent. Most often, the optic nerve is displaced medially by the medial projection of the dome of the aneurysm.

Exposure of the cavernous portion of the aneurysm is first accomplished by incising the dura mater linearly along the presumed axis of the internal carotid artery over the site where the extradural bone was removed. Before this incision is made, a small spatula is used to gently depress the dura mater intended to be cut to make sure that no part of the aneurysm dome lies immediately beneath the site.

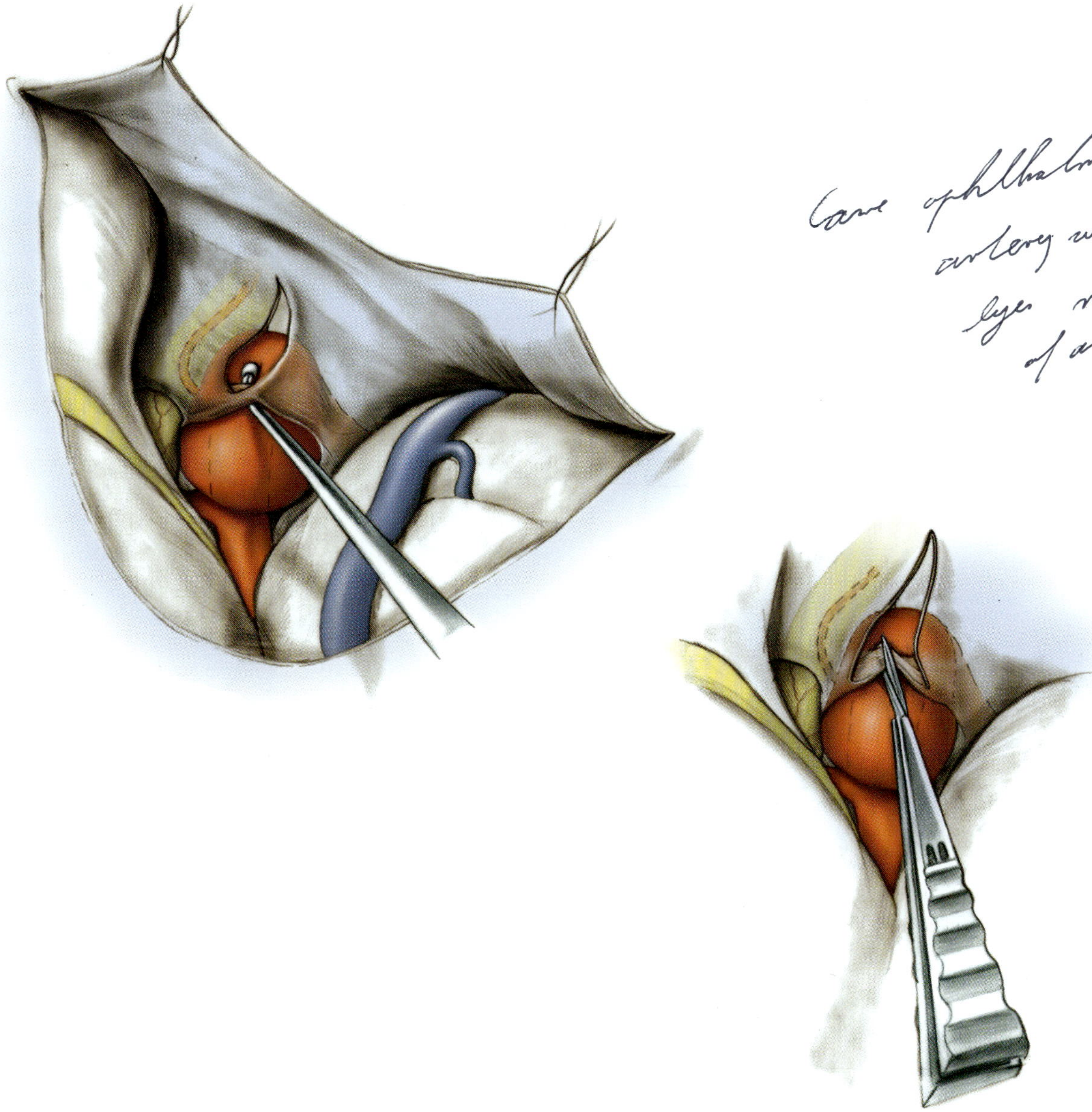

Figure 1–51.

Step 7. A small ball-tip dissector is used to separate the distal dural ring from the underlying aneurysmal dome. The ball-tip dissector is swept medially to laterally. The freed dural ring is then incised with either a scalpel, micro Potts scissors, or standard straight microscissors. The advantage of either the micro Potts or microscissors is that the dural ring can be lifted off the dome of the aneurysm and cut more easily than with a scalpel.

After the distal dural ring is incised, it is necessary to dissect the medial and lateral portions of the aneurysm. Most often, the dome of the aneurysm is adherent to the lateral portion of the wall of the cavernous sinus. A small spatula can be used to sharply dissect the dome off this wall. It is important to recognize that cranial nerves run in this lateral cavernous wall. At this level, the primary nerve at risk for injury is the oculomotor nerve.

Medially, it is necessary to identify the origin of the ophthalmic artery. Most often, the origin of this artery marks the junction between the aneurysm and the parent carotid artery along the medial border. This is an important landmark because it may be difficult to identify this transition zone. Sometimes, it is not enough to remove the bony optic strut. If so, a small punch can be used to remove more bone to allow a better line of site to identify the junction between the aneurysm and the parent artery.

It also is important to identify the proximal margin of the aneurysm and its point of takeoff from the parent carotid artery. Usually, this proximal neck occurs at the anterior genu of the internal carotid artery, as it starts to curve laterally and deep.

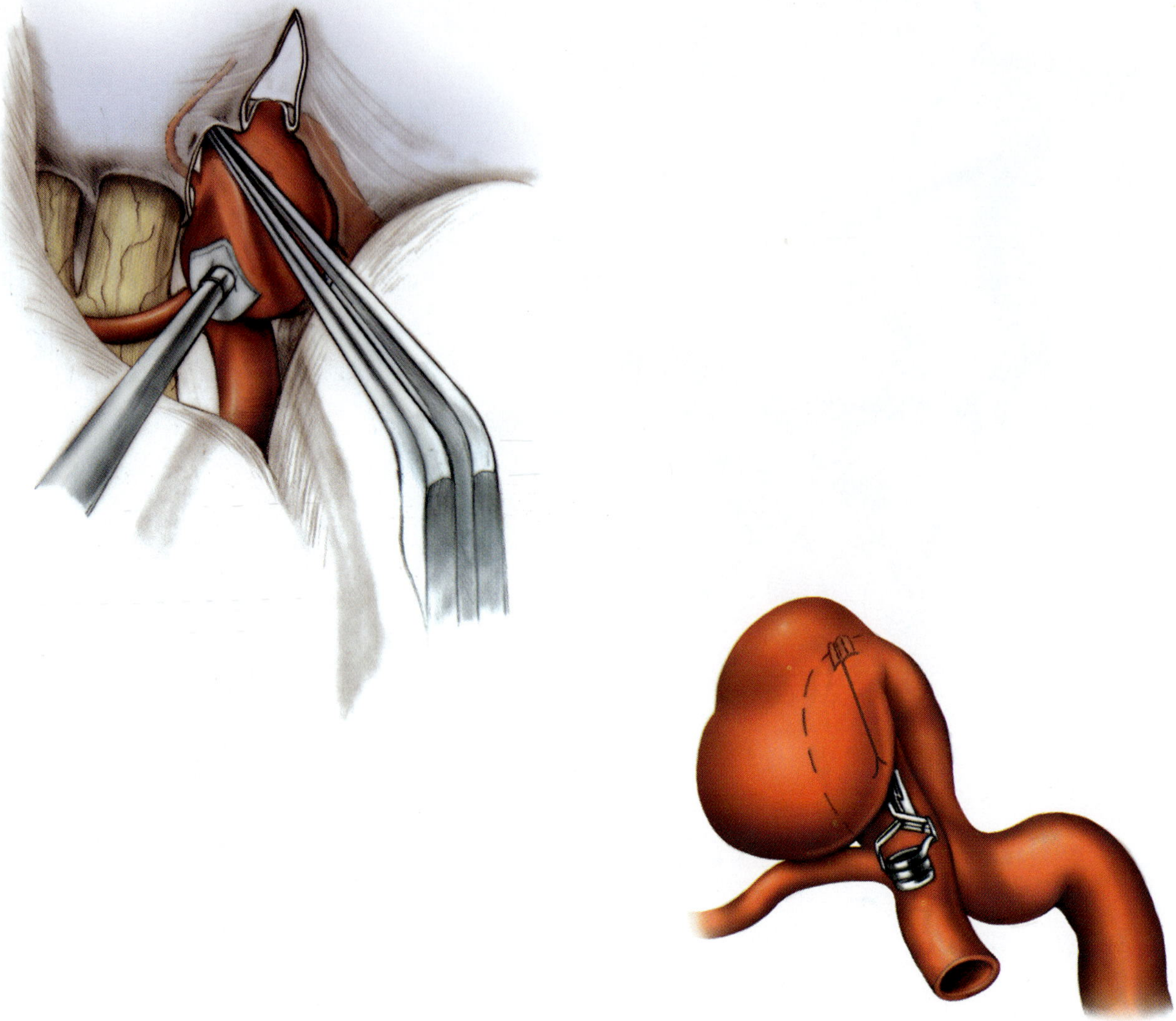

Figure 1–52.

Step 8. The dome of the aneurysm is displaced with a #5 or #7 straight suction tip and cottonoid to allow exact identification of the junction of the ophthalmic artery, parent carotid artery, and medial neck of the aneurysm. The best clip to use for most of the aneurysms is a forward-angled straight clip passed along the long axis of the artery. Helpful visual and tactile guides to use for the initial placement of the clip are the ophthalmic artery medially and the anterior wall of the cavernous sinus. If the clip is placed just above the ophthalmic artery and inserted until there is resistance when the tips of the clip hit the anterior bony wall of the cavernous sinus, it is likely that this initial clip placement will successfully obliterate the neck without compromising the internal carotid artery.

After the location of the jaws of the aneurysm clip have been inspected visually, the dome is aspirated for decompression of the aneurysm. Thereafter, correct placement of the aneurysm clip is reconfirmed. At this point, it is useful to have objective documentation that the aneurysm has been obliterated and that the parent internal carotid artery is not stenosed or occluded. Intraoperative Doppler or ultrasonography of the internal carotid–middle cerebral artery complex is useful. However, currently, intraoperative angiography is the best method of documentation. Therefore, if available, a radiolucent headholder and table should be used. Intraoperative angiography can be performed through either a direct cervical carotid puncture or by femoral artery catheterization.

2

Frontotemporal Approach

Copyright © 1999 Mayo Foundation.

ANATOMIC CONSIDERATIONS

Gross Anatomy

The temporal lobe occupies the anterior portion of the cerebral hemisphere below the lateral, or Sylvian, fissure and anterior to the parietooccipital sulcus (Figure 2–1). The supramarginal gyrus of the parietal lobe caps the Sylvian fissure, and the angular gyrus curves around the end of the superior temporal sulcus. Wernicke's area (the posterior speech area) is located in the region of the supramarginal and angular gyri and the posterior portion of the superior temporal gyrus of the dominant hemisphere. An imaginary line connecting the parietooccipital sulcus and the temporooccipital notch marks the posterior limit of the temporal lobe. The temporal lobe has three surfaces: lateral, inferomedial, and superior. The lateral surface has three longitudinal gyri—the superior, middle, and inferior temporal gyri—separated by the superior and inferior temporal sulci. If the floor of the middle cranial fossa is not exposed during a craniotomy, often only the first two gyri will be visualized. The superior temporal sulcus is parallel with the Sylvian fissure, and its ascending ramus ends in the angular gyrus.

The inferior temporal gyrus curves onto the inferomedial surface of the temporal lobe. From lateral to medial on the inferomedial surface are the inferior temporal gyrus, the fusiform (or lateral occipitotemporal) gyrus, and the parahippocampal gyrus. The fusiform gyrus occurs only in the posterior half of the temporal lobe and is set off by the occipitotemporal sulcus laterally and the collateral sulcus medially. The posterior end of the parahippocampal gyrus curves around the splenium and becomes the cingulate gyrus. The portion of this gyrus that is immediately posterior and inferior to the splenium is called the "isthmus" of the cingulate gyrus. The anterior end of the parahippocampal gyrus curves medially and turns posteriorly to form the uncus. Deep to the parahippocampal gyrus lies the convoluted hippocampal formation.

The superior surface of the temporal lobe (the opercular surface) contains the transverse gyrus of Heschl, or auditory cortex. Posterior to this gyrus is the planum temporale.

Auditory cortex (Brodmann areas 41 and 42) is tonotopically organized, with low frequencies represented anterolaterally and high frequencies posteromedially. Damage to auditory cortex is associated with subtle auditory impairment (mainly, impaired ability to localize sound in space), because the auditory cortex in each cerebral hemisphere receives input from both ears. In addition, areas 41 and 42 are connected with the corresponding areas in the opposite hemisphere through the corpus callosum. Area 22, primarily responsible for the comprehension of spoken language, is located on the lateral temporal surface adjacent to areas 41 and 42. It receives projections from auditory cortex.

Because of the bilaterality of the projections in the auditory system, including projections through the corpus callosum, deafness in one ear does not produce aphasia. However, destruction of area 22 in the dominant cerebral hemisphere can result in auditory aphasia, as can bilateral destruction of areas 41 and 42. Injury to an area inferior and adjacent to area 22 can produce anomia (amnesic aphasia), the inability to recall names.

It is important to recognize that the location of eloquent language cortex in both the temporal and frontal lobes can vary from patient to patient. For surgical procedures in which potential injury of these cortical areas is a concern, preoperative mapping or awake surgery with intraoperative mapping is necessary.

Part of the visual system is also contained in the temporal lobe, specifically, Meyer's loop of the geniculocalcarine tract (visual radiations). Meyer's loop is the portion of the geniculocalcarine tract that extends forward into the temporal lobe and curves around the tip of the temporal horn of the lateral ventricle. These visual fibers represent the superior quadrant of the visual field. Temporal lobectomy may involve Meyer's loop. However, the degree of visual impairment depends on how far posteriorly the resection extends. Resections that extend more than 9 cm from the tip of the temporal lobe produce a complete homonymous hemianopia. The temporal lobe also contains visual association cortex important in the recognition of shapes, including faces.

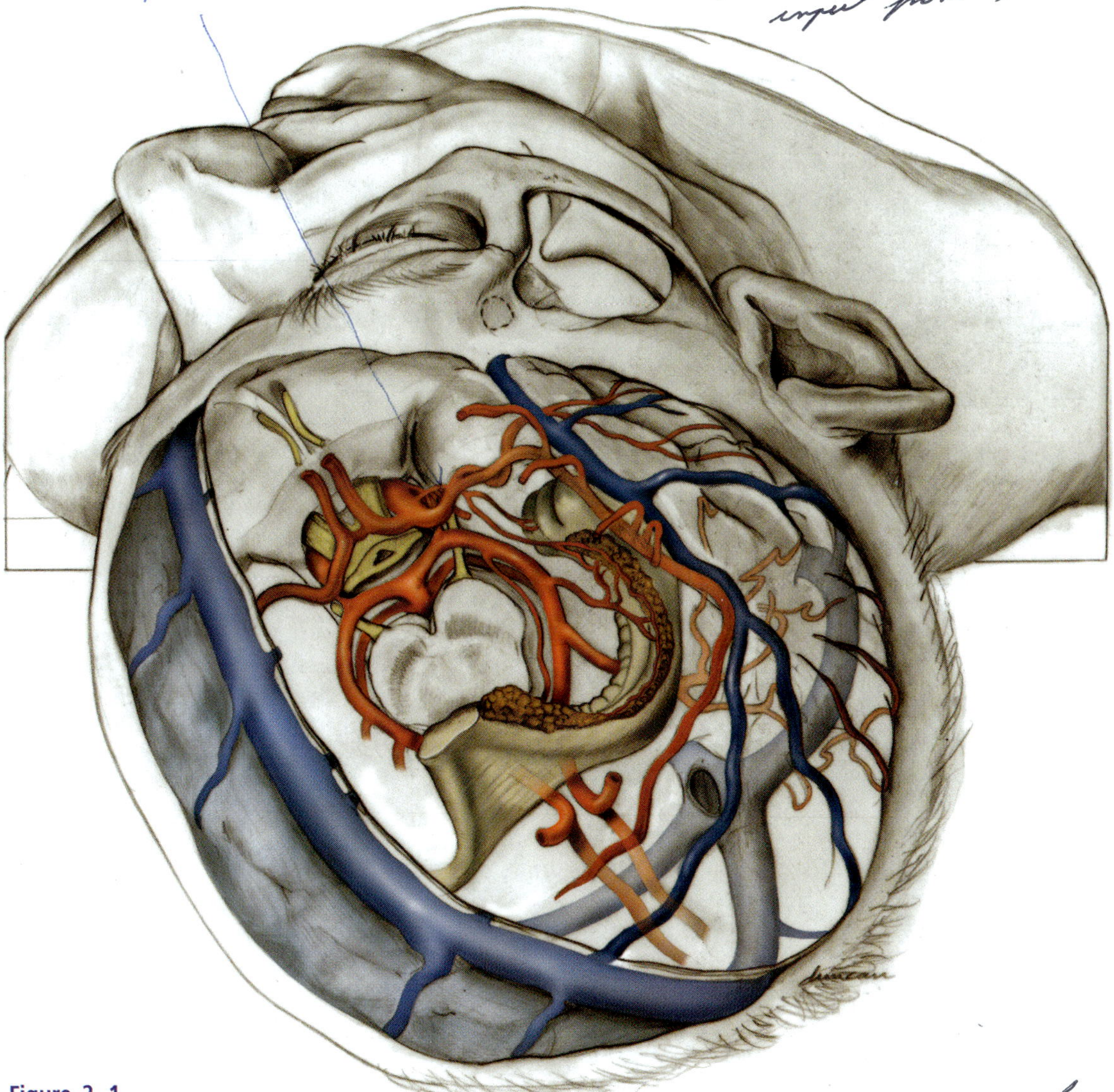

Figure 2–1.

THE HIPPOCAMPUS

Structure

The hippocampal formation is a special area of cerebral cortex and consists of the dentate gyrus, the hippocampus proper (also called "Ammon's horn" and usually referred to as "hippocampus"), and the subiculum and presubiculum. The subiculum and presubiculum are part of the parahippocampal gyrus on the inferomedial surface of the temporal lobe. The dentate gyrus and hippocampus form a bulge in the medial wall of the temporal horn of the lateral ventricle, immediately inferior to the choroidal fissure. This bulge extends the length of the temporal horn. Anteriorly, the bulge is prominent and indented and resembles a paw, hence the name "pes hippocampi."

The hippocampus is considered the oldest part of the cerebral cortex and is called "archicortex." Unlike most of the cerebral cortex ("neocortex"), which has six recognized layers, the hippocampus consists of only three layers. The middle layer is composed of the cell bodies of hippocampal pyramidal cells, and the inner and outer layers are composed mainly of dendrites and axons. The major afferents to the hippocampal formation synapse on granule cells in the dentate gyrus, the doorway to the hippocampus. The axons of these granule cells synapse on hippocampal pyramidal cells. Many of the axons of the hippocampal pyramidal cells, in turn, project to the subiculum and presubiculum. Other hippocampal axons enter the fornix. The myelinated axons that join the fornix go to the ventricular surface of the hippocampus and form a thin layer of white matter called the "alveus." The axons of the alveus converge and form the fimbria, a flange of white matter on the superior surface of the hippocampus. Posteriorly, the fimbria becomes the fornix.

On entering the temporal horn of the lateral ventricle, the surgeon sees the prominent pes hippocampi covered by the thin white veil of the alveus and fimbria and the choroid plexus. In the choroid plexus lie the anterior choroidal artery, the inferior choroidal vein (a branch of the basal vein of Rosenthal), and the lateral posterior choroidal artery. If the choroid plexus is retracted superiorly and medially, the ambient cistern is visible. This cistern contains the posterior cerebral artery, the basal vein of Rosenthal, the cerebral peduncles, and the oculomotor and trochlear nerves.

Connections

The hippocampus is connected with a large portion of the rest of the cerebral cortex and with many subcortical areas. The major source of afferents to the hippocampal formation is the entorhinal cortex of the parahippocampal gyrus. Entorhinal cortex receives afferents from areas of sensory association cortex—visual, auditory, and somatosensory. Axons of pyramidal cells in the entorhinal cortex form the perforant path, which ends among the granule cells of the dentate gyrus. The hippocampus and, to a larger extent, the subiculum and presubiculum project back to the entorhinal cortex and, through it, to sensory association cortex. Other axons from the hippocampus and subiculum and presubiculum project to subcortical areas through the fornix.

The Fornix

Near the posterior end of the hippocampus, the fimbria forms a thick bundle of axons called the "fornix." On each side, the fornix arches upward and forward under the splenium of the corpus callosum. This part of the fornix is called the "crux" (plural, crura). The left and right crura are joined by the commissure of the fornix, called the "psalterium." The fornix continues anteriorly under the body of the corpus callosum. This is the "body of the fornix." Anteriorly, at the level of the foramen of Monro, the fornix curves posteriorly and enters the substance of the diencephalon. Some of the axons pass anterior to the anterior commissure; this is the precommissural component of the fornix. These axons are distributed to the septal nuclei, the preoptic area, and the anterior portion of the hypothalamus. The rest of the fornix curves posterior to the anterior commissure, forming the postcommissural component. These axons are distributed to the anterior and intralaminar nuclei of the thalamus, the medial nucleus of the mammillary body, and the midbrain reticular formation.

Functional Importance

The dentate gyrus, hippocampus, subiculum, presubiculum, and entorhinal cortex are of central importance in declarative memory function, that is, the formation and the recall of memories of facts and places. Lesions of subcortical areas associated with the fornix, especially the dorsomedial nucleus of the thalamus and the mammillary bodies of the hypothalamus, have been implicated in the memory loss that is part of Korsakoff syndrome, or amnestic confabulatory syndrome, a sequela of Wernicke's encephalopathy.

THE AMYGDALA

Structure

The amygdala is a collection of nuclei located in the anteromedial part of the parahippocampal gyrus, deep to the region of cerebral cortex called the "uncus." The amygdala is incompletely separated from the pes hippocampi by the tip of the temporal horn of the lateral ventricle. The amygdala is divided into a basolateral group and a corticomedial group of nuclei separated by the central nucleus.

Connections

The olfactory system is a major source of afferents to the corticomedial group of nuclei. The basolateral group receives most of its afferents from the cerebral cortex, especially sensory association cortex.

The basolateral group of nuclei project back to the cerebral cortex through the entorhinal cortex, thus influencing function in sensory association cortex. In addition, the basolateral group sends axons to the central nucleus, which is the origin of many subcortical projections from the amygdala, especially through the stria terminalis. The amygdala also projects to subcortical areas through the ventral amygdalofugal pathway. The subcortical areas that receive axons from the amygdala include the thalamus, hypothalamus, and brain stem.

Functional Importance

It has been demonstrated experimentally in animals and, to a lesser extent, in humans that the amygdala affects a wide range of behavioral, visceral, and endocrine functions roughly grouped into "flight" and "fight" behaviors. For example, electrical stimulation of unanesthetized animals can lead to intense behavioral arousal that begins with the arrest of all ongoing activity, the so-called freezing reaction. This reaction may represent the initial phase of flight or fight behavior. Also, stimulation of relatively discrete areas of the amygdala can produce specific reactions, including pupillary dilatation, piloerection, and disturbances of awareness. The basolateral group of nuclei appear to be especially important in learning associations between unconditioned and conditioned stimuli, for example, learning to associate a buzzing sound with a damaging blast.

Bilateral destruction of the amygdala produces profound emotional disturbances. Animals become placid and do not evince reactions of rage, aggression, or fear. Similar changes have been observed in humans after bilateral damage to the amygdala.

Vascular Supply

The temporal lobe is supplied by three arteries: the middle cerebral artery, the anterior choroidal artery, and the posterior cerebral artery. The predominant blood supply is from the middle cerebral artery, which supplies the superior and lateral surfaces of the temporal lobe. The middle cerebral artery is divided into four segments: M_1, from the origin of the middle cerebral artery to the bottom of the Sylvian fissure; M_2, from the bifurcation-trifurcation of the artery in the Sylvian fissure to the distal edge of the insula; M_3, the opercular segment; and M_4, the cortical segment distal to the operculum. Typically, three to five small perforating vessels originate from the proximal M_1 segment; these are the lenticulostriate arteries. The size of the medial group of lenticulostriate arteries is inversely related to the size of the ipsilateral recurrent artery of Heubner and the medial lenticulostriate arteries from the anterior cerebral artery. The middle cerebral artery may have either a bifurcation or trifurcation. Two or three large perforating branches usually originate just proximal to the bifurcation of the middle cerebral artery and go medially into the insular region to supply lateral and posterior lenticular structures (lateral lenticulostriate arteries). Often, no perforating branches arise from the trunk of the middle cerebral artery between the origin of the medial and lateral lenticulostriate arteries. Therefore, this short length of segment M_1 is fit for temporary occlusion of the middle cerebral artery if necessary. Approximately 50 percent of patients have a branch off the proximal portion of the M_1 segment that runs lateral to the anterior temporal lobe.

The anterior choroidal artery arises from the internal carotid artery approximately 2 mm distal to the origin of the posterior communicating artery. It runs lateral to the posterior communicating artery, parallel with the optic tract. This vessel varies considerably in diameter and may arise as more than one vessel; it is duplicated in 4 to 30 percent of patients. Occasionally, it can originate from either the middle cerebral artery or the posterior communicating artery. The anterior choroidal artery is divided into a cisternal segment and a plexal segment. The cisternal segment is the source of perforating branches that go medially to supply the uncus, optic tract, lateral geniculate body, cerebral peduncle, anterior perforated substance (putamen and internal capsule), hippocampus, and pulvinar. The plexal segment enters the choroidal fissure to supply the choroid plexus. Several branches usually originate from the proximal trunk of the plexal segment to supply the hippocampus.

The posterior cerebral artery is the source of two arterial supplies of the temporal lobe. First, approximately three to four branches of the P_2 segment of the posterior cerebral artery supply the hippocampus; these vessels enter the hippocampus through the choroidal fissure. Second, the posterior temporal artery arises at the junction of segments P_2 and P_3. This artery goes along the floor of the middle cranial fossa underneath the temporal lobe and perfuses the inferior surface and adjacent lateral surface of the temporal lobe.

Venous drainage of the temporal lobe includes the deep venous and superficial systems. The superficial system involves the Sylvian vein, which has connections with the inferior and superior great anastomotic veins posteriorly and the cavernous sinus and sphenoparietal sinus anteriorly. The deep venous system involves the deep Sylvian vein, which drains into the basal vein of Rosenthal. The anterior hippocampal vein, the uncal veins, the anterior and posterior longitudinal hippocampal veins, the inferior ventricular vein, and the inferior choroidal vein all drain into the basal vein of Rosenthal. The basal vein of Rosenthal drains into the internal cerebral vein. Cortical polar veins often come off the tip of the temporal lobe and drain directly into the sphenoparietal sinus.

TEMPORAL LOBECTOMY

Conceptually, there are two types of temporal lobectomy, depending on the goals of the operation. One, temporal lobectomy often is performed on patients with a temporal lobe neoplasm to provide evidence for diagnosis, to produce decompression, and to decrease the risk of uncal herniation. As much neocortical tissue as needed is removed to afford maximal decompression. Two, temporal lobectomy performed in combination with resection of the amygdala and hippocampus is the primary means of treating intractable partial seizures originating in the temporal lobe. As little neocortex as possible is removed to gain access to the hippocampus. Subsequently, an aggressive resection of medial temporal structures is performed.

Surgeons debate about the maximal length of temporal neocortex that can safely be resected, as measured from the temporal tip. In the left temporal lobe, it should be less than 6.0 cm; in the right temporal lobe, a 7- to 8-cm length of neocortex can be removed with a minimal risk. For both temporal lobes, the more posterior the resection, the greater the risk of producing a contralateral homonymous hemianopia. Resection of a length longer than 9.0 cm results in complete homonymous hemianopia. With resection of a 5-cm length of neocortex, the risk of superior quadrantanopia is about 10 to 15 percent. When operating on the left temporal lobe, the primary concern is the risk of language dysfunction. When performing a standard left temporal lobectomy to resect a glioma, it is prudent to limit the extent of the superior temporal resection to 3.5 cm. The posterior margin can be angled back to remove 6 cm of the inferior temporal gyrus. With these cortical margins, the risk of significant permanent language dysfunction is less than 5 percent.

It is important to consider the vascular structures at risk during temporal lobectomy. Along the Sylvian fissure, the middle cerebral artery complex can be injured, and along the tentorial notch, the anterior choroidal and posterior cerebral arteries can be injured. More posteriorly, adjacent to the edge of the tentorium cerebelli, the posterior cerebral artery can be harmed. The best means of preventing vascular injury is to respect the overlying arachnoid along the Sylvian fissure and the basal cistern. Therefore, it is best to perform a subpial resection of the superior temporal and parahippocampal gyri. A Penfield #1 dissector or fine spatula can be used to peel the superior temporal gyrus off the Sylvian fissure. One or two small arteries probably will need to be cauterized and divided. Otherwise, any bleeding or oozing originating from the arachnoid of the Sylvian fissure should be controlled with hemostatic fabric (Surgicel). It is important never to cauterize along the Sylvian fissure because it can cause dissection or thrombosis of the middle cerebral artery. Also, it is important to peel the uncus out of the tentorial notch without violating the arachnoid. This not only protects the underlying anterior choroidal and posterior cerebral arteries but also prevents blood from seeping into the basal cistern.

The cranial nerves at risk during temporal lobectomy include the oculomotor, the trochlear, and the trigeminal nerves. The oculomotor nerve may be injured if the arachnoid over the tentorial notch is violated. This nerve is exquisitely vulnerable to manipulation. In fact, irrigation of the operative bed with cold saline may result in the patient temporarily experiencing blurred vision. The trochlear nerve may be injured if the edge of the tentorium cerebelli is manipulated. The trigeminal nerve may be injured if the dura mater along the middle cranial fossa is excessively cauterized. Often during temporal lobectomy, bleeding occurs from veins and sinuses along the dura mater. Bleeding from these small vessels within the dura mater of the middle cranial fossa is best controlled with bits of absorbable gelatin sponge (Gelfoam) instead of cauterization. In fact, cauterization may lead to retraction of the dura mater along these venous channels and make hemostasis more difficult.

The operation described below is performed for intractable right temporal lobe seizures. Therefore, the anterior neocortex of the temporal lobe is removed to provide access to the hippocampus. It often is easier to perform this resection in two steps instead of performing an en bloc resection.

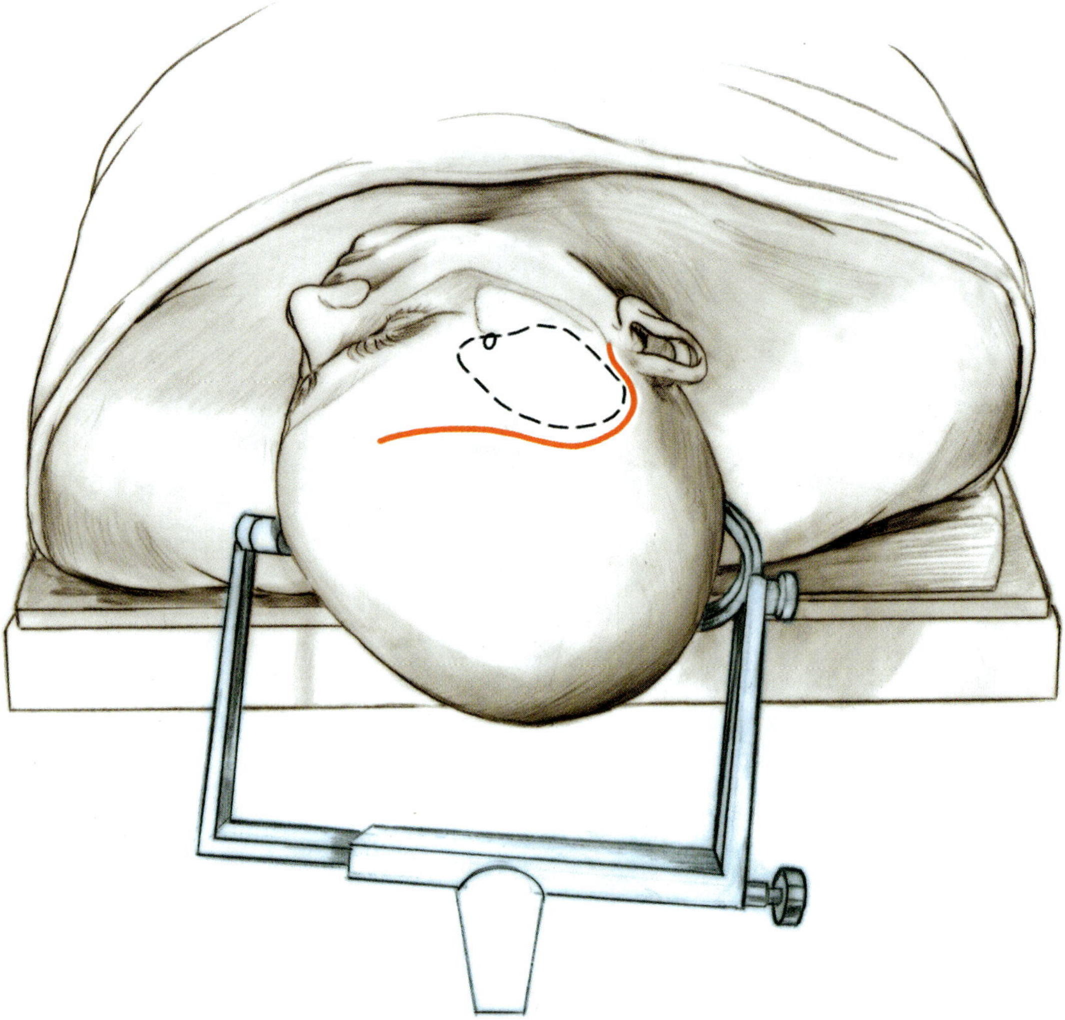

Figure 2–2.

Step 1. Diagram of the position of the patient's head, the incision, and the craniotomy. The position of the head that is advocated is not that of a standard temporal lobectomy, in which the head is parallel to the floor. Instead the head is angled, as illustrated here, to allow the surgeon to look down the long axis of the hippocampus. In this way, the hippocampus can be resected back to the level of the tectal plate or atrium. It is important to have the craniotomy extend low down along the middle cranial fossa to facilitate resection of the inferior temporal and fusiform gyri.

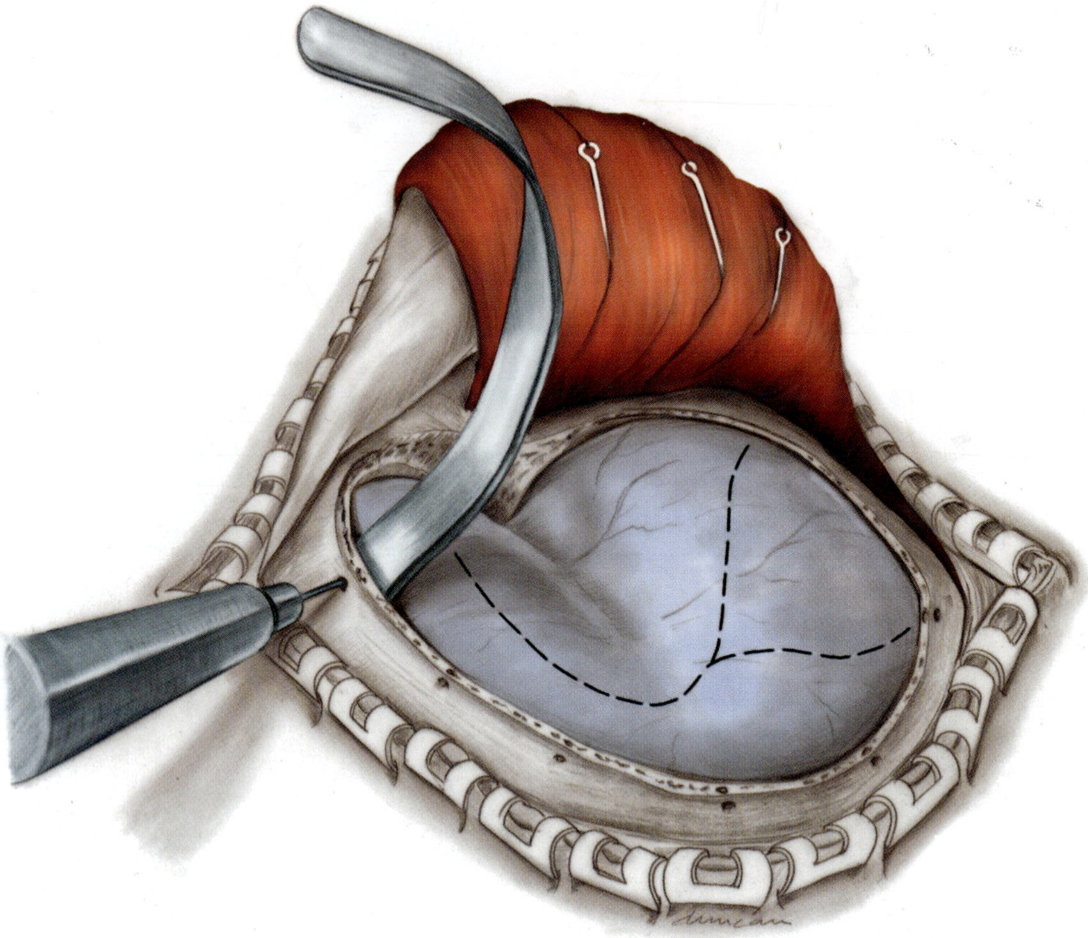

Figure 2–3.

Step 2. After the craniotomy, the dura mater is tacked to the margins of the bone and muscle and then opened so that only the cerebral cortex destined for removal is exposed. In this example, intraoperative electrocorticography will be performed. Accordingly, part of the inferior frontal lobe is exposed to facilitate placement of the strip electrode.

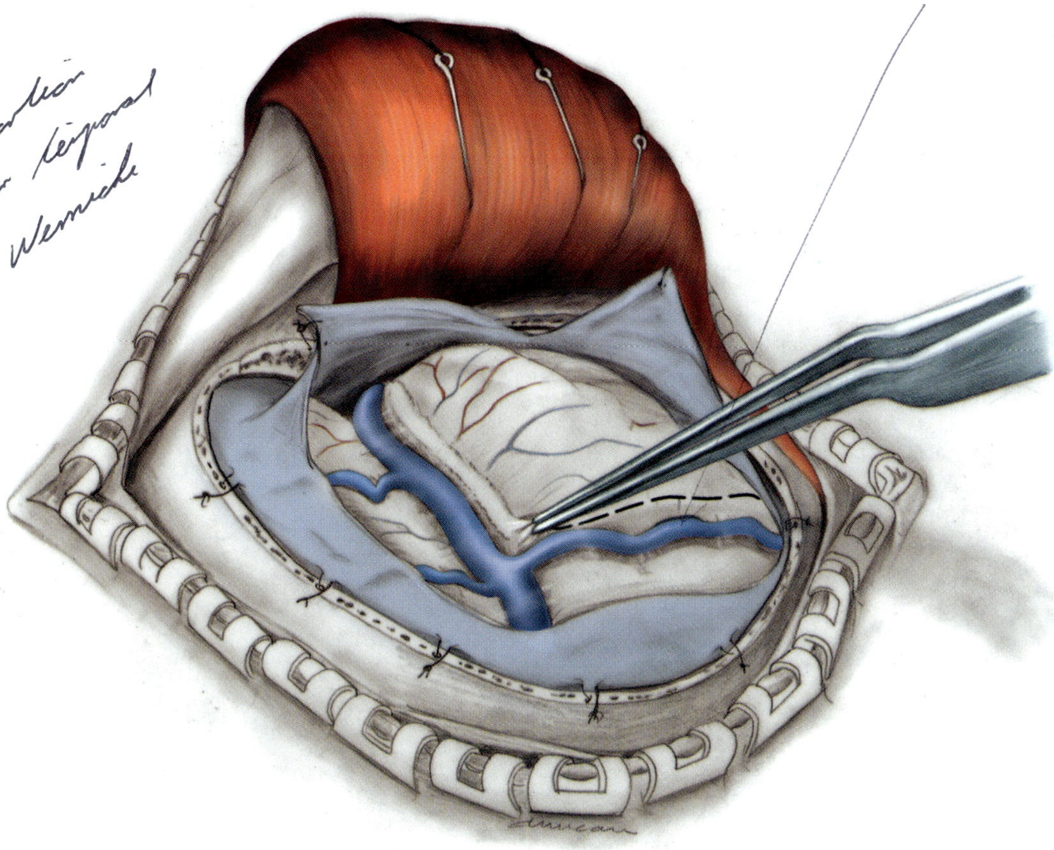

Figure 2–4.

Step 3. Before the neocortex is resected, it is best to examine the surface anatomy. In this illustration, a large anterior vein runs from the lateral fissure to the inferior surface of the temporal lobe. A major vein such as this may be an anterior vein of Labbé, which must be preserved. Also, before resection, it is best to take a Penfield #1 dissector and determine the exact length from the tip of the temporal lobe to the cut margin of the dural opening. In this way, the exact length of the neocortical resection can be determined. Surface inspection often reveals one or two branches of the middle cerebral artery that emanate from the Sylvian fissure or the superior temporal sulcus and run posteriorly. These arteries should be preserved during neocortical resection, especially in the left temporal lobe, to decrease the risk of language dysfunction caused by vascular injury of the posterior portion of the superior temporal gyrus. Before commencing the lobectomy, it is useful to take into account these surface observations and to outline the margins of the proposed resection with a bipolar cautery.

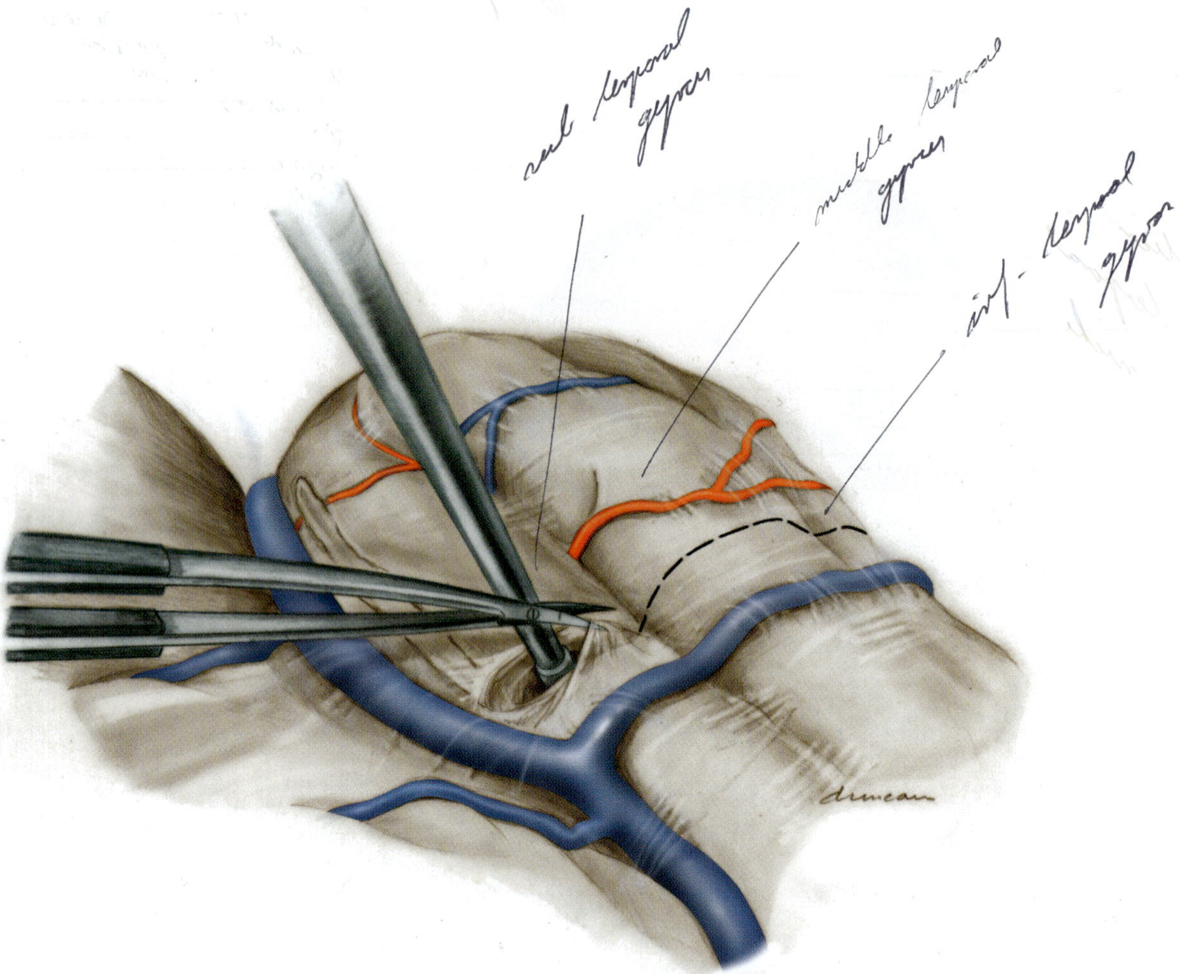

Figure 2–5.

Step 4. Resection of the temporal lobe begins along the posterior margin, extending from the superior temporal gyrus to the inferior temporal gyrus. A #5 or #7 straight suction tip should be the primary instrument for removing the neocortex along the junction of the posterior resection line with the incision of the superior temporal gyrus. In patients with intractable epilepsy, there typically is atrophy of the temporal lobe, and the middle cerebral artery may be more superficial than expected. Use of the straight suction tip instead of the bipolar cautery to divide the white matter at this junction limits the risk of inadvertently injuring a more superficially located middle cerebral artery. After the Sylvian fissure or the middle cerebral artery has been identified, a cottonoid (Americot) is placed for protection.

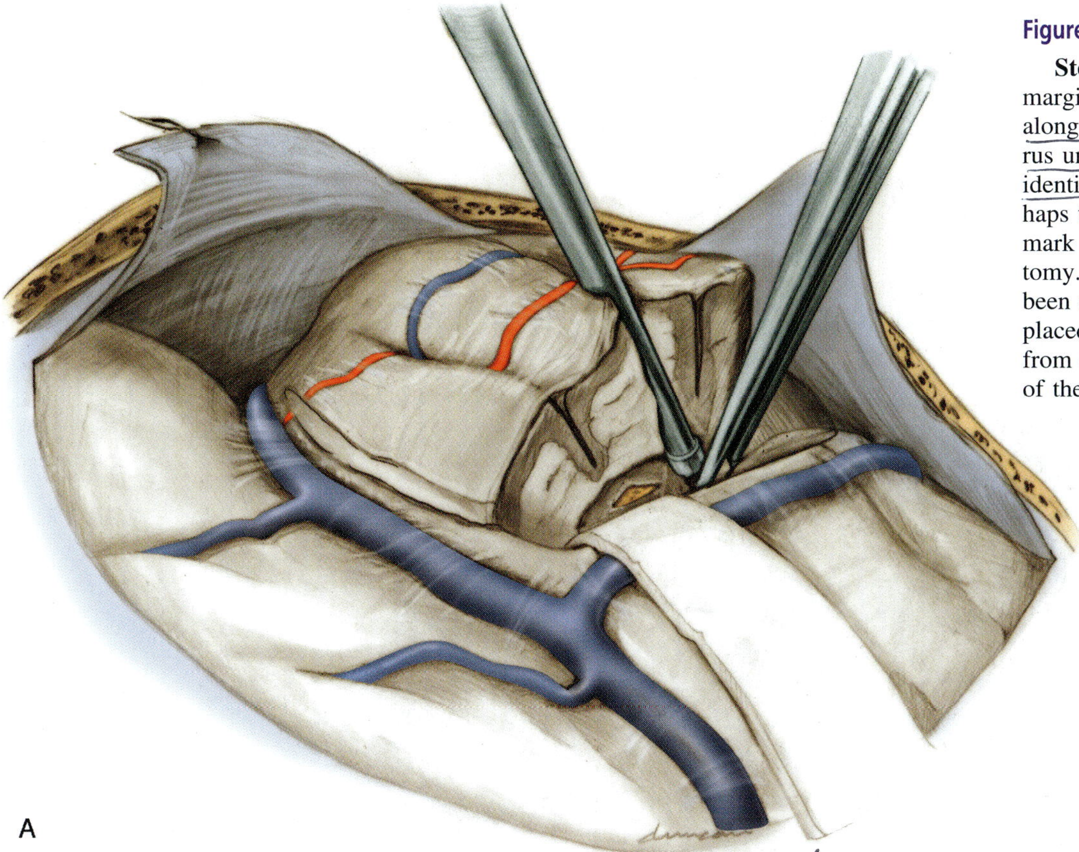

Figure 2–6.

Step 5. *A*, The posterior margin incision is deepened along the middle temporal gyrus until the lateral ventricle is identified. The ventricle is perhaps the most important landmark during temporal lobectomy. After the ventricle has been entered, a cottonoid is placed in it to prevent blood from entering the occipital horn of the lateral ventricle.

B, The resection line is extended inferiorly through the inferior temporal gyrus into the fusiform gyrus. Occasionally, it can be difficult to distinguish among the margins of the inferior temporal gyrus, the fusiform (lateral occipitotemporal) gyrus, and the parahippocampal gyrus. There are always partial sulci between these gyri that contain invaginating arachnoid and several small blood vessels. It is useful to identify the sulci by visualizing the invaginating arachnoid. The resection of the inferior temporal lobe is carried through the fusiform gyrus to the collateral sulcus.

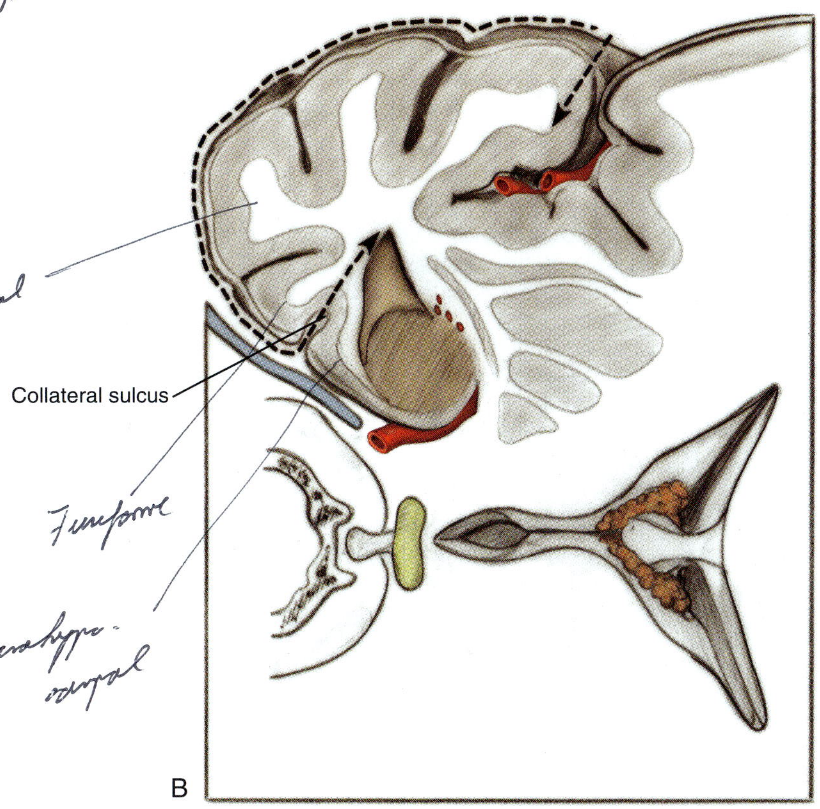

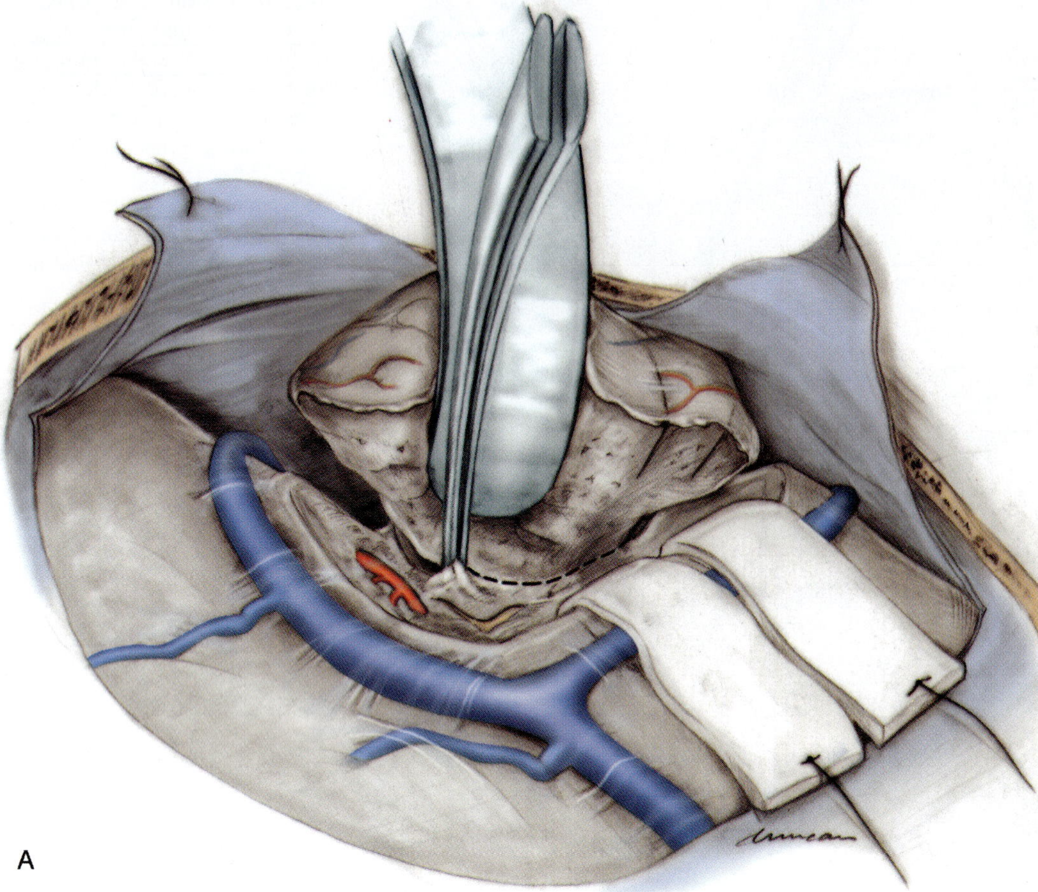

A

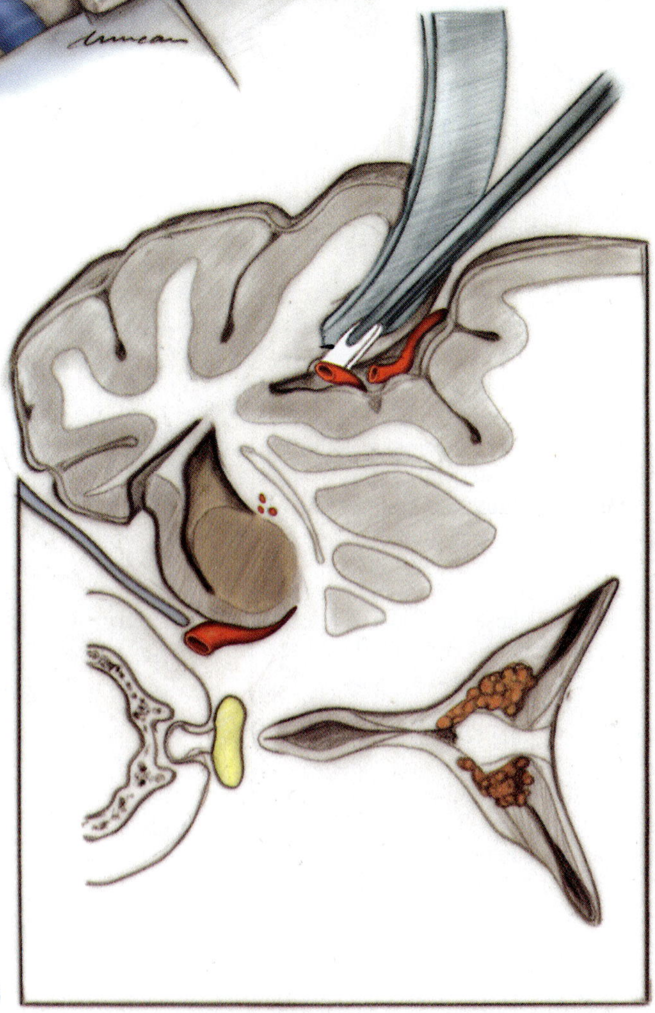

B

Figure 2–7.

Step 6. *A* and *B*, After the resection of the posterior margin down to the collateral sulcus has been completed, the superior temporal gyrus is resected. The arachnoid just lateral to the Sylvian vein is cauterized and incised. A small suction tip is used to remove the underlying superior temporal gyrus off the Sylvian fissure. A small jeweler's forceps can be used to hold the arachnoid of the Sylvian fissure medially to provide countertraction as the suction tip or Penfield dissector is used to pull the superior temporal gyrus off the Sylvian fissure. During this process, it is critical to make sure that the arachnoid over the Sylvian fissure is not violated. After the Sylvian fissure has been identified, cottonoids are placed over it to protect the vascular structures within it. The incision in the superior temporal gyrus is carried progressively deeper from back to front with bipolar cautery. A retractor is placed on the temporal lobe to lift it partially out of the wound to allow better visualization. Resection of this deeper white matter is angled to run over the top of the lateral ventricle toward the collateral sulcus.

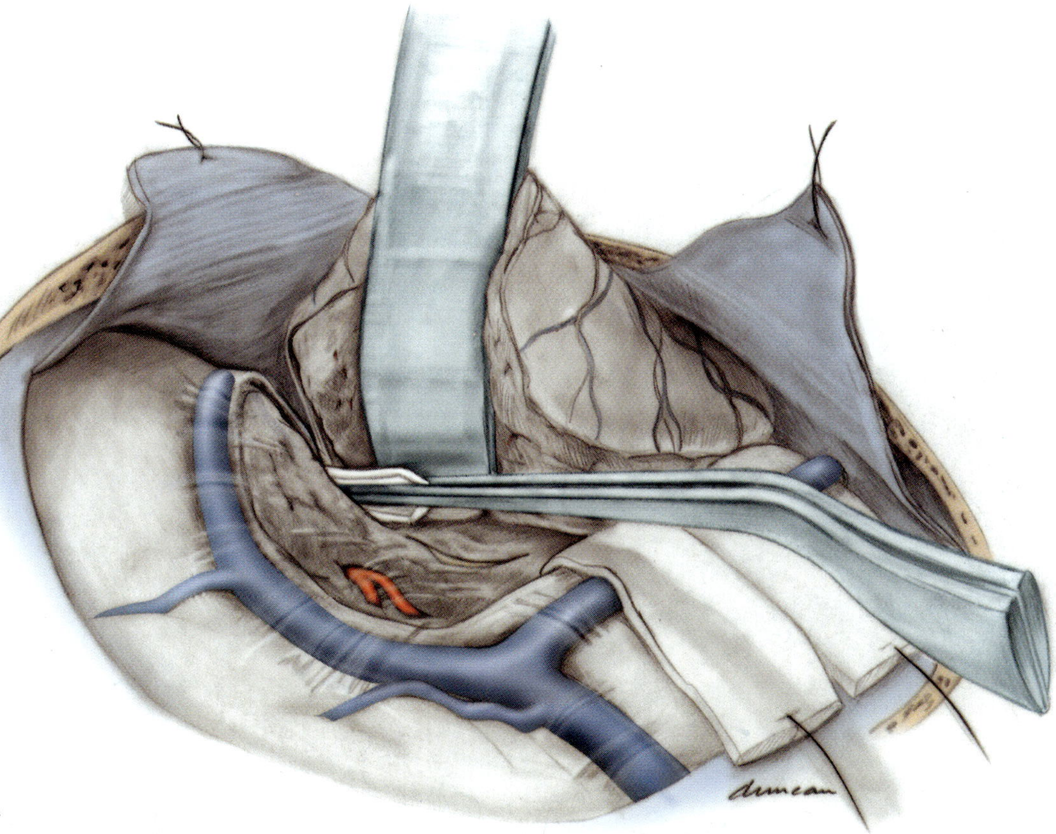

A

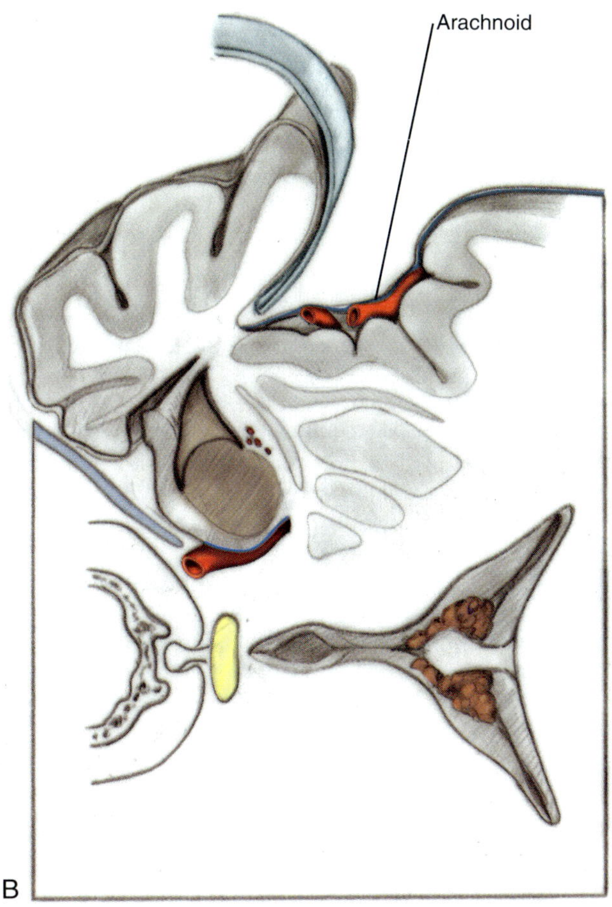

B

Figure 2–8.

Step 7. *A* and *B*, At the depth of the wound along the floor of the middle cranial fossa, the arachnoid along the inferior temporal lobe is cauterized and incised. In fact, a large margin of arachnoid is left intact over the edge of the tentorium cerebelli to protect the neurovascular structures and to prevent blood from entering the basal cistern. At this point, the white matter underlying the fusiform gyrus, which is lateral to the lateral ventricle, is being incised.

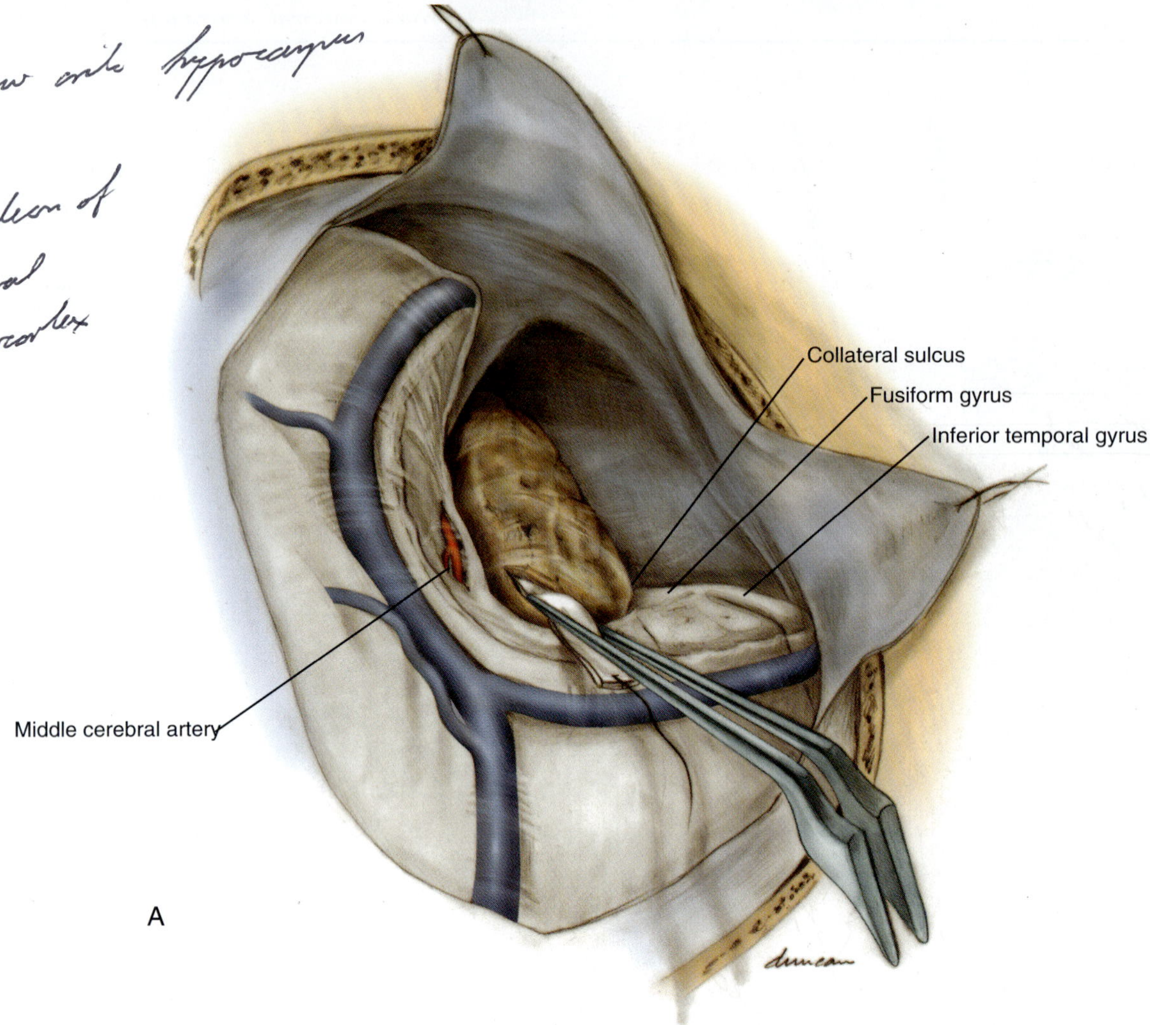

Figure 2–9.

Step 8. *A* and *B*, The neocortex has been removed down to the roof of the temporal horn of the lateral ventricle. This uncapping allows visualization of the hippocampus. The operating microscope is rotated to allow the surgeon to look down the long axis of the hippocampus. A new cottonoid is placed in the lateral ventricle to prevent blood from entering the temporal horn. The posterior margin of the neocortical resection and that along the Sylvian fissure are lined with hemostatic fabric and cottonoids. A Yasargil or self-retaining retractor is placed along the edge of the resection. This retractor is placed under tension to retract the remnant of the temporal lobe in an anterior-to-posterior direction. The temporal lobe tolerates this type of anterior-to-posterior retraction.

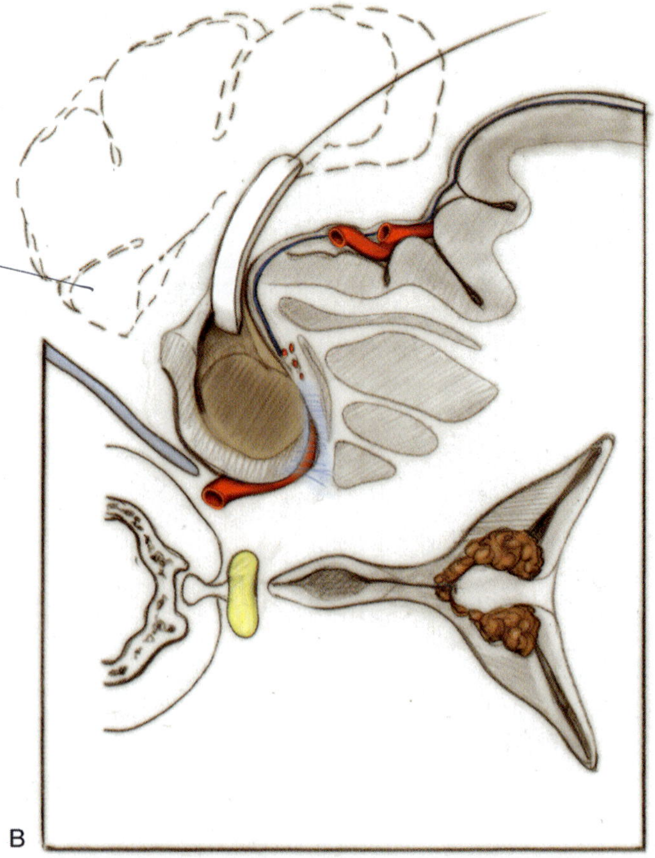

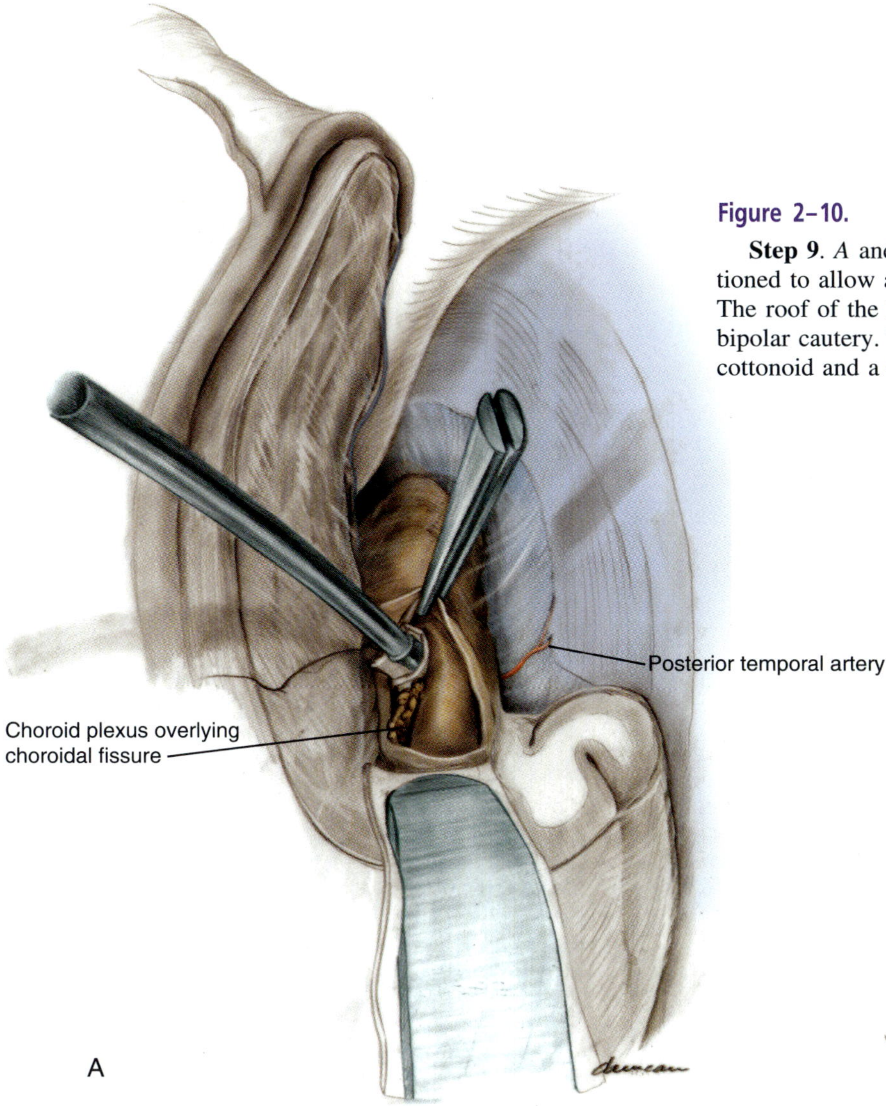

A

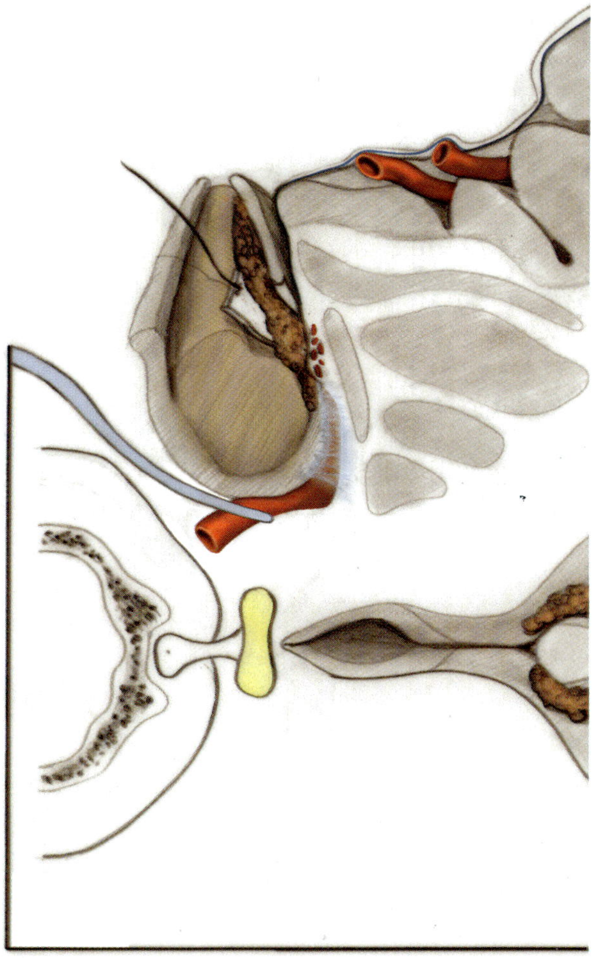

B

Figure 2–10.

Step 9. *A* and *B*, The self-retaining retractor is repositioned to allow a better view of the posterior hippocampus. The roof of the lateral ventricle is opened anteriorly with a bipolar cautery. The choroid plexus is held medially with a cottonoid and a #5 or #7 straight suction tip.

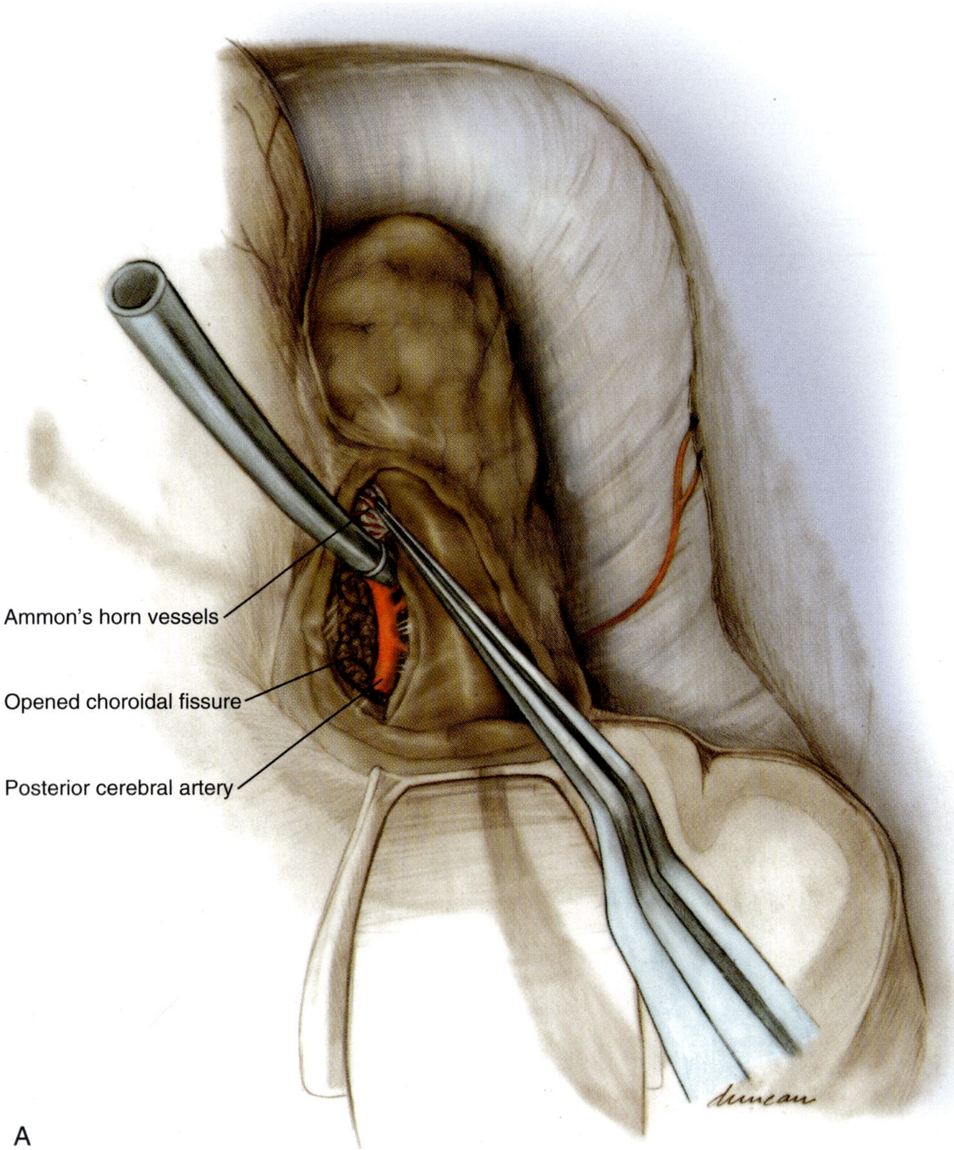

A

Figure 2–11.

Step 10. *A* and *B*, After the roof of the lateral ventricle has been opened anteriorly, the choroidal fissure can be partially identified. It is almost translucent. Usually, four or five small blood vessels penetrate the arachnoid and enter the choroidal fissure to supply the medial side of the hippocampus. These Ammon's horn vessels must be cauterized and divided. They usually are contained in a thin layer of arachnoid as they pass through the choroidal fissure. There-

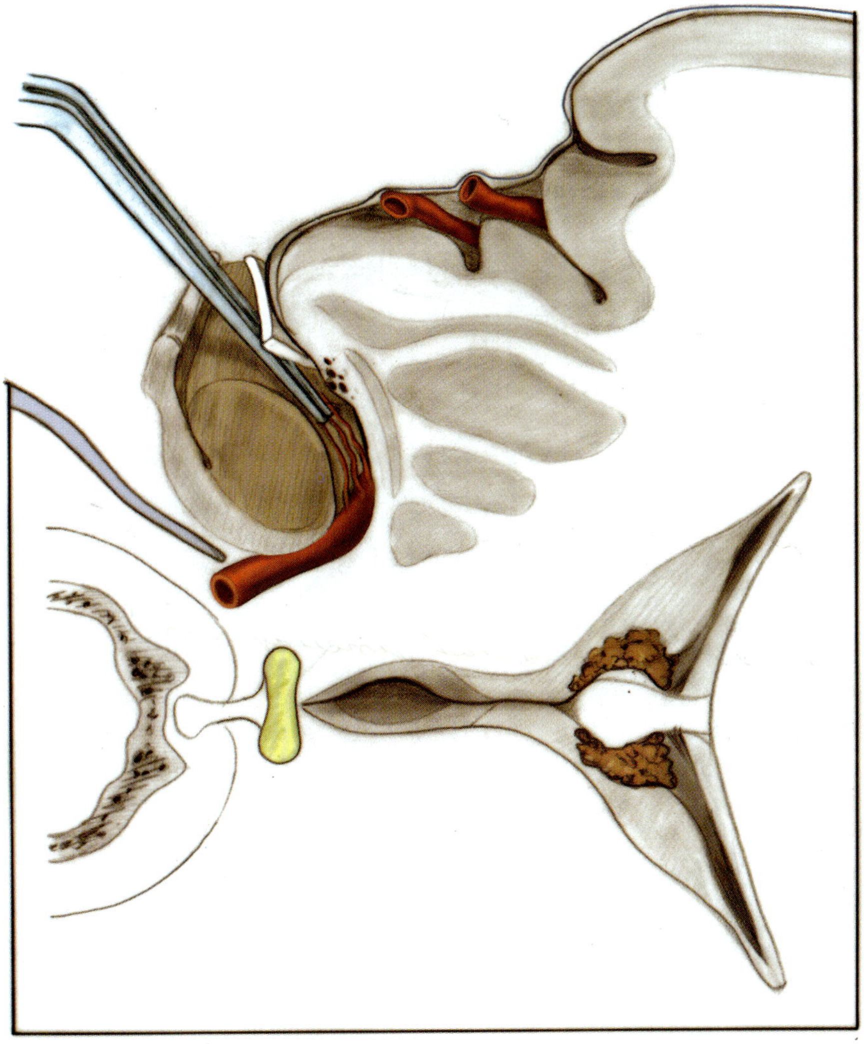

B

fore, there is almost a double layer of triangular arachnoid. This triangular arachnoid and vessels can be displaced medially. A #5 or #7 straight suction tip is used to gently rotate or extract the medial edge of the hippocampus from the curved gutter of arachnoid overlying the posterior cerebral artery. In this way, the arachnoid over the posterior cerebral artery is not violated.

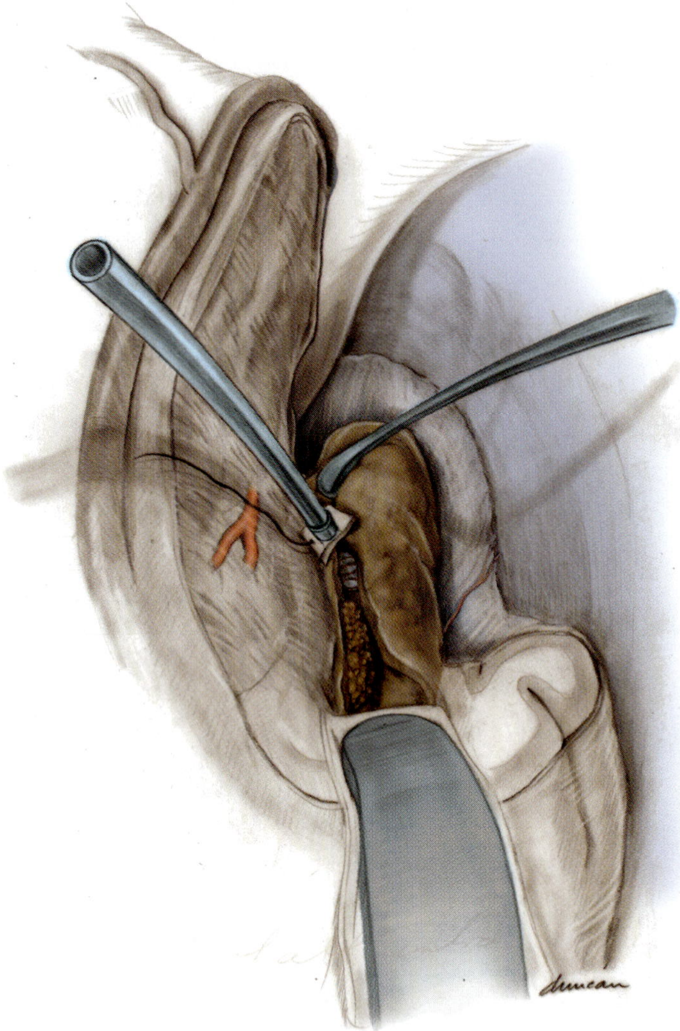

Figure 2–12.

Step 11. The body of the hippocampus is mobilized off the posterior cerebral artery, and the triangular arachnoid containing Ammon's horn vessels is cauterized and displaced medially. The uncus, which contains the amygdala, is pulled out of the tentorial notch with the Penfield #1 dissector and suction tip. Again, the arachnoid over the tentorial notch is not violated. This protects the anterior choroidal and the posterior cerebral arteries. There typically is a small bit of white matter between the uncus and the forward-most cut along the roof of the lateral ventricle that must be removed with suction and bipolar cautery.

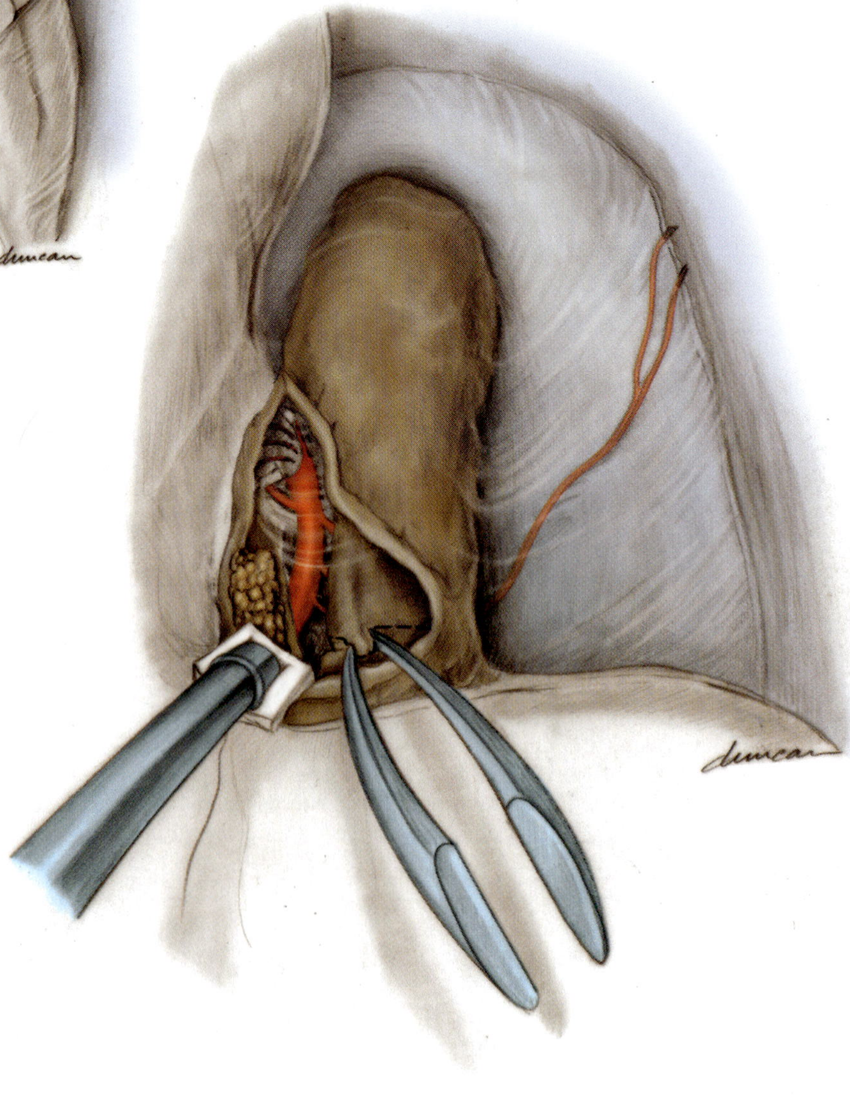

Figure 2–13.

Step 12. At this point, most of the amygdala and hippocampus has been mobilized. The posterior edge of the hippocampus is cauterized and divided. In this way, the hippocampus is removed en bloc. After the hippocampus has been removed, the self-retaining retractor is repositioned along the roof of the lateral ventricle and again retracted in an anterior-to-posterior direction. Typically, a #7 straight suction tip can be used to remove the tail of the hippocampus back to the level of the tectal plate. When removing the tail of the hippocampus, it is important to continue to identify the choroid plexus, which marks the lateral ventricle. The tissue between the lateral ventricle and the collateral sulcus is removed with suction in a subpial fashion. Preserving the tissue lateral to the collateral sulcus decreases the risk of visual field loss.

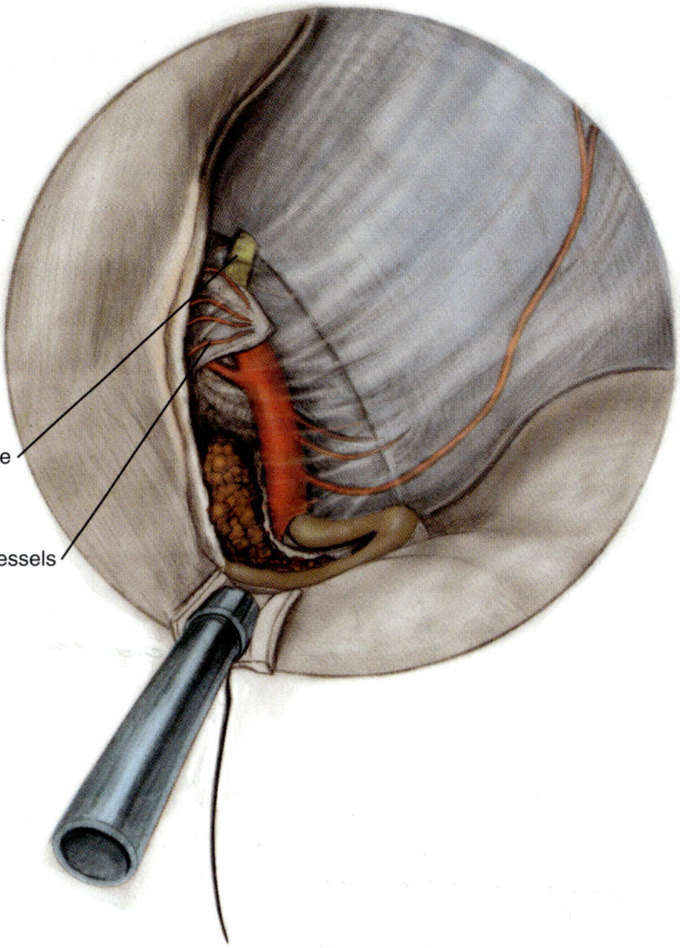

Figure 2–14.

This postresection illustration highlights some of the pertinent arachnoid structures. The deepest arachnoid visualized is that overlying the posterior cerebral artery and the oculomotor nerve. As this arachnoid passes medially, it runs underneath the choroid plexus and turns laterally in a triangular pattern. This contains branches of the posterior cerebral artery, called "Ammon's horn vessels," that feed the hippocampus. The outer layer of this triangular arachnoid continues more superficially and joins the arachnoid over the Sylvian fissure.

MIDDLE CEREBRAL ARTERY ANEURYSM

The most common approach to a middle cerebral artery aneurysm is through a frontotemporal craniotomy with a trans-Sylvian dissection. Some surgeons advocate exposure of these aneurysms through a subpial superior temporal gyrus approach. In the standard trans-Sylvian approach, it is important to remember that the aneurysm usually is located more superficially than expected. This is why a frontotemporal craniotomy is superior to a pterional craniotomy for exposure.

One of the first major decisions the surgeon must make during exposure is whether to start splitting the Sylvian fissure proximally or distally. The advantage of a proximal exposure is that it provides access to the supraclinoid carotid artery and the proximal middle cerebral artery before the aneurysm is dissected. Thus, if inadvertent rupture occurs, a temporary vascular clip can be applied. However, if the patient has had a significant subarachnoid hemorrhage, perhaps associated with a temporal lobe hematoma, the brain may be edematous and obtaining exposure of the proximal or deep Sylvian fissure early may be more difficult than anticipated. The disadvantage of dissecting the lateral Sylvian fissure early in the procedure is that the surgeon comes down on the dome of the aneurysm before achieving proximal control of the blood vessel. A useful rule to follow is that if a hemorrhage has occurred, early proximal splitting of the Sylvian fissure is best (if possible). For aneurysms that have not hemorrhaged, a lateral-to-medial division of the Sylvian fissure can be performed with minimal retraction of the frontal or temporal lobe.

Although middle cerebral artery aneurysms appear to be low risk because of easy access, the reported rate of ischemic stroke complications is high, probably for several reasons. One, many middle cerebral artery aneurysms have a fusiform origin and the takeoff of the M_2 segments may be from the neck of the aneurysm. Accordingly, placement of the clip may compromise the origin of one of these vessels, especially if the base of the aneurysm is partially calcified. Two, often, a lenticulostriate artery originates from the deep side of the middle cerebral artery distally along the M_1 segment close to the bifurcation. This vessel may be occluded inadvertently by the tips of the aneurysm clip. Thus, after the aneurysm clip is placed, it is important to visually inspect the tips of the aneurysm clip and to auscultate the M_2 branches with a micro Doppler probe or ultrasonography, if available.

20% of all intracranial aneurysms!

Early control of proximal (supraclinoid) carotid artery allows early control of bleeding and argues in favour of proximal - distal exposure of sylvian fissure!
If resection from distal - proximal, dome of aneurysm will be encountered before proximal vessel control is gained.

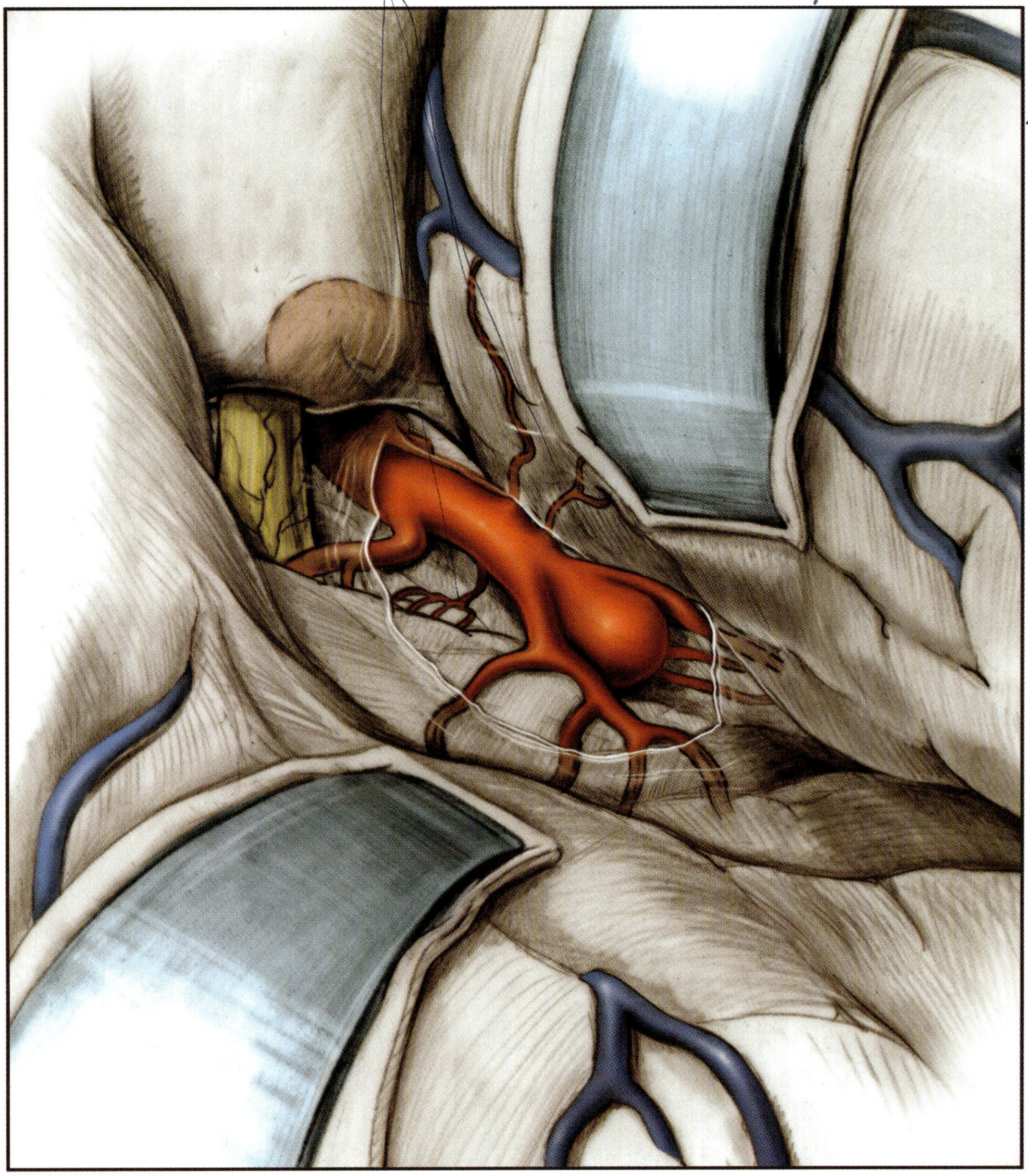

Figure 2–15.

Step 1. In this example, the Sylvian fissure is widely divided. It often is helpful to use a temporal lobe retractor. The retractor should be placed along the medial temporal lobe so that manipulation of the clip and the clip holder is not obstructed if the trajectory of clip placement is horizontal from lateral to medial. This illustration emphasizes the presence of a trifurcation of the middle cerebral artery, with a small branch exiting deep to the dome of the aneurysm. Also, a single lenticulostriate trunk, with its arcade, comes off the medial wall of the M_1 segment.

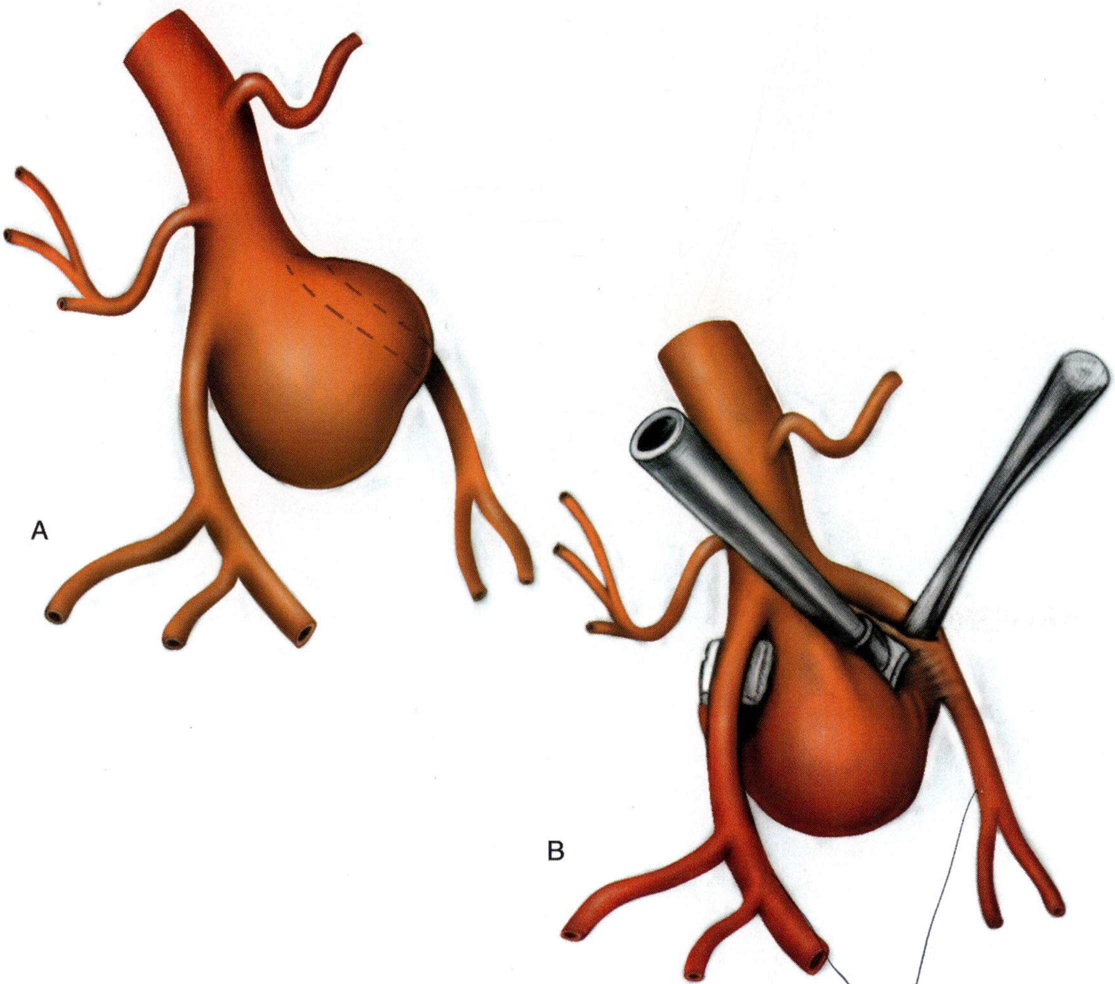

Figure 2–16.

Step 2. *A*, After the Sylvian fissure has been divided, the neck of the aneurysm must be separated from the M_2 branches.

B, Often, part of the neck or dome is adherent to the takeoff of the M_2 branch. A fine spatula is useful in the dissection. After the neck has been identified, placement of a small piece of absorbable gelatin sponge helps protect the takeoff of the M_2 branches. In this illustration, a curved clip has been applied. This is one of the more common trajectories for clip placement for these aneurysms.

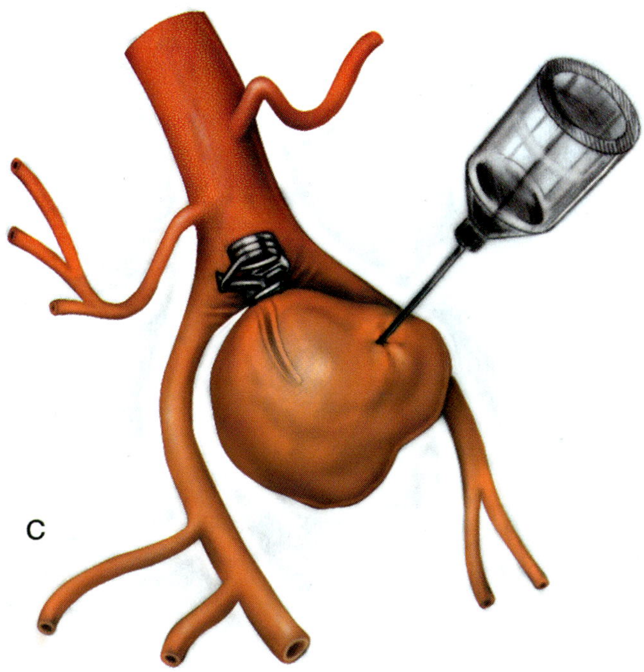

C

C, After the clip has been placed, it is important to aspirate the dome to collapse the aneurysm. Thereafter, the jaws of the clip are inspected to make sure that no vessels are trapped along the back wall. Finally, the M_2 branches should be assessed immediately after clip placement with a micro Doppler probe or ultrasonography.

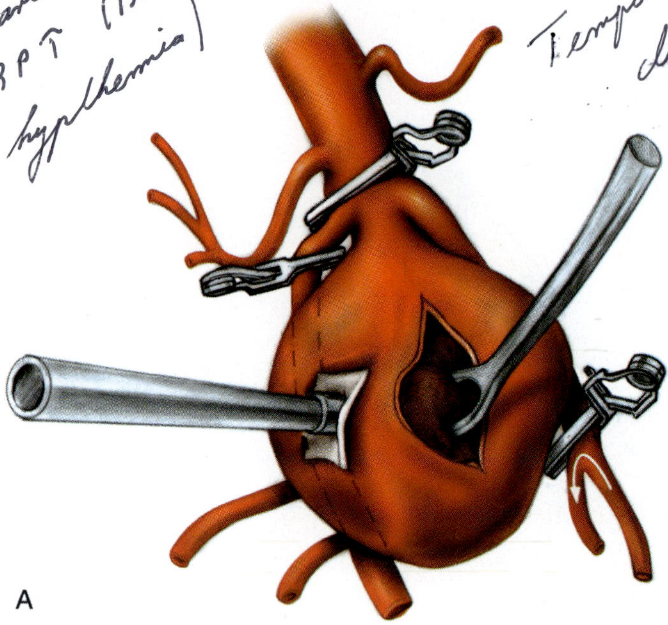

A

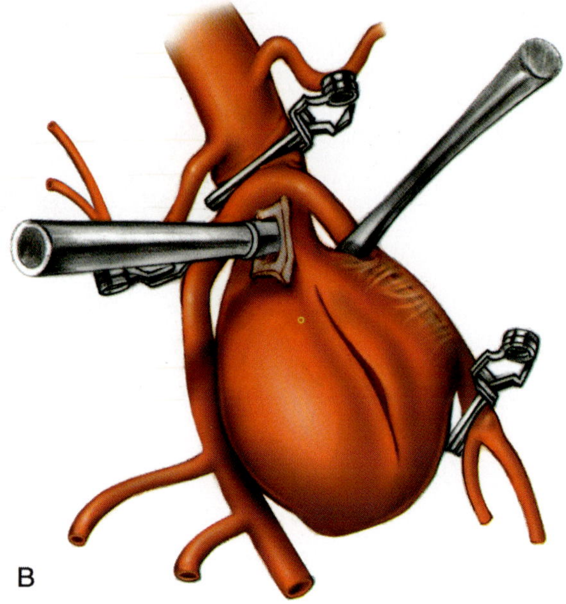

B

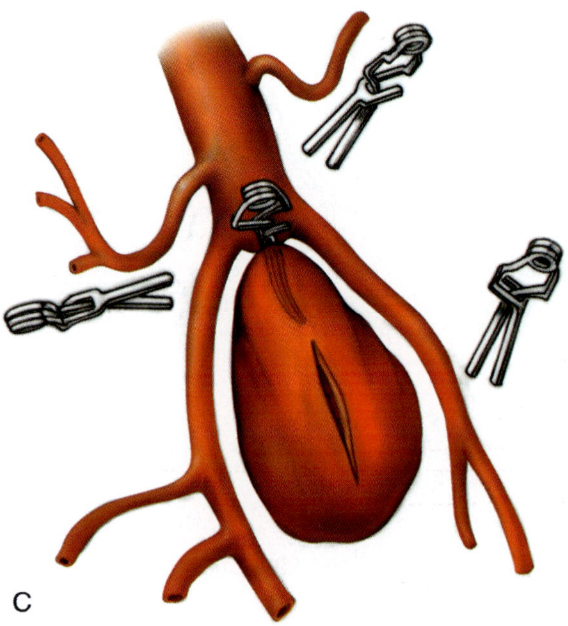

C

Figure 2–17.

A–C, This sequence of drawings illustrates a giant, partially thrombosed aneurysm of the middle cerebral artery. In this situation, partial thrombectomy of the aneurysm is almost always required. Therefore, temporary clips are placed on the distal M_1 segment just proximal to the bifurcation. If possible, the temporary clip should be placed in a way to preserve blood flow to the lenticulostriate arteries that originate from the M_1 segment. Note that a temporary clip has been placed on one branch of the middle cerebral artery just proximal to a bifurcation to allow retrograde collateral blood flow (*curved arrow*). Generally, before the vessels are occluded in this type of aneurysm repair, a metabolic suppressant is administered intravenously, such as thiopental (2 to 3 mg/kg). Also, the patient's systolic blood pressure is increased to 130 to 150 mm Hg to increase leptomeningeal collateral blood flow. Temporary occlusion without reperfusion for less than 10 minutes is safe, with low risk of residual ischemic injury. If major vessels are occluded for more than 20 minutes, the risk of ischemic injury increases, unless there is good collateral blood flow. Currently, the effects of intermittent reperfusion in this type of surgical scenario have not been determined.

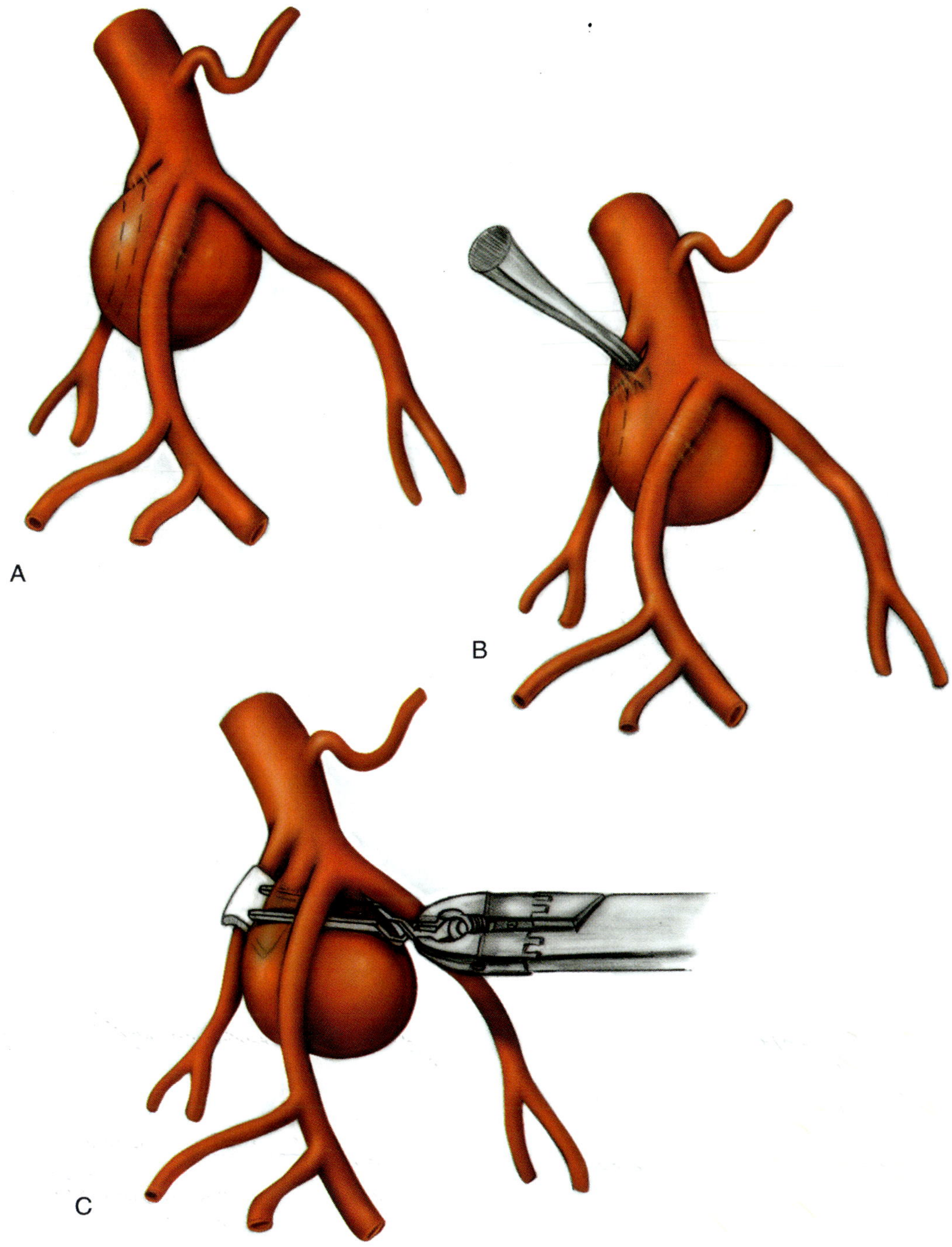

Figure 2–18.

A, A technically difficult middle cerebral artery aneurysm that has dense adhesions with several branches of the middle cerebral artery.

B, After the vessels have been dissected free from the neck of the aneurysm, it is useful to place a small piece of absorbable gelatin sponge when placing the clip.

C, The sponge protects the vessel at risk when the clip is inserted. With complex aneurysms in which the neck is the origin of distal vessels, it is mandatory to have objective evidence that the vessels are patent after clip placement. This evidence can be obtained with Doppler, microultrasonography, or angiography.

TEMPORAL LOBE ARTERIOVENOUS MALFORMATION

When considering surgical resection of an arteriovenous malformation, the surgeon must have a detailed understanding of the three-dimensional anatomy of the lesion, the feeding arteries, and the draining veins. After these relationships are understood, an operation can be devised to minimize the risk of resection. In temporal lobe arteriovenous malformations, the arterial blood supply is derived superficially from the middle cerebral artery along the Sylvian fissure and inferiorly from the posterior cerebral artery and associated branches. The deep blood supply is complicated and derived from branches of the posterior cerebral artery, the anterior choroidal artery, and the middle cerebral artery. The venous drainage is through the Sylvian veins, the parietal veins, and the posterior temporal veins, including the vein of Labbé.

The general approach to a temporal lobe arteriovenous malformation is first to isolate the superficial arterial supply from the Sylvian fissure. Next, the blood supply along the inferior and posterior margins is cauterized and divided. The arteriovenous malformation is then retracted to expose the many arterial feeding vessels along the temporal horn of the lateral ventricle. During the resection, every attempt is made to preserve all the draining veins until after all the arterial blood supply has been isolated and divided. One of the best intraoperative indications that the resection of the arteriovenous malformation is complete is a loss of arterialized venous blood.

General principles of surgery on arteriovenous malformations include the following: one, preoperative embolization is beneficial and should be pursued aggressively if an experienced endovascular interventionalist is available. Embolization significantly decreases the severity of intraoperative bleeding. Also, it allows a graded accommodation of the surrounding brain tissue and blood vessels to changes in blood flow, thereby decreasing the risk of a postoperative hyperperfusion syndrome and hemorrhage. If embolization is performed, it is important that surgery not be delayed too long; otherwise, the deeper and more inaccessible blood supply to the arteriovenous malformation increases and is more difficult to control. Two, it is beneficial to tightly regulate the patient's blood pressure for approximately 48 hours postoperatively, depending on the size of the lesion. The larger the lesion, the greater the risk of a postoperative hyperperfusion syndrome. Tight regulation of blood pressure decreases this risk. With large arteriovenous malformations, the author prefers to keep systolic blood pressure less than 100 mm Hg for 48 hours postoperatively. Three, during resection of an arteriovenous malformation, it is important to preserve all surrounding veins. Veins that have arterialized blood may drain both the malformation and normal brain, and the inadvertent sacrifice of these veins can result in hemorrhagic infarction postoperatively. Four, irrigating bipolar cautery and small wire microclips are most helpful in obliterating small arterial feeding vessels along the ventricular surface. Five, postoperative imaging is needed to confirm complete resection of the arteriovenous malformation unless the surgeon is absolutely certain that this has been accomplished. If a small residual of arteriovenous malformation is left untreated, the risk of future hemorrhage is significant.

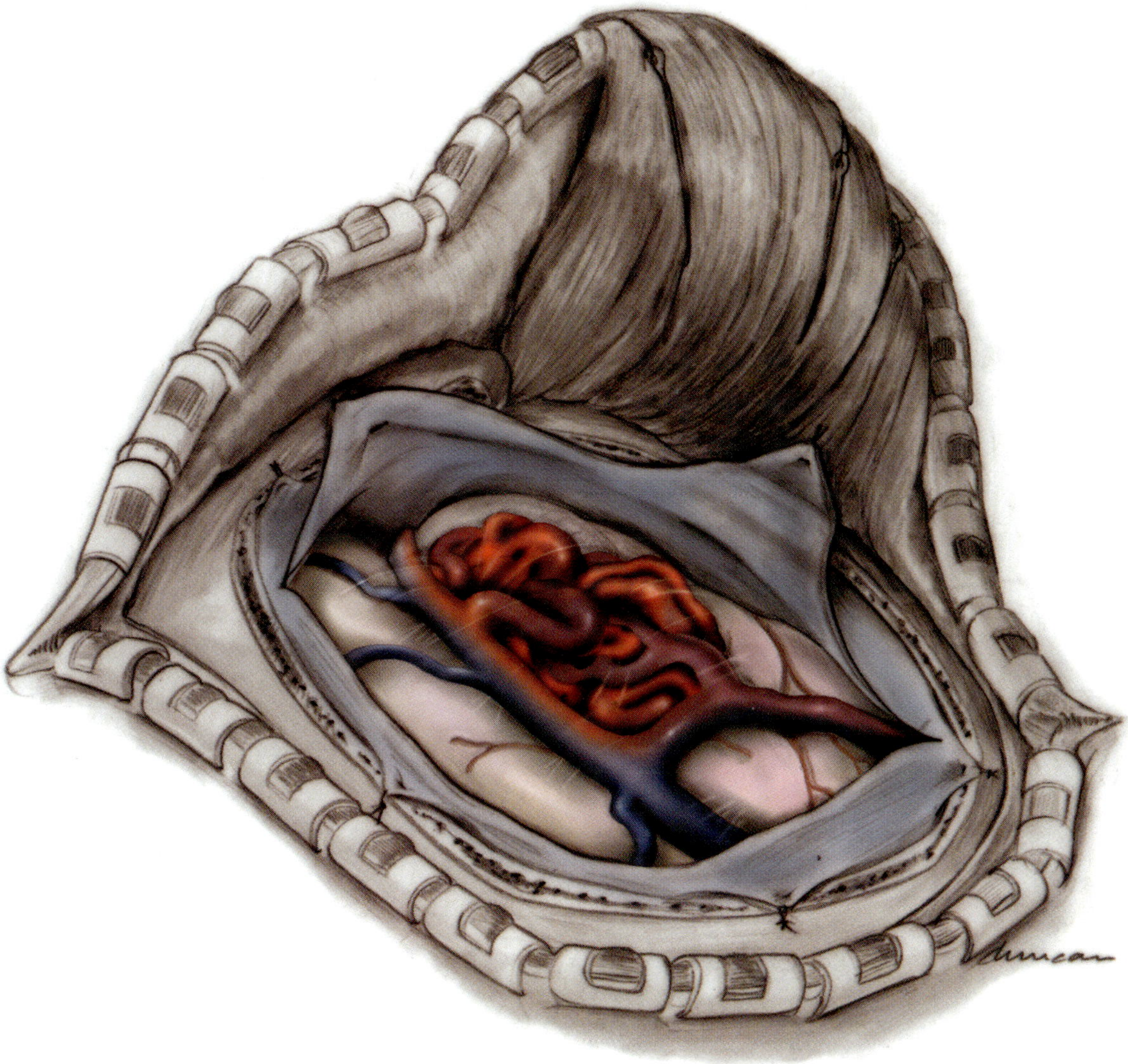

Figure 2–19.

Step 1. Both the craniotomy and the opening of the dura mater must be performed with caution to avoid any inadvertent tearing of the arteriovenous malformation, especially venous varices that may have eroded partially through the dura mater. After the dura mater has been opened, the first step is to examine the arteriovenous malformation to understand its surface anatomy. It is important to identify the draining veins, including those that drain both the malformation and normal brain. It often can be difficult to distinguish between an arterialized vein and a feeding artery. A useful tip is to follow the vessel in question distally along the cortical surface. Often, the smaller branches or ramifications assume the characteristics associated with a thicker walled arteriole or a thin-walled venule.

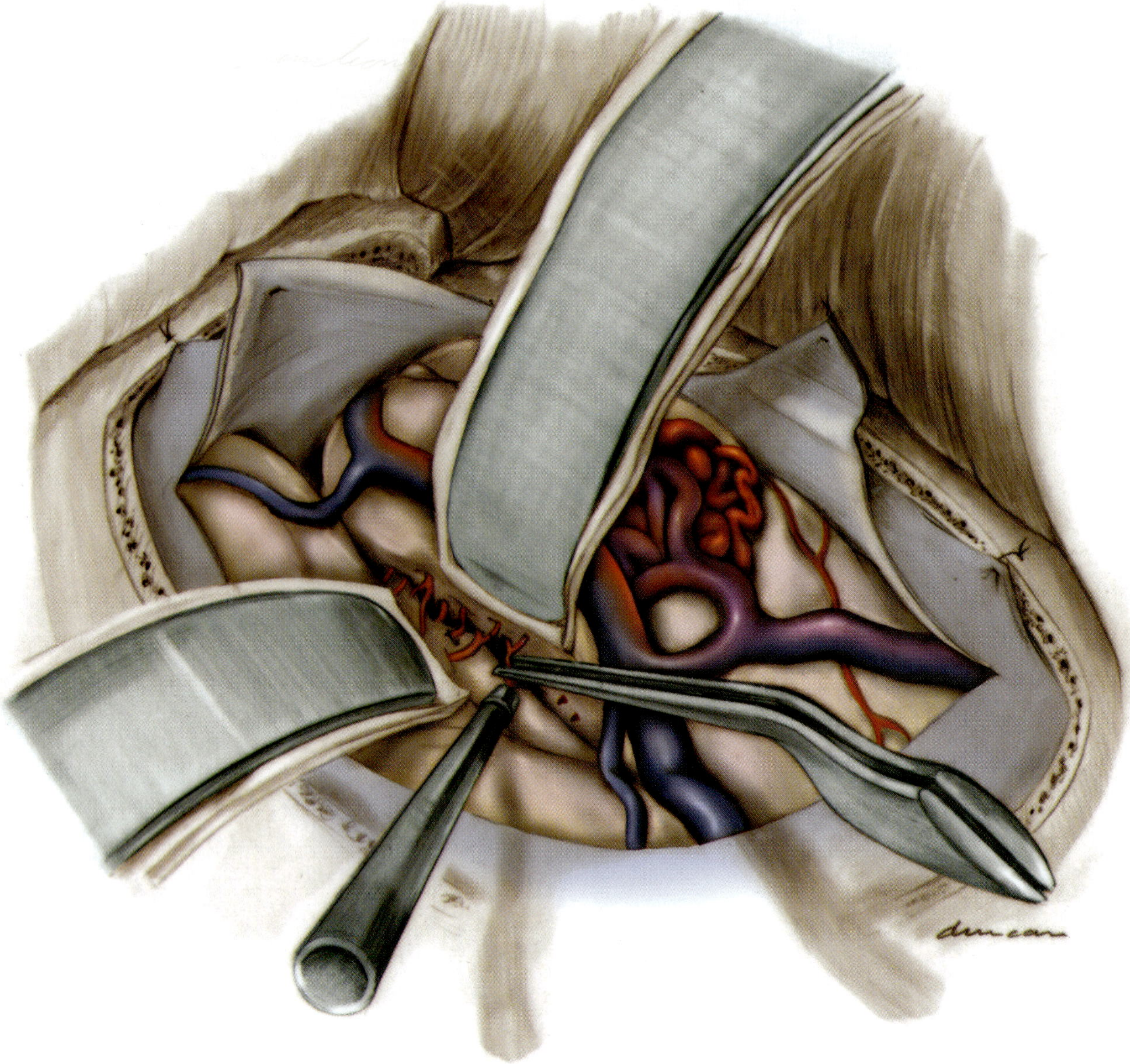

Figure 2–20.

Step 2. In this example, a large partially arterialized Sylvian vein makes it difficult for the surgeon to enter the Sylvian fissure. Therefore, the arachnoid over the Sylvian fissure is divided and the vein is retracted laterally. Many small arteries usually run out of the Sylvian fissure into the substance of the arteriovenous malformation. Each of these should be cauterized and divided.

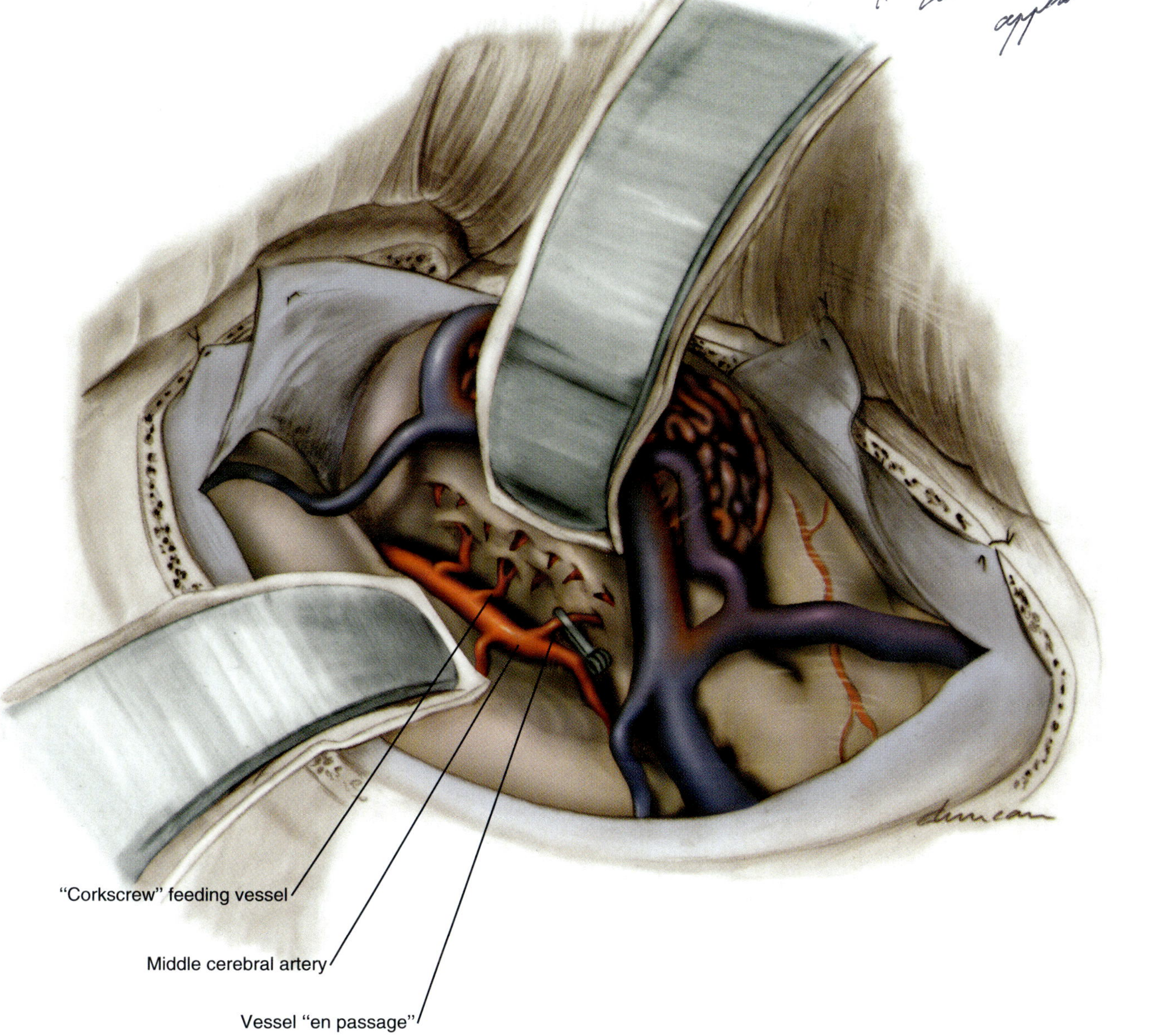

Figure 2–21.

Step 3. As the division of the Sylvian fissure is extended, some larger branches of the M_1 and M_2 segments become apparent. Some of these clearly may enter the arteriovenous malformation; they can be cauterized. However, for other vessels, it may not be clear that they contribute to the malformation; in fact, they may be vessels "en passage." Vessels that may not feed the arteriovenous malformation can be occluded temporarily with small microclips until their anatomy has been defined more completely. A useful visual clue for identifying feeding vessels of an arteriovenous malformation is that their origin from the middle or posterior cerebral artery often has a corkscrew shape.

Normally the brain tissue between the vessels of a AV malformation is gliosis and non functioning

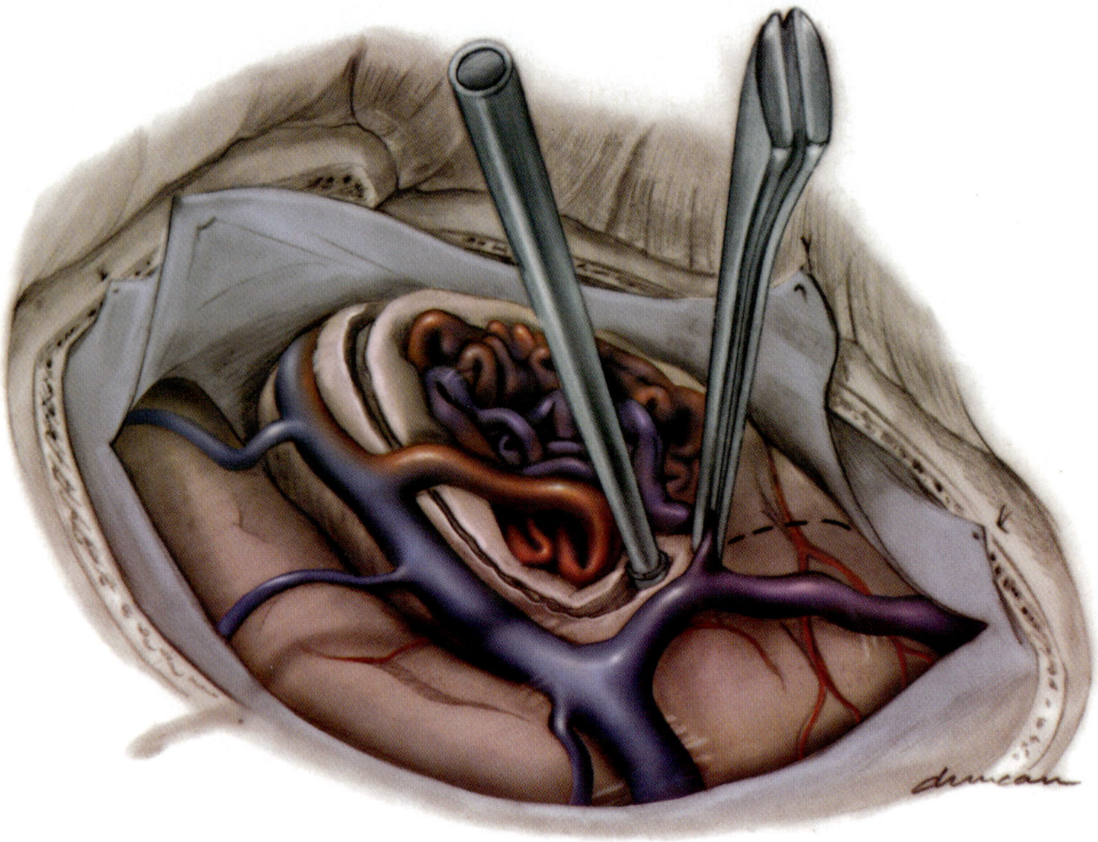

Figure 2–22.

Step 4. After potential feeding vessels from the Sylvian fissure have been cauterized or temporarily clipped, an incision is made in the cerebral cortex just posterior to the arteriovenous malformation. In the example shown here, the arteriovenous malformation has two obvious draining veins. The posterior draining vein has been cauterized and divided to facilitate rotation of the arteriovenous malformation.

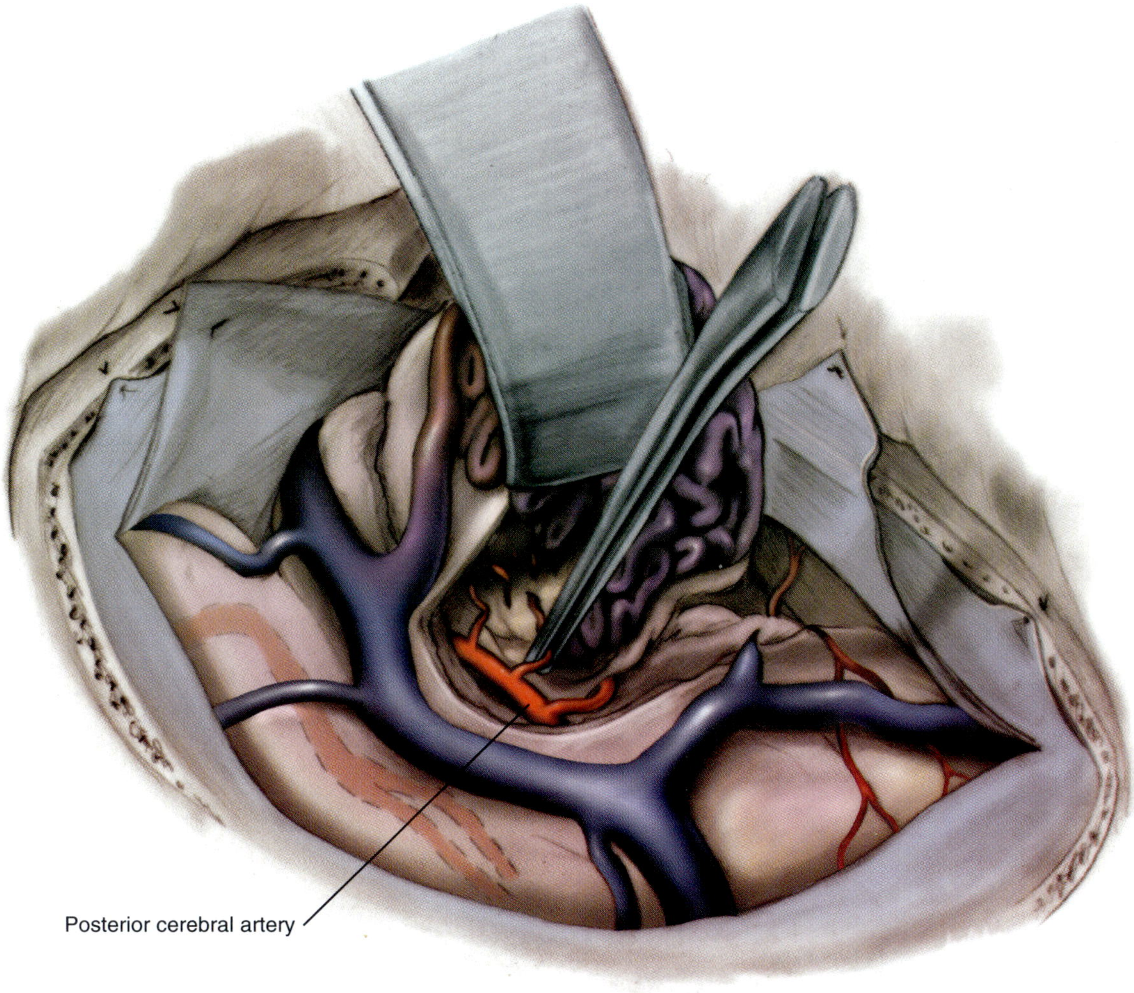

Figure 2–23.

Step 5. A retractor is placed gently on the arteriovenous malformation as the dissection is carried deeper. There are always several branches from the posterior temporal artery, a branch of the posterior cerebral artery. These branches run underneath the temporal lobe and enter the arteriovenous malformation laterally, along the floor of the middle cranial fossa. Also, enlarged Ammon's horn vessels usually feed the arteriovenous malformation. They should be cauterized and divided. To protect the posterior cerebral artery, every attempt should be made to preserve the arachnoid overlying the artery.

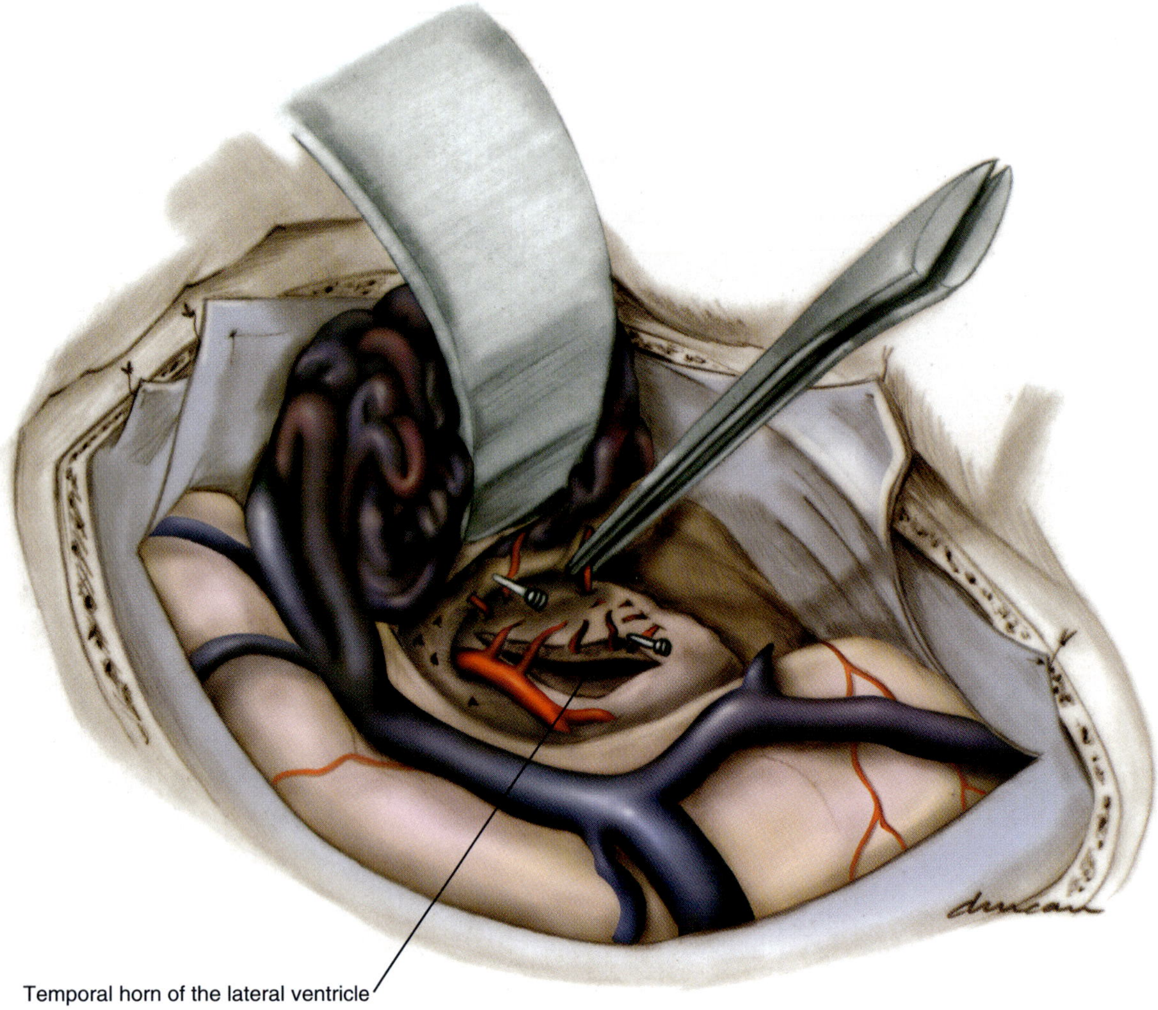

Figure 2–24.

Step 6. The apex of most arteriovenous malformations, regardless of location, is periventricular. Small arteries along the ependymal surface of the ventricle always feed the arteriovenous malformation. These arteries are extremely thin walled and, thus, exceedingly difficult to cauterize. Patience, an irrigating bipolar, and microclips are the best tools.

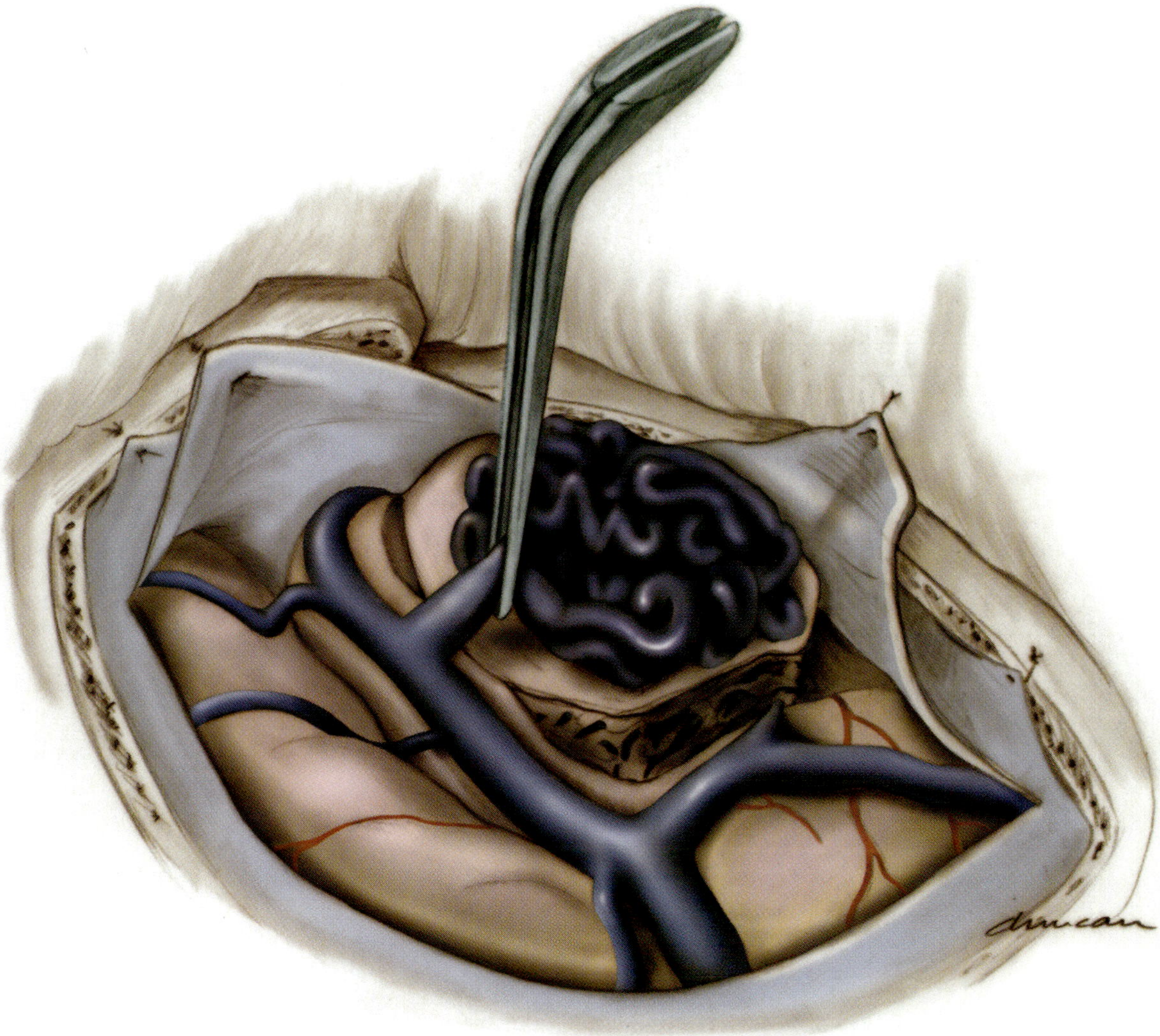

Figure 2–25.

Step 7. After ensuring that all the arterial blood supply to the arteriovenous malformation has been obliterated, the last draining veins can be safely cauterized and divided. After the arteriovenous malformation has been resected, it is important to inspect visually, with the operating microscope, all the surface veins to make sure that there is no residual arterialized blood. The presence of arterialized venous blood indicates that some of the malformation was not resected.

3

Frontal Approach

Copyright © 1999 Mayo Foundation.

ANATOMIC CONSIDERATIONS

The lateral surface of the frontal lobe has three serpentine gyri: the superior, middle, and inferior frontal gyri (Figure 3–1). The superior frontal gyrus (Brodmann areas 6, 8, and 9) extends from the frontal pole to the precentral gyrus, a distance of 10 to 11 cm. Anteriorly, it merges with the middle frontal, orbital, and rectus gyri. Approximately 8 to 10 transverse gyri interdigitate with the middle frontal gyrus. The medial surface of the superior frontal gyrus is also called the "medial frontal gyrus" (Brodmann areas 6, 8, 9, 10, 11, 12, and 32). It is adjacent to the parolfactory sulcus. It extends ventrally toward the frontal pole and curves posteriorly around the cingulate gyrus. The cingulate sulcus separates the medial frontal gyrus from the cingulate gyrus. There usually are several intertwining transverse gyri between the medial frontal and cingulate gyri.

The middle frontal gyrus (Brodmann areas 6, 8, 9, and 10) is inferior to and parallel with the superior frontal gyrus and extends from the frontal pole to the precentral gyrus. Several transverse sulci divide this gyrus.

The inferior frontal gyrus (Brodmann areas 44, 45, and 47) is just above the Sylvian fissure, overlying the anterior half of the insula. It forms the "W-shaped" frontal operculum, which is divided into three segments (pars orbitalis, pars triangularis, and pars opercularis) by ascending rami of the Sylvian fissure and the inferior precentral sulcus. The pars orbitalis (Brodmann area 47) fuses superiorly with the anterior segment of the middle frontal gyrus and anteriorly with the lateral orbital gyrus. The pars triangularis (Brodmann area 45) is demarcated by the ascending rami of the Sylvian fissure and merges anteriorly with the orbital gyri and posteriorly with the pars opercularis. The pars opercularis (Brodmann area 44) lies between the pars triangularis anteriorly and the inferior precentral and inferior frontal sulci posteriorly.

Anatomically, the pars opercularis corresponds to Broca's area (Brodmann area 44). However, intraoperative cortical stimulation indicates that the pars triangularis (Brodmann area 45) should be included within Broca's area. This cortical region has many convolutions with tremendous variability. Also, deep within the sulci are transverse gyri that are not visible with inspection of the surface.

The precentral gyrus is perpendicular to the superior, middle, and inferior frontal gyri and incompletely separated from them by the precentral sulcus. The posterior boundary of the gyrus is the central sulcus. The precentral gyrus extends from the cingulate sulcus on the medial surface of the hemisphere (where it comprises the anterior portion of the paracentral lobule) to the Sylvian fissure on the lateral surface. A useful tip for identifying the precentral gyrus on magnetic resonance images is to follow the superior frontal sulcus, which terminates posteriorly in two ramifications that form a "T." This "T" (part of the precentral sulcus) abuts the precentral gyrus.

The precentral gyrus is the primary motor cortex (Brodmann area 4), which traditionally is considered the cortical area for voluntary movement. As shown with electrical stimulation of the cortical surface, the muscles of the body are represented systematically (but disproportionately) along the gyrus. This topographic organization is epitomized in the so-called motor homunculus of Penfield. Muscles of the throat (including the pharyngeal muscles) are represented in the most inferior part of the gyrus, the part abutting the Sylvian fissure. Proceeding superiorly are the representations of the muscles of the face, thumb, fingers, hand, distal arm, proximal arm, and shoulder. The muscles of the trunk and hip are represented near the superior edge of the hemisphere, where the gyrus continues onto the medial surface of the hemisphere. The representations of the muscles of the leg, feet, and toes are on this medial surface of the gyrus, as are the representations for the muscles of the bowel and bladder.

Immediately anterior to the primary motor cortex is the premotor cortical area (Brodmann area 6). The portion on the lateral surface of the hemisphere is called the "premotor cortex" and that on the medial surface is the "supplementary motor cortex." Electrical stimulation of the primary motor cortex usually elicits contraction of only one or a few muscles on the opposite side of the body. In contrast, electrical stimulation of the premotor areas produces a more complicated reaction that may consist of the contraction of several muscles on both sides of the body, causing movement of several joints.

The blood supply to the medial frontal lobe is from branches of the anterior cerebral artery (Figure 3–2). These branches include the orbitofrontal, frontopolar, anterior internal frontal, middle internal frontal, and posterior internal frontal arteries. The blood supply to the lateral frontal lobe is from branches of the middle cerebral artery, including the orbitofrontal, operculofrontal, and central sulcus arteries.

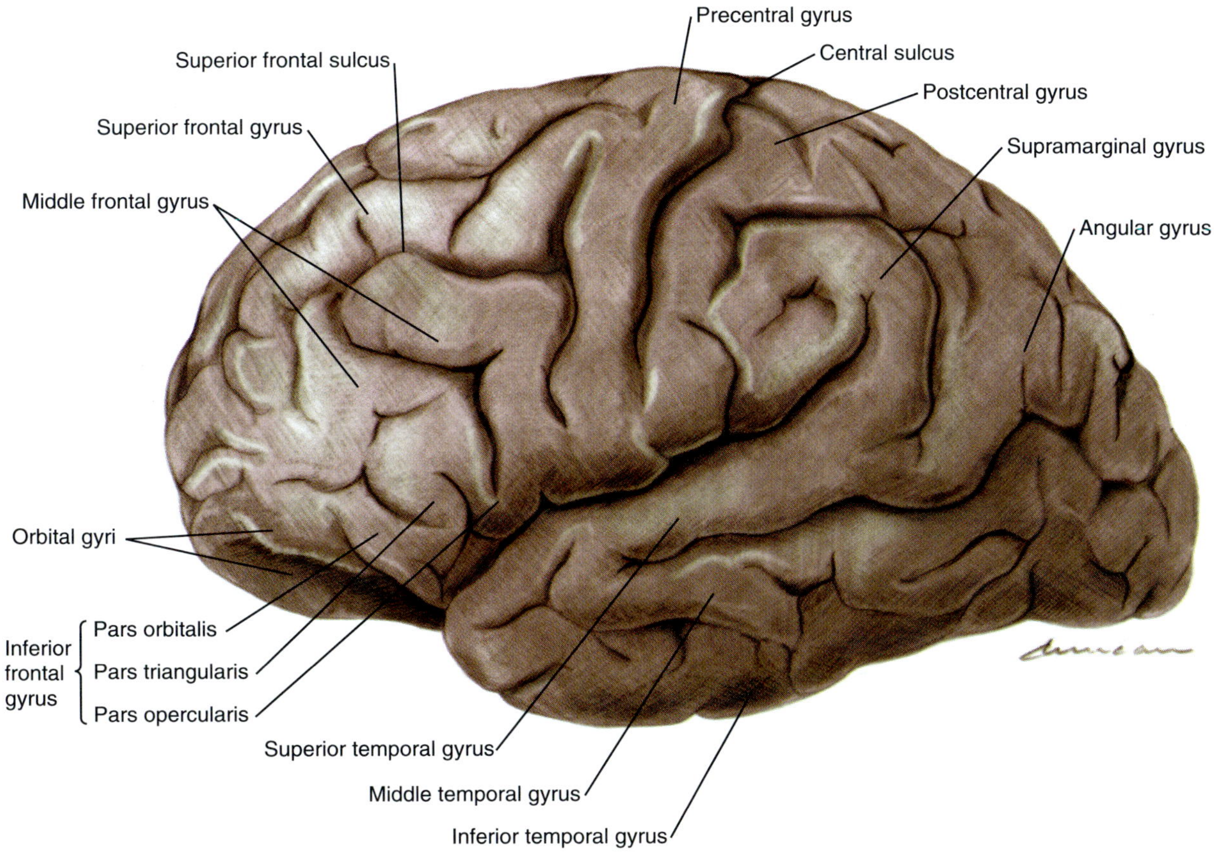

Figure 3–1.

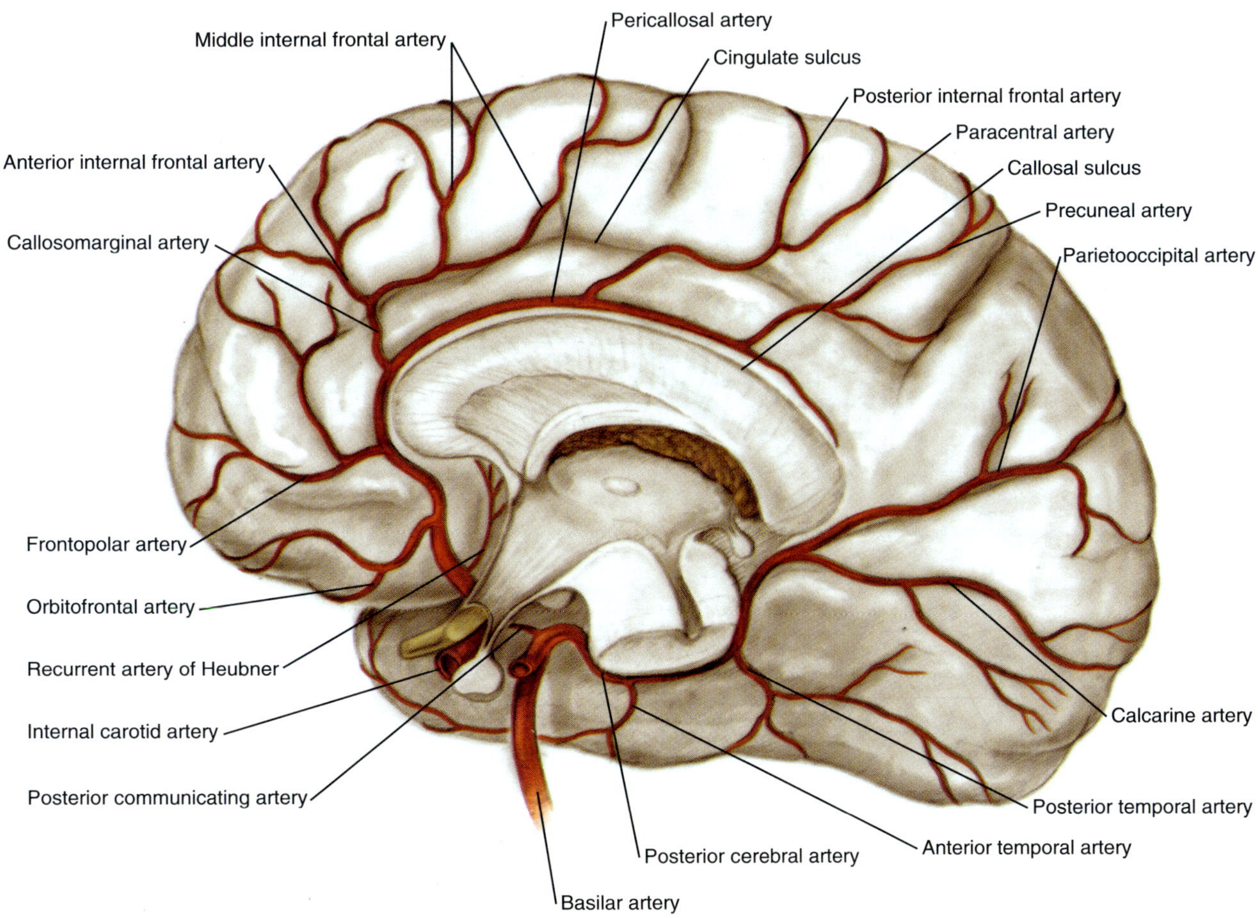

Figure 3–2.

FRONTAL LOBECTOMY

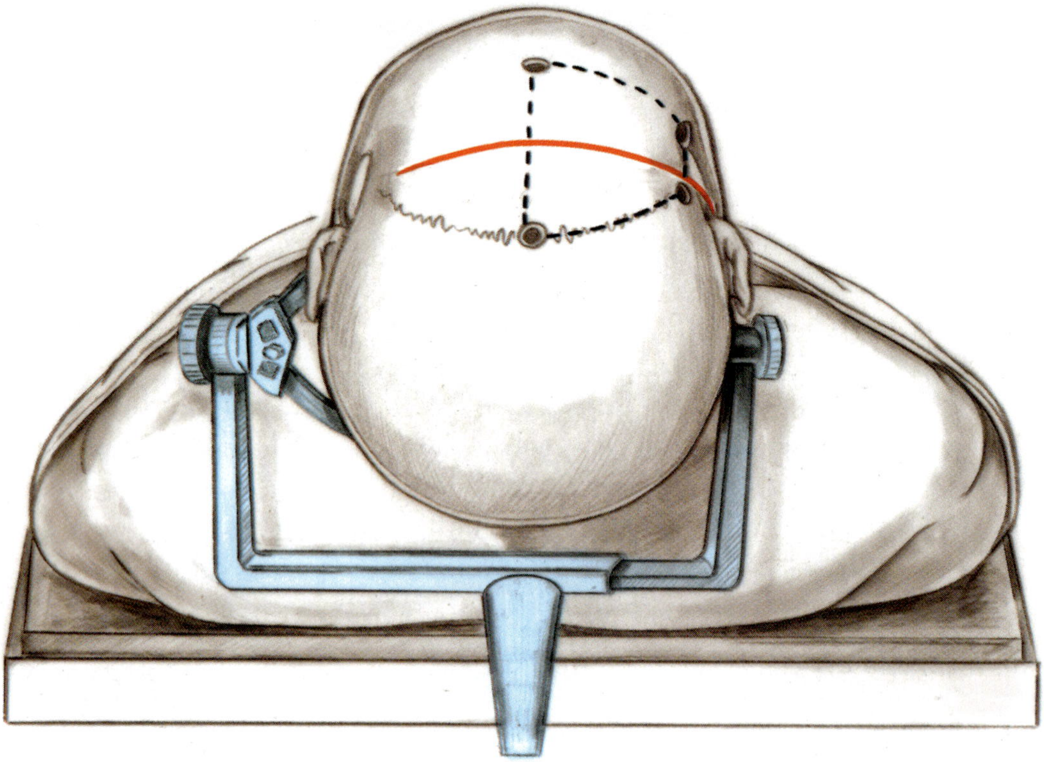

Figure 3–3.

Step 1. The patient's head is held in a donut or fixed in a pinion, as illustrated here. The head should be slightly flexed and higher than the heart to promote venous drainage. To prevent partial kinking of the internal jugular veins, it is important not to overflex the head. The incision is a standard bicoronal incision. The medial edge of the bone flap should be along the superior sagittal sinus. This provides easier access to the interhemispheric fissure, with better visualization of the anterior cerebral artery and its branches. The posterior margin of the bone flap is at the coronal suture. The lateral margin extends from the junction of the coronal suture with the superior temporal line to the "keyhole."

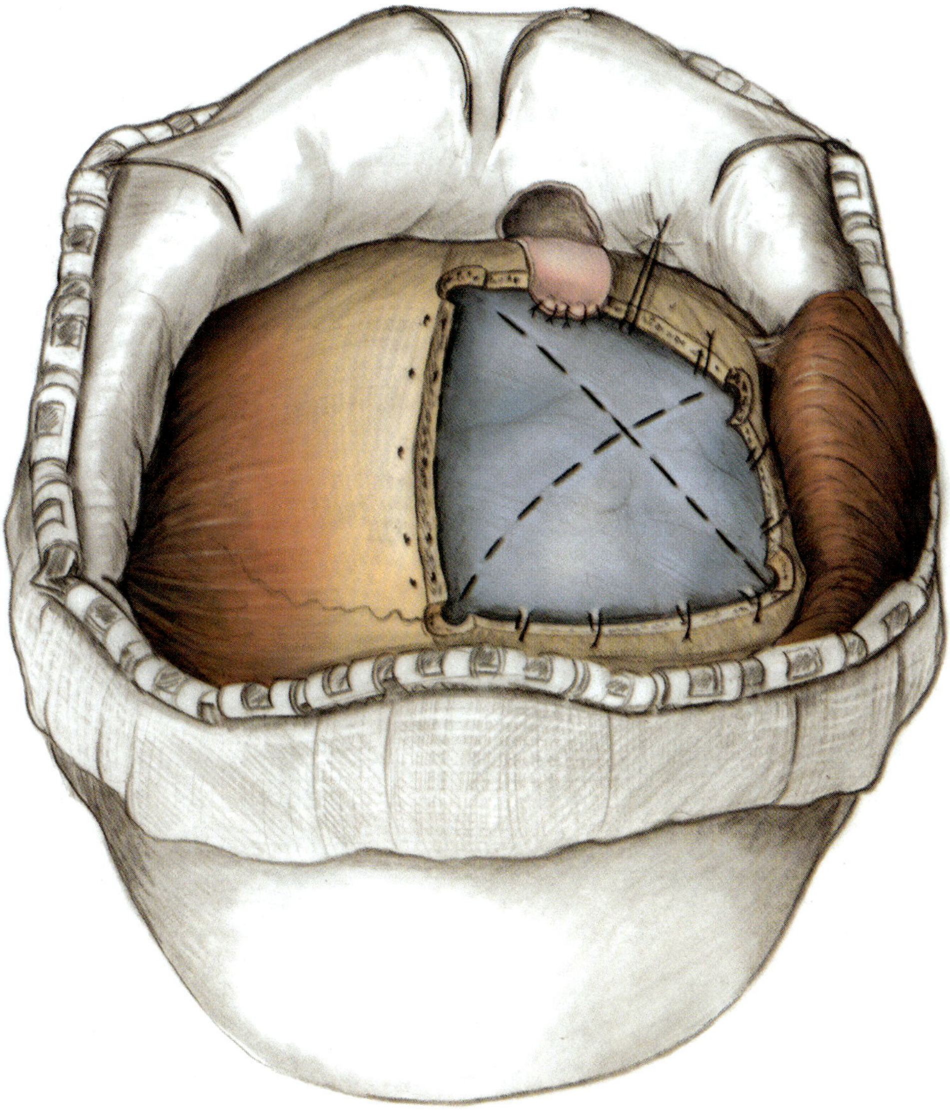

Figure 3–4.

Step 2. After the bone flap has been removed, the dura mater is tacked to the margins of the bone. Ensure that tack holes along the anterior or ventral edge of the bone do not enter the frontal sinus, because if they do, it may be a source of rhinorrhea. Occasionally, the frontal sinus is entered along the medial aspect of the craniotomy. If this occurs, the mucosa should be stripped with a small punch. A piece of temporalis muscle is harvested and used to plug the ostium of the sinus. Thereafter, a small galeal-periosteal flap is rotated with a #11 blade knife and tacked to the adjacent dura mater. This effectively obliterates the sinus.

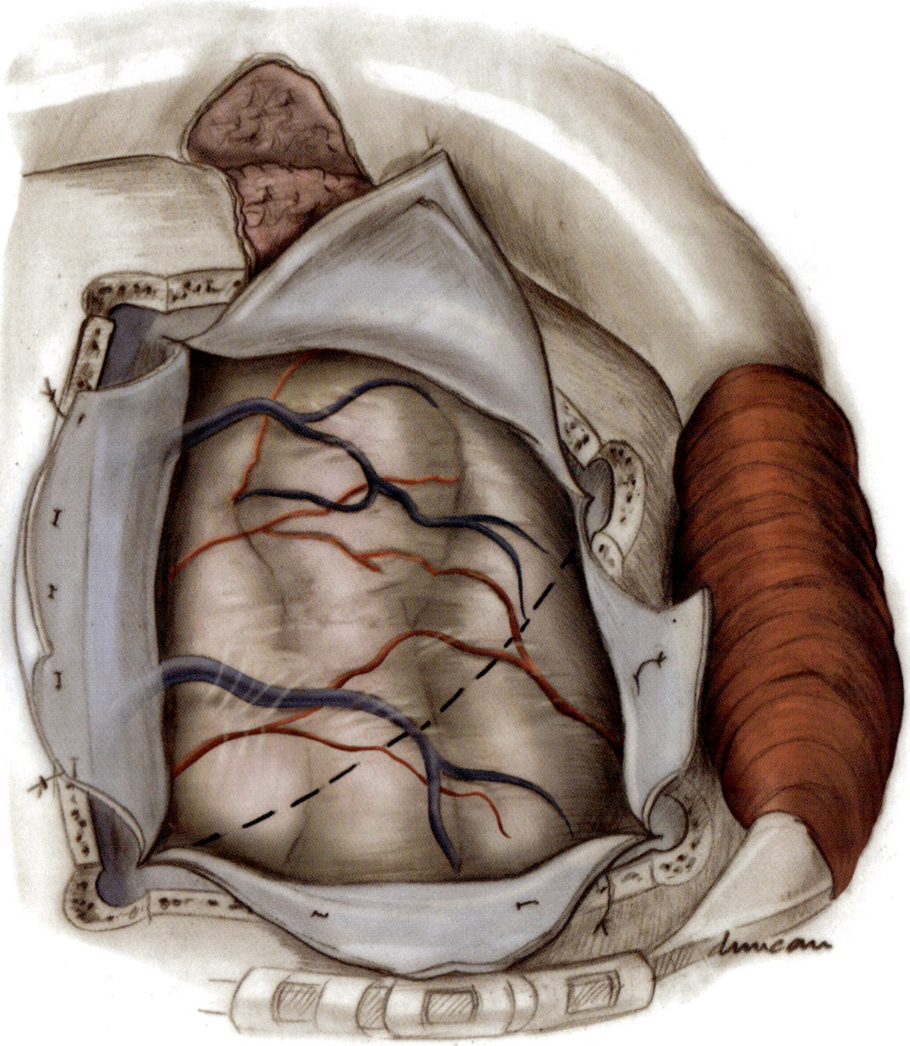

Figures 3–5 and 3–6.

Step 3. The margin of the frontal lobectomy is outlined using bipolar cautery. Some of the brain regions at risk during frontal lobectomy include the precentral gyrus, the frontal operculum, and the deeper basal ganglia. If the operation is performed without preoperative or intraoperative mapping of eloquent brain regions, the following guidelines are useful for preventing neurologic dysfunction postoperatively. The posterior resection line should be approximately 1.0 cm anterior to the coronal suture. This line should project lateral to the sphenoid wing and medial to the olfactory bulb. In a left frontal lobectomy, this will spare the frontal operculum by a safe margin.

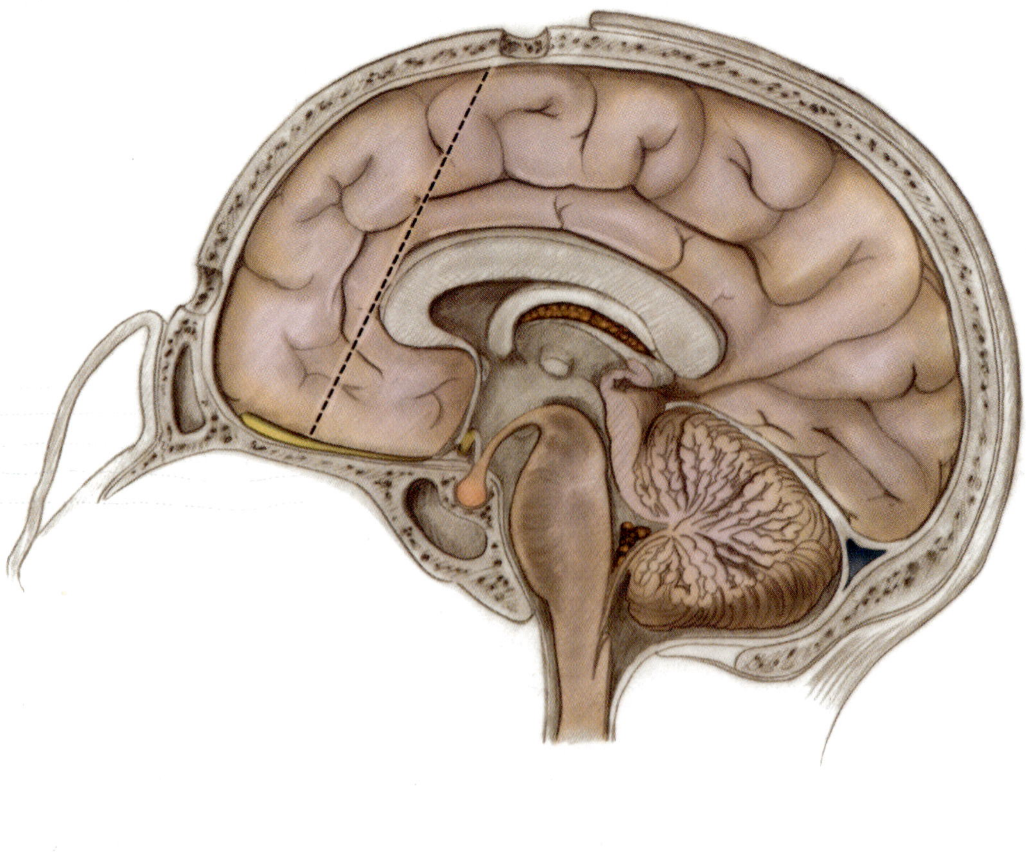

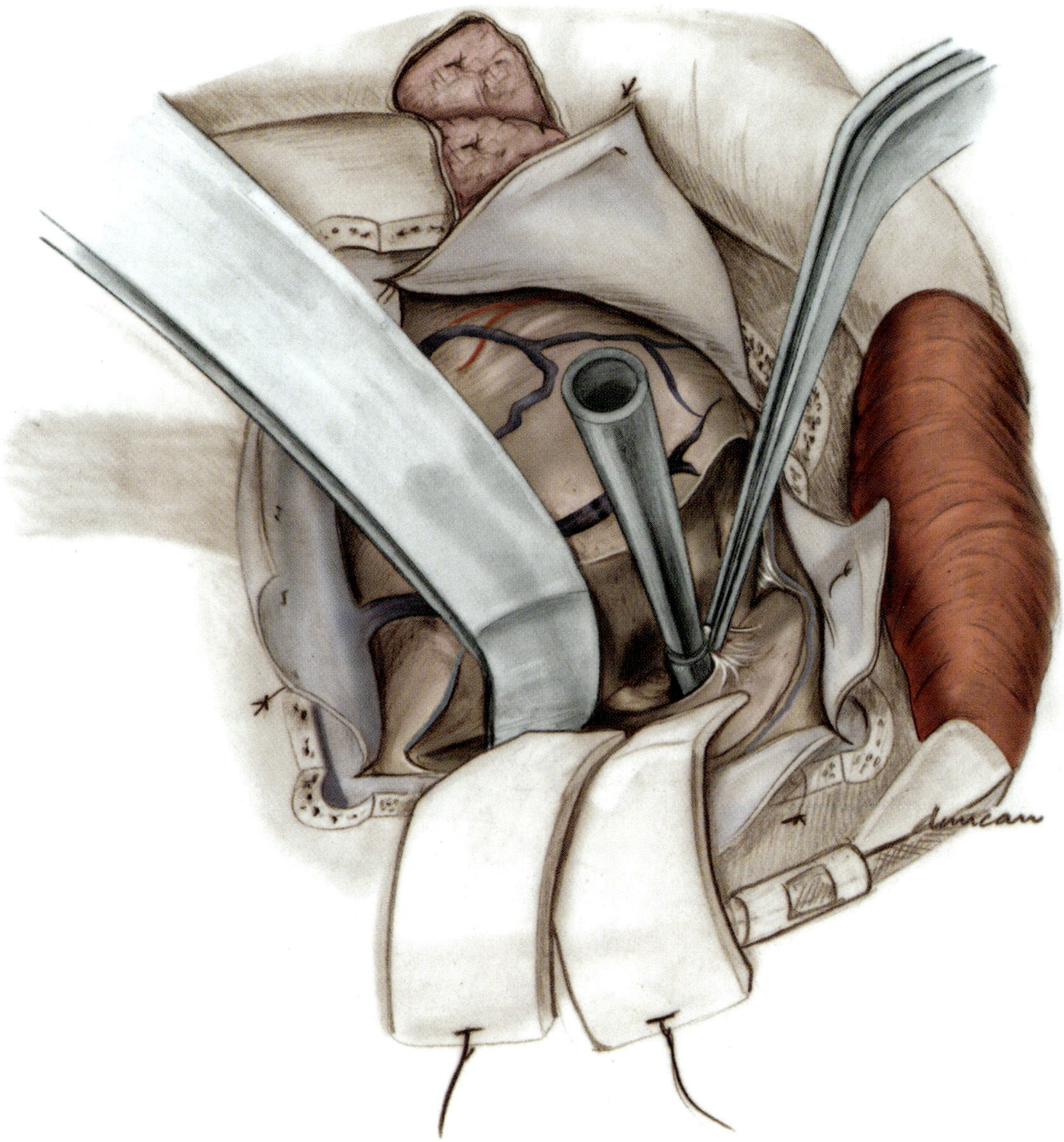

Figure 3–7.

Step 4. The incision is deepened with the use of bipolar cautery and suction. If the operation is performed for treatment of frontal seizures only, there is no need to extend the resection into the deep white matter. After cutting through the cerebral cortex, the surgeon's trajectory can then angle anteriorly to the olfactory bulb. If the operation is performed for tumor debulking for relief of mass effect, it is necessary to extend the resection deeper toward the tip of the frontal horn of the lateral ventricle. Laterally, along the sphenoid wing, it is important to respect the pial barrier, which in turn will prevent inadvertent injury to the middle cerebral artery in the Sylvian fissure.

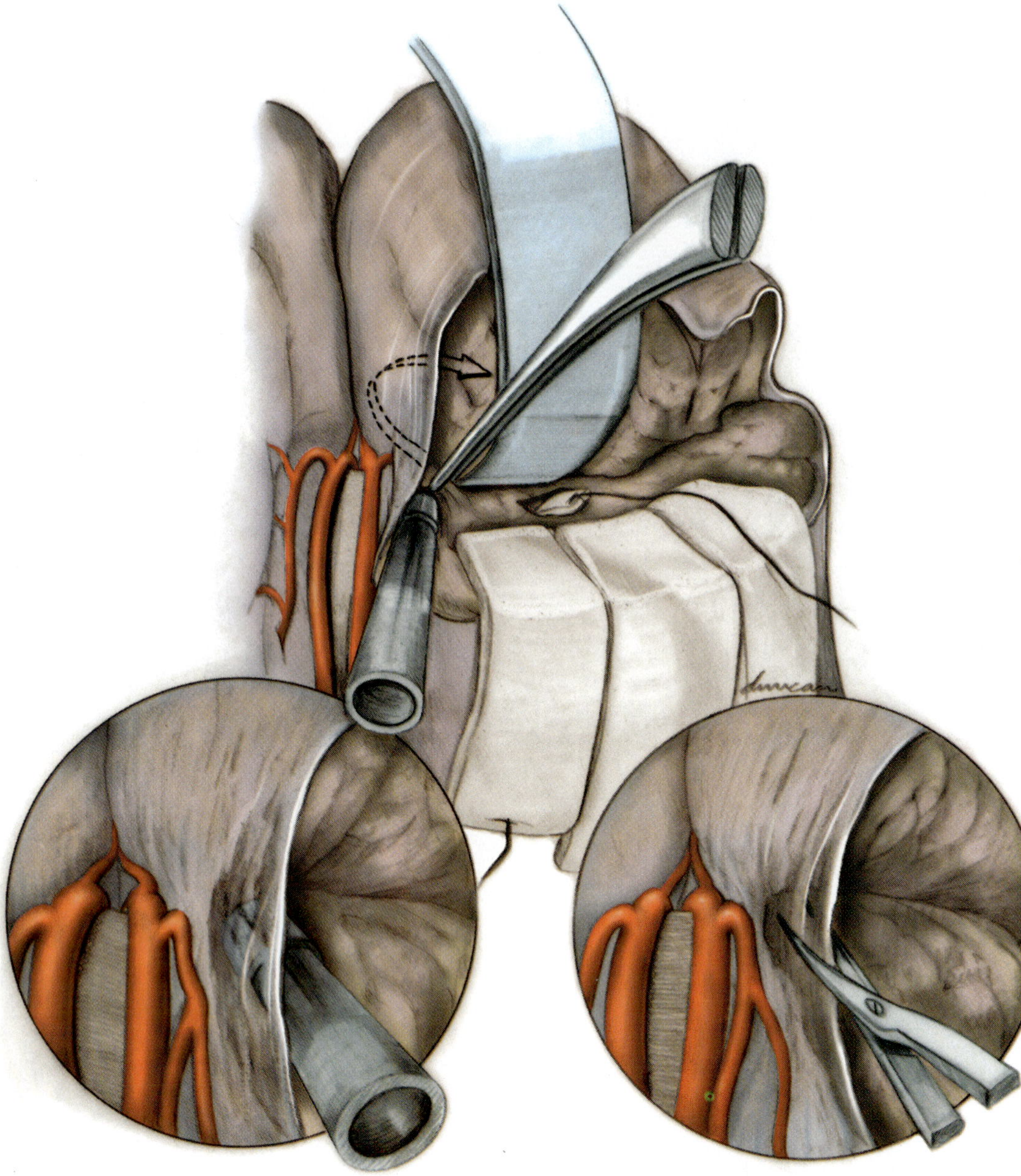

Figure 3–8.

Step 5. At risk medially are the pericallosal and callosomarginal arteries. As in most lobectomies, the best way to prevent vascular injury is to use subpial resection. Specifically, a #7 suction tip is used to remove the cerebral cortex beneath the pia mater. After the pia mater is devoid of blood vessels, it can be cauterized and cut.

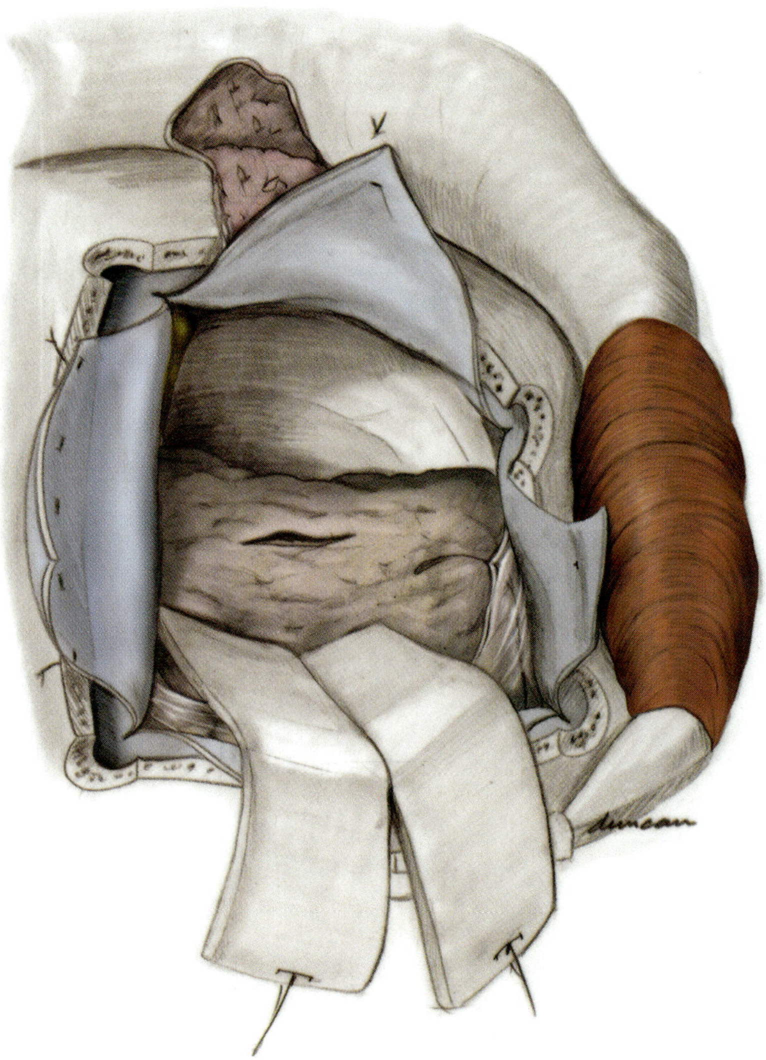

Figure 3–9.

Step 6. In this example, the frontal horn of the lateral ventricle has been entered. A cottonball is used to plug the ventricle while the resection is completed. This helps decrease the amount of blood that seeps into the lateral ventricle. To decrease the risk of postoperative aseptic meningitis, it is important to irrigate the ventricle to flush out blood products.

PERICALLOSAL ARTERY ANEURYSM

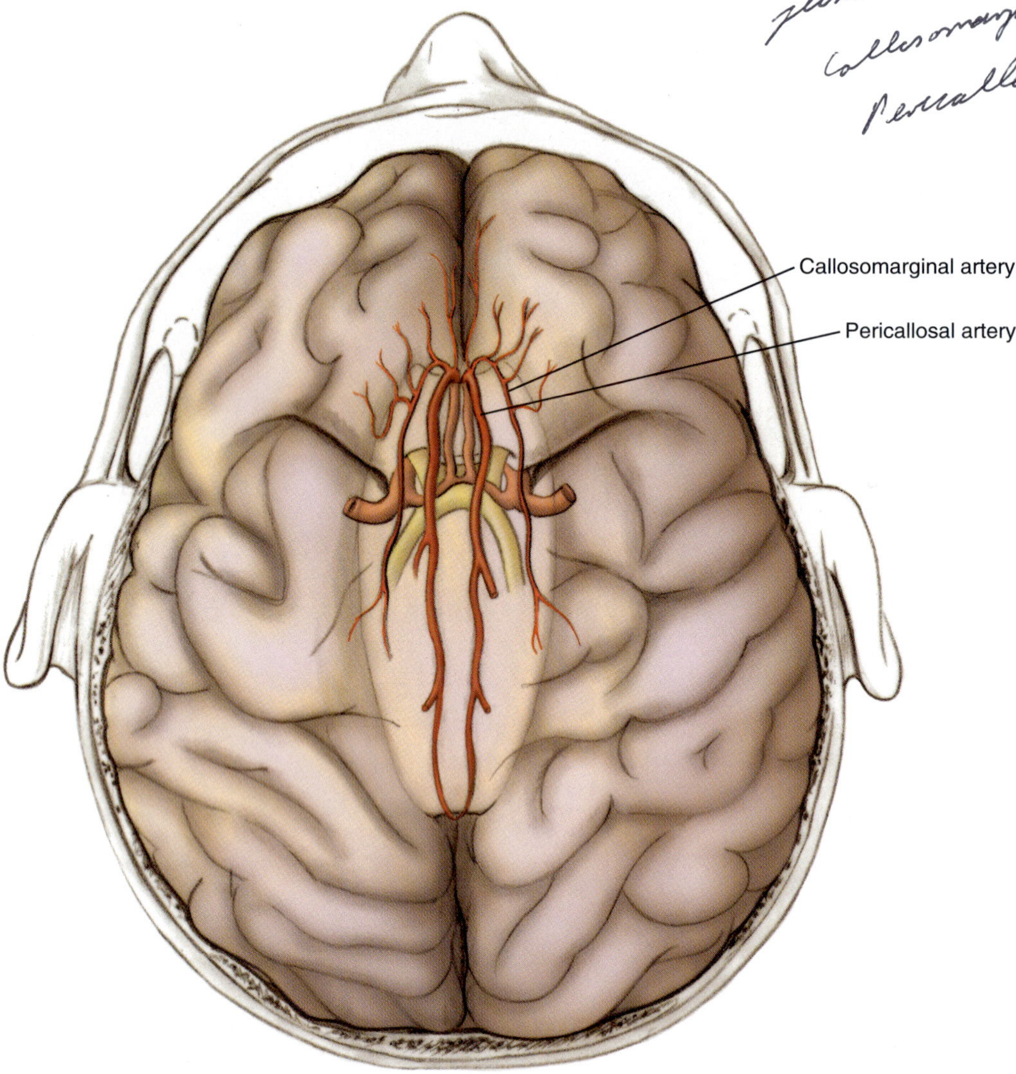

Figure 3–10.

Most pericallosal aneurysms originate at the bifurcation of the callosomarginal and pericallosal arteries. The more frontal the craniotomy, the more likely the surgeon will be to come down upon the neck instead of the dome of the aneurysm.

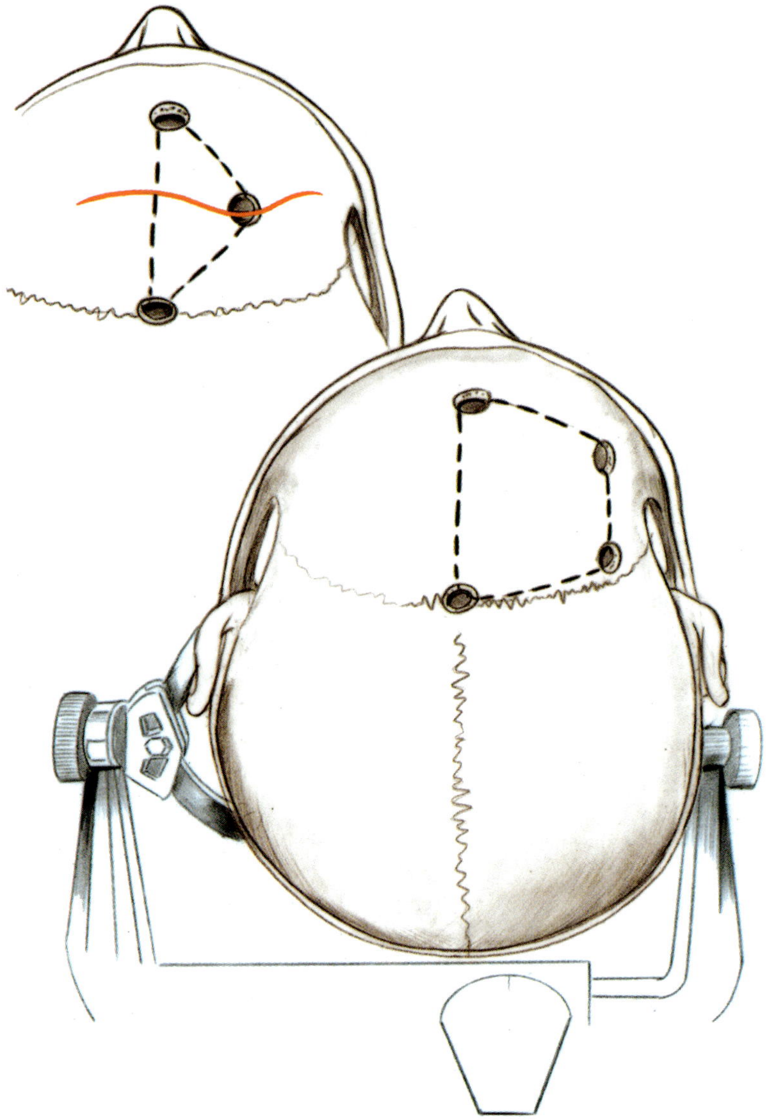

Figure 3–11.

Step 1. As illustrated here, two different types of bone flaps can be used to gain access to the aneurysm. Both of these flaps can also be used to enter the lateral ventricle through an interhemispheric approach and to section the anterior corpus callosum for treatment of certain types of epilepsy. The patient's head is supine and straight up to aid in surgical orientation. The medial edge of the bone flap should be on the superior sagittal sinus; this provides greater access with less retraction of the medial frontal lobe. In patients with pericallosal aneurysms, the venous phase of the angiogram should be studied to determine whether there are major draining veins. If there are, the bone flap can be planned accordingly.

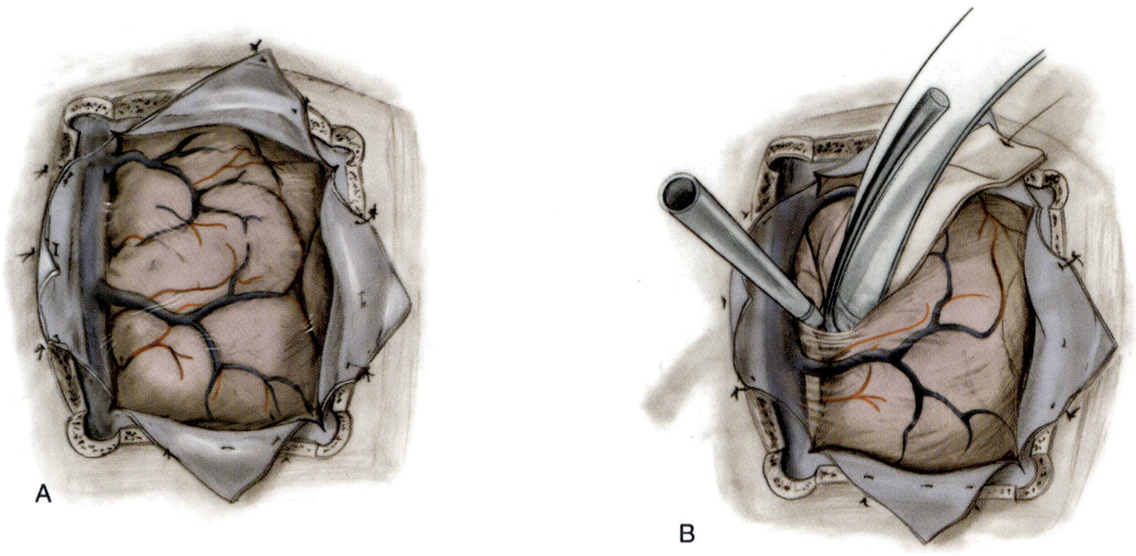

A B

Figure 3–12.

Step 2. *A*, The dura mater has been opened and tacked to the margins of the bone. In this example, a rather large vein crosses the surgical field.

B, Every attempt needs be made to preserve the vein by separating the hemisphere anterior to it. Leaving the enveloping arachnoid intact helps to preserve these bridging veins. In addition, a piece of absorbable gelatin sponge (Gelfoam) can be placed on the vein to act as a buttress. If the hemisphere is swollen because of significant hemorrhage, brain relaxation can be achieved with lumbar or ventricular drainage of cerebrospinal fluid or with mannitol. The square bone flap provides easier access should a ventricular tap be required.

Figure 3–13.

Step 3. *A*, Most pericallosal aneurysms can be approached from the right, thereby eliminating retraction on the medial left (dominant) frontal lobe. The right hemisphere is lined with hemostatic fabric (Surgicel) and cottonoids (Americot) and gently retracted. The thin bridging arachnoid between the two hemispheres can easily be divided with a dissector or a bipolar forceps. As true for most aneurysm surgery, it is best to first identify the proximal parent artery.

B, Placement of a small piece of absorbable gelatin sponge around the neck of the aneurysm will facilitate placement of the clip.

C, After the aneurysm has been clipped, the dome is aspirated and the jaws of the clip reinspected.

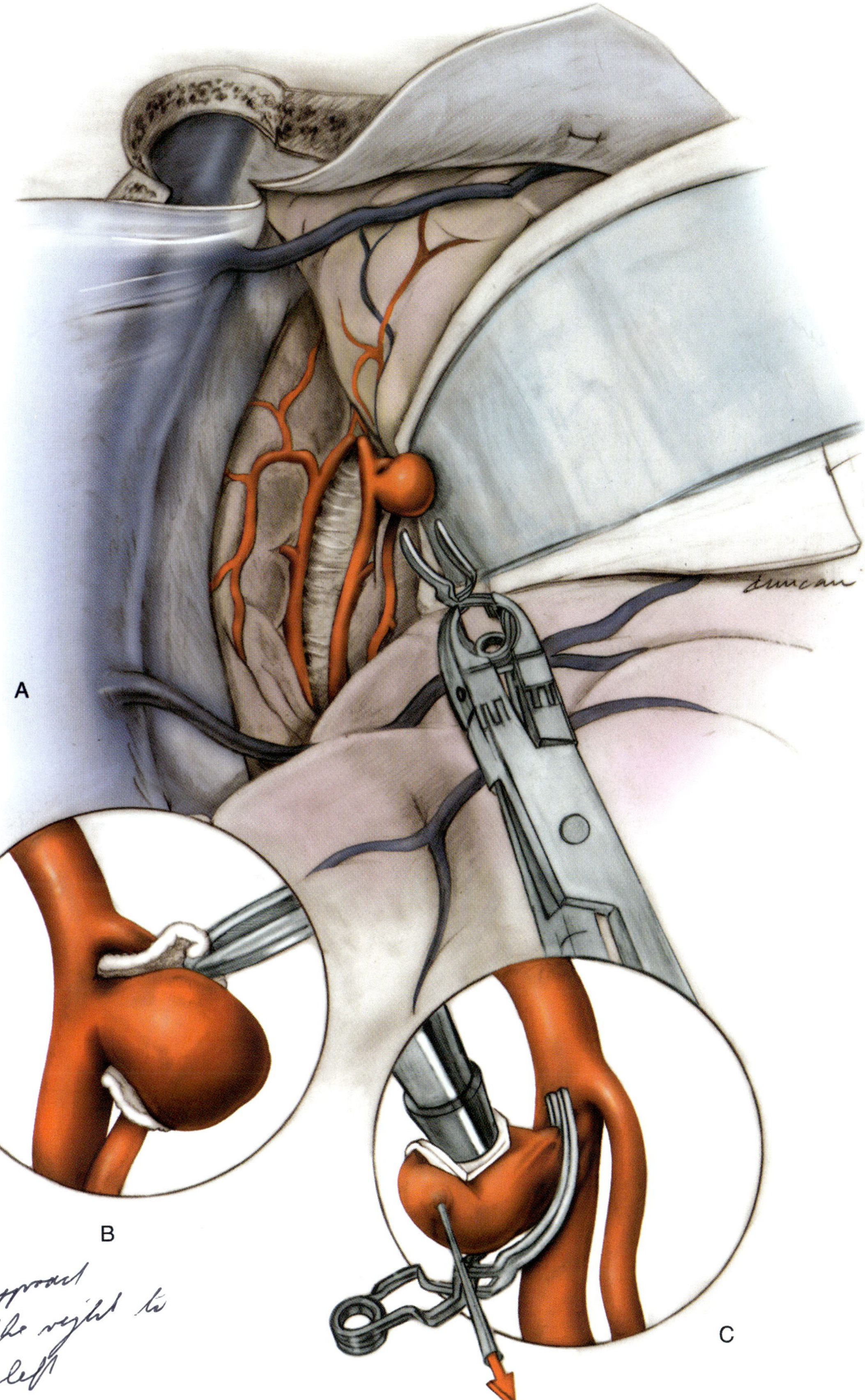
A
B
C

THIRD VENTRICULAR COLLOID CYST —INTERHEMISPHERIC APPROACH

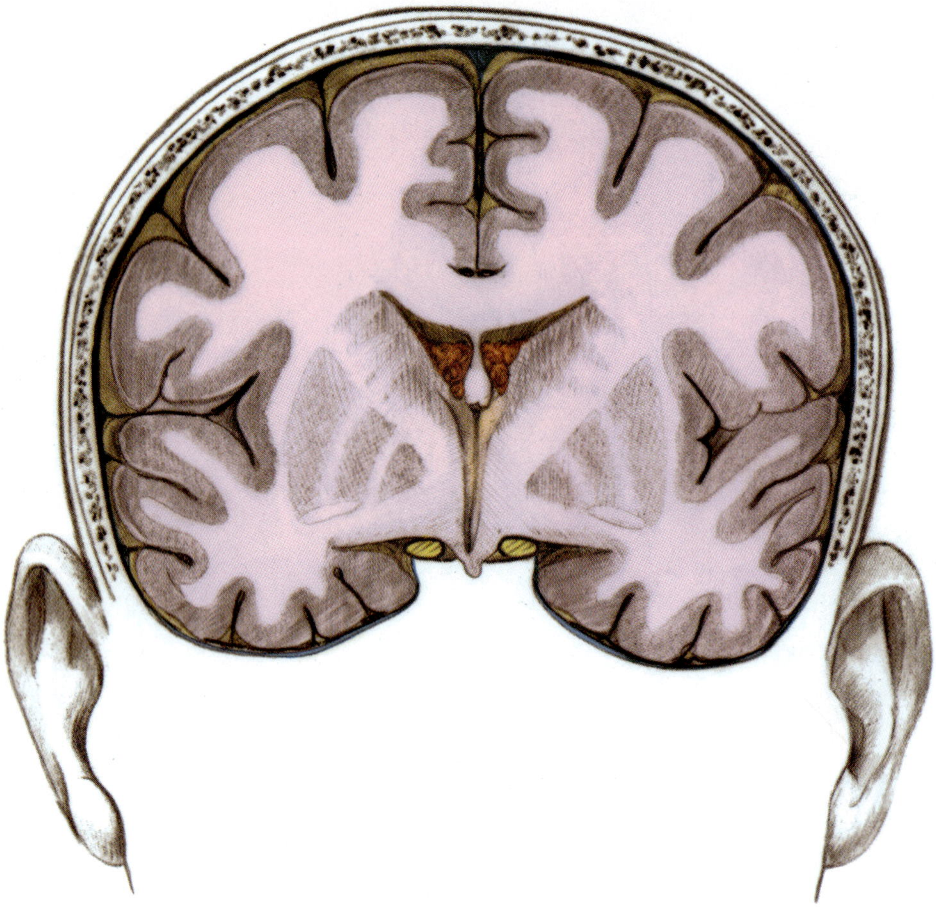

Figure 3–14.

A standard coronal section through the brain at the level of the foramen magnum highlighting the relationship of the fornix and choroid plexus with the foramen of Monro.

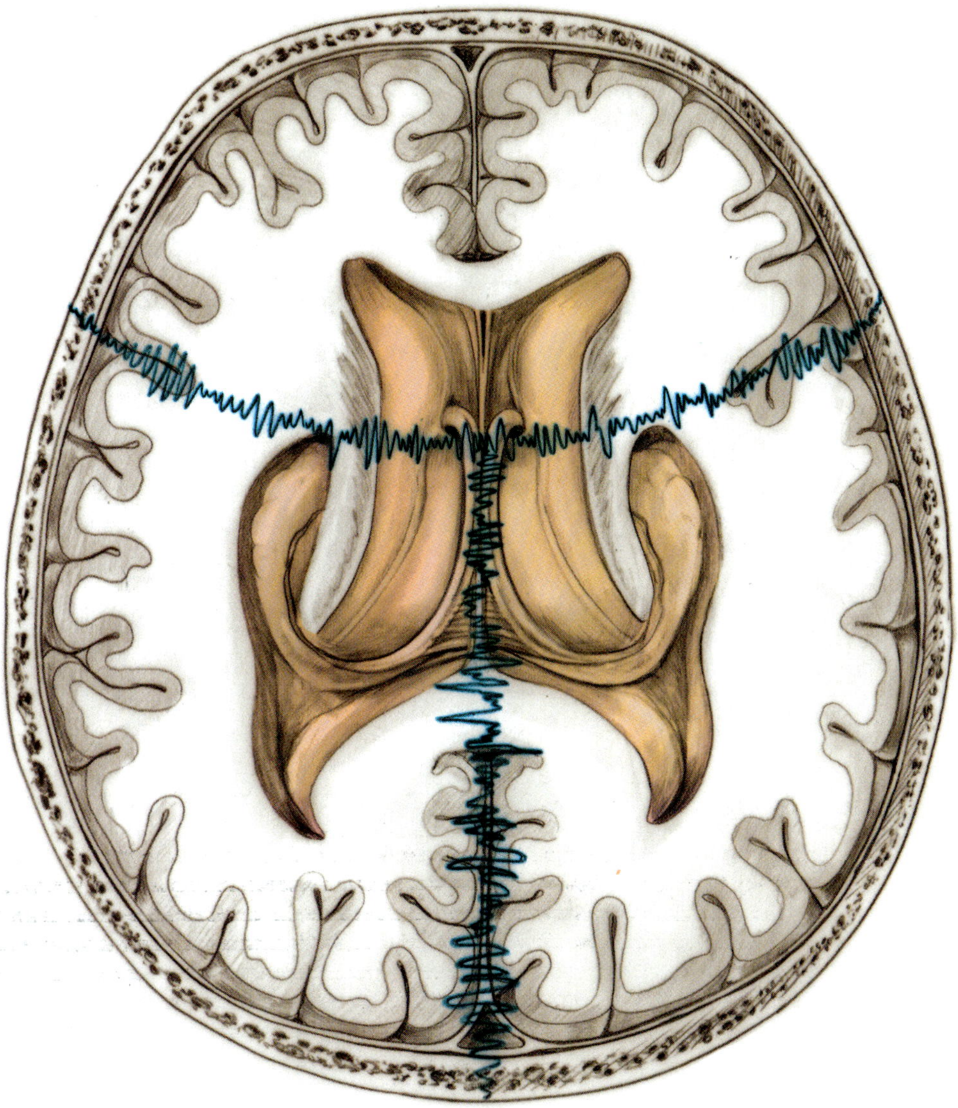

Figure 3–15.

This axial section depicts the relationship of the coronal suture to the lateral ventricle and the foramen of Monro.

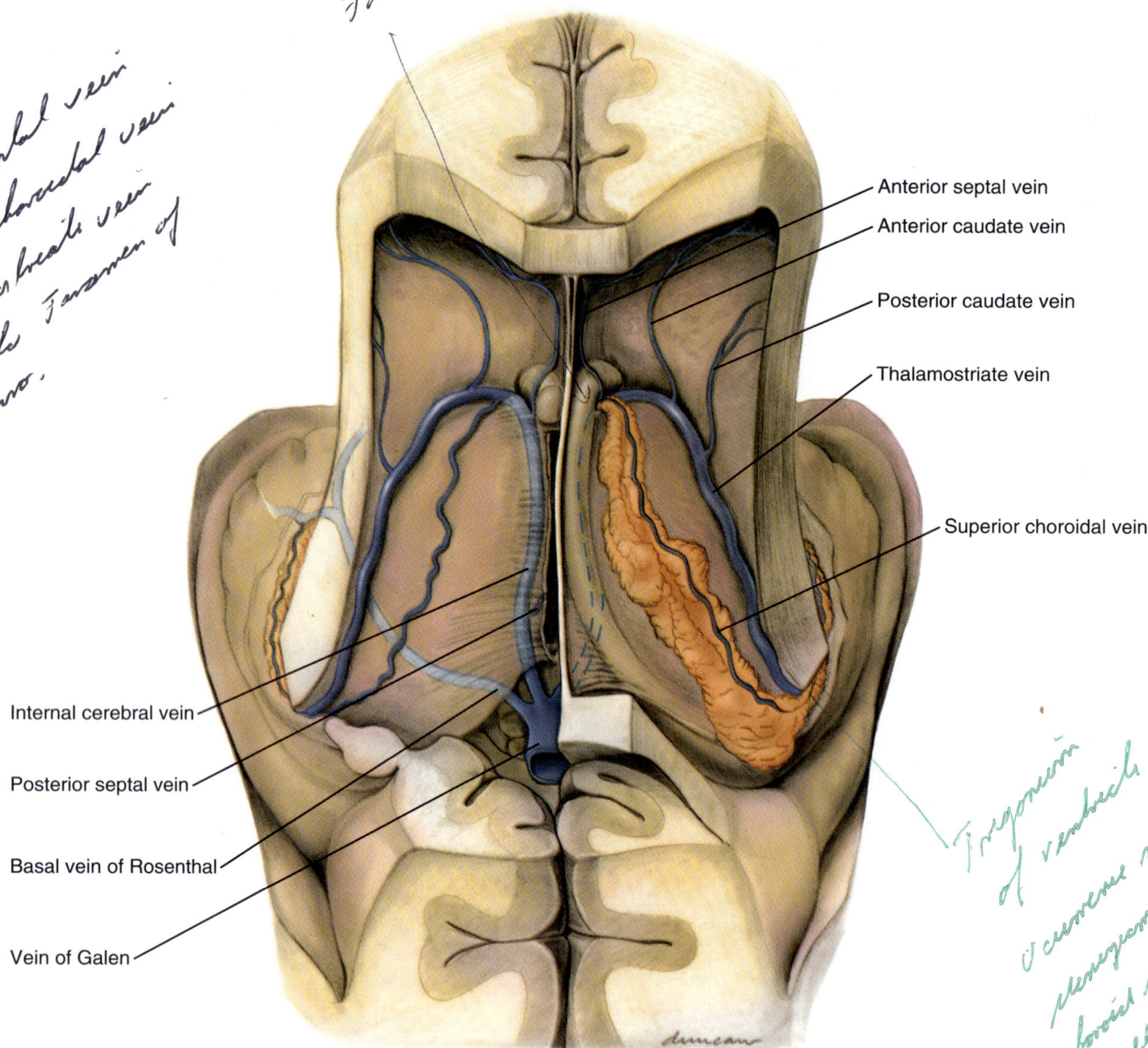
Anterior septal vein
Anterior caudate vein
Posterior caudate vein
Thalamostriate vein
Superior choroidal vein
Internal cerebral vein
Posterior septal vein
Basal vein of Rosenthal
Vein of Galen

Figure 3–16.

This figure emphasizes the pertinent neurovascular anatomy of the lateral ventricle. The first landmark the surgeon visualizes on entering the lateral ventricle is the choroid plexus, which overlies the choroidal fissure. Typically, a small vein called the "superior choroidal vein" runs on top of the choroid plexus. This choroid plexus sits between the body of the fornix and the thalamus. Lateral to the choroid plexus is the convex surface ("bulge") of the thalamus, which forms the floor of the lateral ventricle. The next structure observed is the thalamostriate vein, which has two major tributaries: the anterior caudate and the posterior caudate veins. The thalamostriate vein is the largest contributor to the internal cerebral vein. The thalamostriate vein runs in the groove between the caudate nucleus and the thalamus, above the stria terminalis. At the foramen of Monro, the thalamostriate vein curves around the anterior tubercle of the thalamus and joins the internal cerebral vein. In the frontal horn of the lateral ventricle, the anterior septal vein runs along the septum pellucidum and crosses the fornix to join the internal cerebral vein. A small posterior septal vein may be seen posteriorly in the body of the lateral ventricle. The posterior septal vein also runs along the septum pellucidum and goes around the fornix to enter the midportion of the internal cerebral vein. This figure does not show the small veins in the atrium of the ventricle that pass through the choroidal fissure to enter the basal vein of Rosenthal, the internal cerebral vein, and the vein of Galen.

The paired internal cerebral veins originate at the foramen of Monro and go posteriorly in the velum interpositum. As they go posteriorly, they curve up over the superolateral aspect of the pineal gland and follow the curve of the inferior surface of the splenium of the corpus callosum. The left and right internal cerebral veins join at the posteroinferior surface of the splenium to form the vein of Galen.

The basal vein of Rosenthal begins at the level of the anterior perforated substance and runs posteriorly between the midbrain and the temporal lobe. It drains blood from the medial temporal lobe and the midbrain. In the posterior incisural space, it joins the internal cerebral veins and vein of Galen.

In the midline is the septum pellucidum, which may contain a space called the "cavum septi pellucidi." Deeper (along the inferior edge of the septum pellucidum) is the fornix, which consists of axons that originate in the hippocampal formation, extend around the thalamus, and end in the mammillary bodies in the floor of the third ventricle. The fornix is divided into four parts. Near its origin in the hippocampal formation, the axons form the fimbria. The fimbria passes posteriorly to form the crus (plural, crura) of the fornix. Each crus goes anteriorly along the posterior surface of the pulvinar. At the level of the atrium and body of the lateral ventricle, the two crura join and form the body of the fornix, which continues anteriorly along the medial wall of the lateral ventricle. At the level of the foramen of Monro, the body of the fornix splits into two columns, each of which forms the anterior margin of the foramen of Monro. Each column enters the substance of the brain and goes posteriorly through the hypothalamus to end in the ipsilateral mammillary body.

By using a midline approach and dividing the septum pellucidum, the surgeon will encounter the fornix, a thin layer of tela choroidea, the internal cerebral veins, and then another layer of tela choroidea.

When the surgeon enters the lateral ventricle, the junction of the anterior septal vein, the thalamostriate vein, and the choroid plexus point to the foramen of Monro. Occasionally, the surgeon may be confused about which ventricle has been entered. The pulsating septum pellucidum can be used as the medial landmark for orientation.

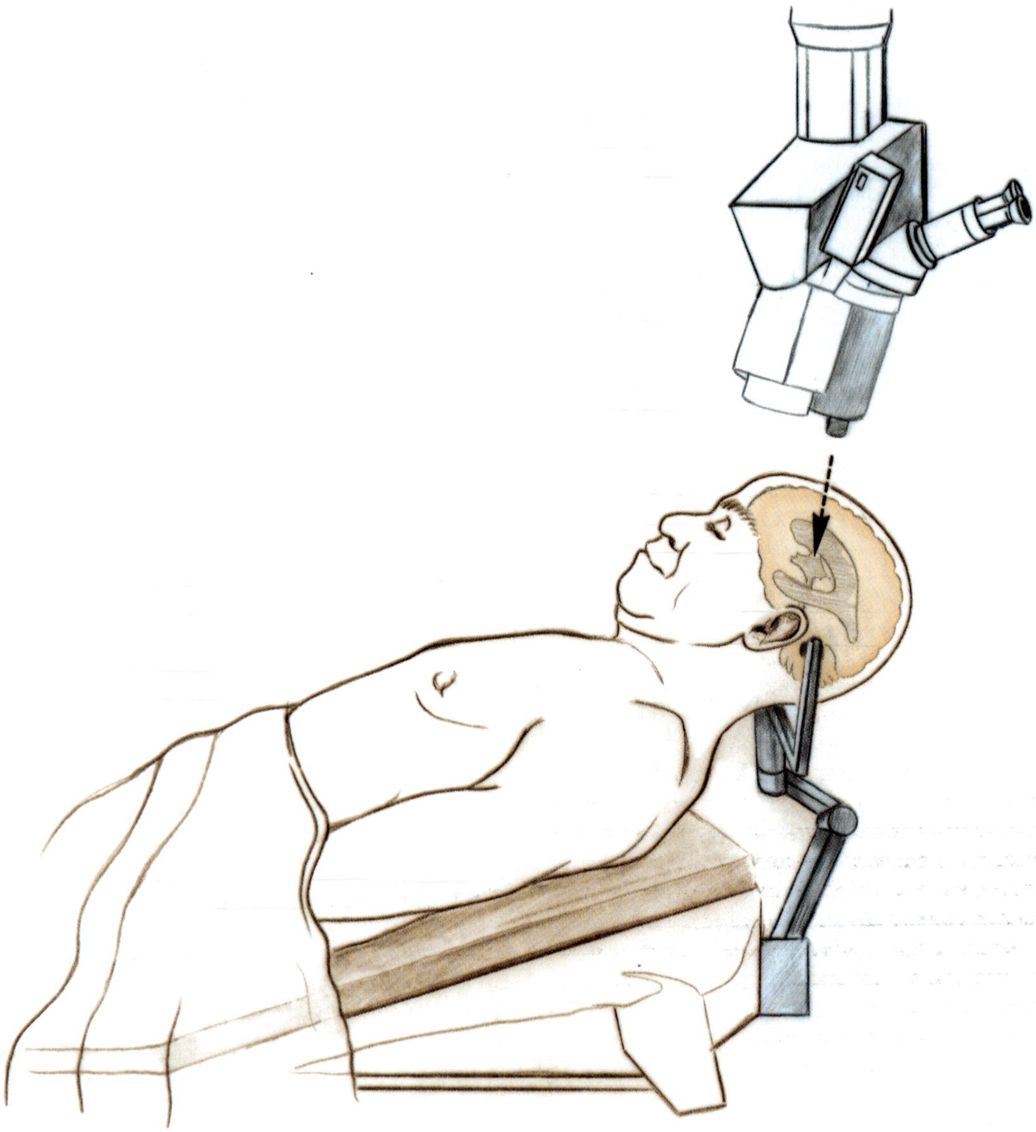

Figure 3–17.

Step 1. The patient's head is fixed in a pinion. Note that the head is at 0 degrees for orientation and slightly flexed and elevated above the level of the heart to decrease intracranial pressure.

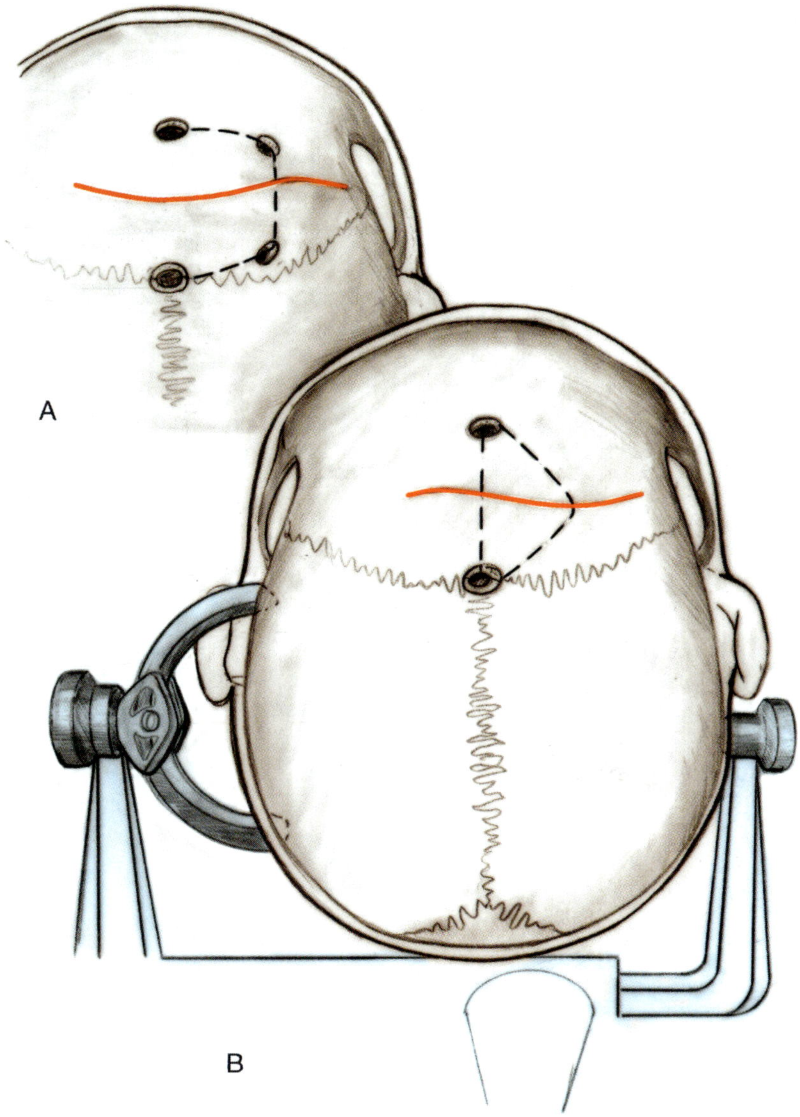

Figure 3–18.

Step 2. Two basic craniotomies, square (*A*) and triangular (*B*), can be used. The square craniotomy provides slightly more room for retraction. However, either craniotomy is excellent for an interhemispheric approach. If angiography was performed preoperatively, the bridging veins should be identified on the angiogram and the bone flap positioned accordingly.

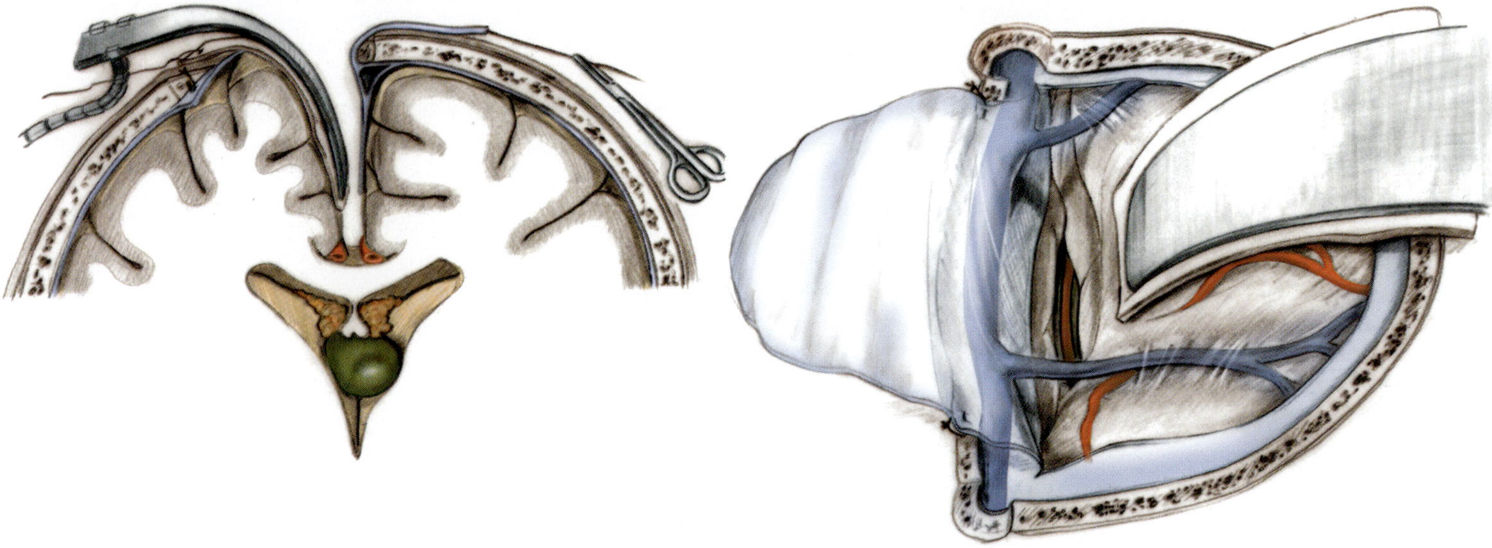

Figure 3–19.

Step 3. The dura mater is opened, reflected over the superior sagittal sinus, and tacked to the margins of the bone. After the right frontal lobe has been protected with hemostatic fabric and cottonoids, it is gently retracted. The arachnoid over any bridging veins should be preserved to reinforce these vascular structures.

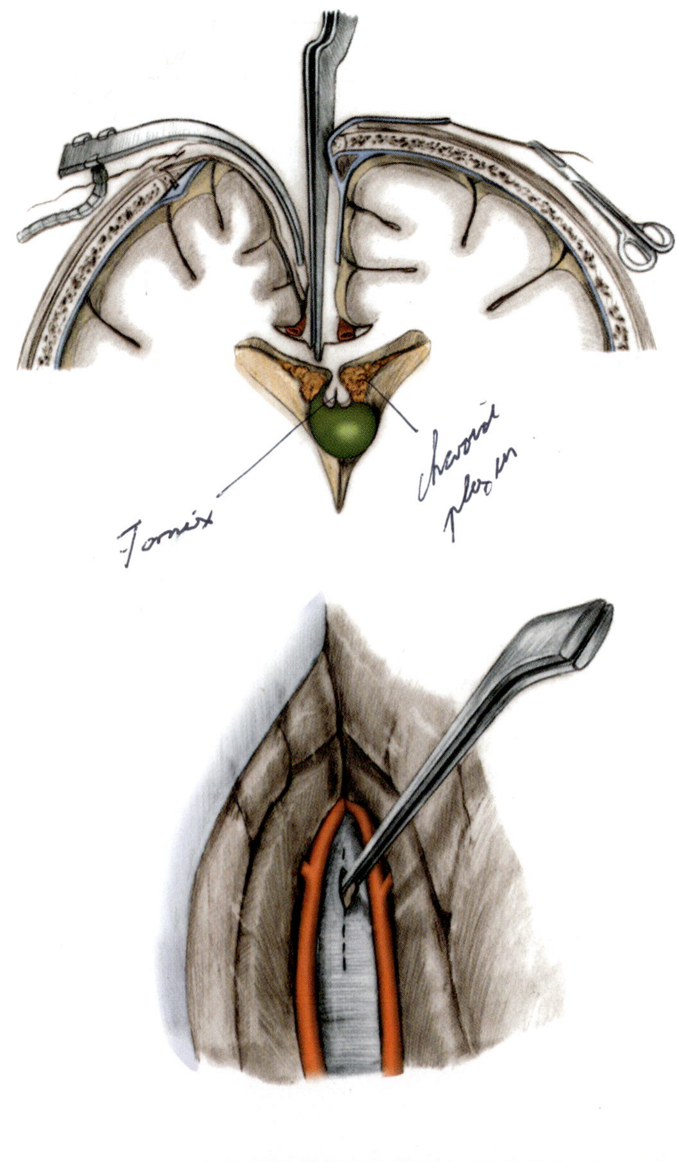

Figure 3–20.

Step 4. The author prefers to approach third ventricular colloid cysts from the right lateral ventricle instead of using an interforniceal approach. In this way, there is less risk of injury to the fornix. The corpus callosum is identified by its whitish appearance. The incision in the corpus callosum is approximately 1.5 cm long.

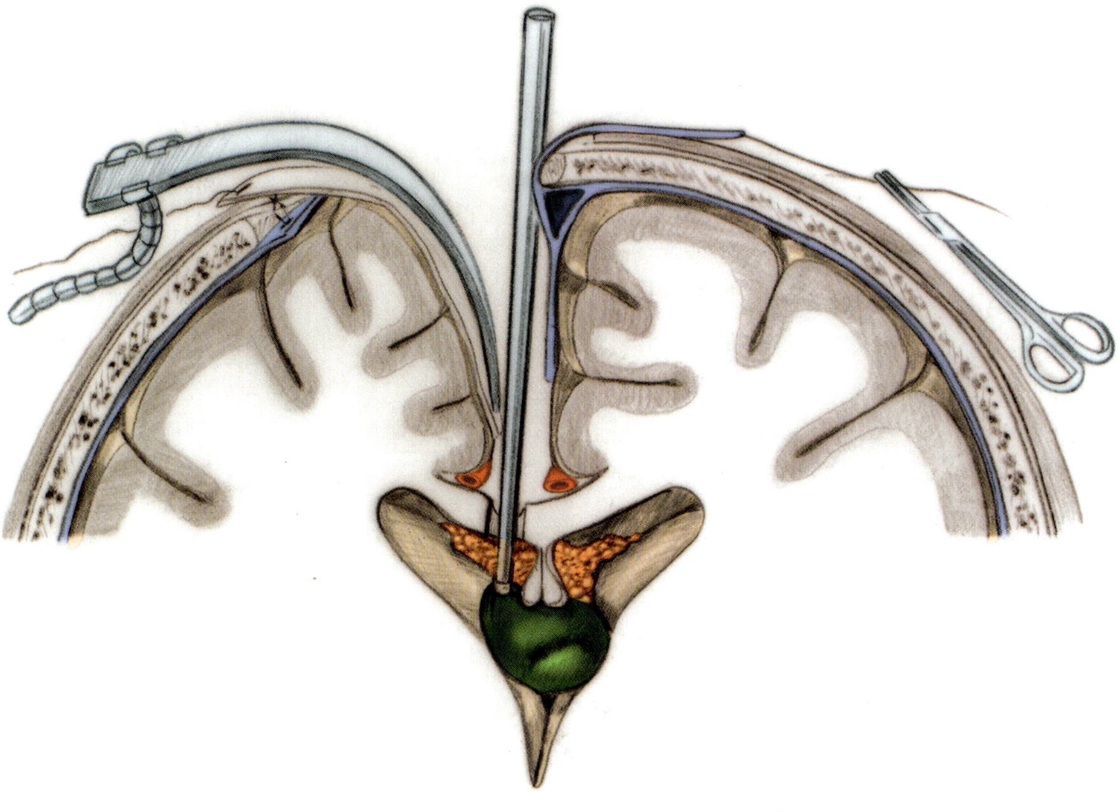

Figure 3–21.

Step 5. The primary means of removing a colloid cyst is decompression with suction.

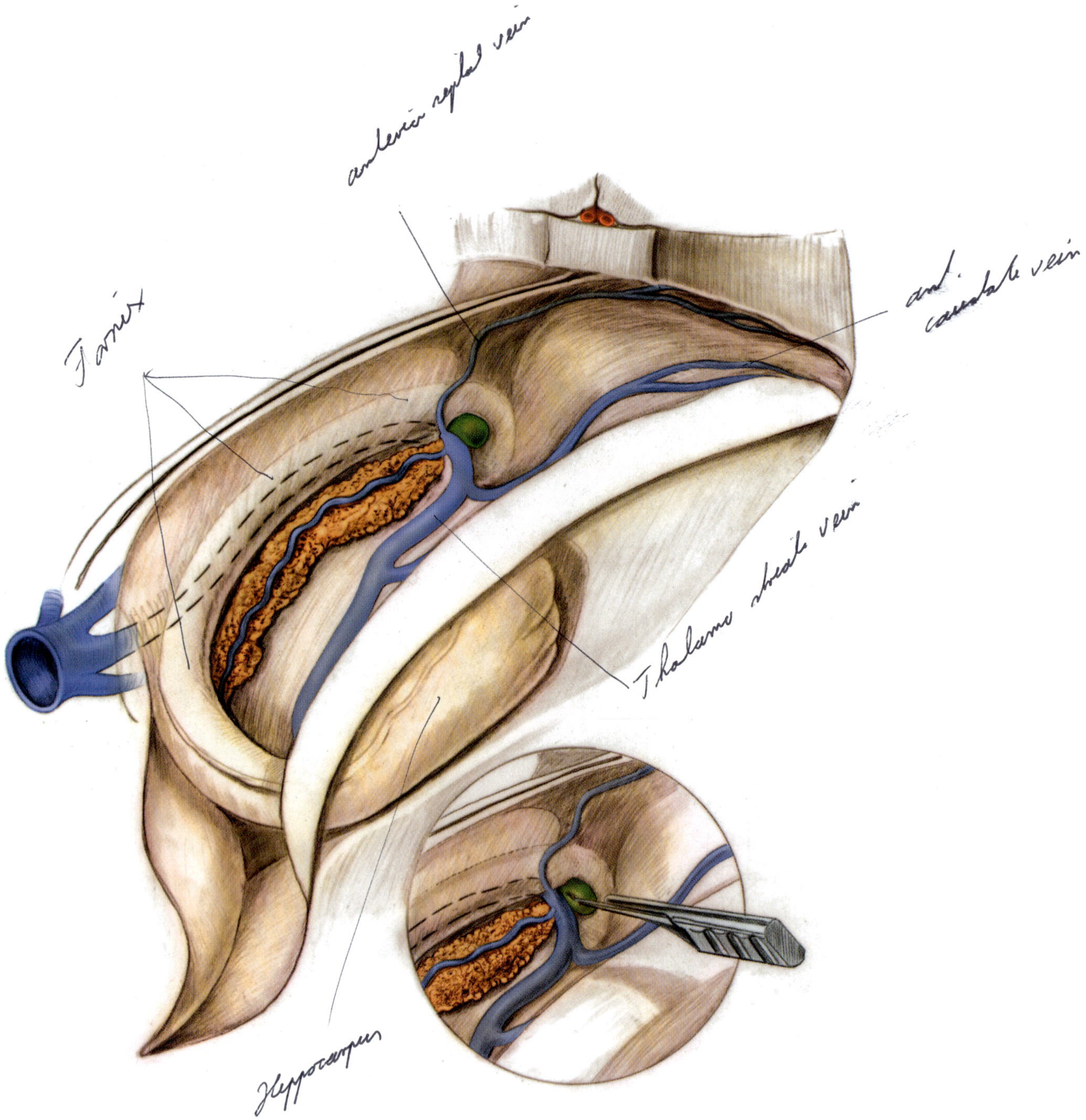

Figure 3–22.

Step 6. After the lateral ventricle has been entered, it is mandatory that the surgeon find the pertinent structures, which include the choroid plexus, the thalamostriate vein, the anterior septal vein, and the anterior caudate vein. Although the bulge of the colloid cyst will be apparent, it is helpful to identify these structures to become oriented and to identify the fornix. Afterward, an incision is made in the colloid cyst bulging through the foramen of Monro.

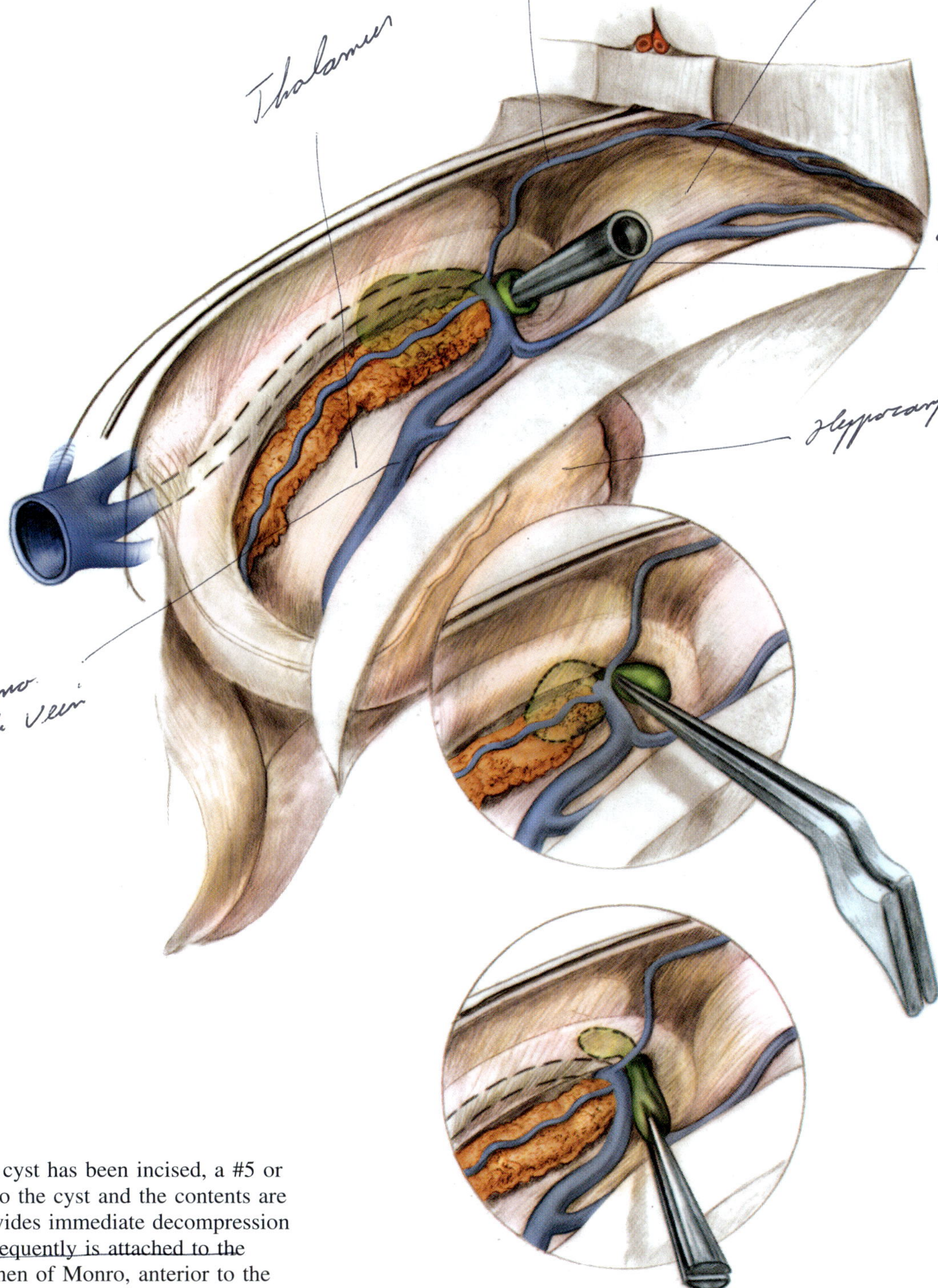

Figure 3–23.

Step 7. After the colloid cyst has been incised, a #5 or #7 suction tip is inserted into the cyst and the contents are evacuated. This usually provides immediate decompression of the cyst wall. The cyst frequently is attached to the posterior aspect of the foramen of Monro, anterior to the internal cerebral vein. It usually is necessary to gently cauterize and then to cut this attachment before extirpating the wall.

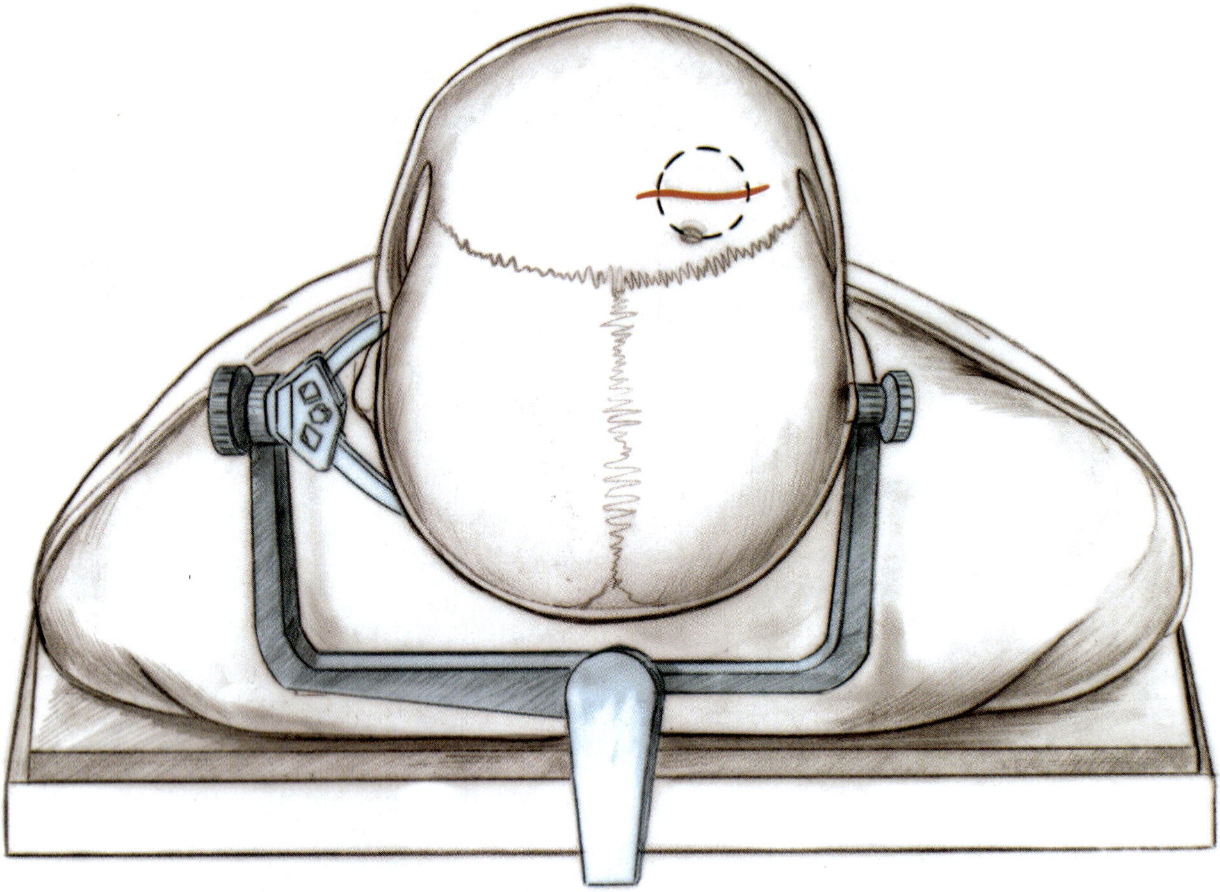

Figure 3–24.

An alternative to an interhemispheric approach is the transcortical route through the middle frontal gyrus. This can be achieved through a small trephine type craniotomy that is 3 cm from the midline and 2 cm in front of the coronal suture. This is the same location for placing an external ventricular drain into the right frontal horn of the lateral ventricle.

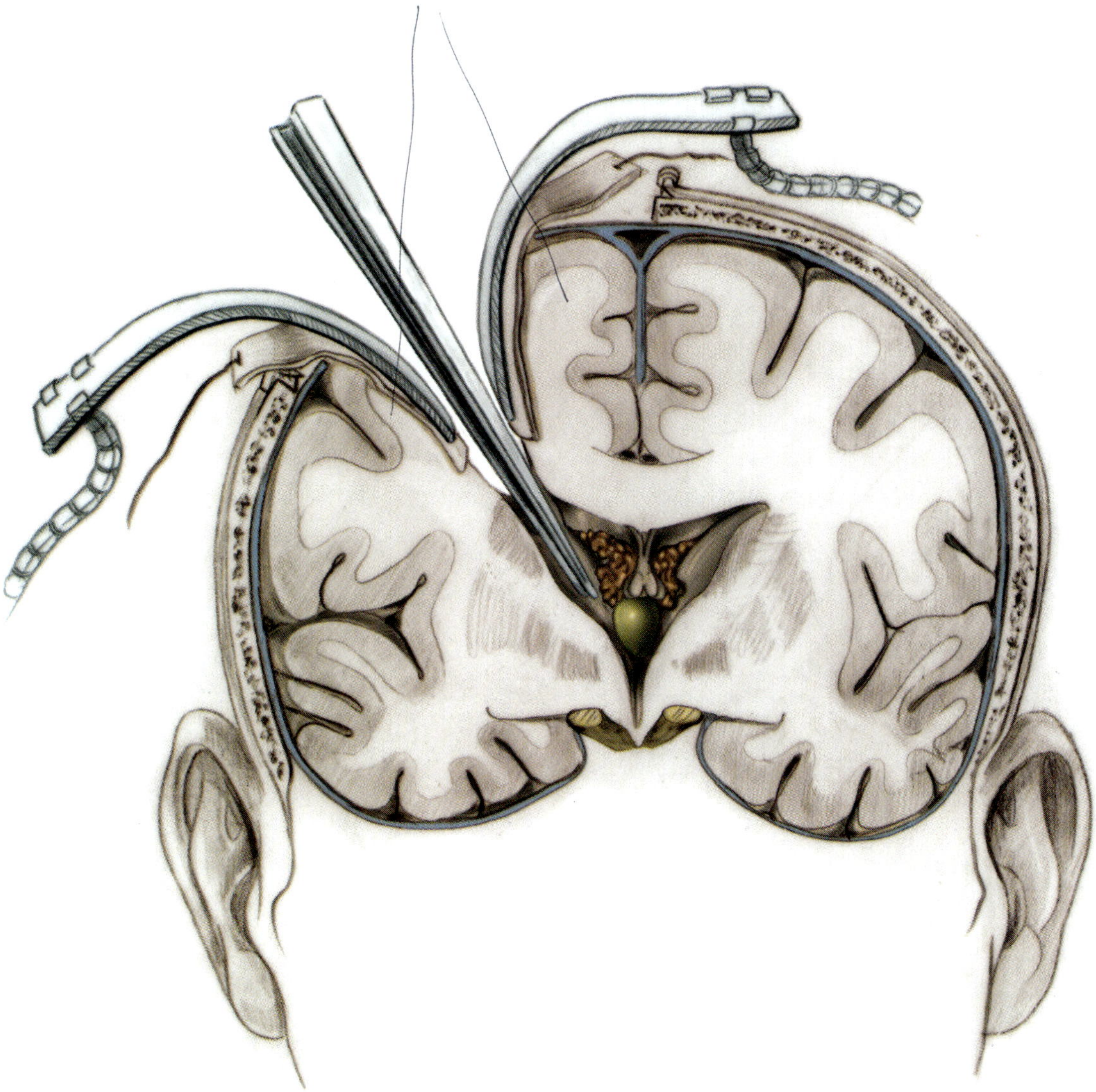

Figure 3–25.

A transcortical approach provides excellent access to the colloid cyst because of the angle. However, the disadvantage of this approach is the cortical incision that must be made and the small risk of postoperative seizures.

CRANIOPHARYNGIOMA—SUBFRONTAL APPROACH

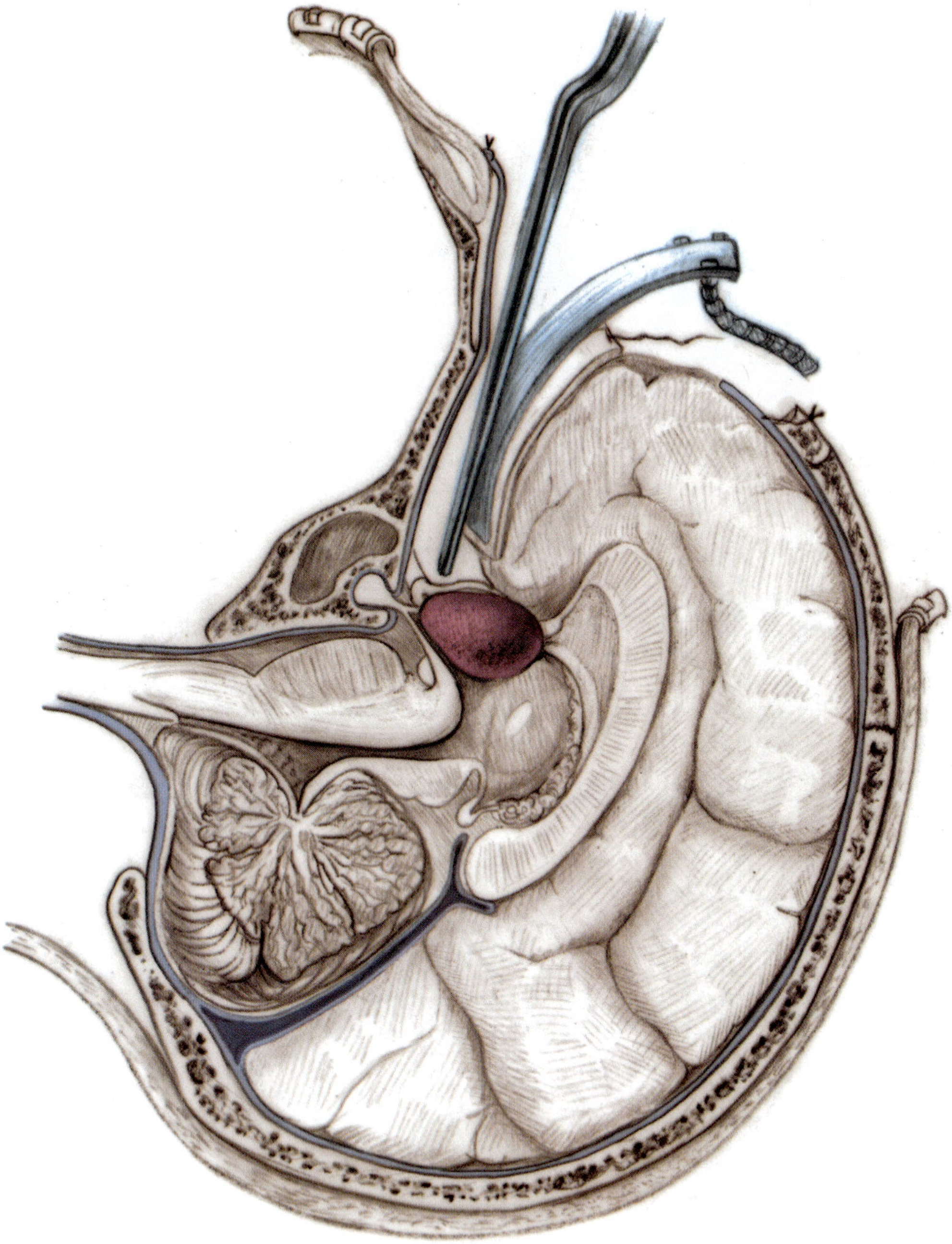

Figure 3–26.

A subfrontal approach for resection of a craniopharyngioma is useful, especially when there is a large extension of the tumor into the third ventricle. In comparison with a standard pterional craniotomy (described in Chapter 1), the subfrontal approach, with removal of the orbital rim, provides a better angle for access to the rostral portion of the tumor. Although removing the orbital ridge increases the surgical time for performing the craniotomy, it is worthwhile.

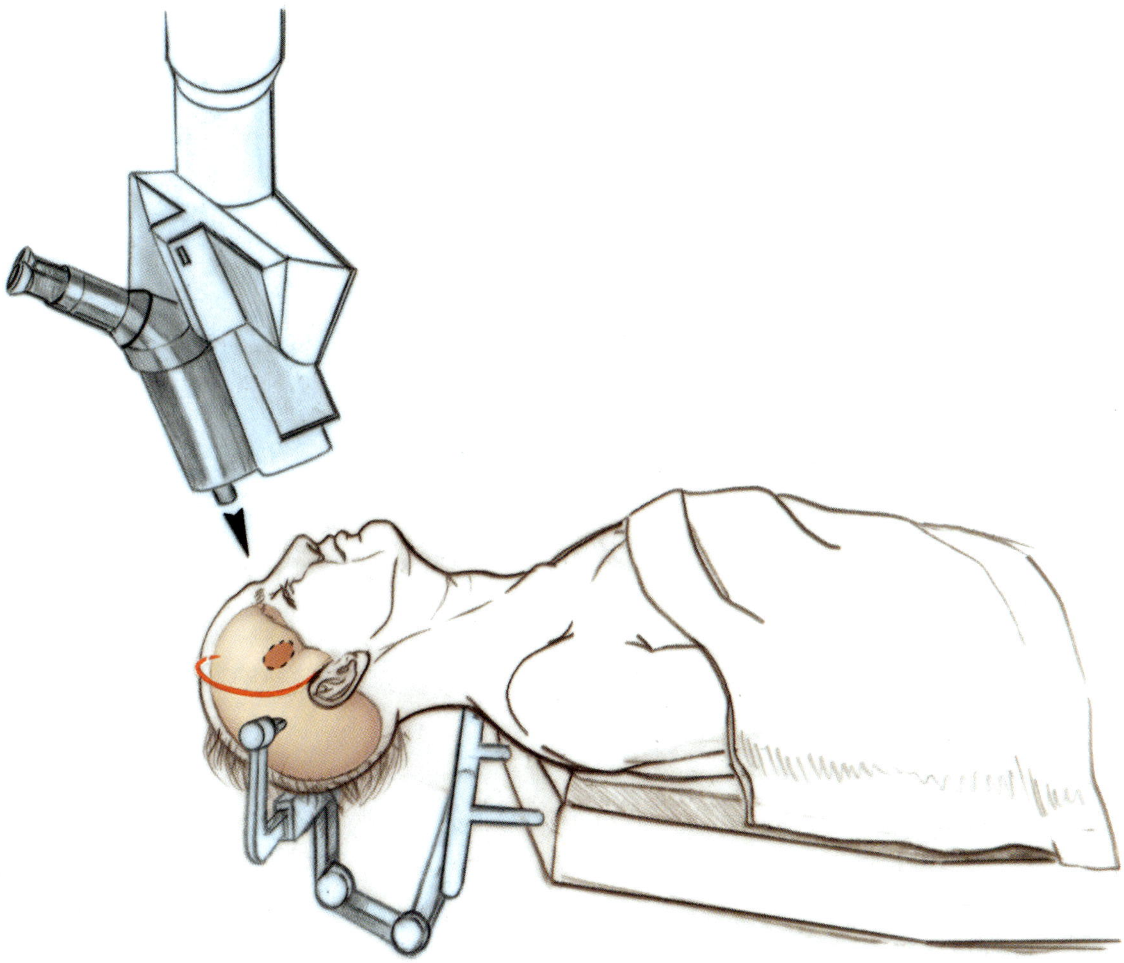

Figure 3–27.

Step 1. The patient's head is extended to decrease the need for frontal lobe retraction. Despite the head being extended, the chest is still angled to promote venous drainage from the brain.

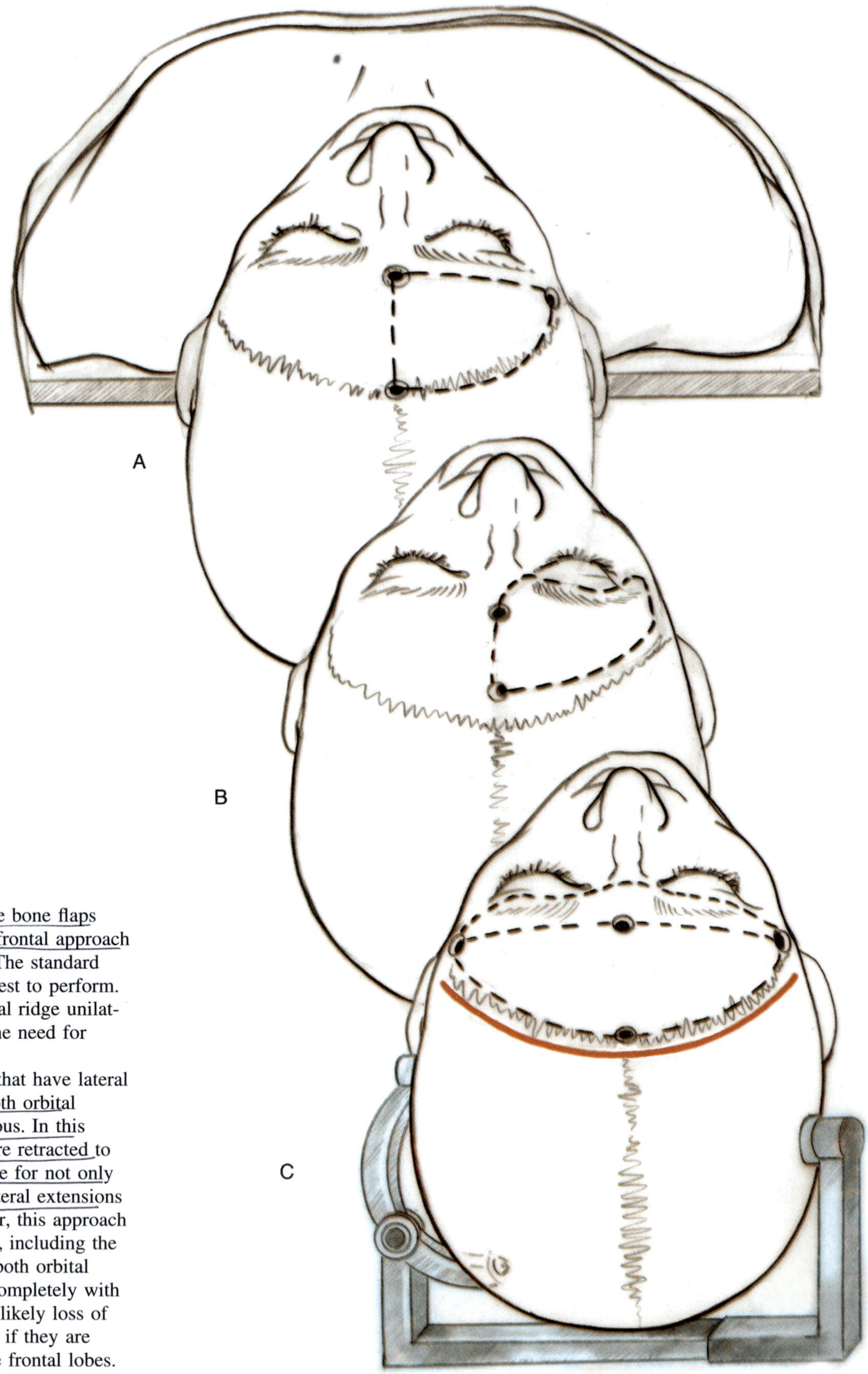

Figure 3–28.

Step 2. There are three bone flaps that can be used in a subfrontal approach to the third ventricle. *A*, The standard frontal craniotomy is easiest to perform.

B, Removing the orbital ridge unilaterally greatly decreases the need for frontal brain retraction.

C, In massive tumors that have lateral extensions, removal of both orbital ridges may be advantageous. In this case, both frontal lobes are retracted to provide excellent exposure for not only the rostral but also the lateral extensions of the neoplasm. However, this approach has several disadvantages, including the time required to remove both orbital ridges, the need to deal completely with the frontal sinus, and the likely loss of both olfactory tracts even if they are carefully dissected off the frontal lobes. All three craniotomies can be achieved through a bicoronal incision.

Figure 3–29.

Step 3. The craniotomy is achieved through two bone flaps. First, a standard frontal bone flap is performed, with its medial margin along the superior sagittal sinus. The outlines of the orbital removal are indicated by the dashed line.

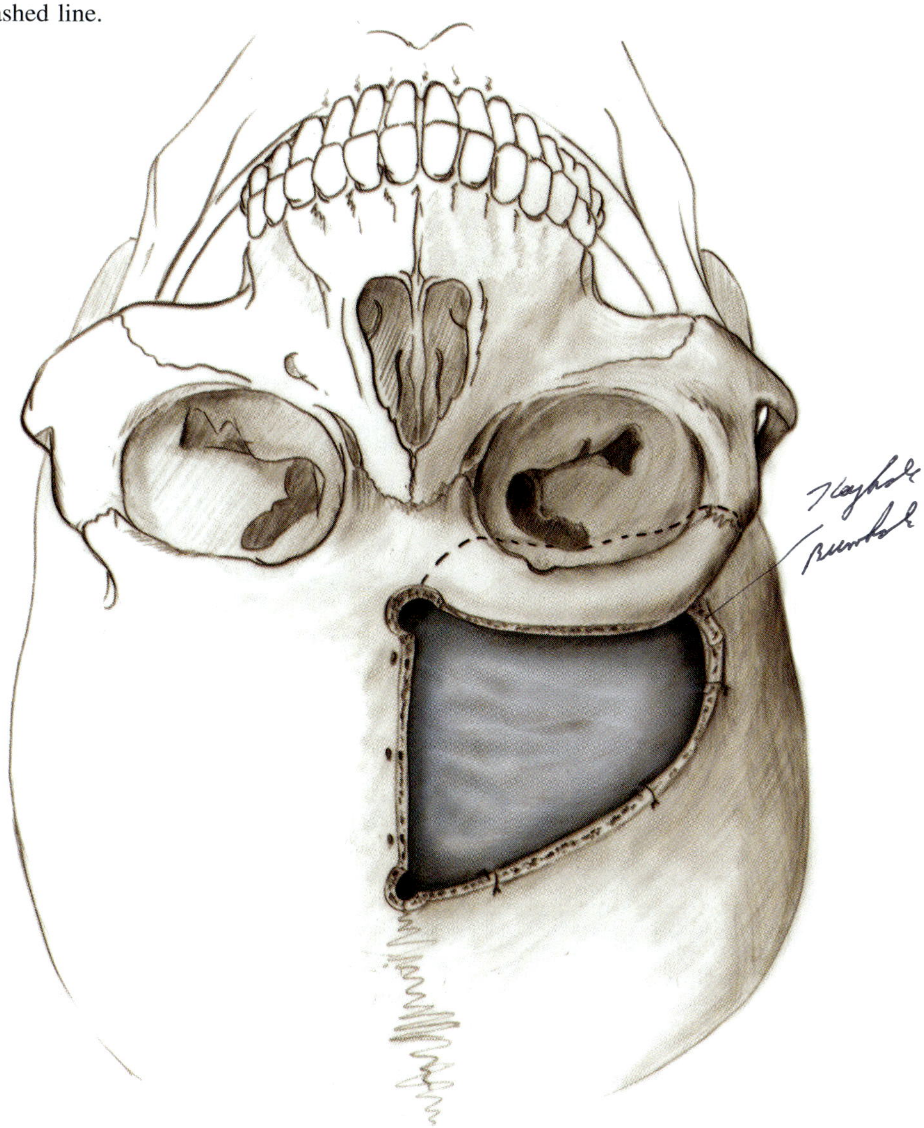

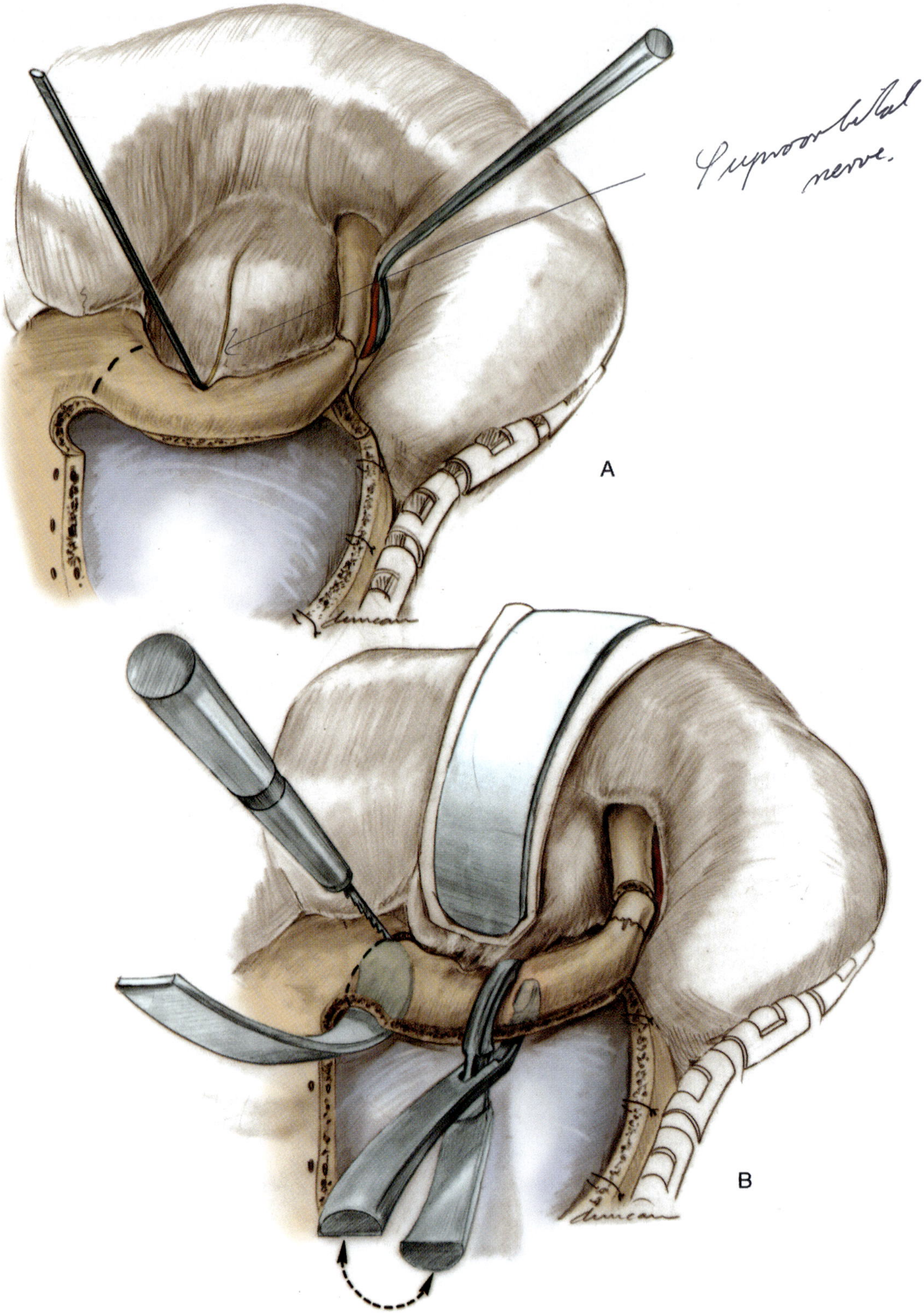

Figure 3–30.

Step 4. *A*, It is important to preserve the supraorbital nerve. Often, the supraorbital foramen is a notch, and a small spatula can be used to dissect the nerve out of its foramen and preserve it with the skin flap. Occasionally, the inferior rim of the foramen must be removed with a small rongeur. The dura mater, the temporalis muscle, and the orbital fascia are dissected off the bone with a curved periosteal elevator and a Penfield #1 dissector.

B, Both the medial and lateral bone cuts are made with an oscillating saw. While the bone cuts are being made, it is important to protect the brain and the orbit with spatulas. A sterilized tablespoon is ideal for protecting the orbit. After the two cuts have been completed, an orbital rongeur is used to grab the orbital ridge and to rock it gently. The posterior bone will crack along lines extending to the superior orbital fissure. Any shelves of bone along the inferior surface of the frontal lobe can then be removed with the rongeur.

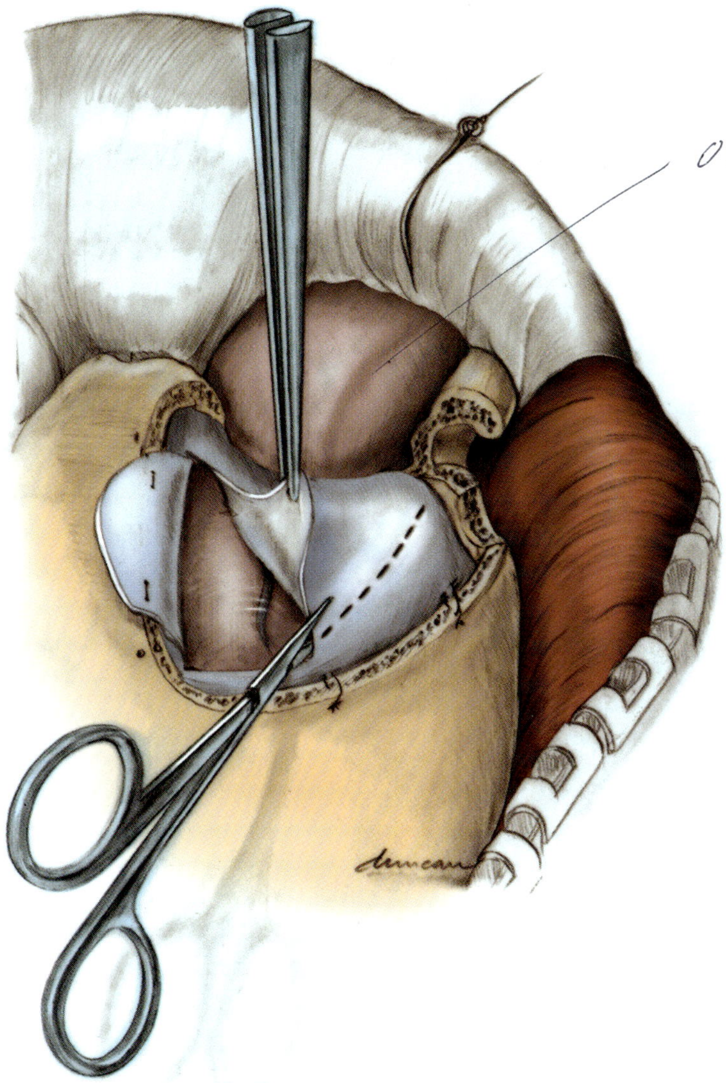

Figure 3–31.

Step 5. Next, the dura mater is opened and folded over the orbit and retracted under tension with fishhooks.

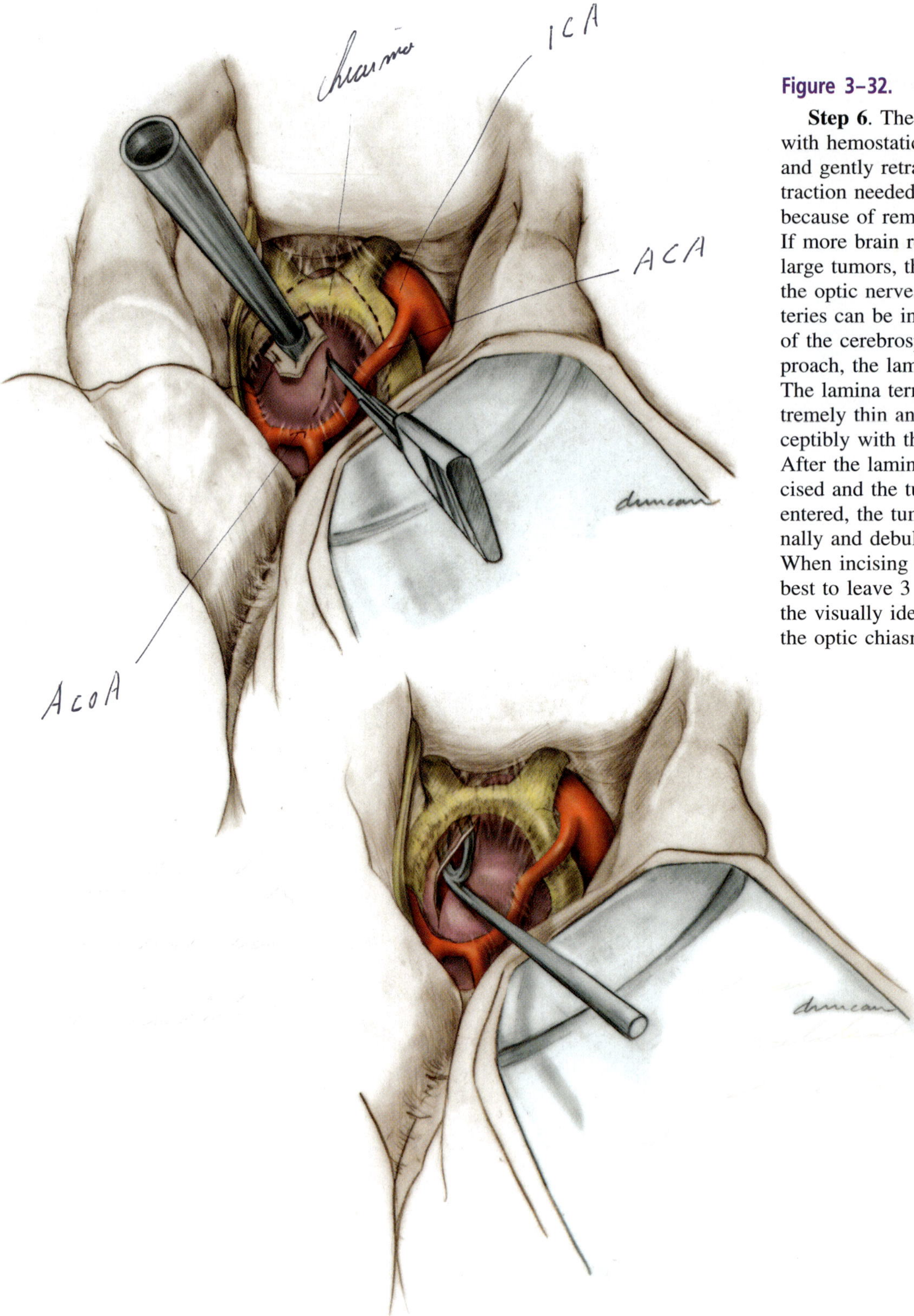

Figure 3–32.

Step 6. The right frontal lobe is lined with hemostatic fabric and cottonoids and gently retracted. The amount of retraction needed is usually quite small, because of removal of the orbital ridge. If more brain retraction is necessary for large tumors, the cisterns that surround the optic nerves and internal carotid arteries can be incised to promote drainage of the cerebrospinal fluid. With this approach, the lamina terminalis is incised. The lamina terminalis usually is extremely thin and merges almost imperceptibly with the capsule of the tumor. After the lamina terminalis has been incised and the tumor capsule has been entered, the tumor is decompressed internally and debulked with ringed curets. When incising the lamina terminalis, it is best to leave 3 to 4 mm of tissue behind the visually identified posterior margin of the optic chiasm.

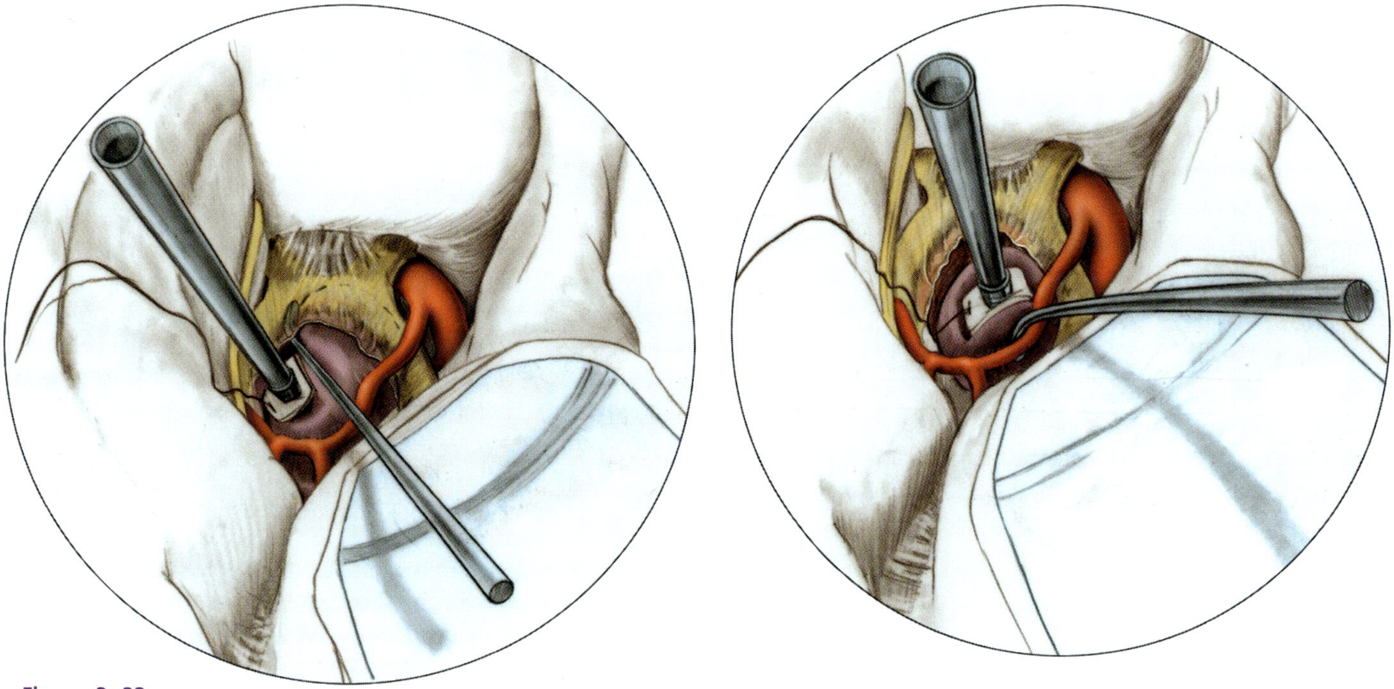

Figure 3–33.

Step 7. After the tumor has been debulked, the capsule is manipulated with a cottonoid and a #5 or #7 suction tip. Fine spatulas or bipolar cautery forceps are used to peel the capsule gently off the optic tracts and optic chiasm. It is important to recognize that deep to the tumor is a layer of arachnoid that overlies the basilar artery and its perforating branches. Laterally, this arachnoid overlies the posterior communicating artery. Preserving this arachnoid will protect these structures.

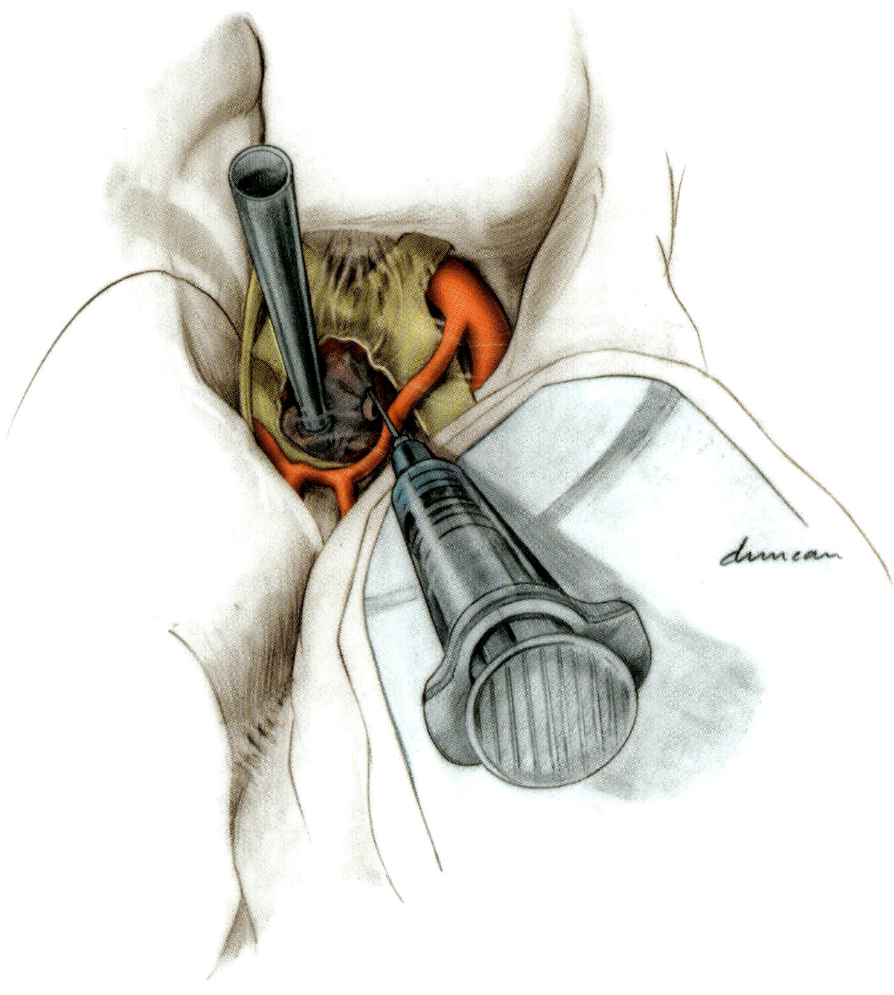

Figure 3–34.

Step 8. After the tumor has been removed, the margins are inspected with small angled Applebaum mirrors or a fiberoptic scope. Do not cauterize any bleeding from the walls of the third ventricle, which at this point are the walls of the hypothalamus. Instead, use gentle irrigation and small pieces of hemostatic fabric to achieve hemostasis. After the resection has been completed, the retractors are withdrawn and the frontal lobe is inspected. The dura mater is closed primarily or with periosteum. The bone flap is repositioned with small metal plates.

OLFACTORY GROOVE–PLANUM SPHENOIDALE MENINGIOMA

Meningiomas that lie in the olfactory groove and extend posteriorly along the planum sphenoidale are resected through a subfrontal approach. A more standard pterional or frontotemporal craniotomy can be used for small tumors and those with a unilateral extension along one orbital roof. If this type of craniotomy is used, it is important to make sure that the bone flap extends to the inner canthus of the eye to facilitate the subfrontal trajectory. The advantage of a unilateral subfrontal approach is that only one cerebral hemisphere is retracted. Also, if the meningioma is posterior along the planum sphenoidale, the opposite olfactory nerve may be preserved.

For large bilateral tumors, a bifrontal craniotomy is advantageous because it facilitates dissection of the lateral and posterior borders of the tumor from the adjacent neurovascular structures. Along those margins, the tumor is intimately related to the optic chiasm, the optic nerves, and branches of the anterior cerebral artery. Bifrontal craniotomy has several disadvantages. One, it is technically more difficult and time consuming. Two, the frontal sinus is often violated and must be exonerated. Three, the superior sagittal sinus must be ligated. Four, the likelihood of the bilateral loss of the olfactory tracts is high. However, with a large tumor along the planum sphenoidale, it is difficult to preserve these tracts regardless of the approach.

For lesions at the base of the frontal skull, such as an esthesioneuroblastoma, a combined otorhinolaryngologic and neurosurgical approach is optimal. With esthesioneuroblastomas, the cribriform plate is eroded. A low frontal trephine or rhomboid-shaped craniotomy is made through a bicoronal incision. The craniotomy extends anteriorly to the nasion and laterally to the orbital roofs. The approach is epidural. Therefore, a periosteal elevator or Penfield #1 dissector is used to dissect the dura mater off the orbital roofs. Eventually, the dura mater is dissected off the crista galli, which is then removed with a bone rongeur. The dura mater is sectioned at the level of the olfactory bulbs. These two rents in the dura mater are oversewn with 4-0 monofilament (Prolene) sutures. The dura mater is continually stripped back along the planum sphenoidale, almost to the tuberculum sella. Subsequently, the frontal lobes protected by dura mater are retracted bilaterally with self-retaining retractors. As the facial surgeon works from below, the neurosurgeon removes the cribriform plate with an orbital rongeur and small angled Kerrison rongeur. Occasionally, a small chisel is needed. This unroofs the sphenoid sinus. Additional bone can be removed posteriorly back to the tuberculum sellae. The neurosurgeon can assist in the dissection of the rostral and caudal extents of the esthesioneuroblastoma sitting in the posterior sphenoid sinus and laterally in the ethmoid sinuses.

Unilateral approach desireable
Bilateral tumours need bilateral approach
In unilateral approach, olfactory bulb can
be preserved contralaterally
and only one lobe needs to
be retracted.

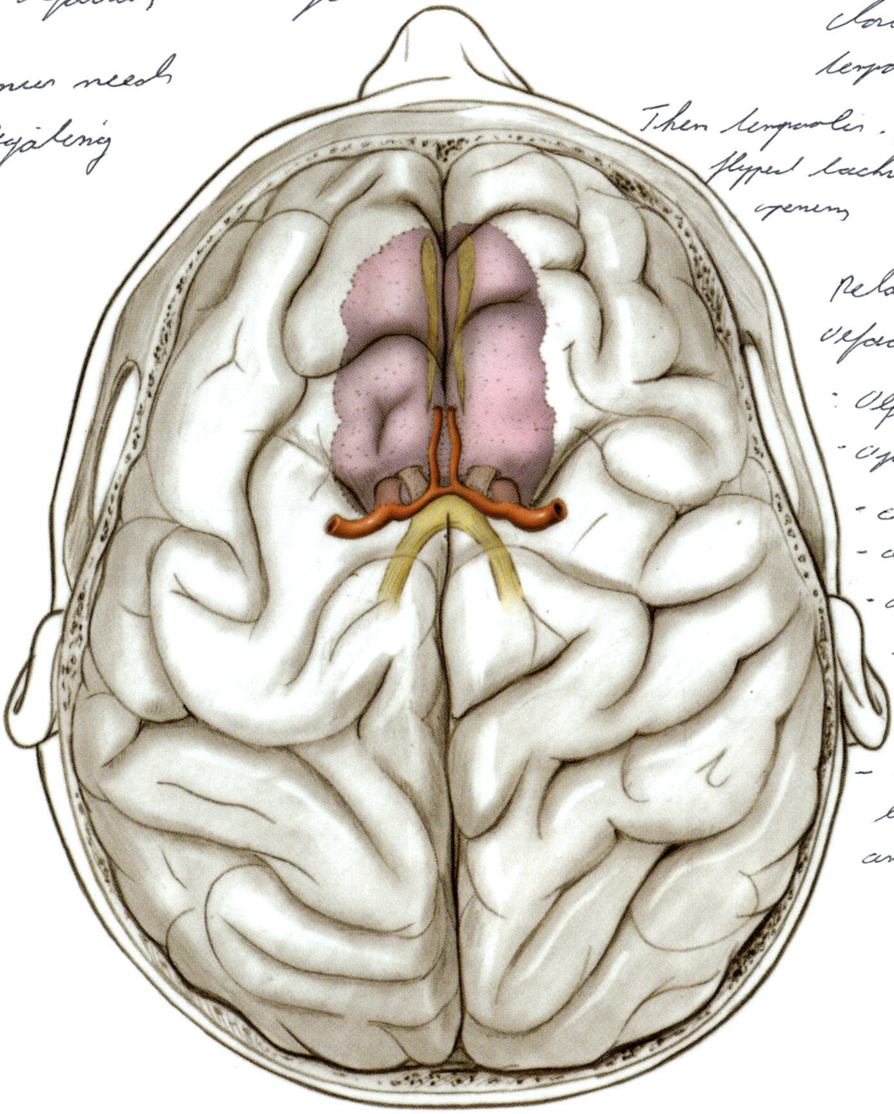

Figure 3–35.

The relationship of the tumor with the olfactory tracts, planum sphenoidale, and neurovascular structures.

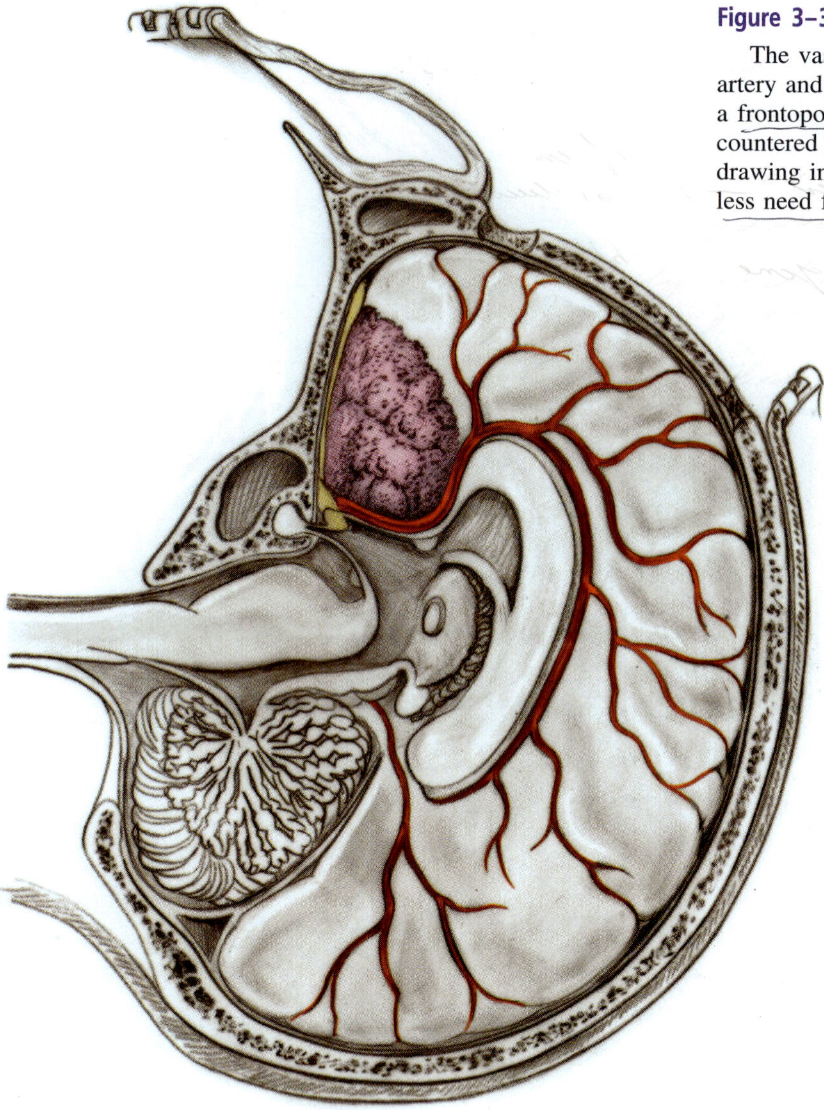

Figure 3–36.

The vascular structures at risk are the anterior cerebral artery and its branches, including the orbitofrontal artery. If a frontopolar artery takes off relatively low, it may be encountered laterally along the rostral part of the tumor. The drawing indicates that the lower the frontal craniotomy, the less need for frontal brain retraction.

Figure 3–37.

Step 1. *A*, The patient's head is fixed in a pinion, and a bifrontal craniotomy is made through a bicoronal incision. Note that in this example both frontal sinuses have been entered. After the mucosa has been stripped from the walls of the sinuses, pieces of temporalis muscle are used to plug the frontal sinuses. A small vascularized periosteal flap can be harvested from the skin flap and sewn over the muscle packing and tacked to the dura mater.

B, The dura mater is tacked laterally to the bone margins and opened low over both frontal lobes. Penfield #1 or small retractor blades are used to separate the mesial frontal lobes off the superior sagittal sinus and the adjacent falx cerebri. The superior sagittal sinus is then ligated with braided 3-0 sutures and severed.

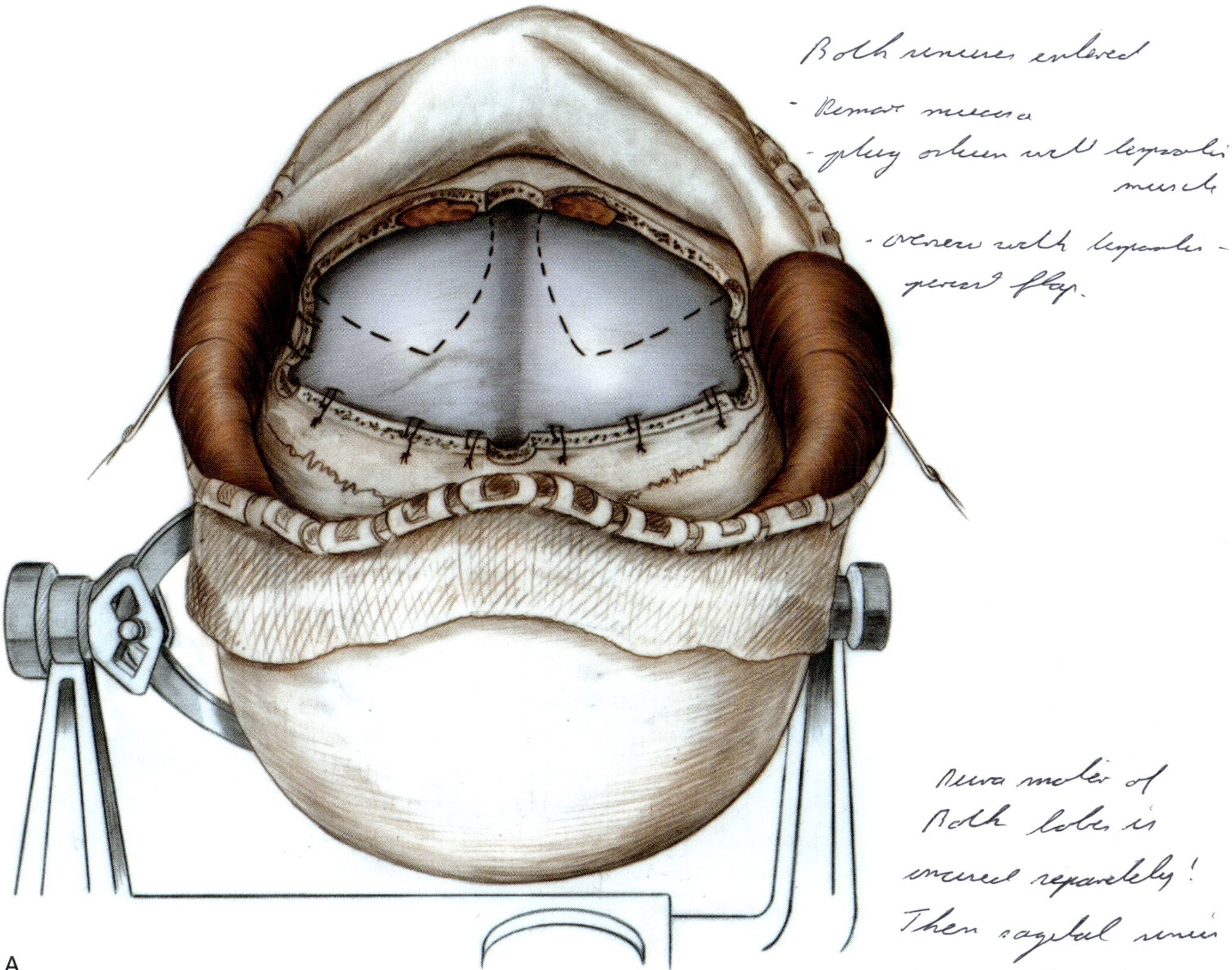
Both sinuses entered
- Remove mucosa
Dura mater of both lobes is incised separately!
Then sagittal sinus is ligated!!

A

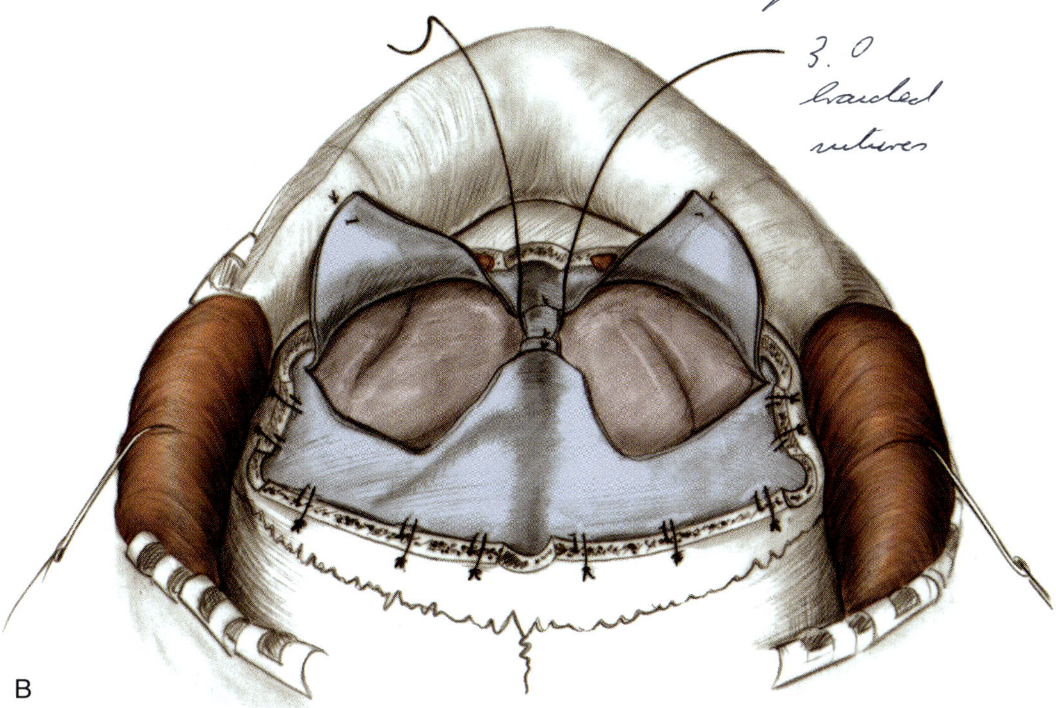
3.0 braided sutures

B

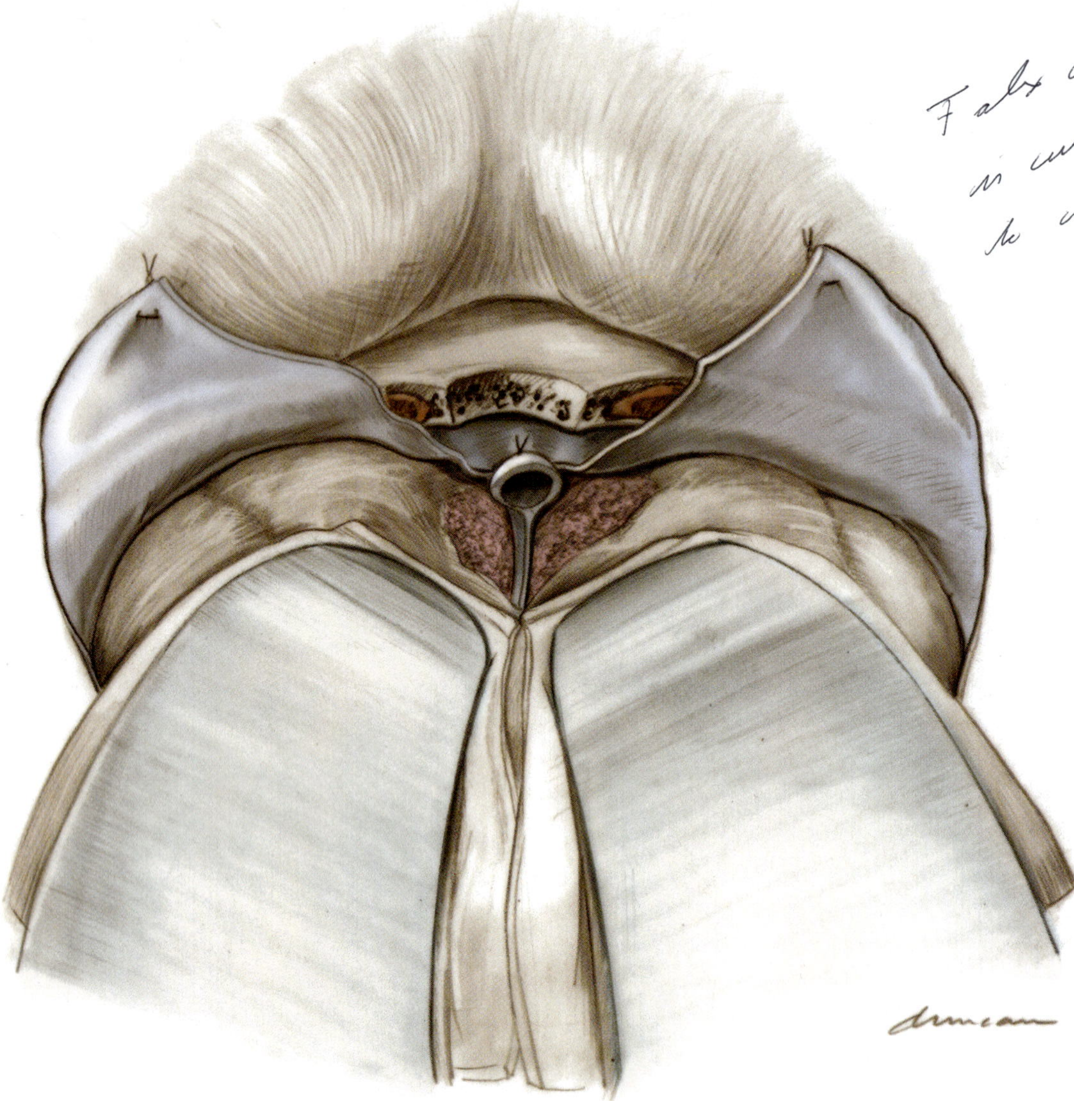

Figure 3–38.

Step 2. The frontal lobes are lined with hemostatic fabric and cottonoids and gently retracted. Next, the falx cerebri is cut posterior to the crista galli.

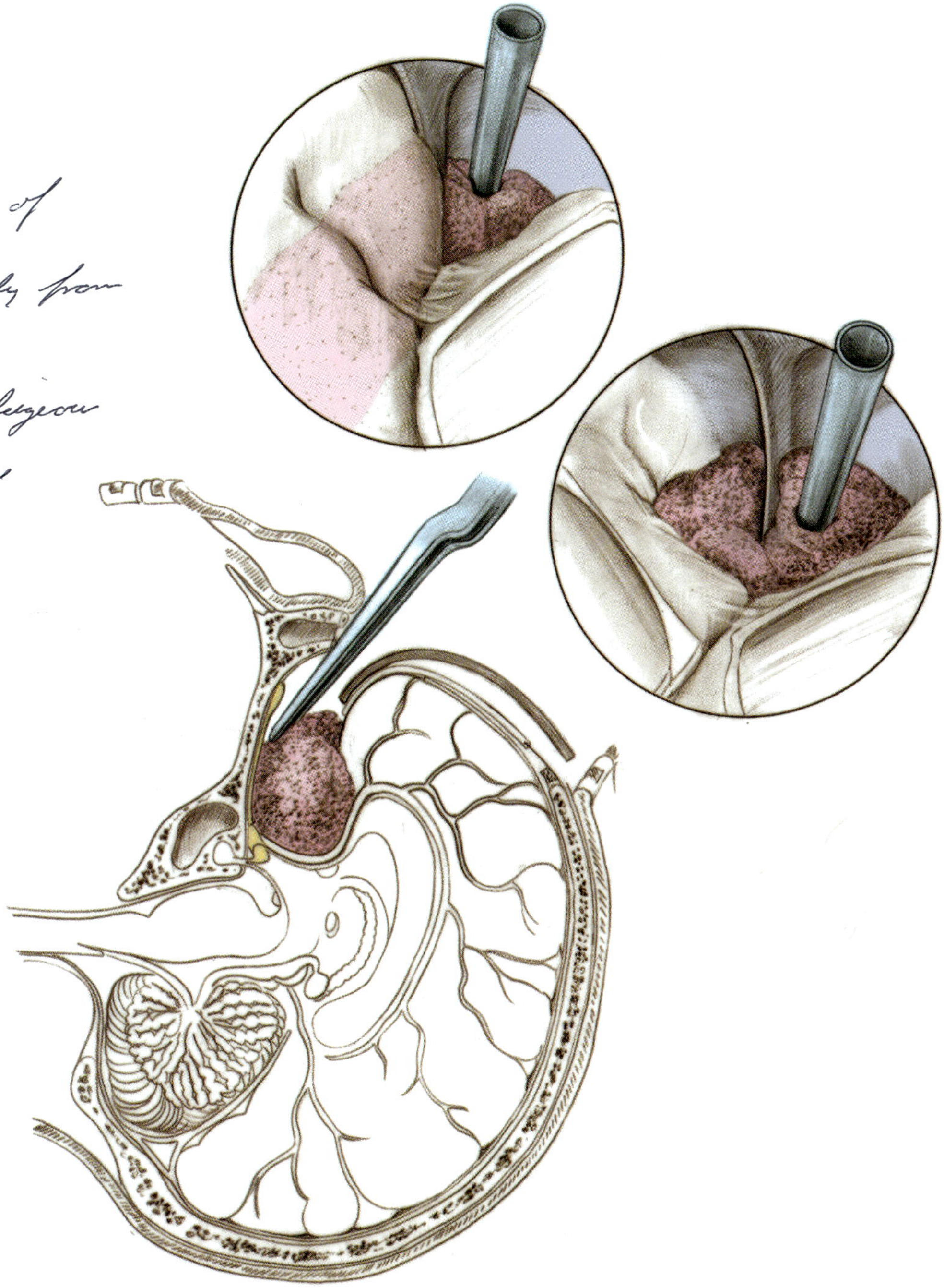

Figure 3–39.

Step 3. As the frontal lobes are retracted, the tumor is encountered. The blood supply to the tumor runs along the underside of the tumor, along the olfactory groove and dura mater of the planum sphenoidale. Therefore, it is advantageous first to dissect the underside of the tumor with bipolar cautery and suction. The tumor then is debulked internally.

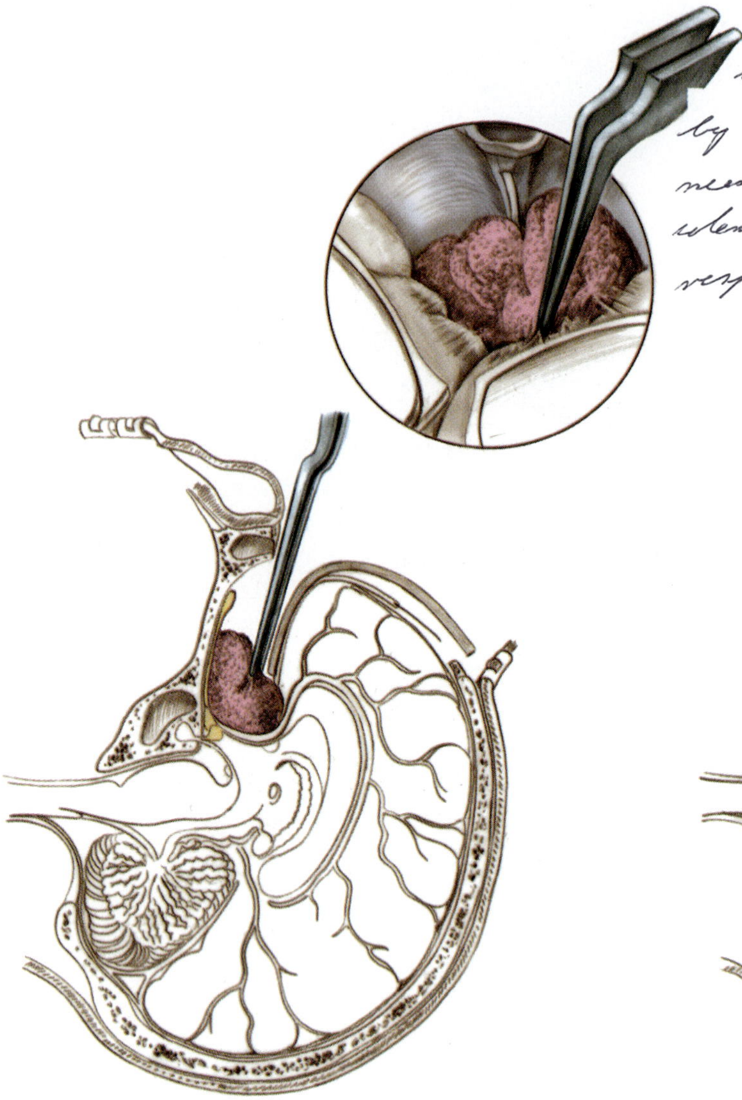

Figure 3–40.

Step 4. The tumor is progressively debulked using bipolar cautery, suction, and an ultrasonic aspirator. Sometimes, dividing the interhemispheric arachnoid may facilitate retraction of one frontal lobe without causing undue traction on the opposite frontal lobe. As true for most operations on meningiomas, it is important to respect the arachnoid plane between the tumor capsule and the cerebral cortex.

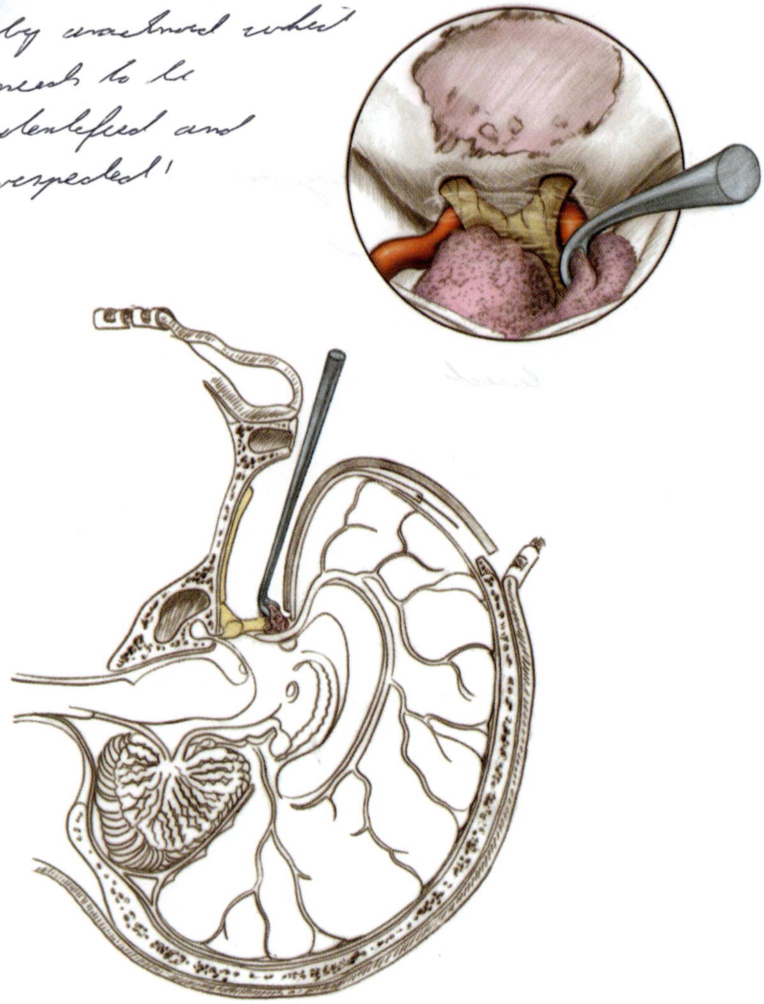

Figure 3–41.

Step 5. The difficult portion of the tumor is its posterior, or deep, extension along the optic chiasm. With very large tumors, the bifurcation of the internal carotid artery is displaced laterally and the optic chiasm is pushed posteriorly. A layer of arachnoid along the anterior clinoid process overlies the optic nerves, the optic chiasm, and the internal carotid arteries. Because this arachnoid plane separates the tumor from these neurovascular structures, it is important to identify this arachnoid. The tumor usually can be retracted with a #5 or #7 suction tip and cottonoid, while the tumor capsule is separated off the arachnoid with a small dissecting spatula.

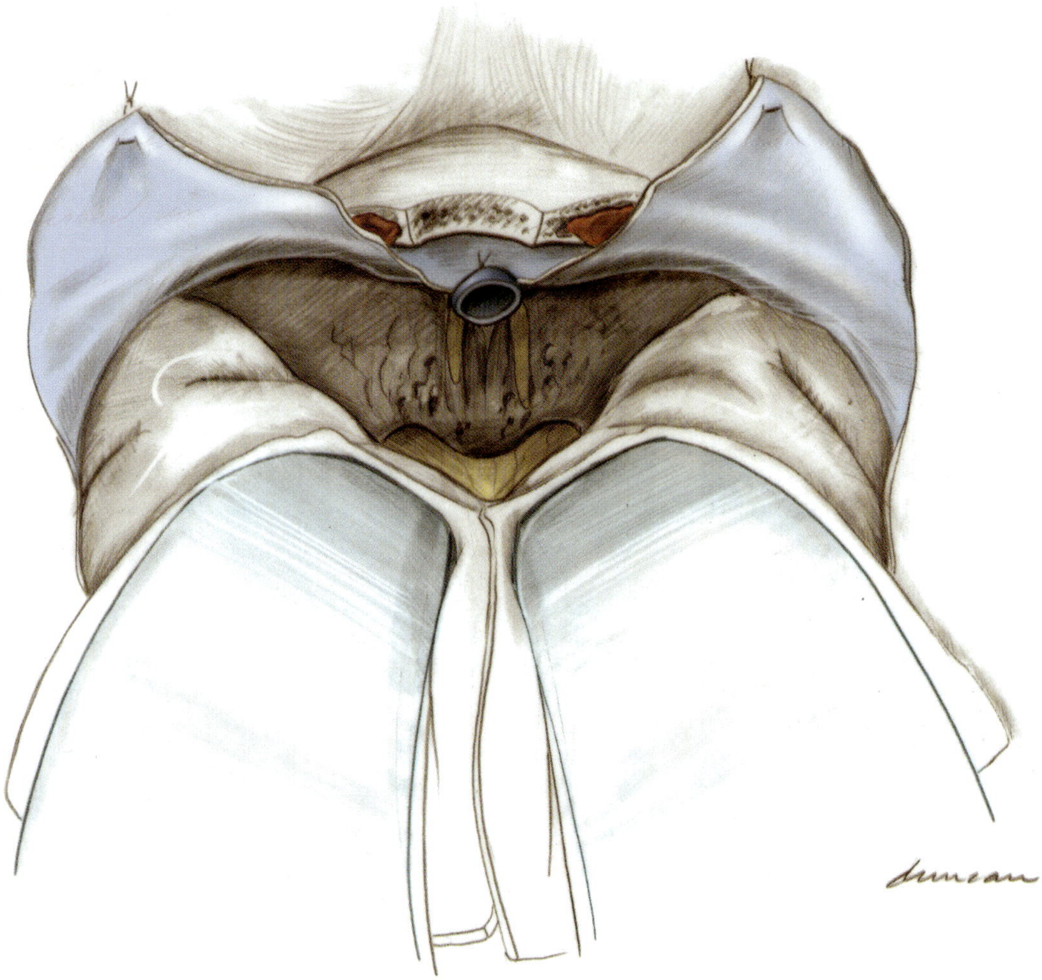

Figure 3–42.

This postoperative view demonstrates that both olfactory tracts were lost. It is better to control bleeding from the olfactory bulb with absorbable gelatin sponge than with cautery. It is important to cauterize the dura mater along the planum sphenoidale.

4

Parietal Approach

Copyright © 1999 Mayo Foundation.

ANATOMIC CONSIDERATIONS

Central Lobe

The demarcation between the frontal and parietal lobes is the central sulcus. However, many anatomists and surgeons prefer to describe a "central lobe" that consists of the precentral, postcentral, and paracentral gyri. Thus, the central lobe sits between the frontal and parietal lobes. The rationale for a central lobe is based partly on the integrated sensorimotor function of these gyri.

The precentral gyrus (Brodmann area 4) begins at the middle third of the Sylvian fissure and runs vertically toward the interhemispheric fissure. Medially, it is continuous with the anterior part of the paracentral lobule. Near the midportion of the precentral sulcus, the precentral gyrus abuts the middle frontal gyrus. Posteriorly, the precentral gyrus is separated from the postcentral gyrus by the central sulcus. Within the central sulcus are several transverse gyri that interdigitate with the postcentral gyrus. The precentral gyrus is 10 to 12 cm long and 10 to 15 mm wide, and its cerebral cortex is 3.5 to 4.5 mm thick. This gyrus is considered to be responsible primarily for skilled voluntary movements. Cortical mapping studies have demonstrated that despite moderate variability there generally is a topographic representation of movements ("motor map") along the precentral gyrus. Commencing with the most inferior part of the precentral gyrus adjacent to the Sylvian fissure and going toward the interhemispheric fissure, cortical stimulation causes movements of the jaw, lips, upper face, thumb, fingers, wrists, elbows, and shoulders.

The postcentral gyrus (Brodmann areas 1, 2, and 3) is separated from the precentral gyrus by the central sulcus. Medially, it extends into the paracentral lobule. Several incomplete sulci partially divide the postcentral gyrus.

The paracentral gyrus (Brodmann areas 1, 2, 3, 4, and 5 on the medial surface of the hemisphere), or lobule, is a rectangular region that contains the medial interhemispheric aspect of both the precentral and postcentral gyri. It is separated anteriorly from the medial frontal gyrus by the paracentral sulcus and posteriorly from the precuneus by the marginal limb of the cingulate sulcus. The paracentral gyrus often has several incomplete sulci. Stimulation of the anterior portion of the paracentral gyrus elicits movements of the lower extremity. This region is also involved with bowel and bladder functions.

Parietal Lobe

The parietal lobe consists of four lobules (Figures 4–1 and 4–2): the precuneus and the superior, inferior, and middle parietal lobules. The precuneus (Brodmann areas 7 and 31) is located on the medial surface of the parietal lobe between the cingulate gyrus and the superior parietal lobule. Anteriorly, it is separated from the paracentral lobule by the marginal limb of the cingulate sulcus, and posteriorly, it is separated from the cuneus (of the occipital lobe) by the parietooccipital sulcus. Grossly, the precuneus appears to consist of obliquely running gyri that are continuations of the cingulate gyrus, especially the isthmus of the cingulate gyrus. On the lateral cortical surface, the precuneus is continuous with the postcentral gyrus and the superior parietal lobule.

The superior parietal lobule (Brodmann areas 5 and 7) sits between the interhemispheric fissure and the interparietal sulcus. Anteriorly, it is associated with the postcentral gyrus and medially and superiorly, with the precuneus. Injury to the right parietal lobule can lead to disturbances of space perception, as manifested by dressing apraxia, central extinction, and constructional apraxia.

The inferior parietal lobule (Brodmann areas 39 and 40) is divided into the inferior lobule (supermarginal or circumflex gyrus) and the middle lobule (angular gyrus). They are demarcated by the distal Sylvian fissure, the superior temporal sulcus, and the interparietal sulcus. The middle parietal lobule is posterior to the inferior lobule and merges with the occipital lobe posteriorly.

The arterial supply to the convexity of the central and parietal lobes is from the middle cerebral artery, and the vessels supplying the medial surface and the apical portion of the convexity are primarily from the anterior cerebral artery.

Vascular Supply

The middle cerebral artery gives off five to eight branches along its insular course. The Sylvian triangle is defined angiographically by the following landmarks. The Sylvian point or apex of the Sylvian triangle is established by the most posterior branch of the middle cerebral artery as it exits from the Sylvian fissure. The superior margin is demarcated by the branches of the superior ramifications of the middle cerebral artery. The inferior margin of the Sylvian triangle is outlined by the inferior loops of the middle cerebral artery.

The middle cerebral artery usually has either a bifurcation or trifurcation depending on whether the anterior temporal branch originates at or just proximal to the main bifurcation. The trunk of the middle cerebral artery typically bifurcates to yield an anterior and a posterior group of arteries. The first branch of the anterior division is the orbitofrontal artery, which supplies the inferolateral aspect of the frontal lobe. The second division of the ascending frontal group is the operculofrontal artery, which forms a candelabra of branches. By definition, this group of operculofrontal arteries consists of the arteries anterior to the central sulcus arteries. They supply most of the middle and inferior frontal gyri, including Broca's area and part

Central sulcus divides frontal from parietal lobe. However r.t. a " central lobe " is defined that comprises precentral, postcentral and paracentral lobe as an area of integrated motor function.
This leaves the superior and inferior parietal lobule for the parietal lobe together with the precuneus on the medial side.

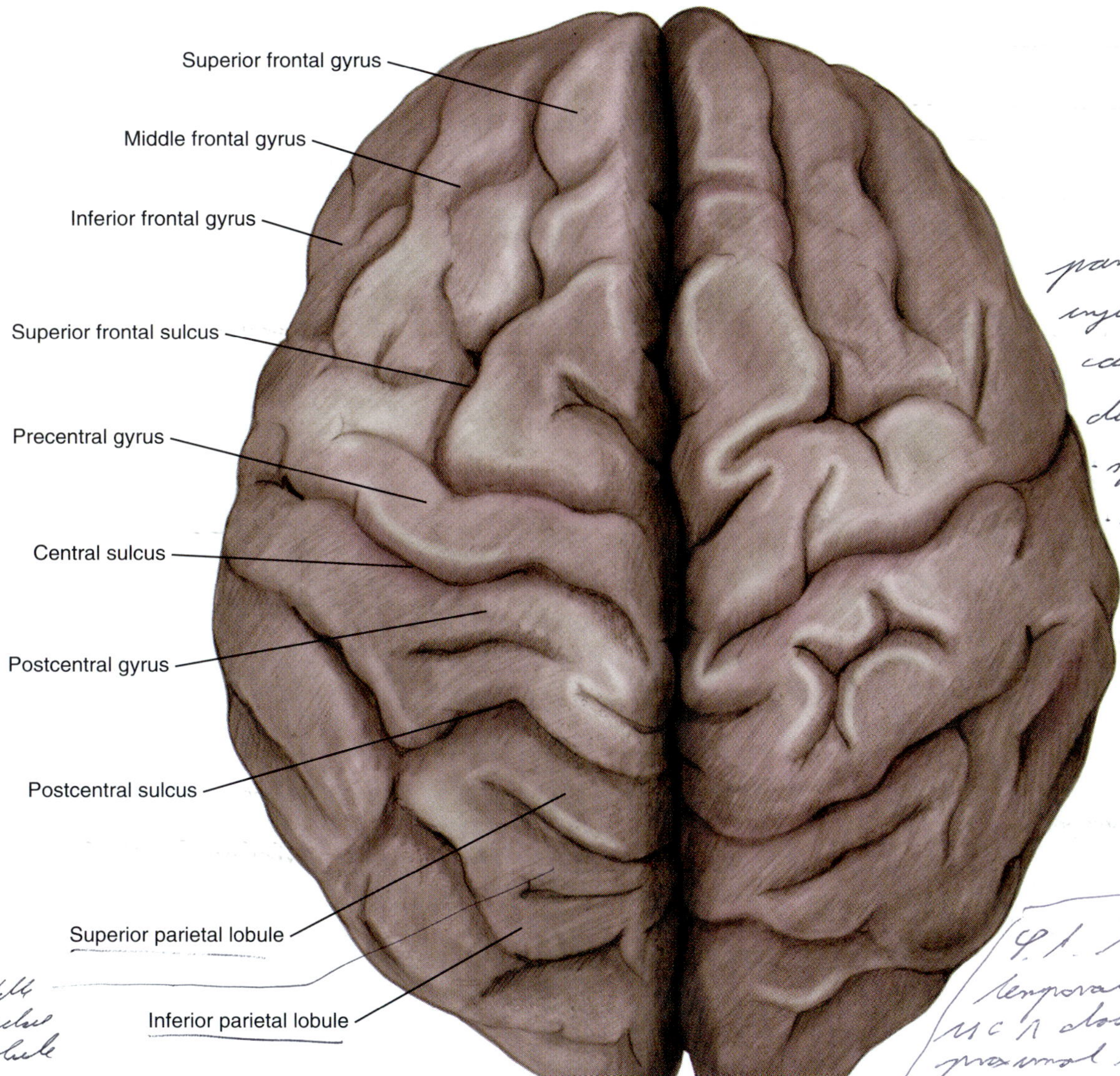

parietal lobe injury R side can cause disturbance of
- space perception
- apraxia
- constructional apraxia

middle parietal lobule

N.B. the anterior temporal branch of the MCA does not emerge proximal to bifurcation ⇒ then trifurcation

Figure 4–1.

Branches of middle cerebral artery (anterior)

- orbitofrontal artery - inferolateral aspect of frontal lobe
- operculofrontal artery - middle + inferior frontal gyrus including Broca's area
- central sulcus arteries (Rolandic) → most of central lobe

of the central lobe through the anterior parietal artery and its ramifications.

There usually are one to two central sulcus arteries (Rolandic arteries), which are the last branches of the anterior bifurcation of the middle cerebral artery. The Rolandic arteries supply much of the central lobe.

The posterior bifurcation of the middle cerebral artery typically has three major branches, which arise in the Sylvian fissure, loop over the insula, and go posterolaterally across the cortical surface. The first major posterior branch is the posterior parietal artery. It supplies most of the parietal lobe posterior to the central lobe. The second major branch is the angular artery, which often has a common trunk with the posterior parietal artery. The angular artery usually is the largest cortical branch of the middle cerebral artery. As it emerges from the apex of the Sylvian fissure, it runs posteriorly and superiorly to supply the posterolateral parietal lobe, the lateral occipital lobe, and the superior temporal gyrus. The third major posterior branch is the posterior temporal artery, which supplies the temporal lobe.

Venous Drainage

The major venous drainage of the central and parietal lobes consists of the vein of Trolard, vein of Labbé, the superficial middle cerebral vein, and several unnamed veins anterior to the vein of Trolard, which run laterally to medially and terminate in the superior sagittal sinus.

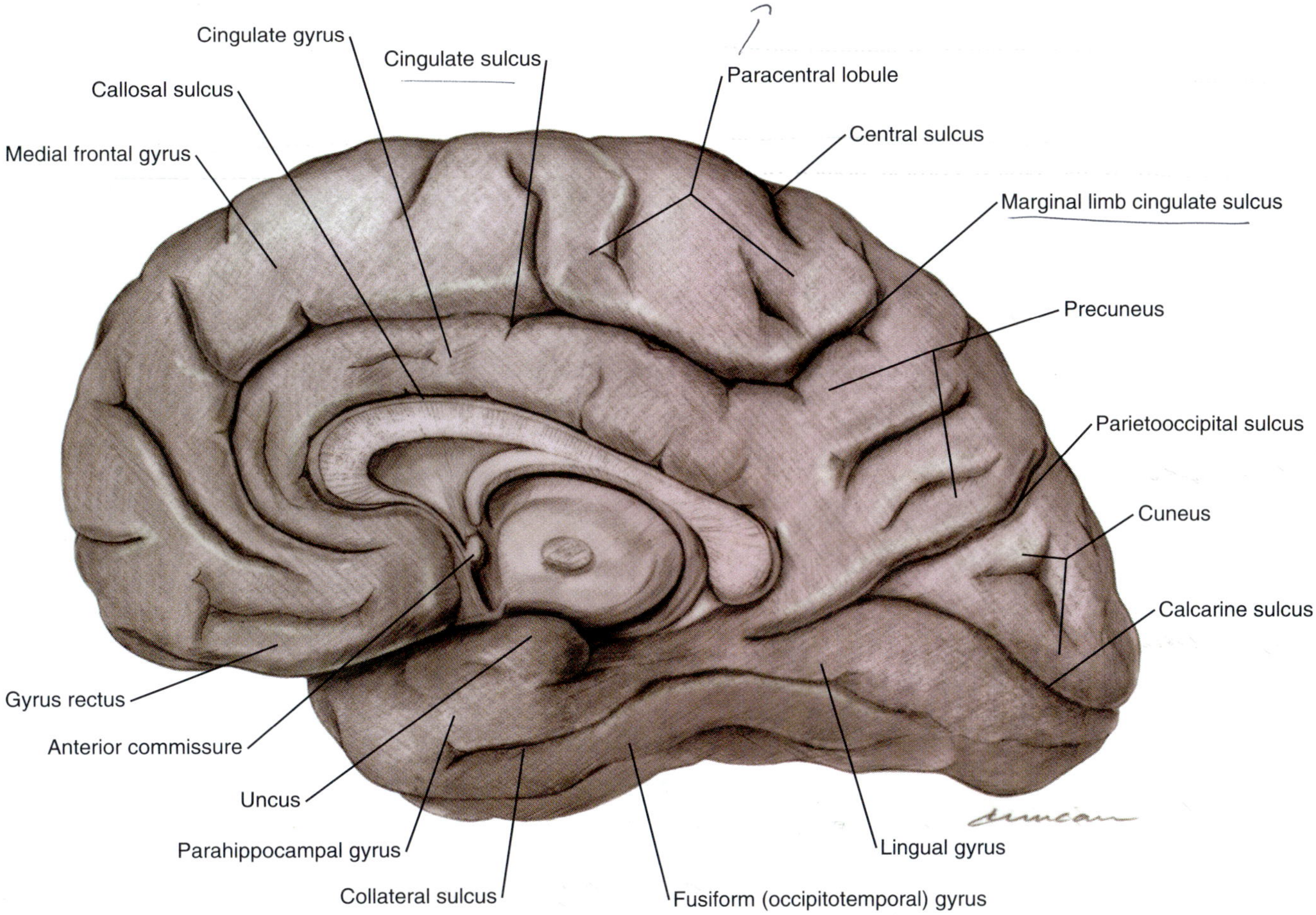
Cingulate gyrus
Cingulate sulcus
Callosal sulcus
Medial frontal gyrus
Paracentral lobule
Central sulcus
Marginal limb cingulate sulcus
Precuneus
Parietooccipital sulcus
Cuneus
Calcarine sulcus
Gyrus rectus
Anterior commissure
Uncus
Parahippocampal gyrus
Collateral sulcus
Fusiform (occipitotemporal) gyrus
Lingual gyrus

Figure 4–2.

FALCINE MENINGIOMA

Falcine meningiomas can occur anywhere along the falx cerebri in the interhemispheric fissure. They may originate along the superior sagittal sinus and invade it, even occlude it. They also may extend inferiorly to involve the inferior sagittal sinus. Some surgeons divide these tumors into outer and inner falcine meningiomas on the basis of whether the epicenter of the tumor arises from the more superficial or deeper aspect of the falx cerebri. The primary blood supply to these tumors is from the dura mater.

Before operating on a falcine meningioma, it is necessary to know the status of the adjacent sagittal sinus. Whether the sinus is patent or thrombosed has serious implications for the surgical management of the tumor. Specifically, if the sagittal sinus is thrombosed because of tumor invasion, complete tumor removal (which requires excision of the involved sagittal sinus) is likely to be tolerated. However, if the tumor has invaded the outer margin of the sinus but the sinus is still intact, the sinus must be preserved. In this circumstance, the outer leaf of the dura mater is cauterized extensively with a bipolar cautery.

In most large falcine meningiomas, a large cortical draining vein inevitably overlies the tumor exposure. It is important to preserve these cortical veins because injury to them can lead to venous hemorrhagic infarction. If the location of the cortical veins can be determined with preoperative imaging studies, a bone flap can sometimes be planned to avoid unnecessary exposure.

It is important to make sure that the bone flap exposes the superior sagittal sinus. This will decrease the amount of retraction needed along the medial surface of the hemisphere. After the superficial aspect of the tumor is exposed, the arterial blood supply originating from the falcine dura mater is cauterized. Thereafter, the tumor is debulked and collapsed into the operative field. An arachnoid plane is usually present between the tumor and the callosomarginal and pericallosal arteries.

Important to know, wether superior sagittal sinus is patent!
If thrombosed → full excision will be tolerated

→ angiography!!

Mostly pericallosal and callosomarginal arteries protected by arachnoid sheath.

4. A. differentiation between inner and outer falx meningioma!

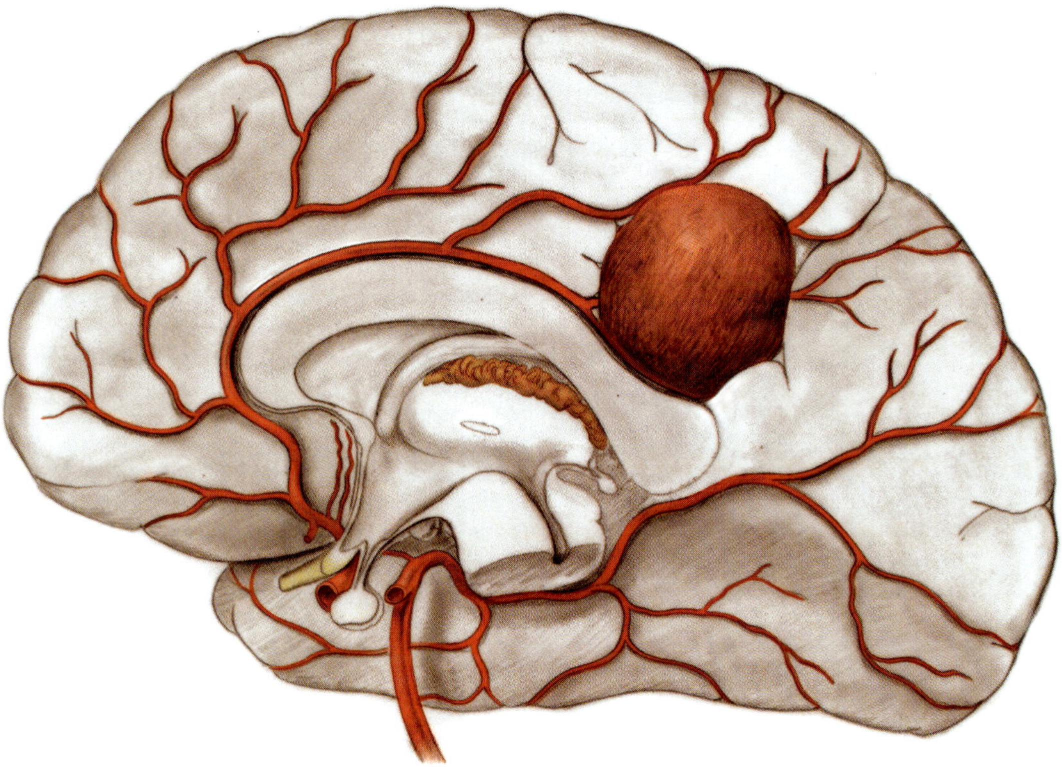

Figure 4–3.

In this example, the epicenter of the meningioma is located along the inferior aspect of the falx cerebri. The precuneus overlies the tumor. The primary blood vessel at risk is the pericallosal artery and its branches.

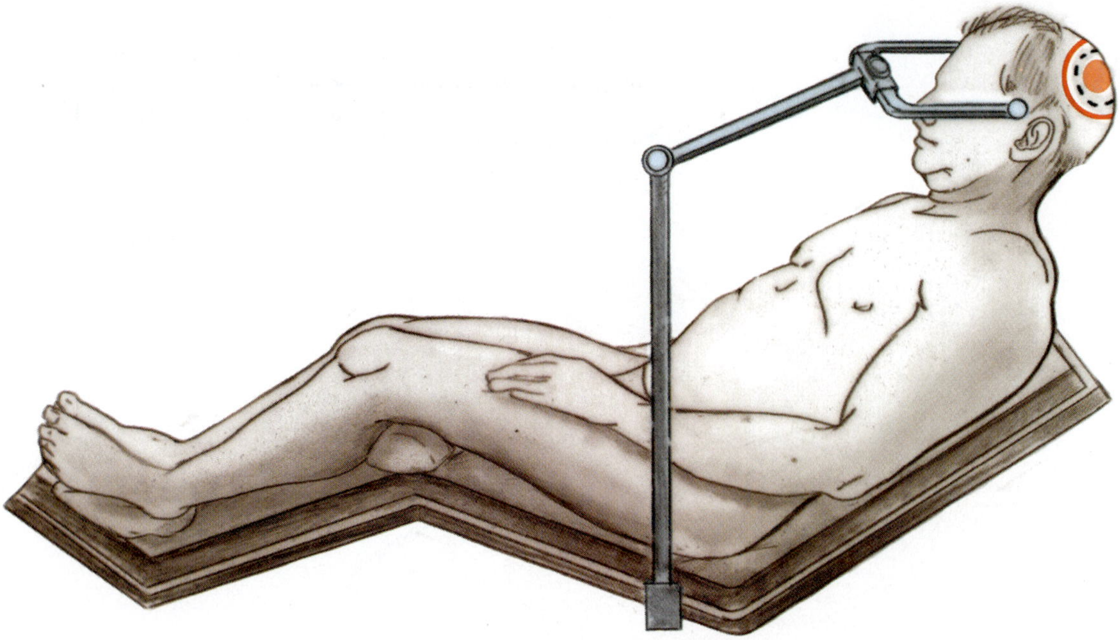

Figure 4–4.

Step 1. Several head positions are good for exposing a posterior falcine meningioma. The slouch position is ideal because it provides good orientation, promotes venous drainage, and provides a good line of sight for visualizing the relationship between the superior sagittal sinus, dura mater, and tumor, thereby minimizing the need for lateral retraction of the brain. An alternative position is the prone position, with a slight-to-moderate reverse Trendelenburg position to promote venous drainage.

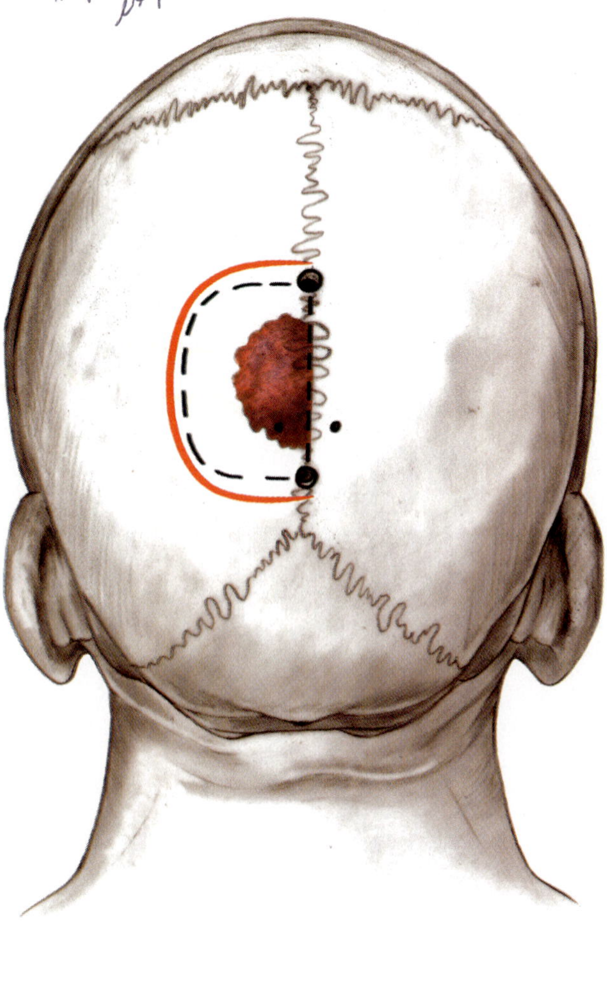

Figure 4–5.

Step 2. It is important to make sure that the bone flap *(dashed line)* is far enough medial to expose most of the width of the superior sagittal sinus. There are several options for making this medial bone cut. As illustrated here, two bur holes are made. A Penfield #3 dissector is used to dissect the dura mater off the underside of the bone flap. The cut can be made with a craniotome, a Gigli saw, or a high-speed air drill with a diamond bur. This medial cut should be made last, so that if an inadvertent tear is made in the superior sagittal sinus the bone flap can be removed quickly to achieve hemostasis.

Figure 4–6.

Step 3. It is important to tack the dura mater to the margins of the surrounding bone. Any oozing of the blood from the superior sagittal sinus is best controlled by placing a piece of absorbable gelatin sponge (Gelfoam) or muscle on top of the sinus and holding it in place by tacking a reflected flap of dura mater.

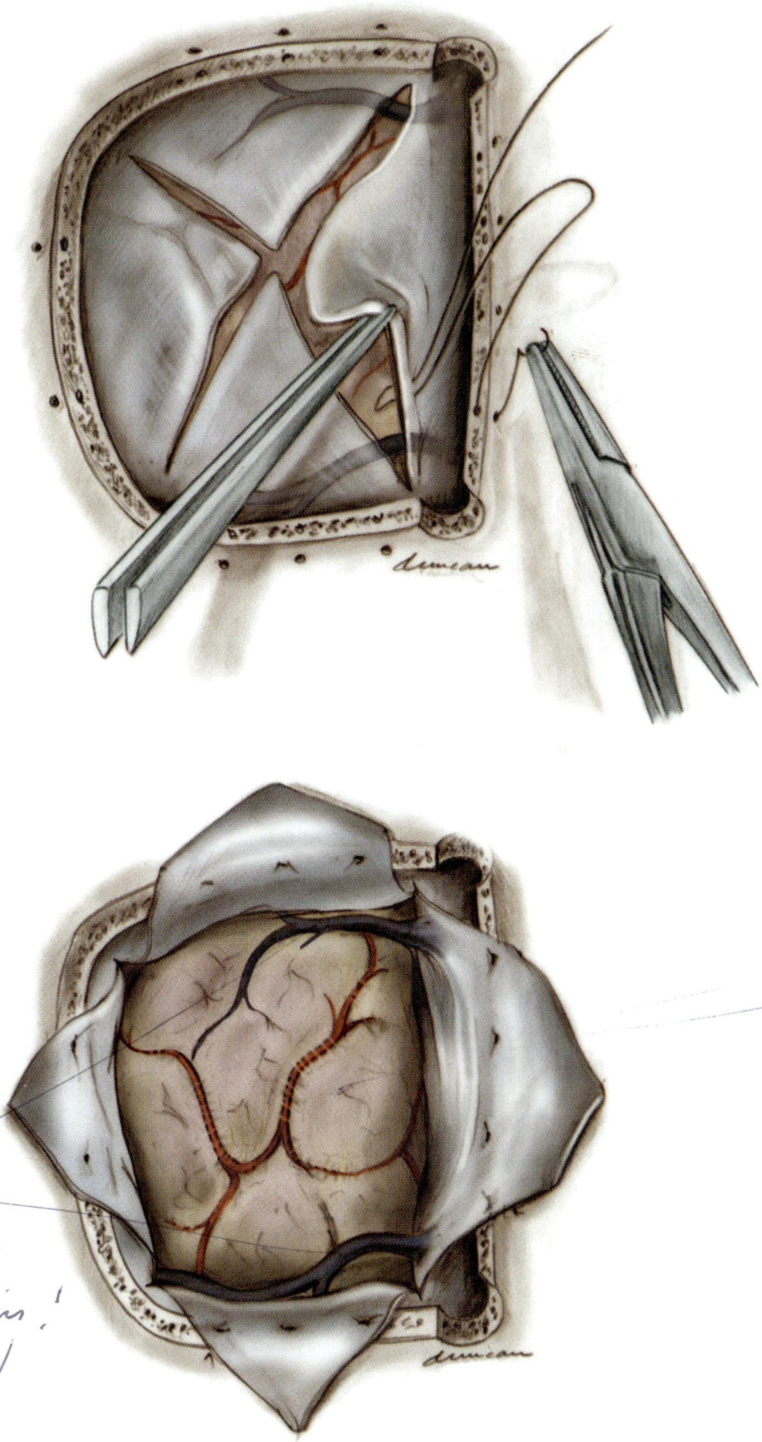

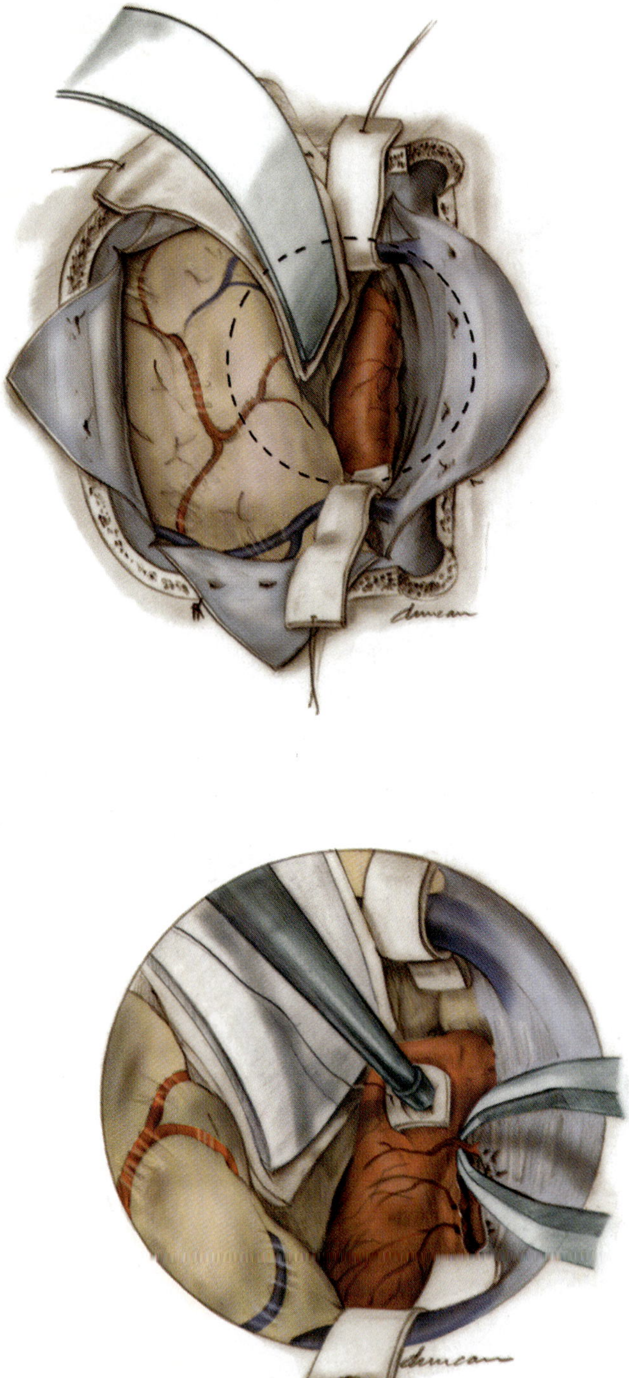

Figure 4–7.

Step 4. In this example, the line of sight to the tumor lies between two cortical surface draining veins, which must be protected. The ensheathing arachnoid should be left intact. A piece of absorbable gelatin sponge can be placed around the junction of the vein with the sagittal sinus to buttress it. The medial hemisphere is lined with hemostatic fabric (Surgicel) and cottonoids (Americot) and then gently retracted laterally.

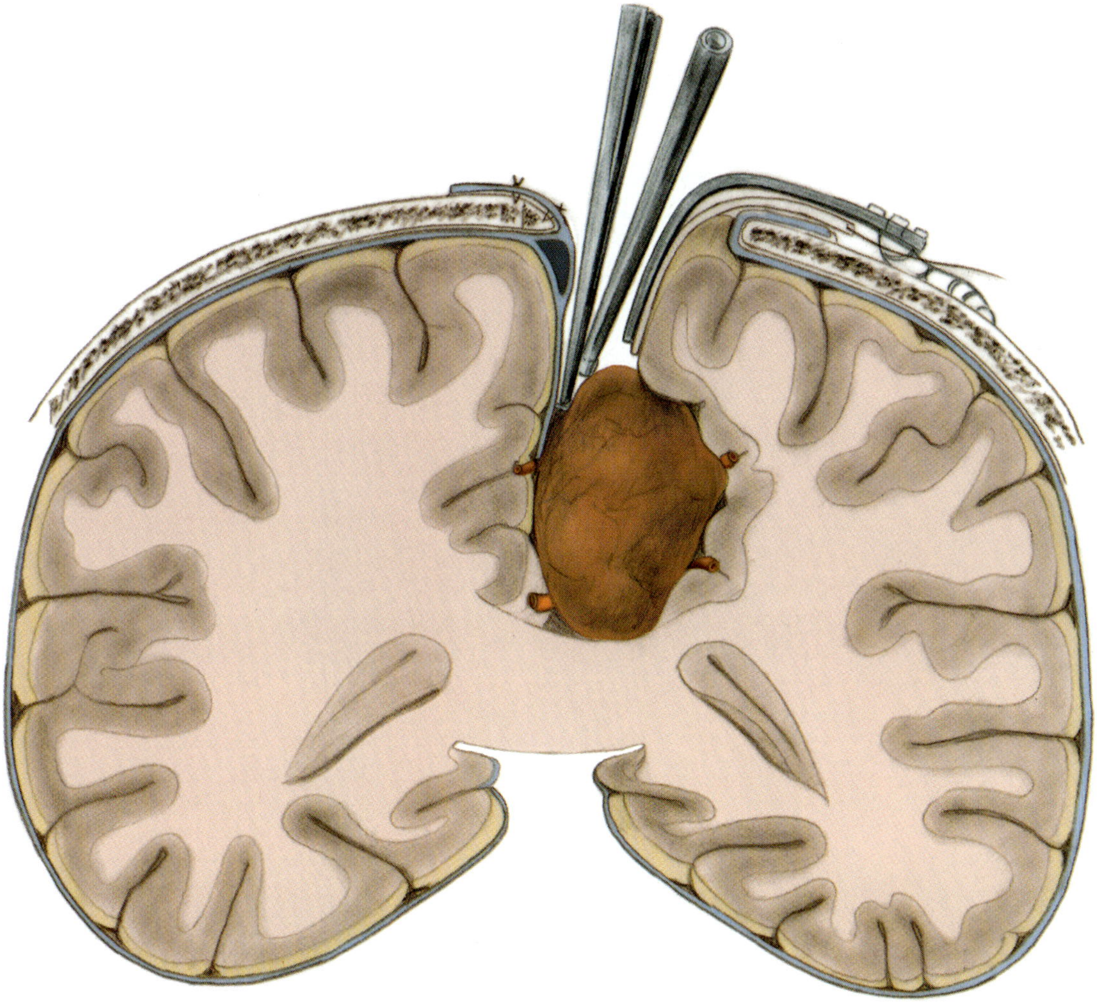

Figure 4–8.

Step 5. The blood supply to the meningioma from the falx cerebri is cauterized with a bipolar cautery.

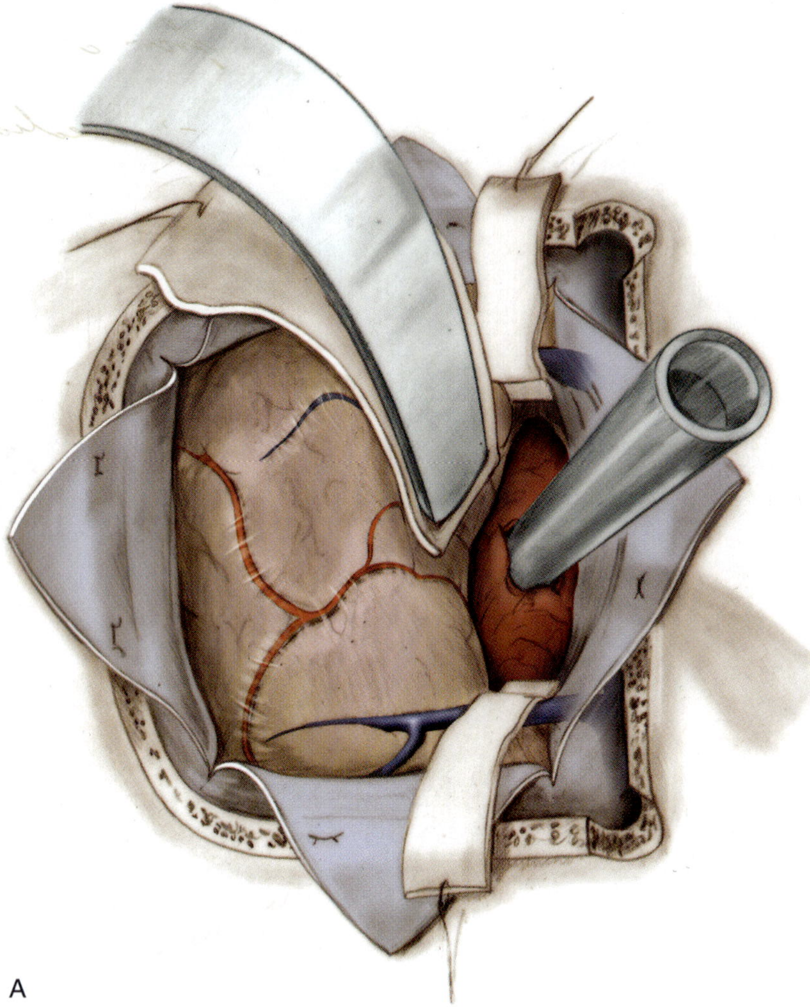

A

Figure 4–9.

A–C, The tumor is debulked with a bipolar cautery, curets, and Ultrasonic aspirator. Next, the tumor is collapsed into the operative field. This will lessen the degree of hemispheric brain retraction. Arachnoid usually overlies the pericallosal artery and its branches. Respecting this arachnoid will help preserve these vessels.

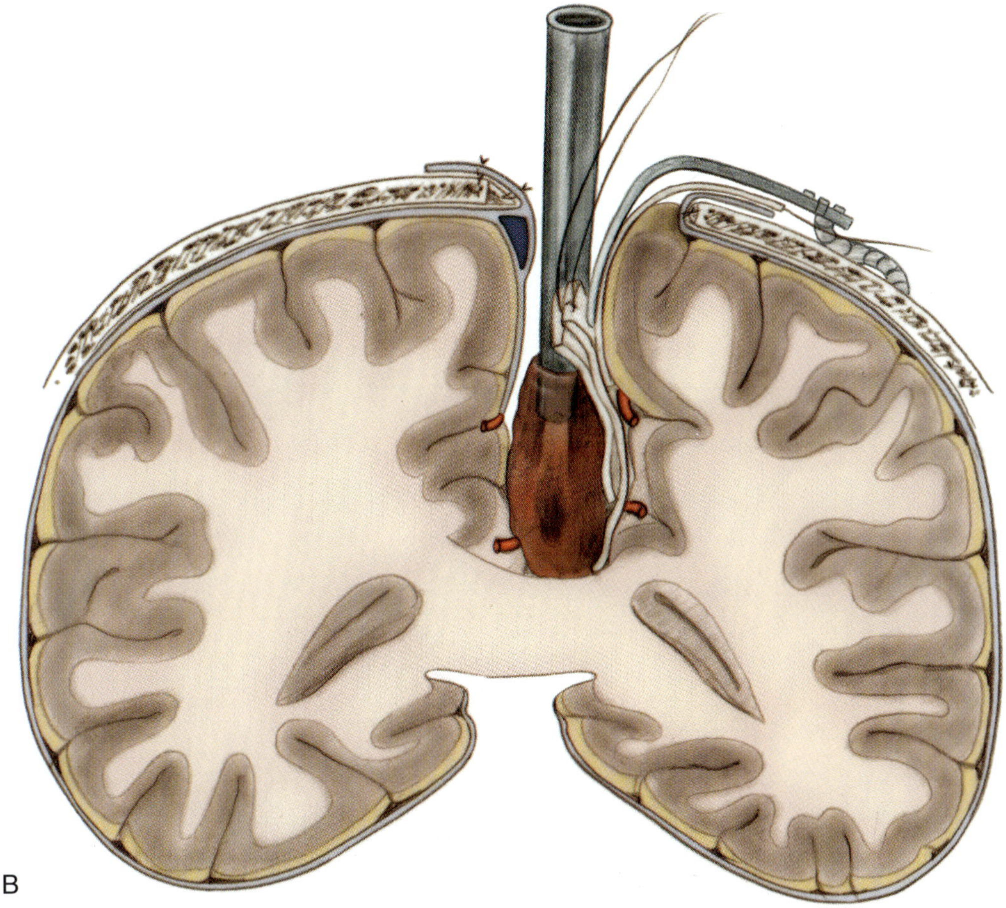

B

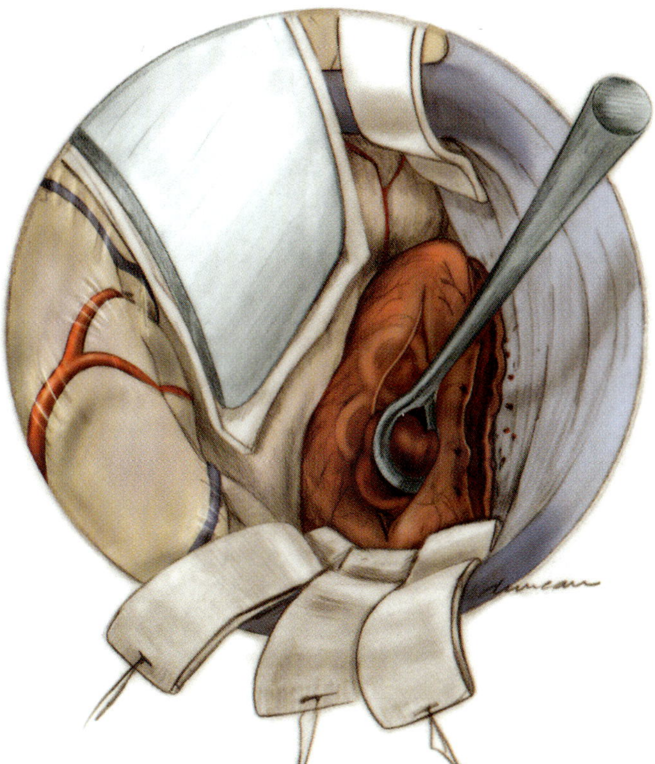

C

Figure 4–9 *Continued*

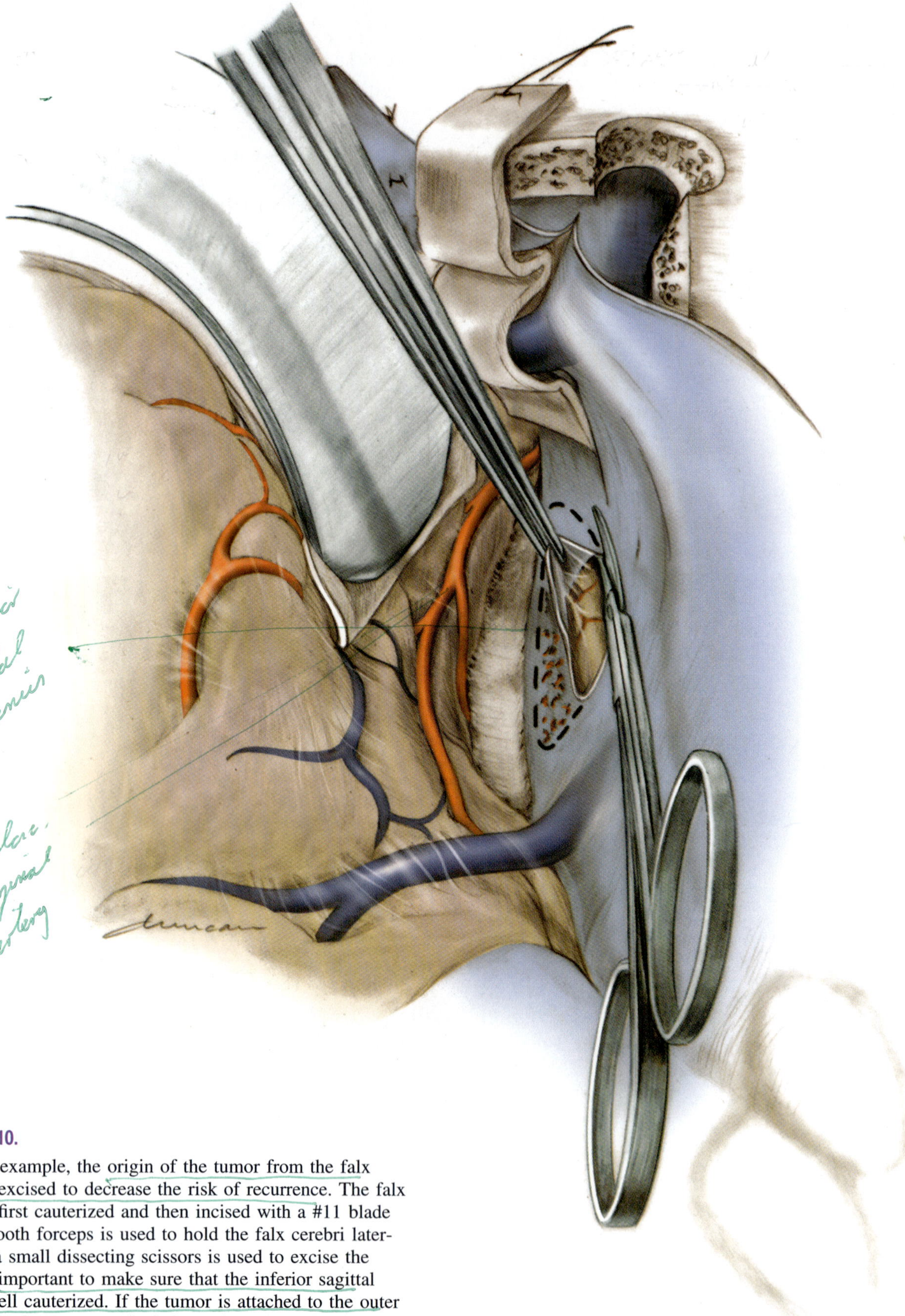

Figure 4–10.

In this example, the origin of the tumor from the falx cerebri is excised to decrease the risk of recurrence. The falx cerebri is first cauterized and then incised with a #11 blade knife. A tooth forceps is used to hold the falx cerebri laterally, and a small dissecting scissors is used to excise the falx. It is important to make sure that the inferior sagittal sinus is well cauterized. If the tumor is attached to the outer dura mater of a patent sagittal sinus, the only option is aggressive bipolar cauterization.

CONTRALATERAL APPROACH TO FALCINE MENINGIOMA

Rarely, a large cortical vein may overlie the middle of the operative field, putting the vessel at high risk during tumor removal. In this circumstance, the surgeon may consider a contralateral approach to the tumor. The advantage of the contralateral approach is that the major cortical draining vein will be protected. However, this approach has at least two disadvantages. First, both cerebral hemispheres are placed at risk, because to achieve exposure the opposite hemisphere must be retracted. Second, the relationship of the tumor to the pericallosal and callosal marginal arteries is less well visualized than with an ipsilateral approach.

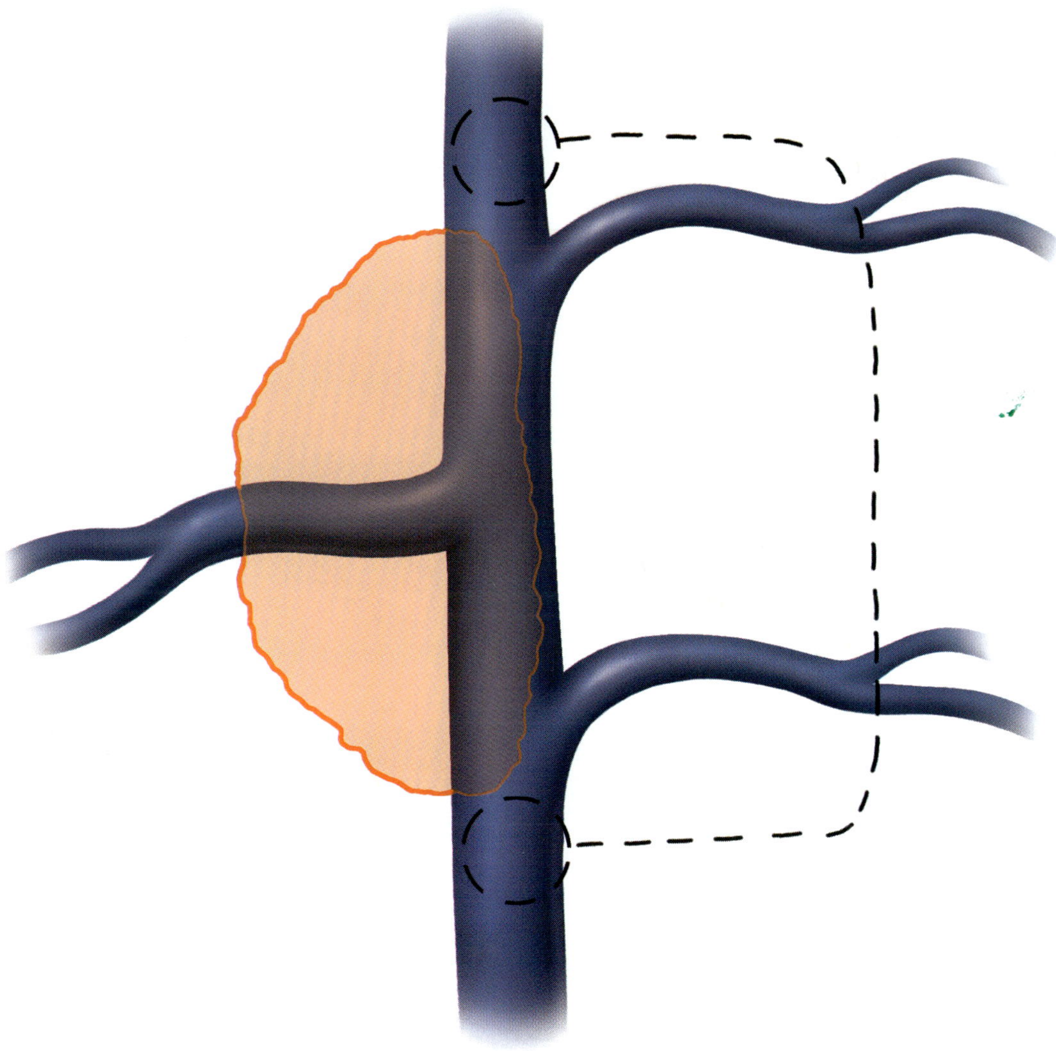

Figure 4–11.

The bone flap has been planned to consider all three cortical draining veins.

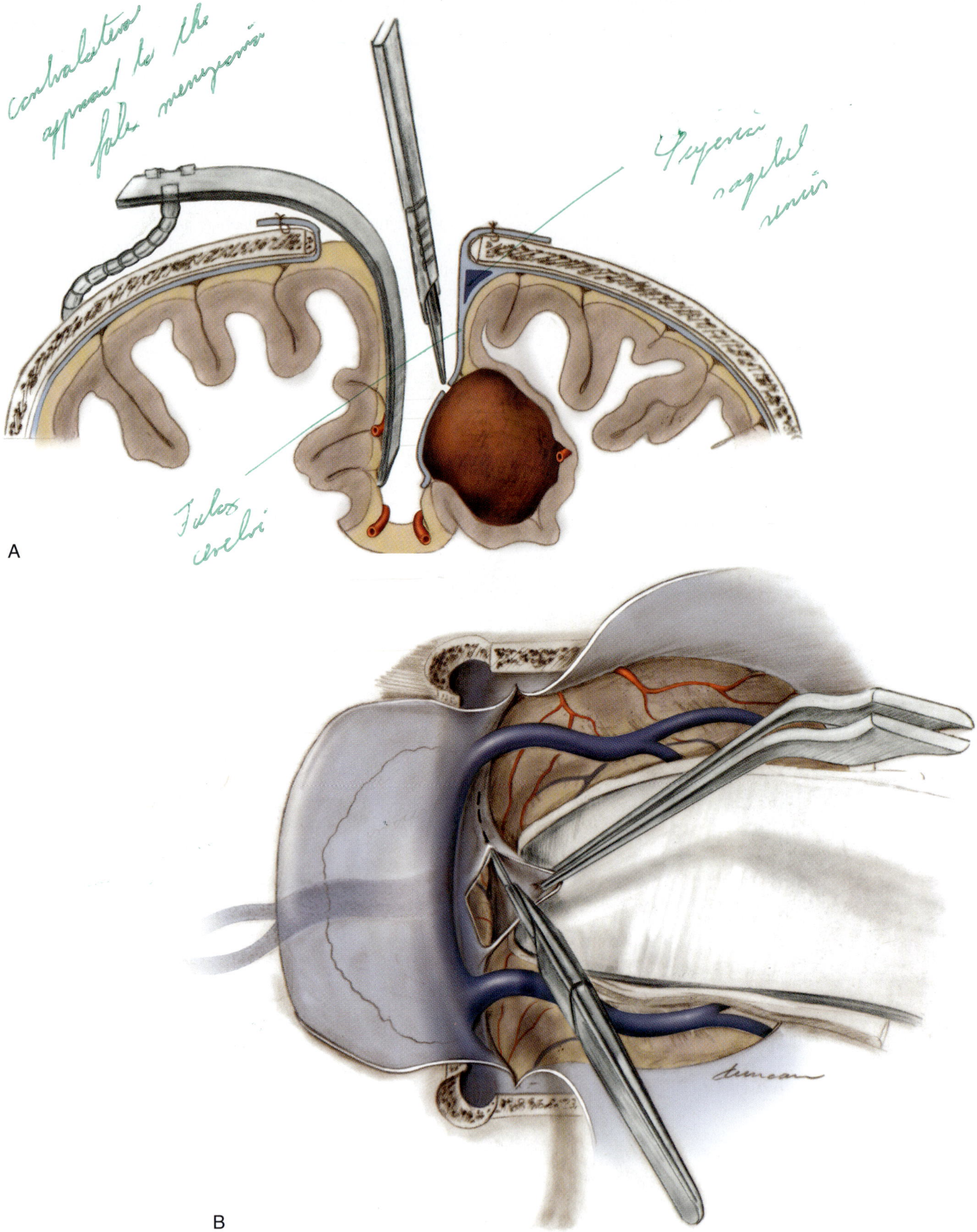

Figure 4–12.

A and *B*, The contralateral hemisphere is gently retracted. The falx cerebri is incised below the superior sagittal sinus. Typically, the falx cerebri is red and vascular. Palpating the falx cerebri with a small spatula will give the surgeon a tactile sense about where the tumor is located. The falx cerebri is cauterized and incised with a #11 blade knife. A bipolar cautery is used to sever the attachments and the blood supply between the tumor and the falx cerebri.

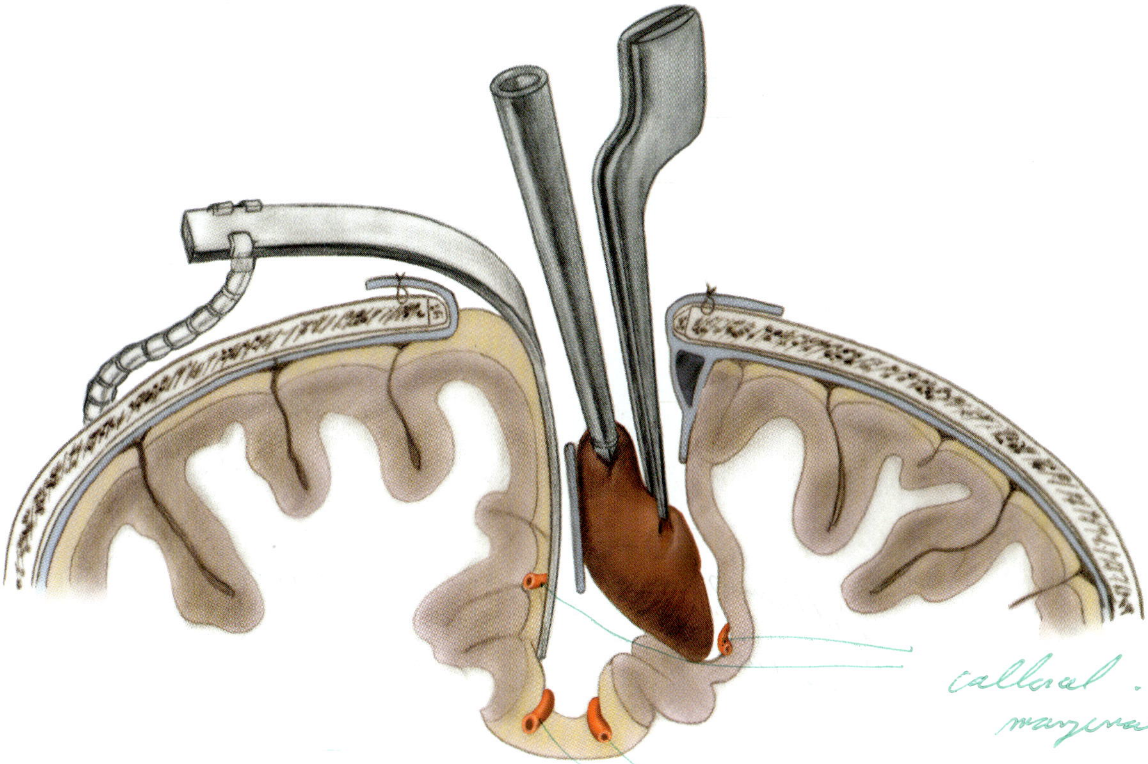

Figure 4–13.

As with all meningiomas, it is important to debulk the tumor and to collapse the tumor capsule into the operative field. Although the final "surgical specimen" is less impressive in size than the original tumor, aggressive debulking minimizes the need for brain retraction.

TRIGONE VENTRICULAR TUMOR

The most common neoplasms of the trigone of the lateral ventricle are meningiomas and choroid plexus papillomas. Other tumors, including gliomas of all types, subependymomas, and giant cell astrocytomas, are more frequent more anteriorly in the body of the ventricle. Still more anteriorly, adjacent to the septum pellucidum and the foramen of Monro, colloid cysts and central neurocytomas are more frequent.

Meningiomas originate from the arachnoid cap cells of the choroid plexus and tela choroidea. The most common site for an intraventricular meningioma is the trigone, although this tumor may rarely arise in the third ventricle or, least commonly, in the fourth ventricle. Choroid plexus papillomas, in comparison, occur most commonly in the fourth ventricle, with extensions into the cerebellopontine angle, or in the trigone.

The primary blood supply of both meningiomas and choroid plexus papillomas is derived from the anterior and posterior choroidal arteries. Three surgical approaches can be considered for gaining access to tumors in the trigone. The first and oldest is through the middle posterior temporal gyrus. The advantage of this approach is that it allows the surgeon good access to the anterior blood supply of the tumor along the choroid plexus. A disadvantage is that an incision in the posterior left temporal lobe has the risk of causing language dysfunction. Also, significant brain retraction must be applied to visualize the posterior aspect of the trigone.

The second approach is through the superior parietal lobule. This is described in the sequence of illustrations shown here. The disadvantage of this approach is that a cortical incision must be made in the parietal lobe. A cortical incision in and retraction of the left superior parietal lobule is well tolerated, with little risk of injury; however, a significant incision in or retraction of the right superior parietal lobule can cause the patient marked spatial disorientation postoperatively. Another disadvantage is that it is more difficult to access the anteriorly located blood supply of the tumor.

The third approach is an interhemispheric-splenial approach through a parietooccipital craniotomy, with an incision in the junction between the precuneus and the splenium of the corpus callosum. The advantage of this approach is that it does not require an incision in the temporal or parietal cortex. The disadvantage is that moderate lateral retraction of the cerebral hemisphere may be required to access both the lateral margin of the tumor and the anterior and inferior blood supply from the choroid plexus.

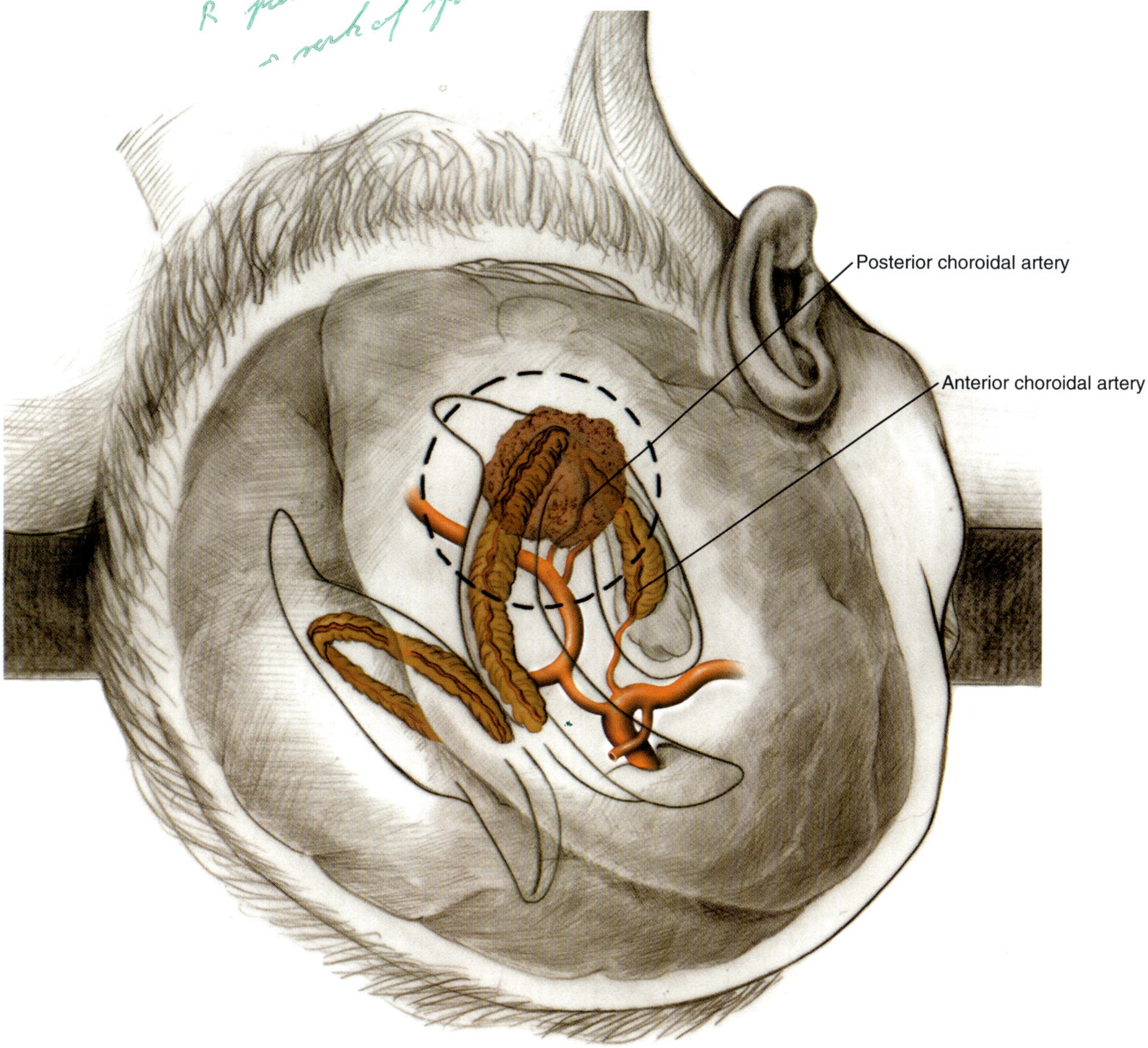

Figure 4–14.

This drawing shows a tumor in the trigone and its relationship with its arterial blood supply from the anterior and posterior choroidal arteries. The surgical approach chosen for this tumor is a stereotactic craniotomy through the left superior parietal lobule.

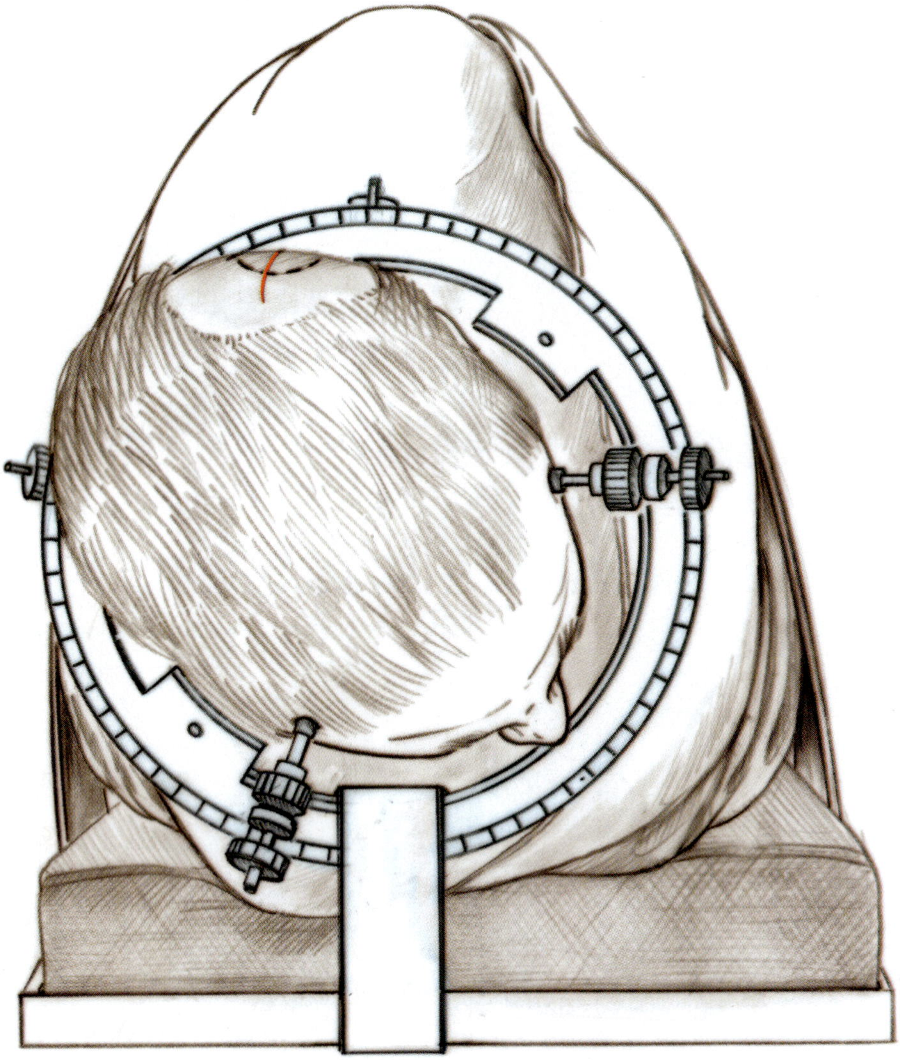

A

Figure 4–15.

Step 1. The use of stereotaxis, either frame (*A*) or frameless (*B*), allows the surgeon to plan many surgical approaches that allow the best line of sight for the surgeon with the least amount of brain retraction and cortical disruption.

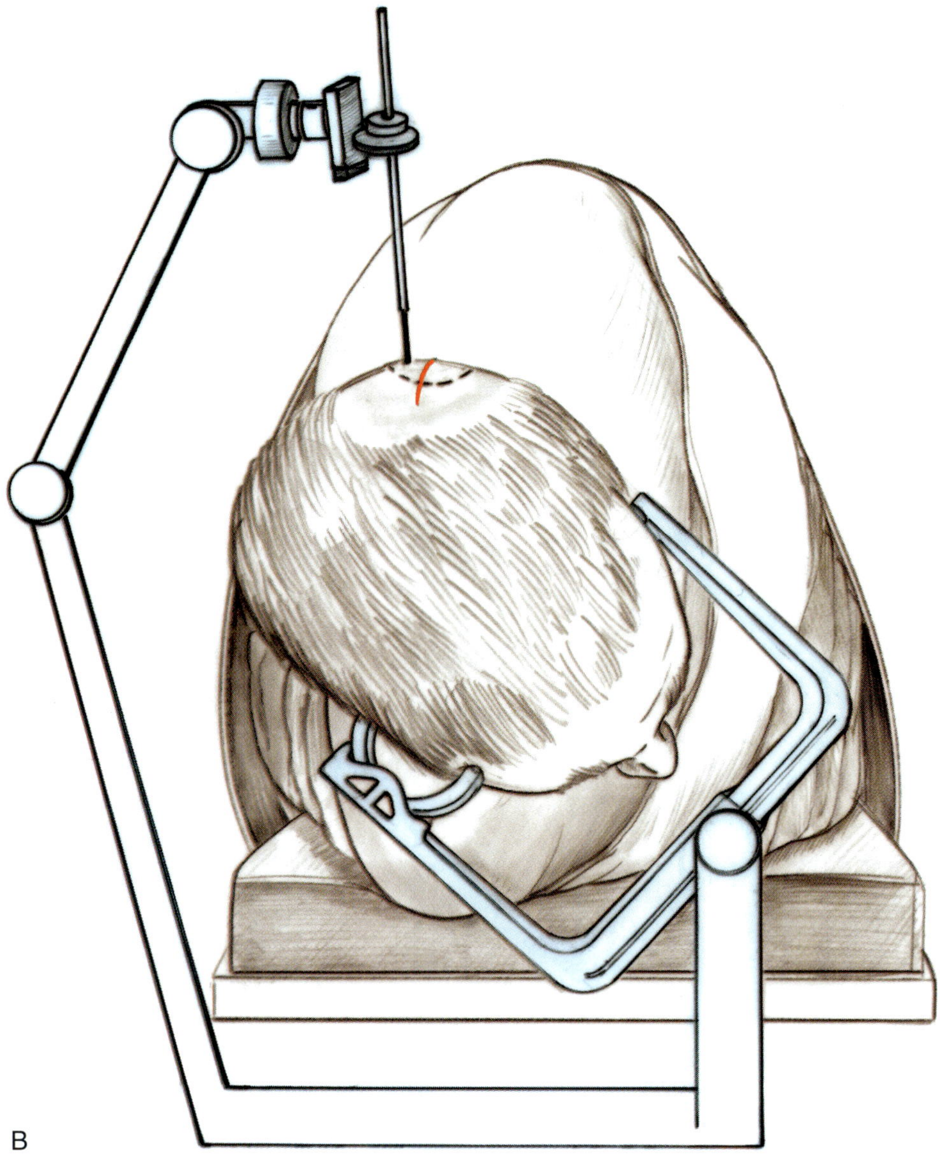

B

Figure 4–15 *Continued*

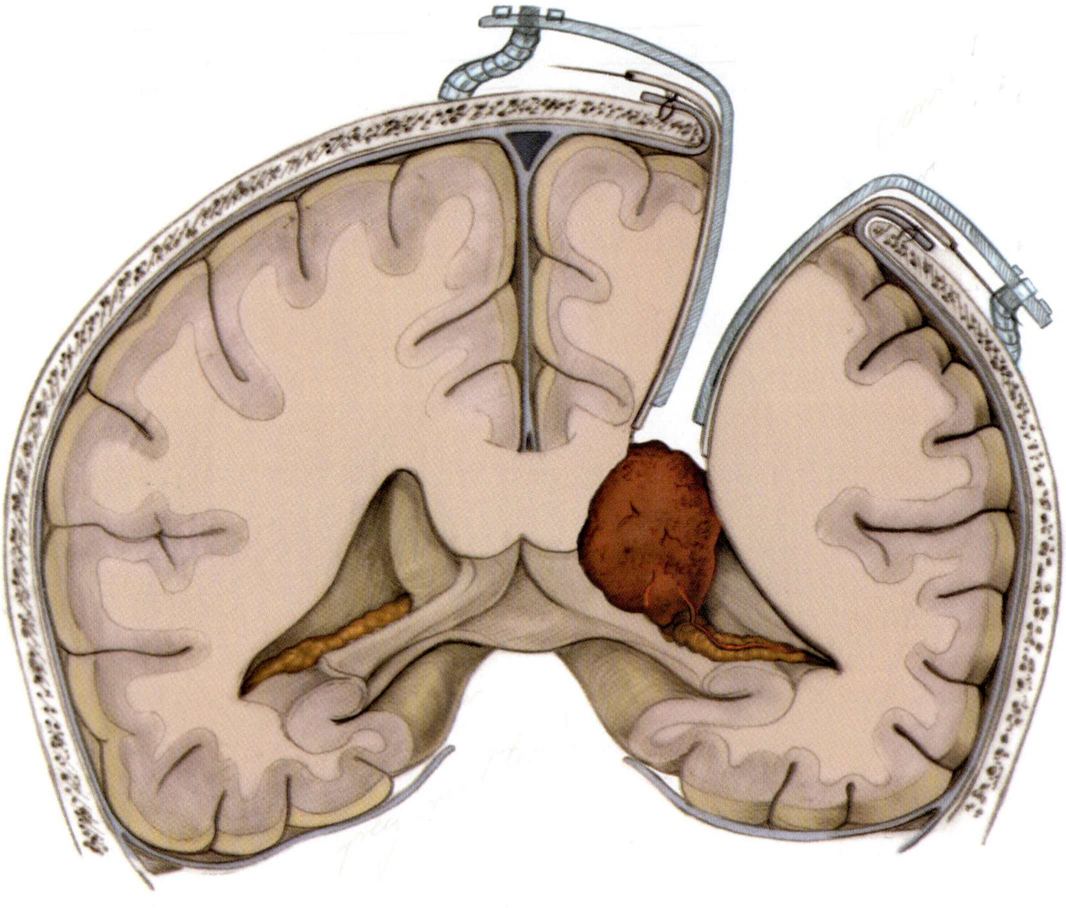

Figure 4–16.

Step 2. When planning a stereotactic approach through the superior parietal lobule, the surgeon can often see on magnetic resonance imaging a deep or enlarged sulcus around the planned trajectory. If such a sulcus is present, the surgeon should use it during the approach to the lateral ventricle. This intrasulcal approach lessens the degree of cortical injury. As depicted here, the disadvantage of the superior parietal approach is that the arterial blood supply of the tumor is deep and more difficult to access than it is with the traditional middle temporal gyrus approach.

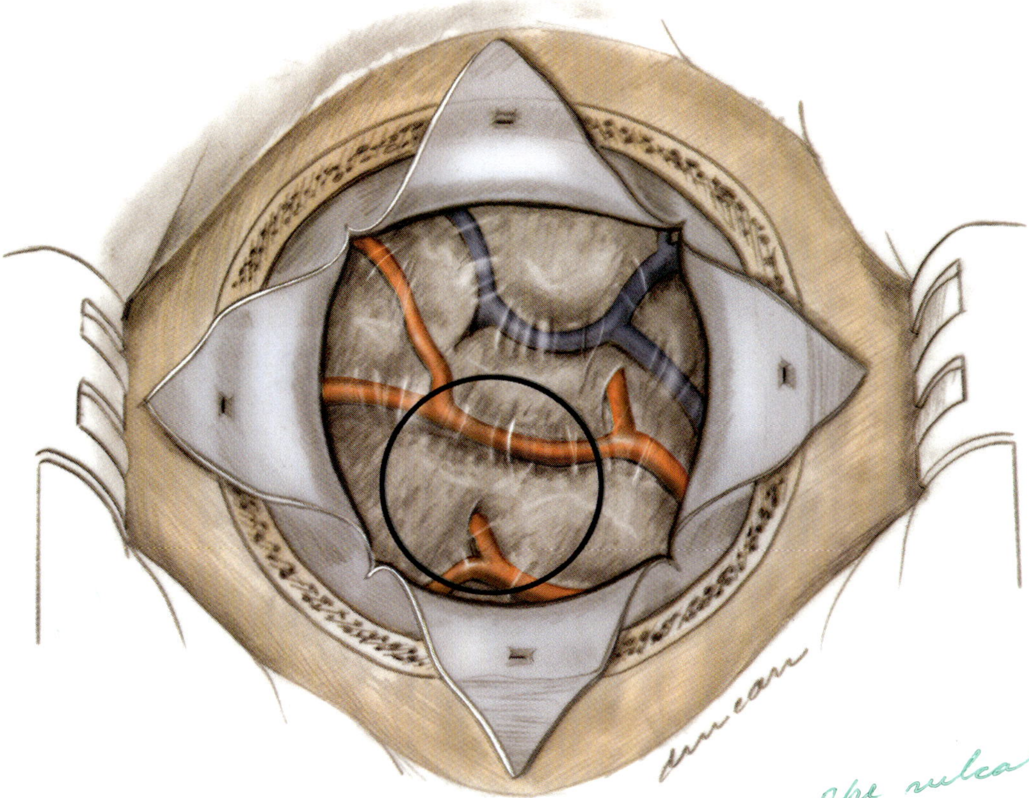

A

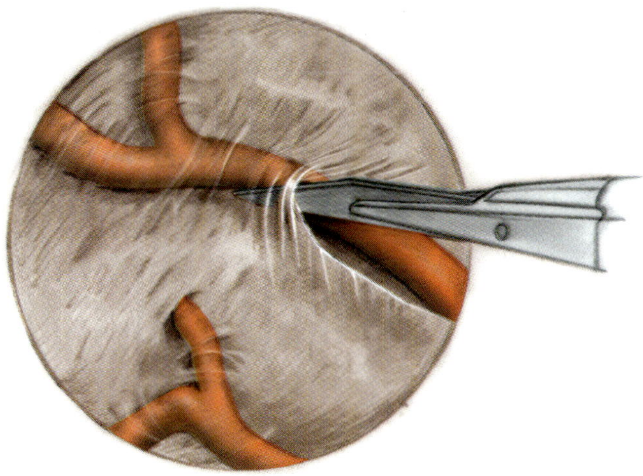

B

Figure 4–17.

Step 3. *A*, A trephine craniotomy is shown: with the use of an operating microscope, the sulci are inspected for an intrasulcal approach. In this example, there is an appropriate sulcus just posterior to a cortical vessel. All the cortical arteries and veins in this region should be protected. Opening the sulcus is similar to dividing the Sylvian fissure.

B, A sharp #11 blade knife is used to stab the arachnoid and to lift it up as it is severed. A microscissors can be used to continue the cut in the arachnoid that overlies the sulcus. Usually, about a 1.5-cm length of sulcus has to be exposed to obtain adequate exposure of the lateral ventricle.

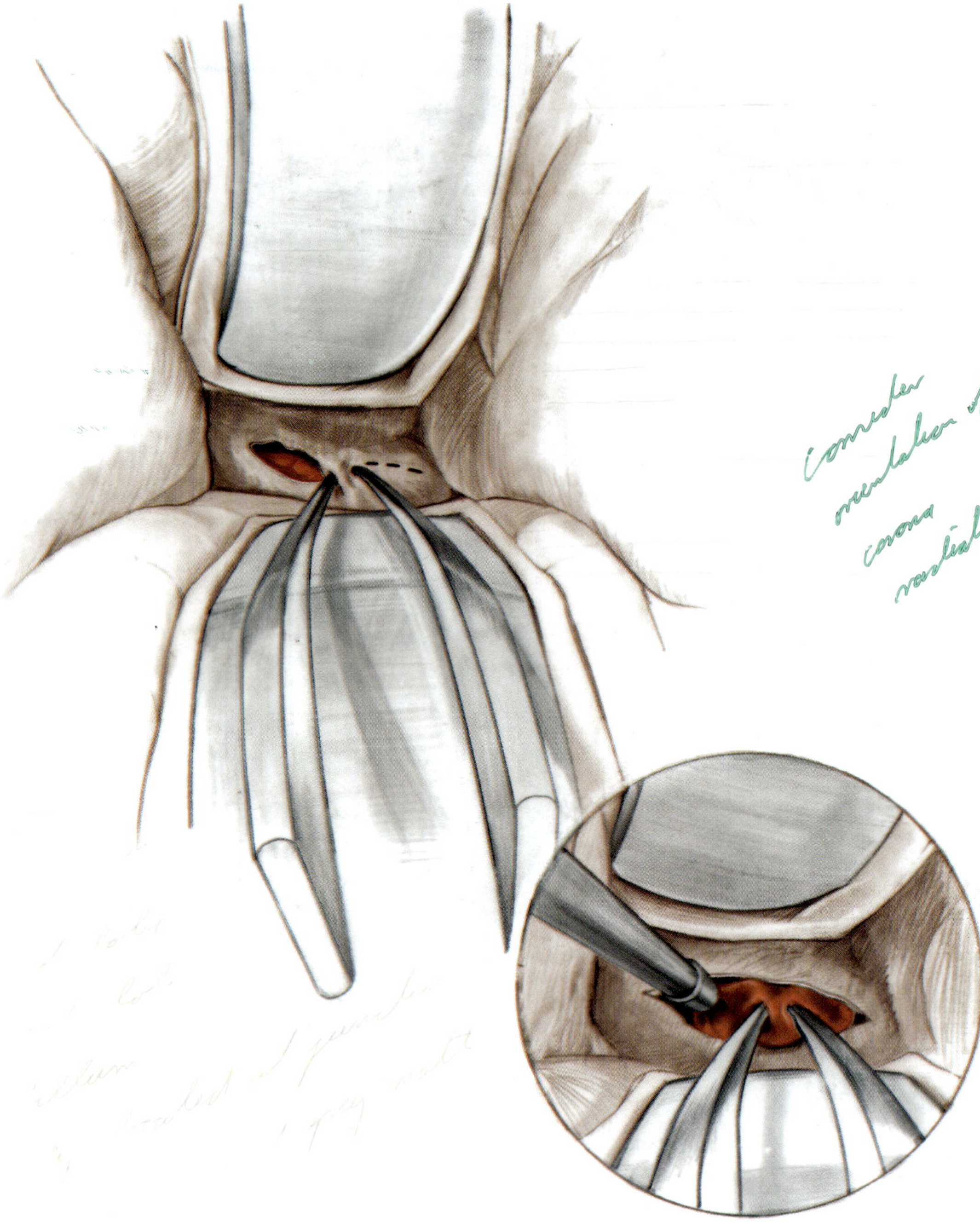

Figure 4–18.

Step 4. After the arachnoid has been incised, bipolar cautery is used to spread the sulcus until the deeper arcuate fibers ("U fibers") of the white matter are encountered. Two self-retaining retractors are used to retract the adjacent gyri after they are lined with hemostatic fabric and cottonoids. The white matter is divided using the bipolar cautery and suction. Whenever using an intrasulcal approach to a deep-seated tumor, it is best to consider the direction of the radiations within the corona radiata, which is being entered. Dividing the white matter parallel with, or in the plane of, these radiations will decrease the risk of neurologic injury.

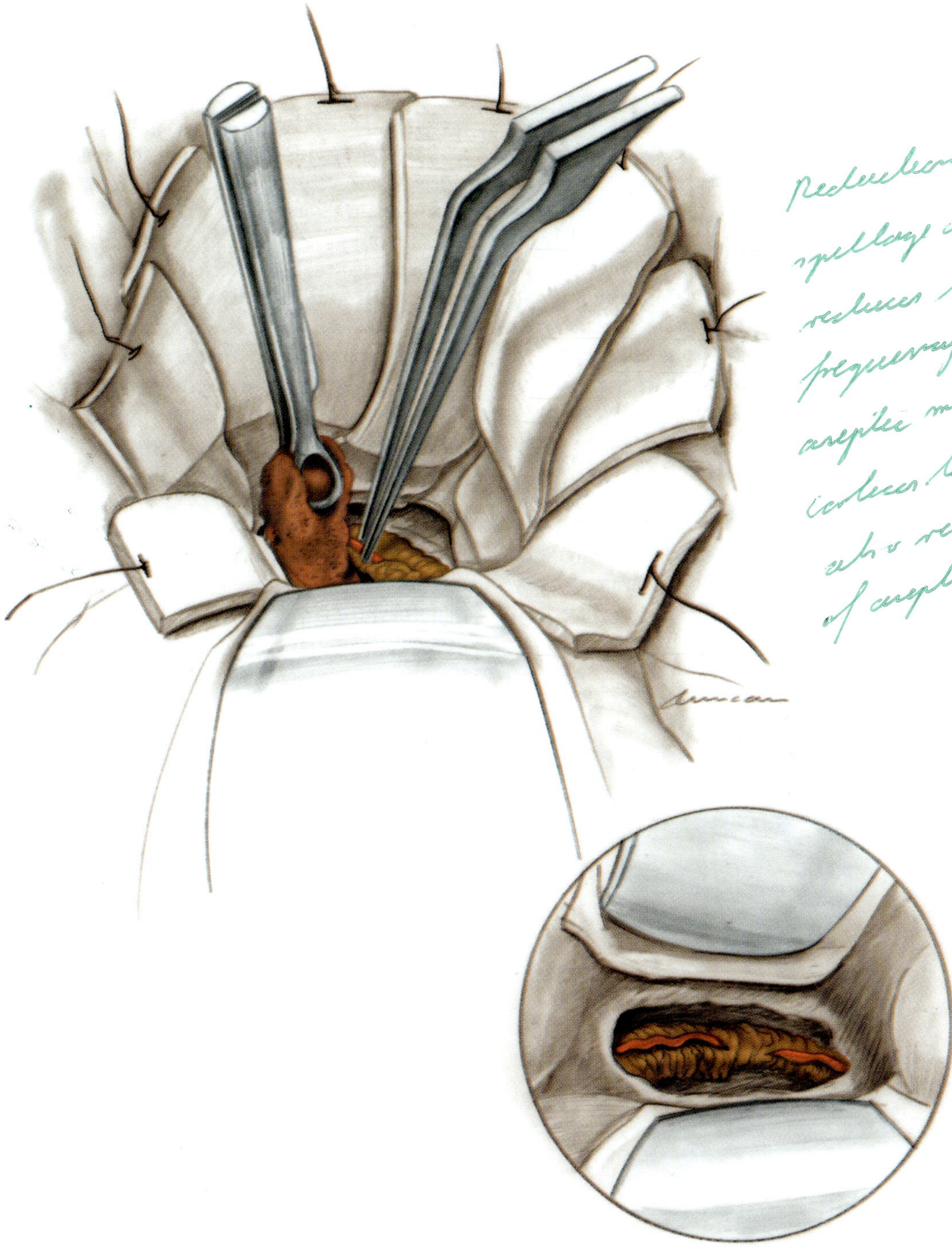

Figure 4–19.

Step 5. As the tumor is approached, the ependyma of the lateral ventricle is seen bulging out into the surgical field; it forms a thin cap over the tumor. After the ependyma has been incised, the tumor capsule becomes visible. The tumor is centrally debulked, using primarily the bipolar cautery and suction. By using the bipolar cautery instead of curets or an ultrasonic aspirator, hemostasis will be earlier and better, which has the advantage of decreasing the amount of blood entering the lateral ventricle. Spilling of blood into the lateral ventricle may cause aseptic meningitis postoperatively. The administration of corticosteroids perioperatively lessens the severity of such aseptic meningitis. After a space has been created between the ependyma and the tumor capsule, cottonballs or cottonoids can be placed deep to help prevent blood from spilling into the lateral ventricle. After the tumor has been resected, it is important to irrigate the lateral ventricle copiously with warm saline solution. After the tumor has been debulked, its capsule is collapsed into the surgical view. The anteroinferior feeding arteries arising from the choroid plexus can be cauterized and divided. The tumor is debulked further and subsequently extracted from the lateral ventricle.

LESIONECTOMY—METASTATIC TUMORS AND CAVERNOUS HEMANGIOMAS

The most common cerebral metastases occur from neoplasms of the lung, breast, skin, kidney, and gastrointestinal tract. Their distribution within the central nervous system mirrors the volume of brain compartments and lobes. Therefore, the most common locations are the frontal lobe, the parietal lobe, and the cerebellum. In the cerebral cortex, these tumors tend to occur at the junction of the gray and white matter and they typically are well circumscribed. Accordingly, a localized stereotactic craniotomy is ideal for resecting these subcortical tumors. In the central or parietal lobe, the major issue is the relationship of the tumor to eloquent cortex.

Cavernous hemangiomas are vascular malformations that at surgery are lobulated and well demarcated; they have a reddish-brownish mulberry appearance. They tend to grow like slow neoplasms and have repetitive microhemorrhages that often cause seizures. Cavernous hemangiomas are found in all lobes of the cerebral cortex, the brain stem (with a propensity to localize to the pons), and the basal ganglia. Surgical resection of cortical lesions usually produces good results; for example, lesionectomy alone produces seizure control in 80 to 90 percent of patients. Surgical resection of cavernous hemangiomas is technically easy because they are well-circumscribed, low-flow lesions that do not have a significant arterial blood supply. Furthermore, there is a good plane of separation between the cavernous hemangioma and the surrounding gliotic plane that results from the repetitive hemorrhages. In large cavernous hemangiomas, the various cysts can be decompressed to collapse the wall of the tumor into a small operative field. The major difficulty with resection of small cortical cavernous hemangiomas is their location and relationship to eloquent cortex. For this reason, use of stereotactic guidance and the intrasulcal approach described below is ideal for resecting both metastatic tumors and cavernous hemangiomas.

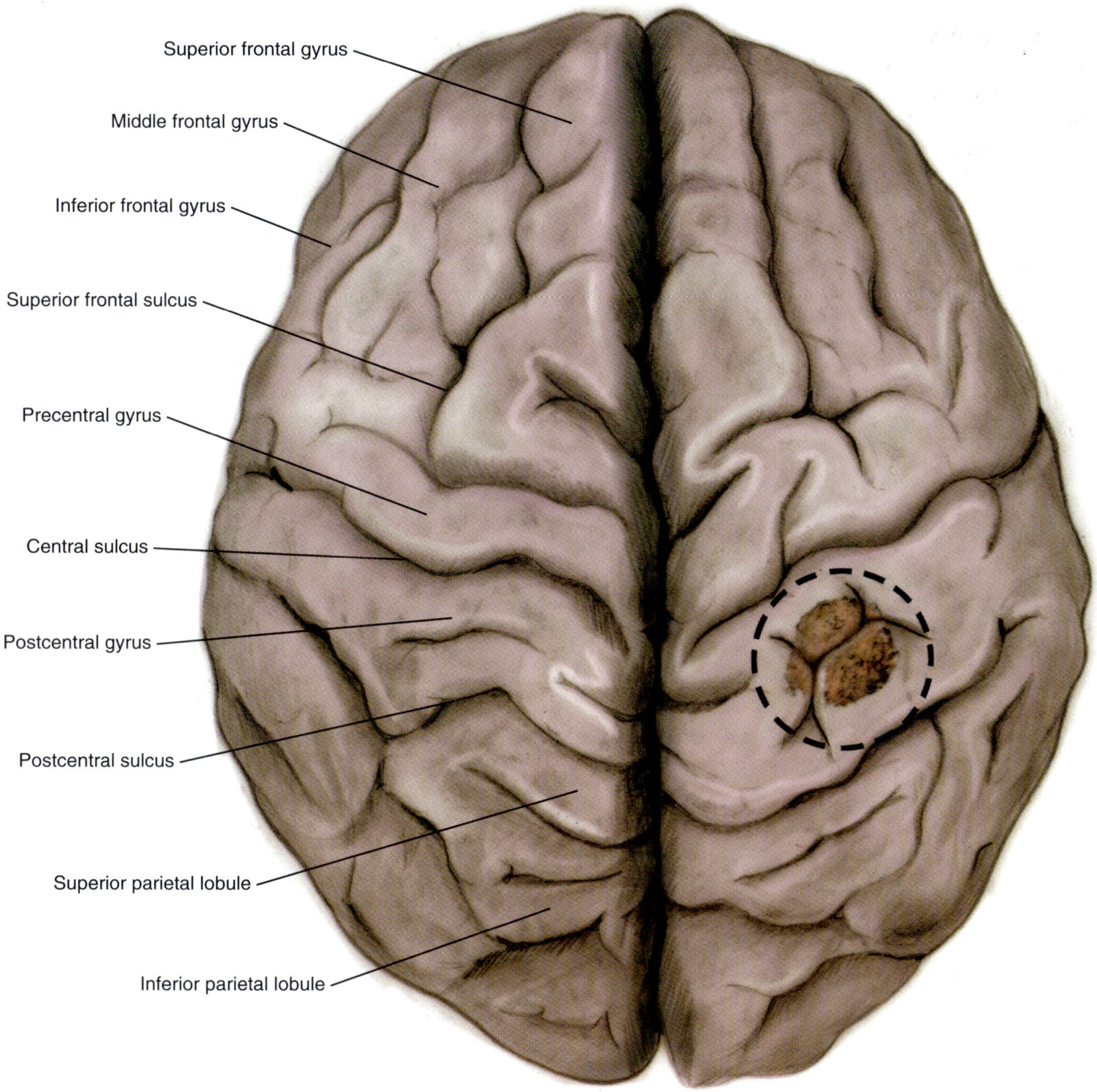

Figure 4–20.

Step 1. A stereotactic trephine craniotomy is made using a frameless system; therefore, the skull is held rigid.

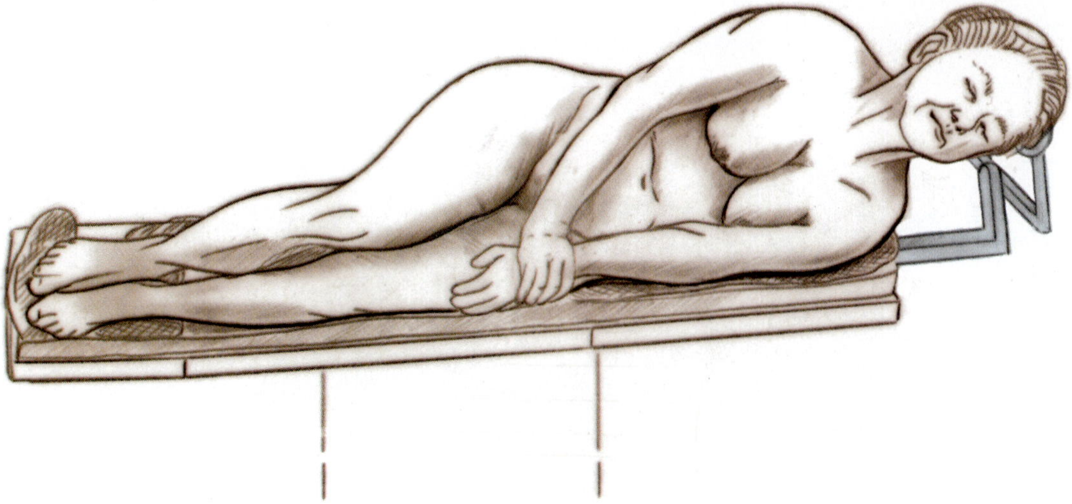

Figure 4–21.

Two good head positions are the lateral decubitus position, with the head parallel to the floor, and the supine position, with the head straight up. Both of these positions are helpful in surgical orientation. If the lateral decubitus position is chosen, it is important to make sure that the neck is not overrotated. Placing towels or blankets under the shoulder relieves tension on the neck.

Figure 4–22.

Step 2. The dura mater is tacked to the bone margins and opened. In most metastases, the subcortical location may be difficult to visualize by inspection of the surface with the operating microscope. Therefore, stereotaxis helps to minimize the size of the craniotomy and brain exposure. Because the exact location of the precentral gyrus usually is not clear, as in this example, somatosensory evoked potential monitoring is used to identify the central sulcus. The wave reversal points to the location of the central sulcus. In this example, electrode "A" is on top of the precentral gyrus, "B" represents the central sulcus, and "C" identifies the postcentral gyrus. An alternative to this type of mapping is direct electrical stimulation of the cerebral cortex with assessment of motor function, with the patient either awake or given general anesthesia without inhalation anesthetics. As preoperative functional imaging improves, this type of intraoperative stimulation or mapping may not be necessary.

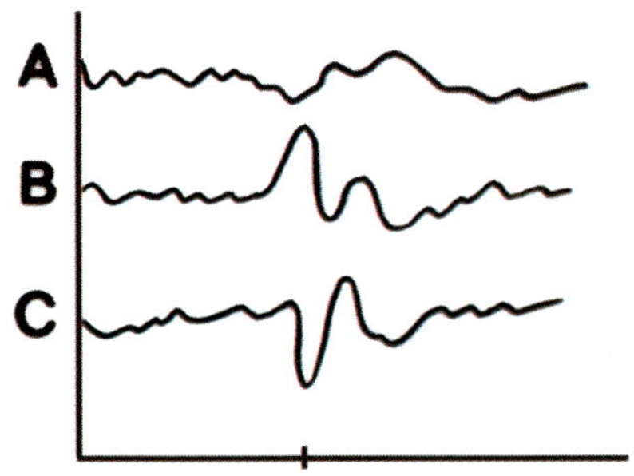
A
B
C

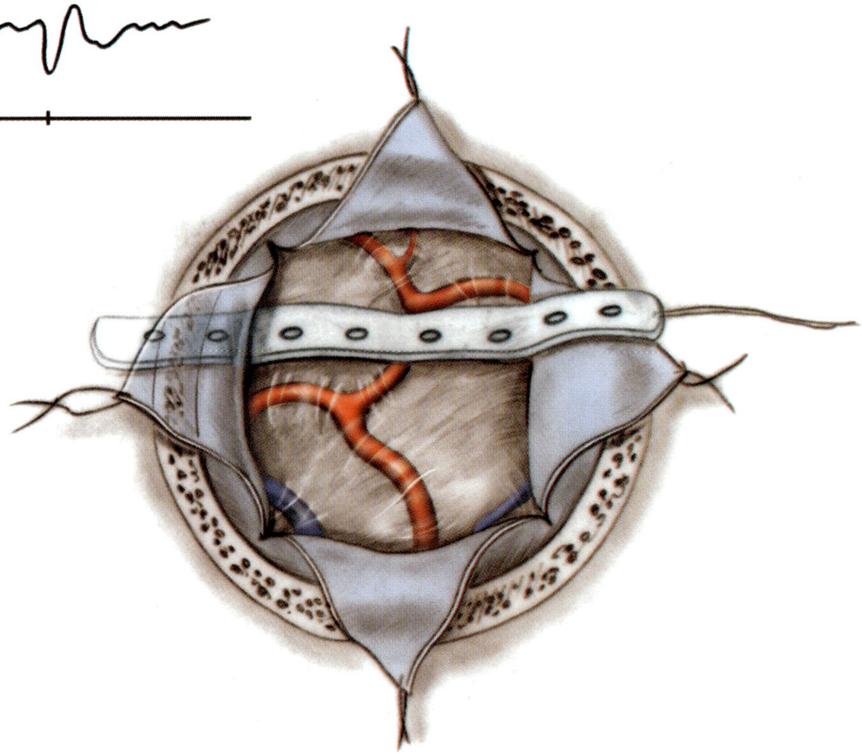

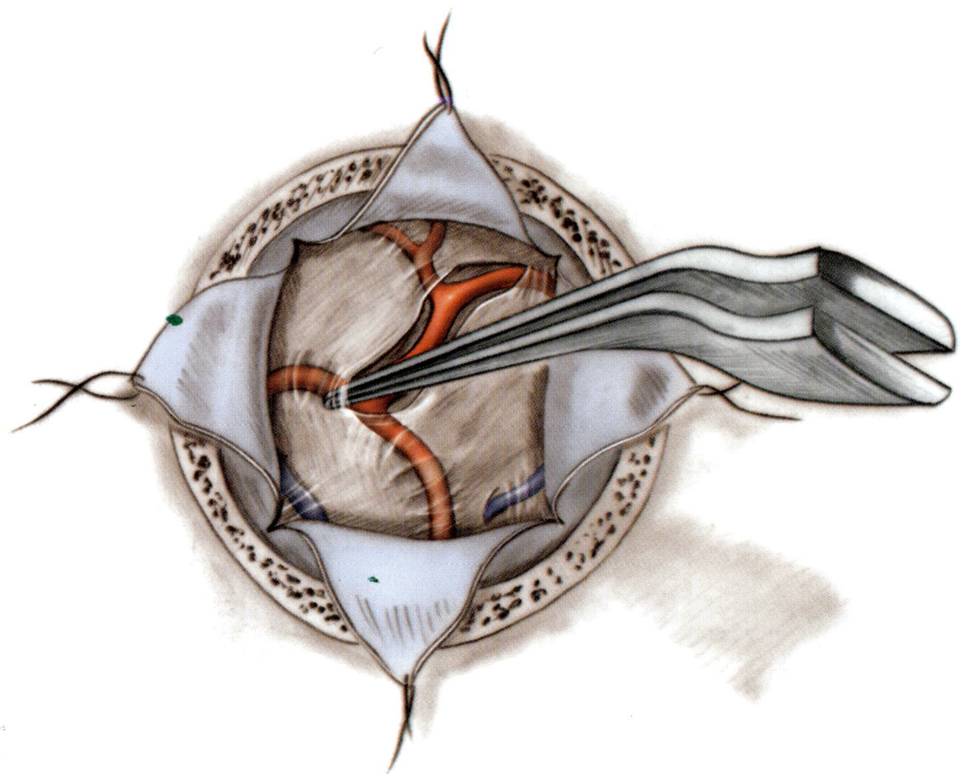

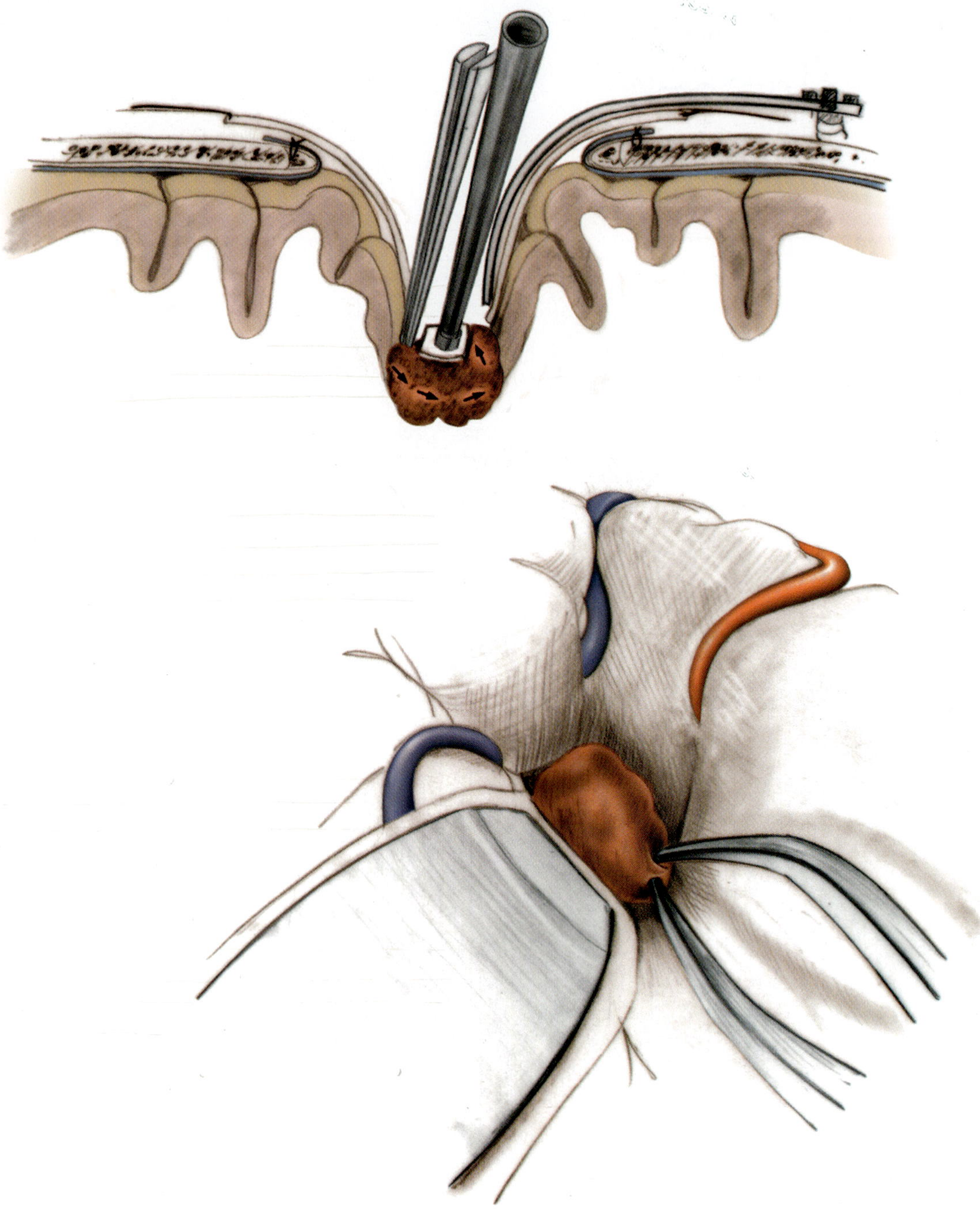

Figure 4–23.

Step 3. An intrasulcal approach to the tumor has been chosen. The arachnoid is incised with a #11 blade knife and spread with the bipolar cautery forceps. The adjacent cortical vein is preserved. The intrasulcal approach is extended down to the "U" fibers, where a metastatic tumor is typically encountered. If necessary, small self-retaining retractors can be used to spread the sulcal opening. A bipolar cautery and suction are used to separate the tumor from the adjacent brain parenchyma.

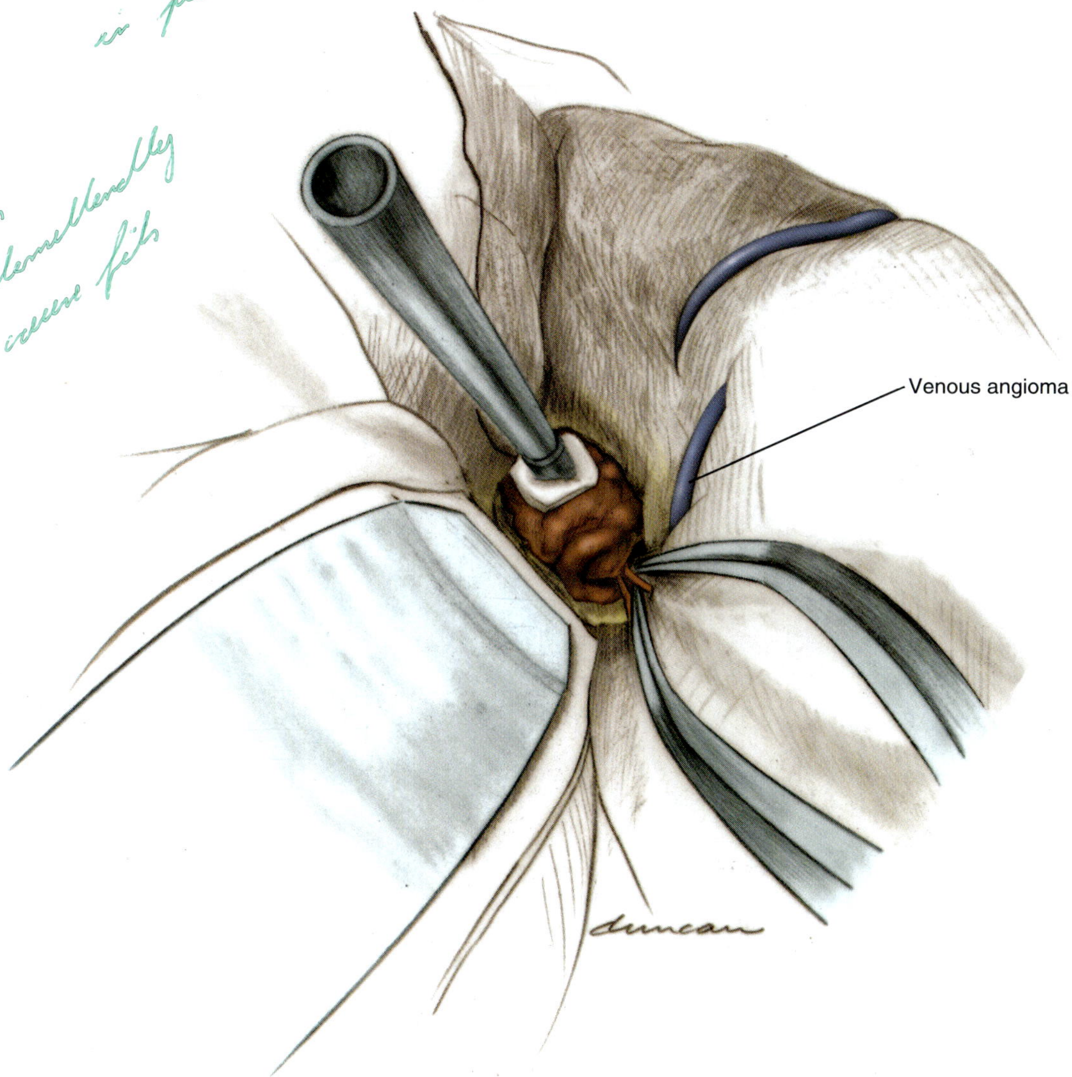

Figure 4–24.

Several small feeding arteries usually enter a cavernous hemangioma. They should be cauterized and divided individually. Remember that irrigating the tips of the bipolar cautery helps while these vessels are being cauterized, as in resection of an arteriovenous malformation. In the example shown here is an adjacent venous angioma that should be preserved.

TRIGONE ARTERIOVENOUS MALFORMATION

Arteriovenous malformations of the trigone and body of the lateral ventricle derive their primary arterial blood supply from the anterior and posterior choroidal arteries and branches off segments P_1, P_2, and P_3 of the posterior cerebral artery. The primary venous drainage is through subependymal veins, which drain into the basal vein of Rosenthal. If the arteriovenous malformation extends into the lateral ventricle, it usually involves the posterior limb of the internal capsule and the thalamus, and the venous drainage also includes the posterior septal and thalamostriate veins, which drain into the internal cerebral vein and the basal vein of Rosenthal. The location of the intraventricular arteriovenous malformation dictates the surgical approach. An arteriovenous malformation or tumor located in the posterior medial quadrant of the trigone can be resected through a posterior transcallosal approach, using a midline parietooccipital craniotomy. A lesion located more laterally or posteriorly in the lateral ventricle can be accessed better through an intrasulcal transcortical approach through the posterior parietal lobe. An inferolaterally located lesion that involves the temporal horn is best approached transcortically through the middle temporal gyrus. In many ventricular arteriovenous malformations, the initial presentation is that of a cerebral hemorrhage, with extension of the blood clot into brain parenchyma. The blood clot can be used to the surgeon's advantage. First, it often dissects some aspects of the margin of the arteriovenous malformation from the surrounding parenchyma. Second, if the hemorrhage approaches the cortical surface, it often provides a route for reaching the arteriovenous malformation with little risk of causing more neurologic injury.

Some general principles need to be followed for all resections of arteriovenous malformations regardless of their location. Yasargil originally emphasized the importance of the location of an arteriovenous malformation, whether it was superficial or deep, supratentorial or infratentorial. Subsequently, Spetzler and Martin introduced a grade I to V classification that considers size, relationship to eloquent cortex, depth, location, and venous drainage.

First, as in any operation, it is mandatory that the surgeon have a realistic assessment of the expected risk of resecting the arteriovenous malformation. This is especially true with the advent of alternative options for treatment, including stereotactic irradiation.

Second, preoperative embolization is beneficial for several reasons. The process of embolization forces the surgeon and interventionalist to thoroughly study and understand the three-dimensional anatomy of the arteriovenous malformation. Selective Amytal injections can help determine vessels "en passage" that perfuse eloquent cortex. There is no doubt that multiple-stage preoperative embolization facilitates intraoperative hemostasis. Also, staged preoperative embolization of a large arteriovenous malformation allows time for the brain vasculature to reequilibrate to alterations in cerebral blood flow. This decreases the risk of postoperative hemorrhage and hyperperfusion complications.

Third, during the surgical resection, it is important to have clean irrigating bipolar cautery. Because blood vessels of an arteriovenous malformation do not have a normal media, cauterization of the smaller vessels is difficult. Small microclips are useful for occluding small blood vessels along the ependymal surface that are difficult to coagulate. Small wire clips are also useful for temporarily occluding suspected "en passage" blood vessels.

Fourth, it is important to inspect the surface anatomy of the arteriovenous malformation before resection and to identify the draining veins. These draining veins contain arterialized blood. The best intraoperative confirmation that an arteriovenous malformation has been completely resected is resolution of this arterialized venous blood. At least one major draining vein should be preserved throughout the resection of the malformation and cauterized last. After the arteriovenous malformation has been resected, the entire operative bed should be thoroughly inspected under the operating microscope. Although some surgeons prefer to resect arteriovenous malformations with the patient mildly hypotensive, it is mandatory that systolic blood pressure be normal when the postoperative bed is inspected.

Fifth, in patients with large arteriovenous malformations, the systolic blood pressure is decreased to approximately 90 mm Hg for 48 to 72 hours postoperatively. Cerebrovascular autoregulation may not be normal in the cerebrovasculature surrounding the resected arteriovenous malformation; therefore, controlling the patient's postoperative blood pressure will decrease the risk of postoperative hemorrhage.

Sixth, in very large complex arteriovenous malformations, it is important to consider performing angiography immediately postoperatively while the patient is still intubated. In the author's experience, intraoperative angiograms do not have the same degree of resolution of angiograms obtained in a formal angiographic suite. Therefore, if angiography is considered immediately postoperatively, the craniotomy should be closed quickly and the patient transported to the angiographic suite while under general anesthesia. Thus, if the postoperative angiogram demonstrates residual arteriovenous malformation, the patient can be taken back immediately to the operat-

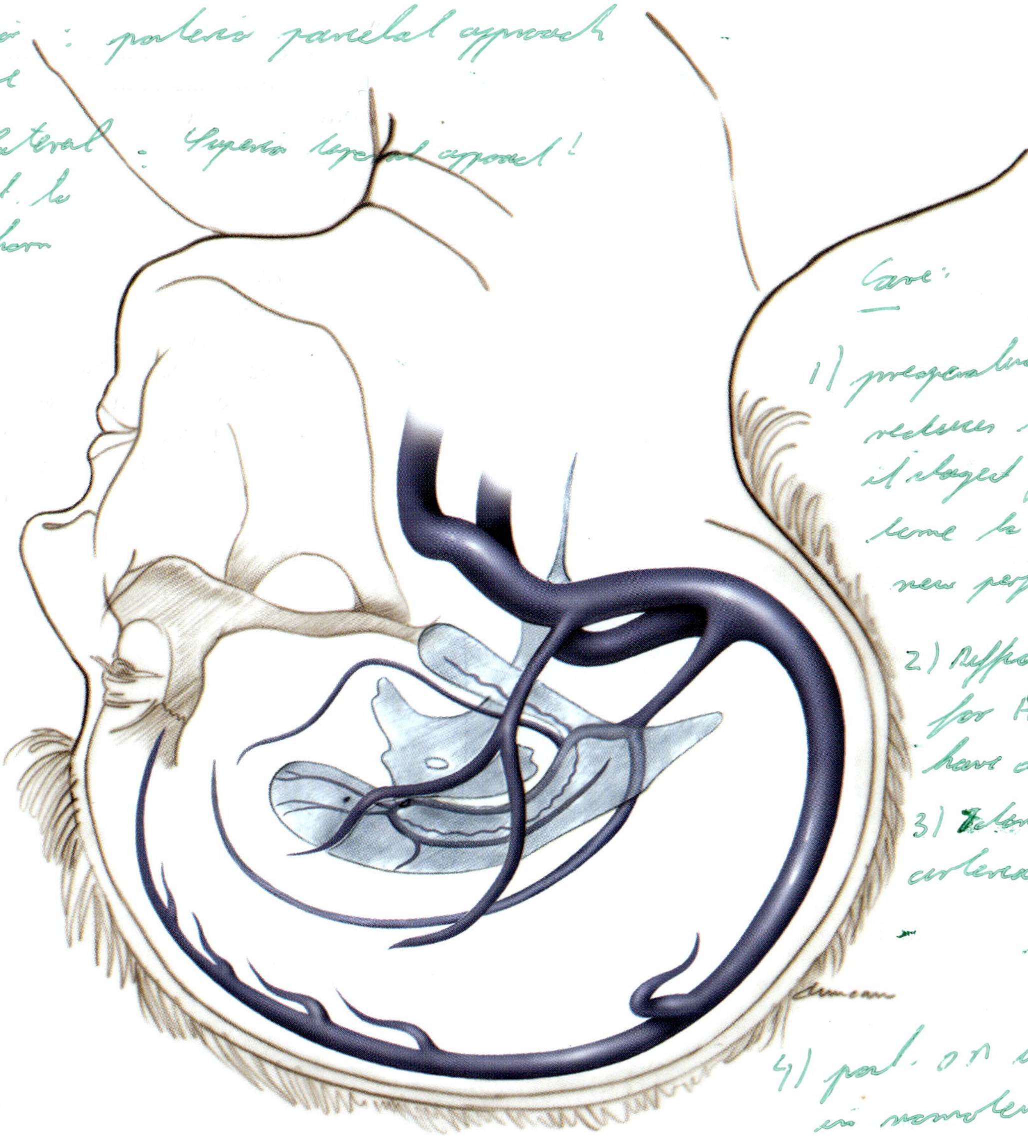

Figure 4–25.

The relationship of the ventricular system with the superficial and deep venous drainage. The primary venous drainage from an arteriovenous malformation in the trigone is the basal vein of Rosenthal and the internal cerebral vein through small subependymal veins, posterior septal veins, and the thalamostriate vein.

ing room, with little waste of time. One must be aware that interpreting an immediate postoperative angiogram is difficult. Often, there is stagnant blood flow or contrast material in draining veins that have been occluded. These should not be mistaken for early draining or shunting veins, which are the hallmark of residual arteriovenous malformation. These early draining veins are best seen in the middle portion of the arterial phase of an angiogram. Any residual arteriovenous malformation must be treated because the risk of hemorrhage is high. If residual arteriovenous malformation is detected in eloquent or difficult to access cerebral cortex, an argument can be made for early postoperative stereotactic irradiation.

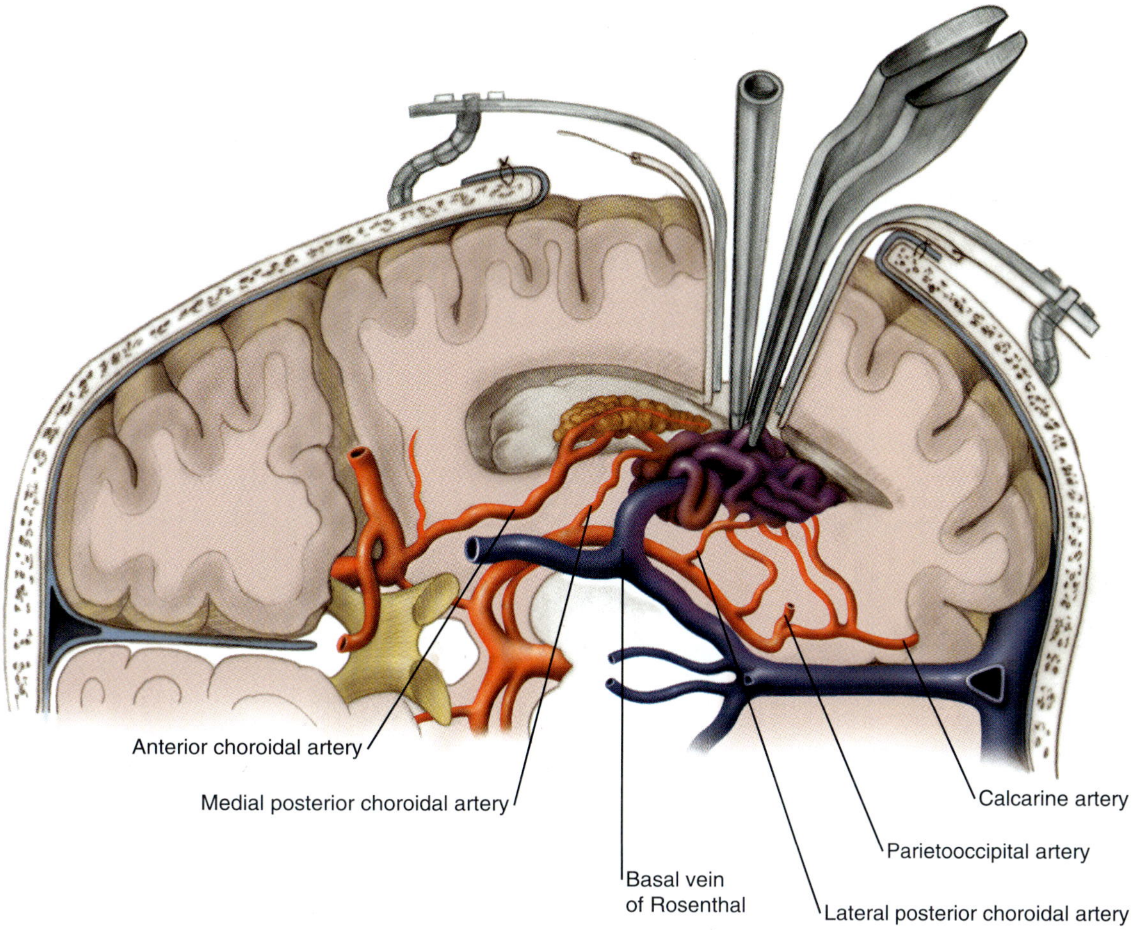

Figure 4–26.

An incision through the posterior middle temporal gyrus provides good access to an arteriovenous malformation that is located in the temporal horn and extends into the trigone. The arterial blood supply is from the anterior choroidal artery, the posterior choroidal artery, and the perforating vessels that come off segments P_2 and P_3 of the posterior cerebral artery. Most of the arterial blood supply is deep to the surgical approach.

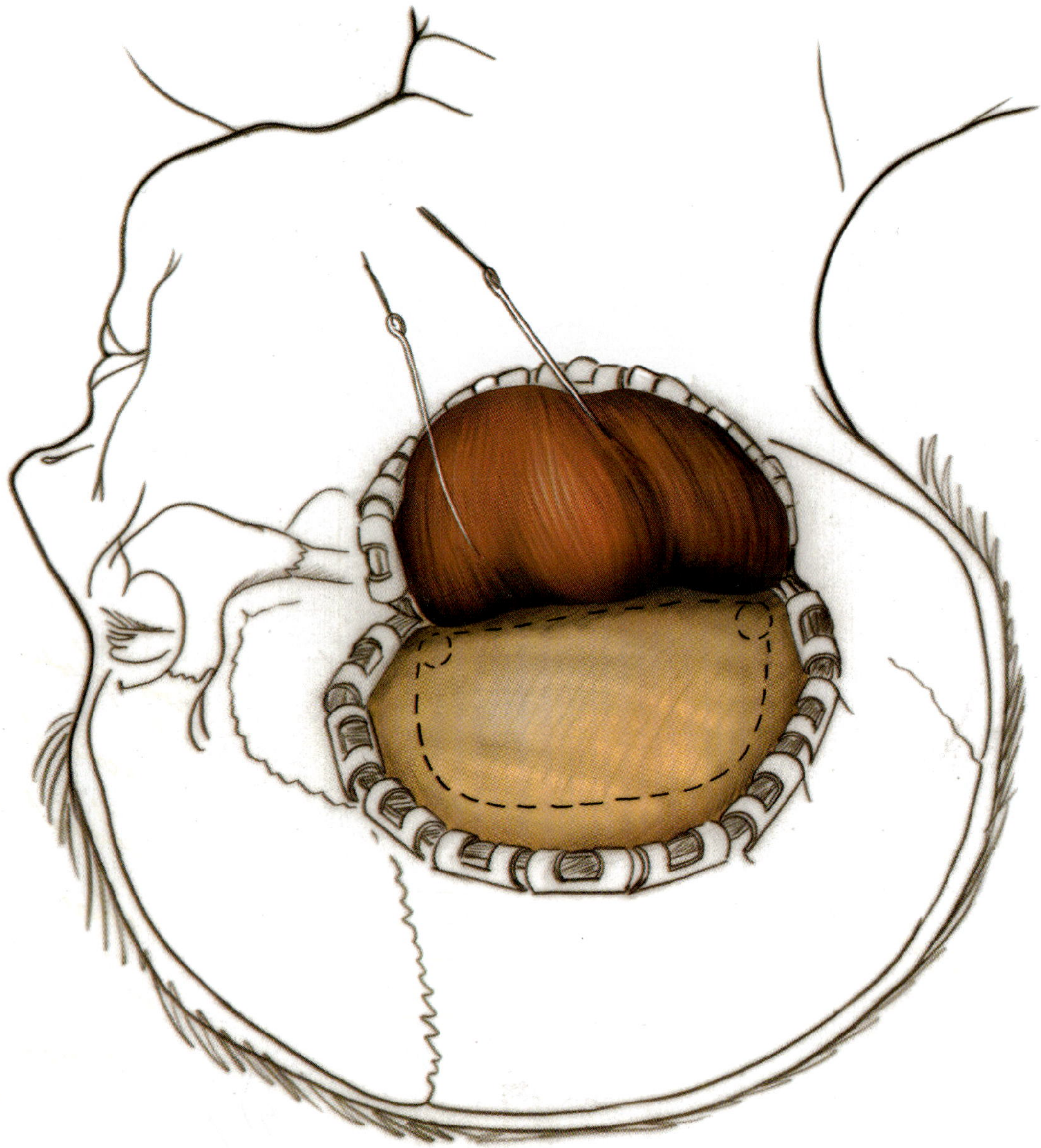

Figure 4–27.

Step 1. A horseshoe-shaped incision centered posterior to the ear provides good access to the posterior temporal lobe. It is important to make the inferior bone cut with care to prevent inadvertent tearing of the transverse sinus. The lower margin of the craniotomy should also be along the floor of the middle cranial fossa. In very large arteriovenous malformations of the trigone with massive branches of the posterior cerebral artery, a subtemporal approach to these feeding vessels can be considered if preoperative embolization was not successful in obliterating them.

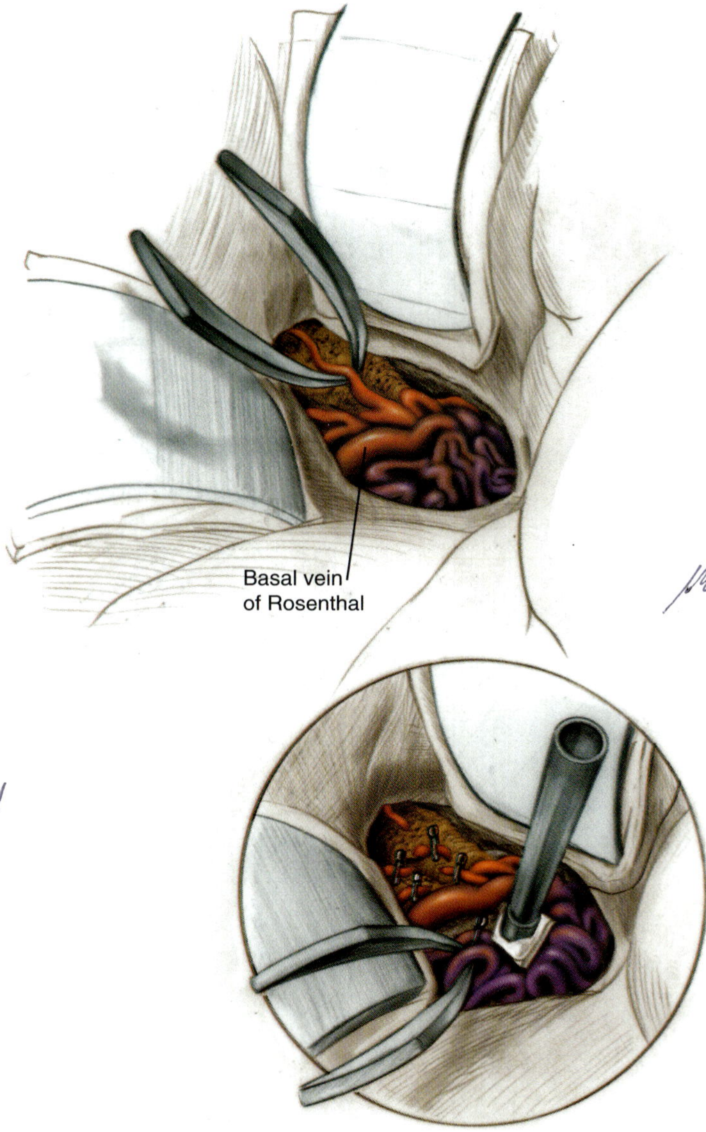

Figure 4–28.

Step 2. A cortical incision is made in the middle temporal gyrus over a length of approximately 2.0 cm. If there is a significant sulcus between the superior and middle temporal gyri, an intrasulcal approach to the lateral ventricle can be attempted. However, the sulci in the posterior temporal lobe usually are not well formed; therefore, an intrasulcal approach offers little advantage. After the lateral ventricle has been entered, two self-retaining retractors are used to retract the ependymal wall. The choroid plexus is identified. Invariably, many arterial feeding vessels come out of the choroid plexus and go to the arteriovenous malformation. They are branches of both the anterior and the posterior choroidal arteries. They should be meticulously cauterized and divided. Microclips may be helpful.

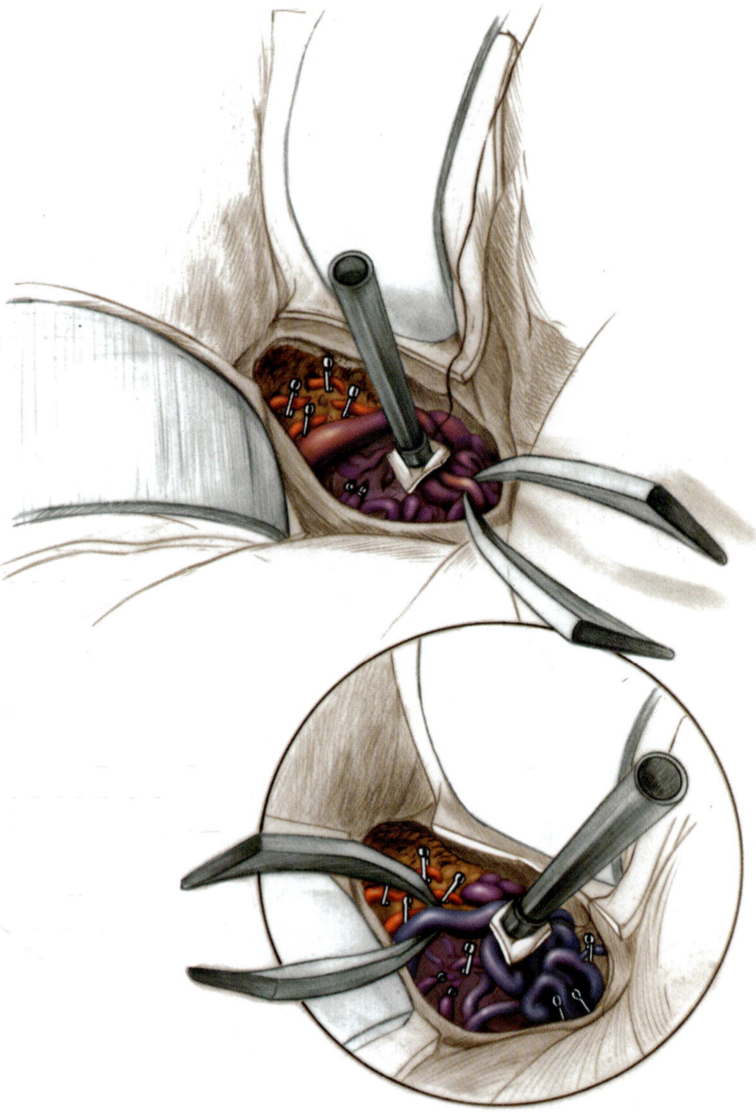

Figure 4–29.

Step 3. The medial, deeper aspect of the arteriovenous malformation is dissected free. This will allow access to the branches that come off the P_2 and P_3 segments. The arteriovenous malformation is gently retracted with a #5 or #7 suction tip and cottonoid. In the example shown here is a large draining vein that presumably goes to the basal vein of Rosenthal. These medial draining veins and arteries enter the lateral ventricle through the choroidal fissure; therefore, there is a layer of arachnoid overlying the posterior cerebral artery. Respecting this arachnoid will help prevent inadvertent injury of this artery. **Step 4**. The arteriovenous malformation is rotated anteriorly to allow exposure and dissection of the posterior feeding arteries and subependymal draining veins. Each is individually cauterized and divided. **Step 5**. After the arteriovenous malformation has been completely isolated from its arterial blood supply, the preserved draining veins should be inspected. If there is arterialized blood, residual arteriovenous malformation is still present and needs to be identified and resected.

5

Occipital Approach and Combined Occipital-Suboccipital Approach

Copyright © 1999 Mayo Foundation.

ANATOMIC CONSIDERATIONS

The occipital lobe forms the posterior part of the cerebral hemisphere. Its lateral surface includes the superior and inferior occipital gyri, which are separated by the lateral occipital sulcus. The major gyrus on the inferior, or tentorial, surface of the lobe is the fusiform, or occipitotemporal, gyrus. The medial surface of the occipital lobe is divided by the calcarine sulcus into two parts, called the "cuneus" and the "lingual gyrus" (or "lingula").

The cuneus (Brodmann areas 17, 18, and 19) is the triangularly shaped area between the parietooccipital sulcus superiorly and the calcarine sulcus inferiorly. The apex of the triangle verges on the isthmus of the cingulate gyrus. The lingual gyrus (Brodmann areas 17, 18, and 19) lies between the calcarine sulcus superiorly and the collateral sulcus inferiorly. It is continuous anteriorly with the parahippocampal gyrus of the temporal lobe. The lingual gyrus is separated from the fusiform (occipitotemporal) gyrus by the collateral sulcus.

The optic radiations, also called the "geniculocalcarine tract," project from the lateral geniculate body of the thalamus to the calcarine cortex (Brodmann area 17), which is the primary visual cortex. Calcarine cortex is the cerebral cortex that borders the calcarine fissure. The optic radiations are organized retinotopically. The portion of the radiations that represents the upper retinal quadrants (lower visual field) terminates along the superior bank of the calcarine sulcus, part of the cuneus. The portion that represents the lower retinal quadrants (upper visual field) terminates along the inferior bank of the calcarine sulcus, part of the lingual gyrus. Moreover, the peripheral retina is represented anteriorly in the calcarine cortex and the central retina (macula) is represented posteriorly, including the occipital pole.

ARTERIAL BLOOD SUPPLY

The blood supply to the occipital lobe is from the posterior cerebral artery, which originates at the bifurcation of the basilar artery on the ventral surface of the midbrain. From its origin, the posterior cerebral artery turns laterally and posteriorly and enters the interpeduncular cistern. The P_1 segment of the artery extends from the bifurcation of the basilar artery to the origin of the posterior communicating artery. This segment gives rise to the posterior thalamoperforating arteries, which vary in number and size. They run superiorly in the interpeduncular cistern to supply the posterior limb of the internal capsule, the thalamus, the hypothalamus, and the subthalamic nuclei.

From the interpeduncular cistern, the posterior cerebral artery turns posteriorly into the ambient cistern. This is segment P_2, which extends from the junction between the posterior communicating and the posterior cerebral arteries to the dorsal aspect of the midbrain. The thalamogeniculate arteries originate from segment P_2 and supply part of the posterior limb of the internal capsule, the lateral and medial geniculate bodies, part of the optic tract, and part of the thalamus. Other perforating branches arising from segment P_2 supply the cerebral peduncles. This segment also gives rise to the medial posterior choroidal artery, which occasionally originates from segment P_1. The medial posterior choroidal artery runs anteriorly around the brain stem and turns superomedially to enter the roof of the third ventricle. As it runs anteriorly toward the foramen of Monro, it supplies the pineal body, the choroid plexus of the third and lateral ventricles, and the thalamus. Segment P_2 also gives rise to one or more lateral posterior choroidal arteries. The posterior choroidal arteries may also originate from the proximal segments of cortical branches of the posterior cerebral artery. The lateral posterior choroidal arteries enter the choroidal fissure laterally and curve anteriorly around the pulvinar to supply the choroid plexus, part of the cerebral peduncle, the lateral geniculate body, the posterior limb of the internal capsule, the thalamus, the fornix, and the caudate nucleus.

Four primary cortical branches originate from the posterior cerebral artery. One of these, the inferior temporal artery, often originates from segment P_2. Branches of the inferior temporal artery supply the inferior part of the temporal lobe. These branches are named the "hippocampal," "anterior," "middle," and "posterior temporal arteries." Occasionally, branches of the posterior temporal artery extend posteriorly to perfuse part of the visual cortex.

Segment P_3 of the posterior cerebral artery extends from the quadrigeminal cistern to the calcarine sulcus. It often divides into branches before entering the calcarine fissure. Its cortical branches are as follows: the parietooccipital artery usually originates in the ambient cistern and extends posteriorly along the parietooccipital sulcus. It supplies part of the precuneus, the cuneus, and the superior occipital gyrus. It also may perfuse part of the parietal and central lobes. The calcarine artery runs in the calcarine sulcus and supplies much of the cuneus and lingual gyrus, that is, primary visual cortex (Brodmann area 17). Some small splenial arteries that arise from segment P_3 or the parietooccipital artery supply the splenium of the corpus callosum.

TORCULAR MENINGIOMA

Often, meningiomas that arise along the posterior falx cerebri and tentorium cerebelli are best removed through an interhemispheric approach, using a parietooccipital craniotomy. The blood supply to the tumor originates from the tentorium cerebelli. The relationship of the tumor to

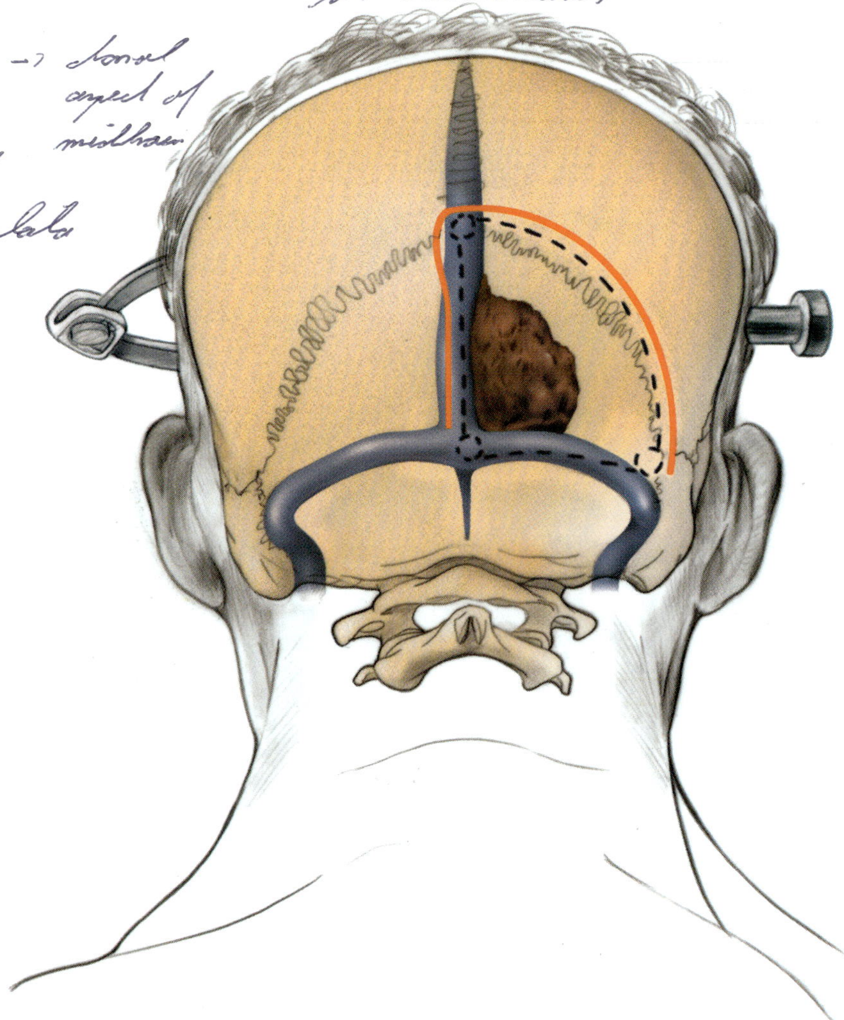

Figure 5–1.

A midline occipitoparietal craniotomy works well for resecting tumors along the falx cerebri and those on or above the tentorium cerebelli. The medial bone cut must be on the superior sagittal sinus, and the inferior cut should extend to the top of the transverse sinus. In this way, there will be less retraction along the occipital pole. The cuts along the superior sagittal and transverse sinuses must be made with care. Placing bur holes and then stripping the dura mater with Penfield #1 and #3 dissectors before making the bone cuts decreases the risk of inadvertently tearing a sinus. If there is significant hyperostosis, it is best to use a high-speed air drill with a diamond bur.

the surrounding venous sinuses and torcular Herophili must be considered. If the tumor invades a patent sinus, the best plan is to create a plane of dissection parallel to the dura mater and sinus using the bipolar cautery. Residual tumor along the wall of the sinus is cauterized aggressively.

Large tumors that have a deep extension into the tentorial notch are more difficult to excise because they are in proximity to the vein of Galen along the midline and to the posterior cerebral arteries laterally. The arachnoid layer between the tumor capsule and these vascular structures must be respected. In tumors that extend caudally, sectioning the tentorium cerebelli is beneficial. An incision is made parallel with and approximately 5 to 10 mm lateral to the straight sinus. For orientation, the vein of Galen and the posterior cerebral arteries are above the tentorium cerebelli, and the superior cerebellar arteries and oculomotor nerves are below it.

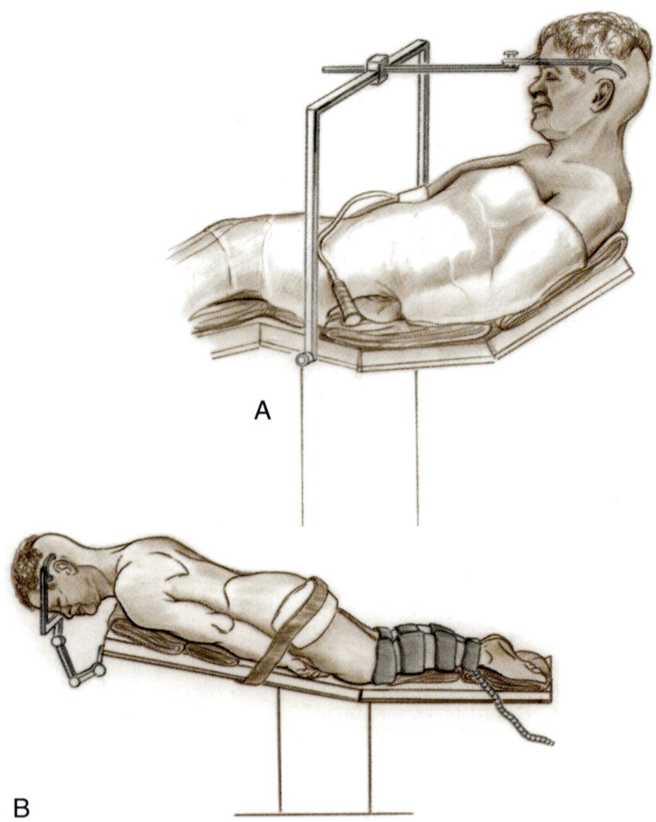

Figure 5–2.

Two patient positions that work well for a midline parietooccipital craniotomy are the semisitting position *(A)* and the prone position *(B)*. The semisitting, or slouch, position affords excellent brain relaxation, with good orientation and surgical access. However, with the head higher than the level of the heart, the risk of air embolism must be considered because the surgeon is working in proximity to the major venous sinuses. Therefore, the anesthesiologist should place both a transesophageal echo and a right atrial catheter. The risk of air embolism may be decreased with the prone position because the head is not elevated above the heart. However, a disadvantage of the prone position is the risk of increased intracranial pressure because of decreased venous drainage from the brain. If the prone position is used, it is important to make sure that the chest rolls are placed correctly to decrease intrathoracic pressure. A reverse Trendelenburg body position combined with head flexion promotes venous drainage. In *B*, note that intermittent compression boots have been placed to help decrease the risk of postoperative deep thrombosis, which is a recognized complication after operations on intracranial meningiomas.

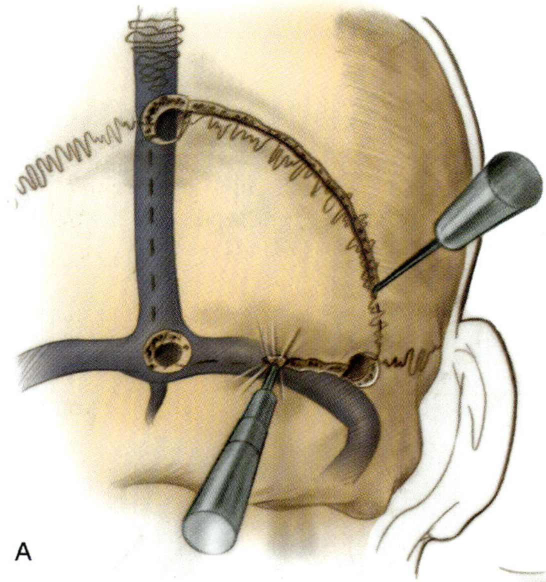

A

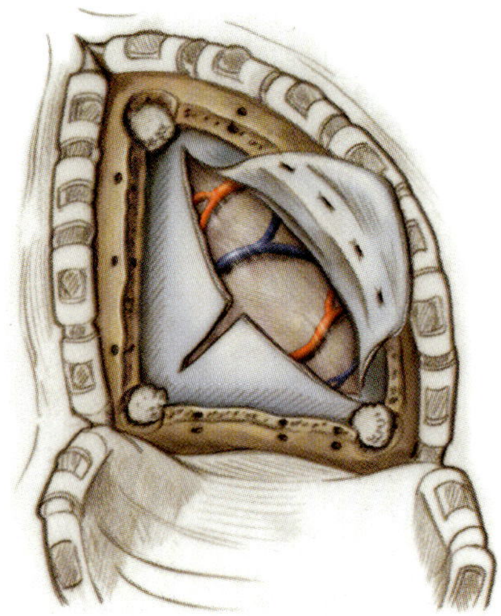

B

Figure 5–3.

Step 1. *A*, A U-shaped flap is used for exposure. Because the broad flap is supplied by branches of the occipital artery, there is no risk of ischemic scalp necrosis. As illustrated here, three bur holes are made over the transverse and sigmoid sinuses. A Penfield #3 dissector is used to dissect the dura mater off the underside of the bone flap. A craniotome is used to make the outer cut. The author's preference is to use a high-speed air drill with a diamond bur to make the medial and inferior cuts over the sinus.

Step 2. *B*, The dura mater is opened and reflected over the transverse and sigmoid sinuses and tacked to the margins of the bone. By exposing the bone over the superior sagittal sinus and then tightly tacking the dura mater, the sinuses are retracted slightly to provide greater exposure.

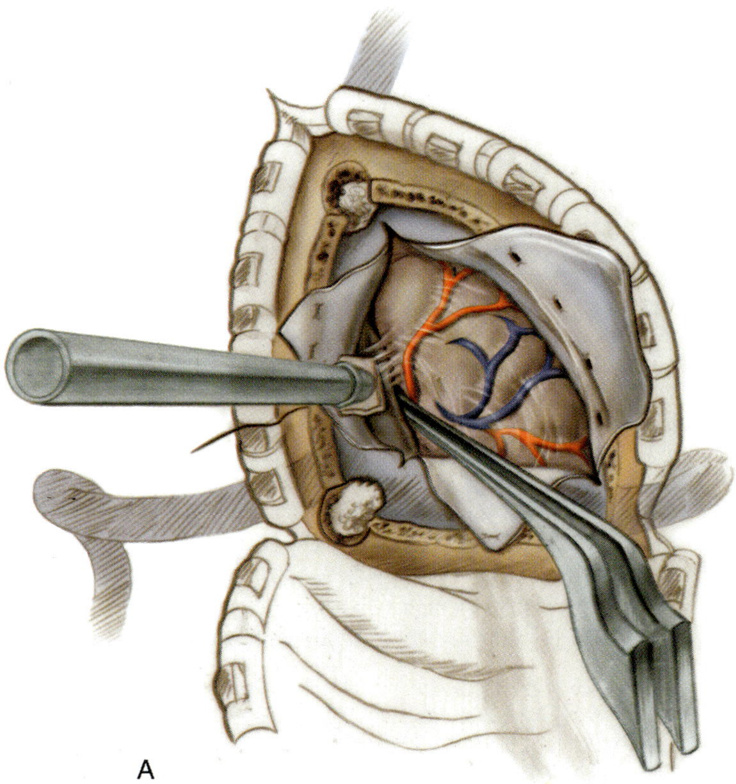

A

Figure 5–4.

Step 3. *A*, A #5 or #7 suction tip and a bipolar cautery are used to investigate the plane between the capsule of the tumor and the occipital pole. As true for most meningiomas, an arachnoid-pial plane separates the tumor from the enveloping cerebral cortex.

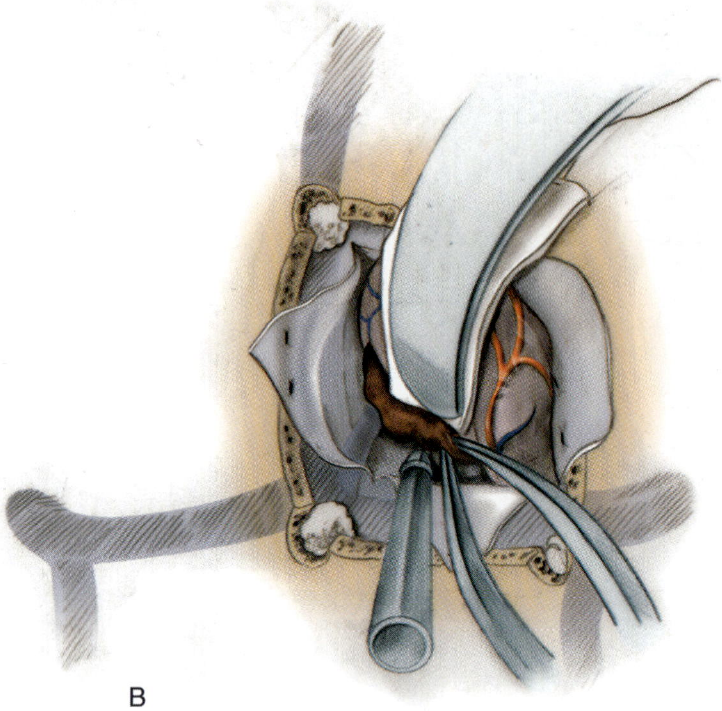

B

Step 4. *B*, The occipital lobe is retracted gently. The base of the tumor along the tentorium cerebelli is sharply divided using a bipolar cautery. Similarly, the attachment of the tumor to the falx cerebri is also cauterized. There usually is an intimate relationship between the base of the tumor and the straight sinus. Bleeding from the straight sinus usually can be controlled with absorbable gelatin sponge (Gelfoam).

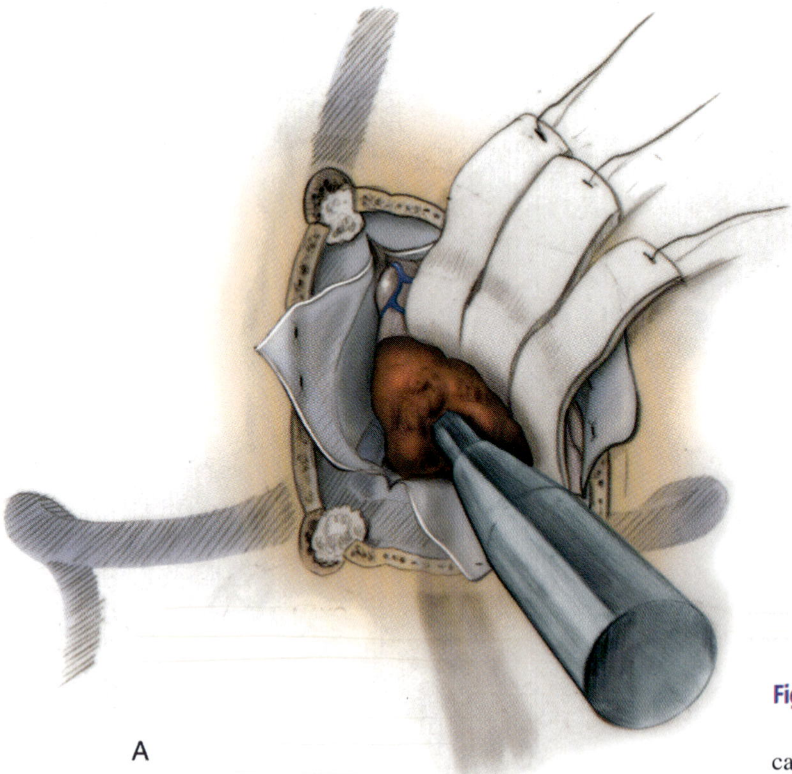

A

Figure 5–5.

Step 5. *A*, The tumor is debulked using the bipolar cautery, suction, ultrasonic aspirator, or cutting loops. Aggressive debulking of the tumor allows large lesions to be removed with little retraction of the brain.

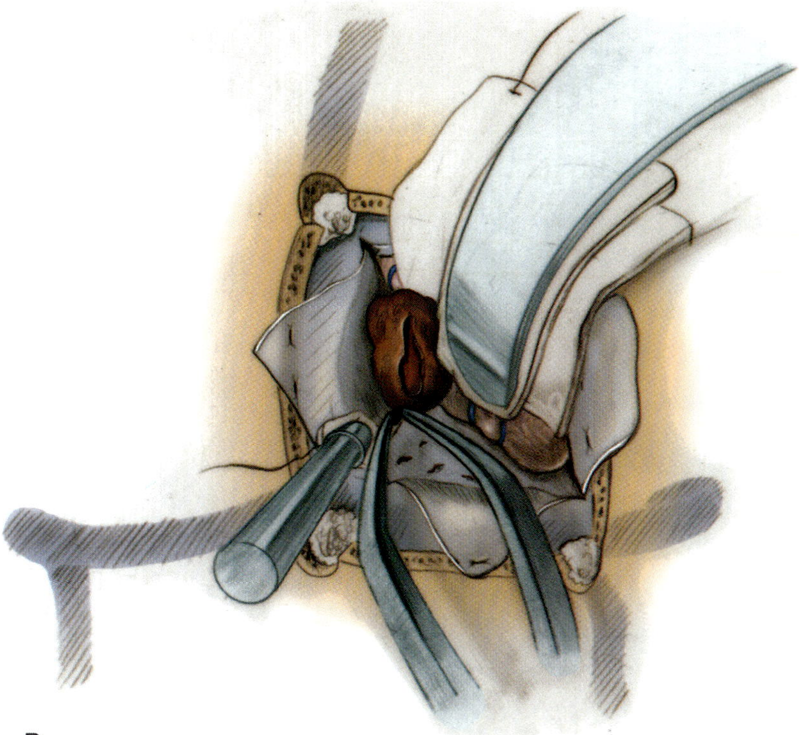

B

Step 6. *B*, The most medial and deep aspect of the tumor is cauterized. Occasionally, along the edge of the tentorium cerebelli, there are unexpectedly large arterial branches from the internal carotid artery.

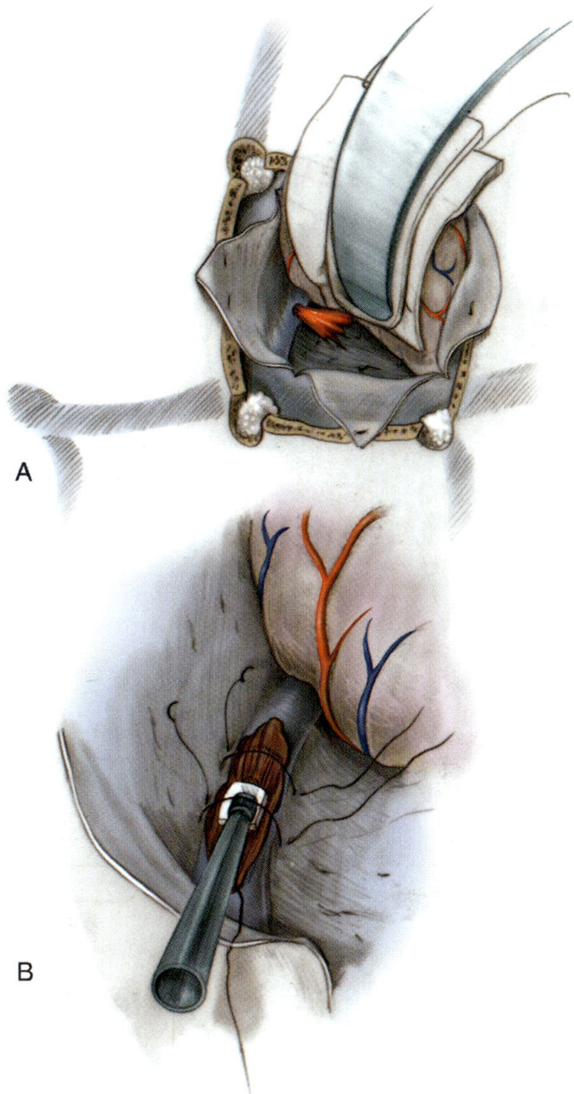

A

B

Figure 5–6.

A, There is a tear in the straight sinus. For all sinus tears, the best way to control hemostasis is first to place a piece of absorbable gelatin sponge and a cottonoid (Americot) with tamponade. Next, the surgical assistant harvests a piece of muscle from the skin flap, which is used to replace the absorbable gelatin sponge.

B, The muscle is sewn in place with several permanent 3-0 tacking sutures. A braided suture such as silk is better than monofilament. When tying the surgical knot, the first two ties should be thrown in the same direction. This allows the surgeon to cinch down the knot on top of the muscle plug. The third tie is thrown in the opposite direction to lock the knot.

PINEAL TUMOR

The parietooccipital transtentorial interhemispheric approach to pineal tumors may be advantageous if the neoplasm has a significant caudal extension toward the fourth ventricle. If the majority of the tumor lies above the tentorium cerebelli, a suboccipital approach is superior. In particularly large tumors, both a parietooccipital and a suboccipital craniotomy can be performed to allow multiple angles for removing the tumor.

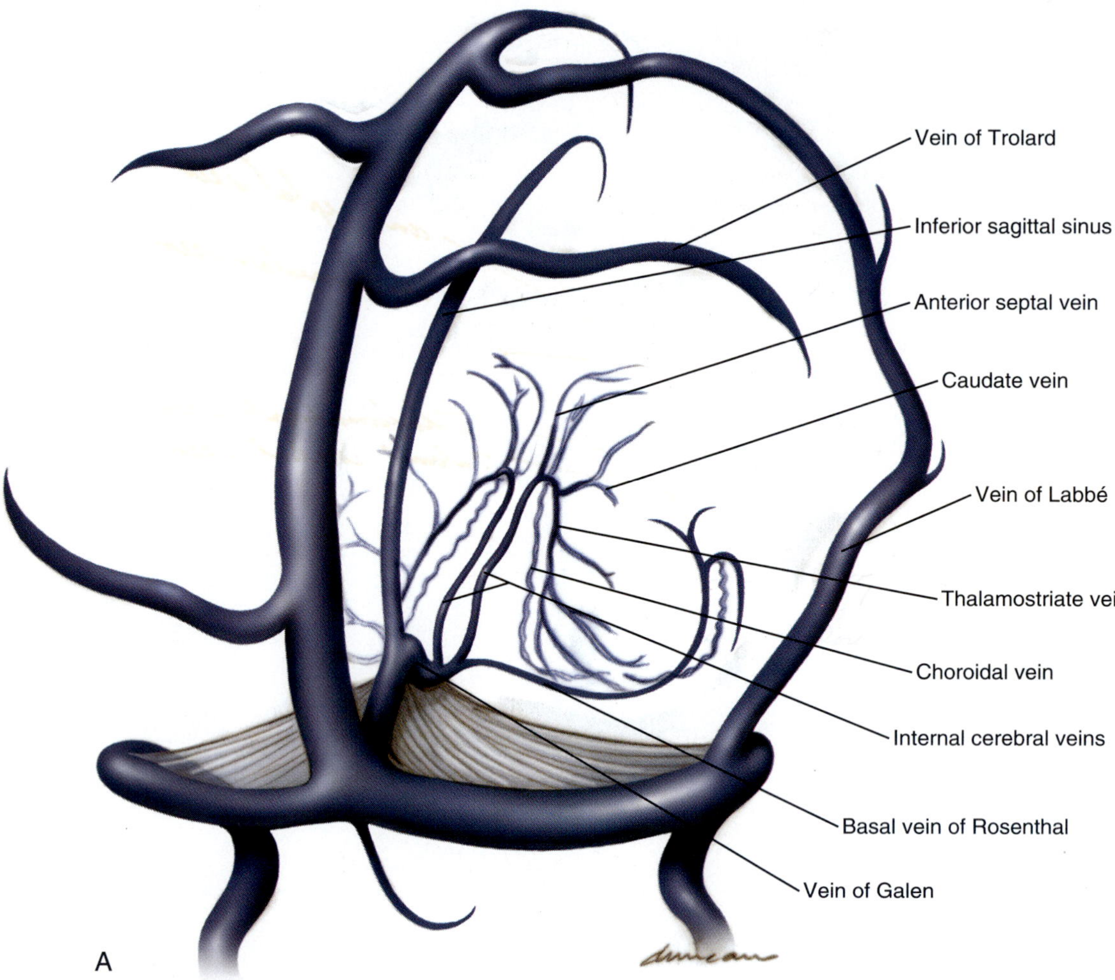

Figure 5–7.

The intracranial venous system. *A* and *B* illustrate the pertinent anatomy of the intracranial venous system that needs to be considered when approaching a tumor in the region of the pineal body. The basal vein of Rosenthal is formed by the anterior and deep middle cerebral veins and small branches from the insula and cerebral peduncles. As the basal vein of Rosenthal goes posteriorly around the cerebral peduncle, it receives tributaries from the temporal horn and the medial temporal lobe and is joined by the inferior striate veins, which drain part of the basal ganglia. The basal vein of Rosenthal may also receive blood from the lateral mesencephalic vein. The basal vein of Rosenthal curves posteriorly around the cerebral peduncle and collicular (tectal) plate to join the vein of Galen.

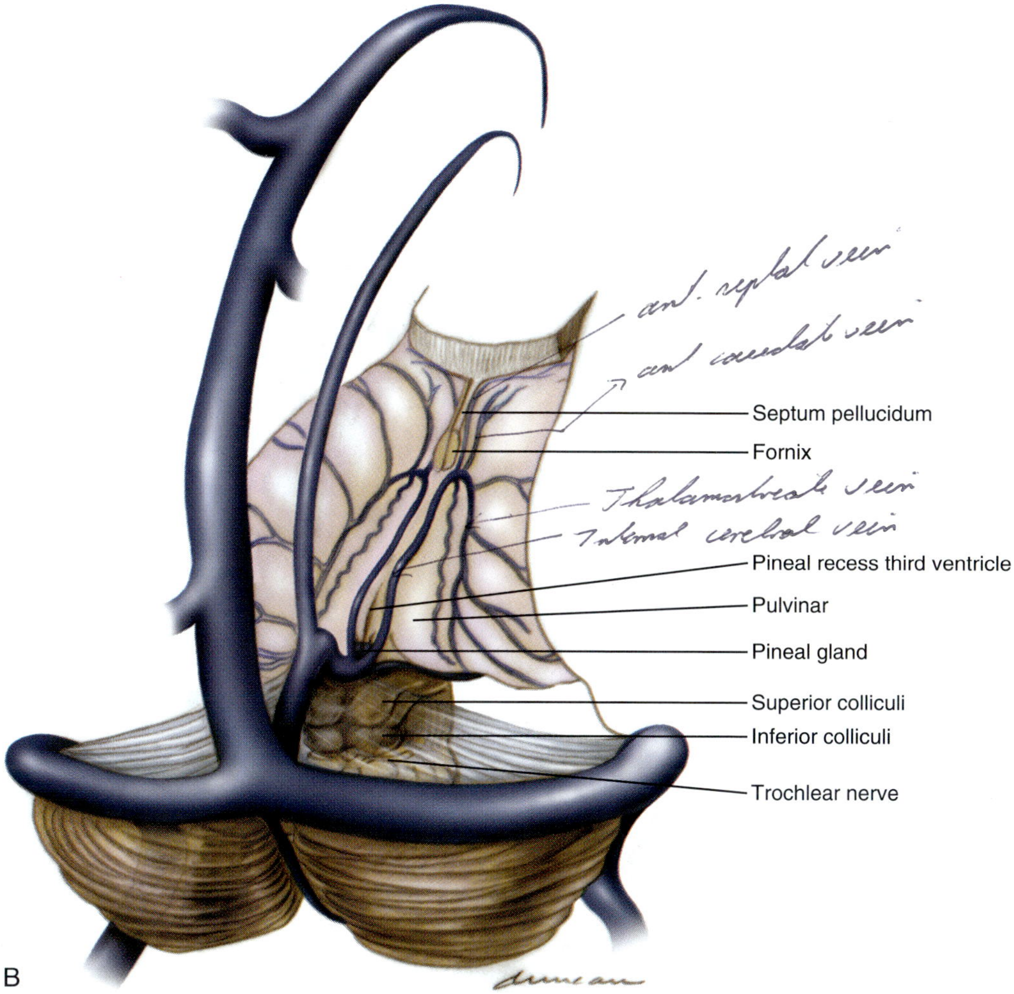

B

The septal and thalamostriate veins join along the inferior aspect of the foramen of Monro to form the paired internal cerebral veins. Each internal cerebral vein penetrates the subarachnoid space to run just lateral to the midline in the velum interpositum. As the vein goes posteriorly, small subependymal veins and the posterior septal veins join it. Just inferior to the splenium of the corpus callosum, the pair of internal cerebral veins join the pair of basal veins of Rosenthal to form the vein of Galen.

The vein of Galen is short and U-shaped as it curves posteriorly and superiorly around the splenium. The vein of Galen ends at the apex of the tentorial notch by joining the inferior sagittal sinus to form the straight sinus. The vein of Galen also receives small venous tributaries from the occipital lobe, the corpus callosum, the mesencephalon, and the cerebellum. An important landmark is the midline precentral vein that extends from the cerebellum to the underside of the vein of Galen.

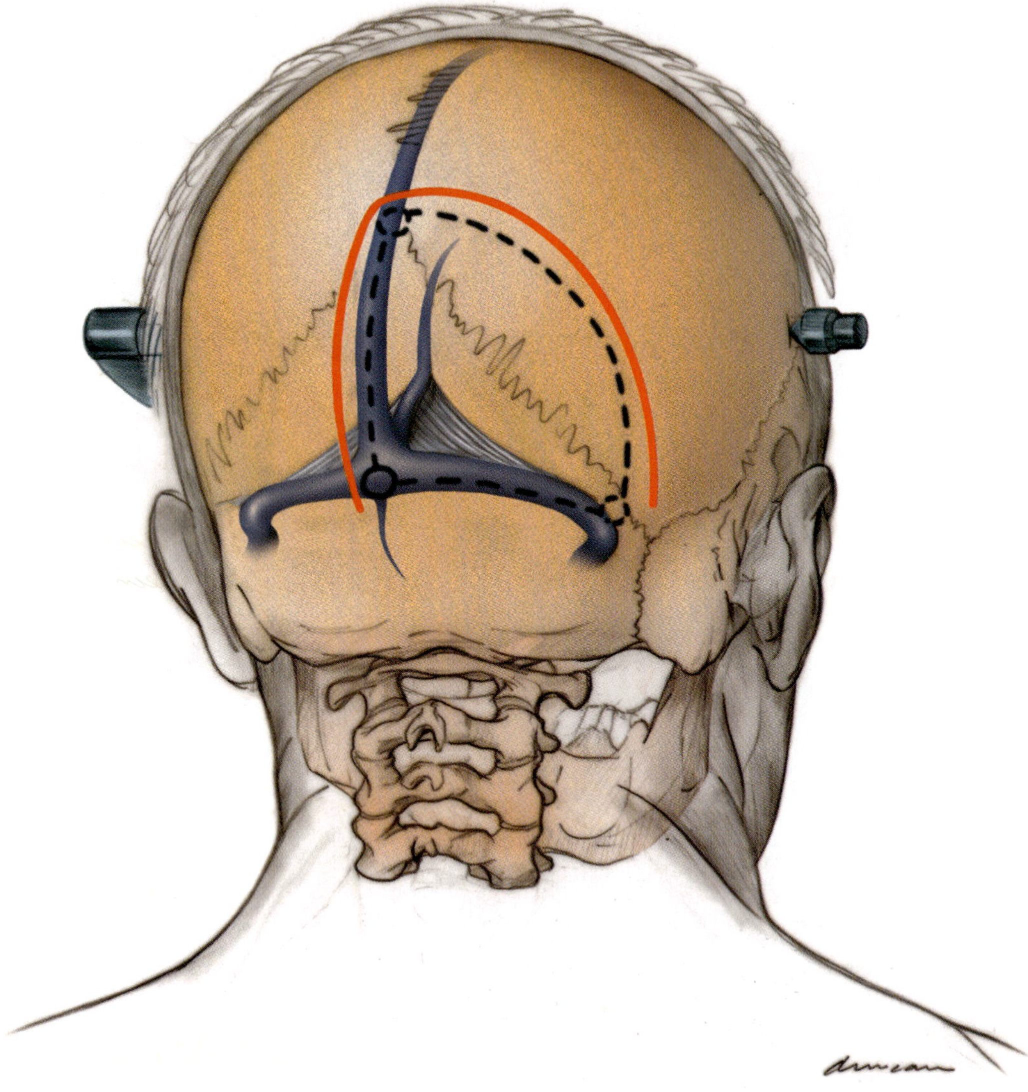

Figure 5–8.

Step 1. A U-shaped incision is made for this exposure. The midline and inferior cuts should be along the superior sagittal and transverse sinuses, respectively. Note that the head is rotated slightly to the right to allow the surgeon a better line of sight. For pineal tumors with large lateral, eccentric extensions, head rotation can be used accordingly. For example, if the patient has a large tumor extending far right, the head should be rotated slightly to the left. Alternatively, a left-sided craniotomy can be performed to allow a "crosscourt" approach. The degree of head flexion is not as pronounced as it is for a suboccipital approach.

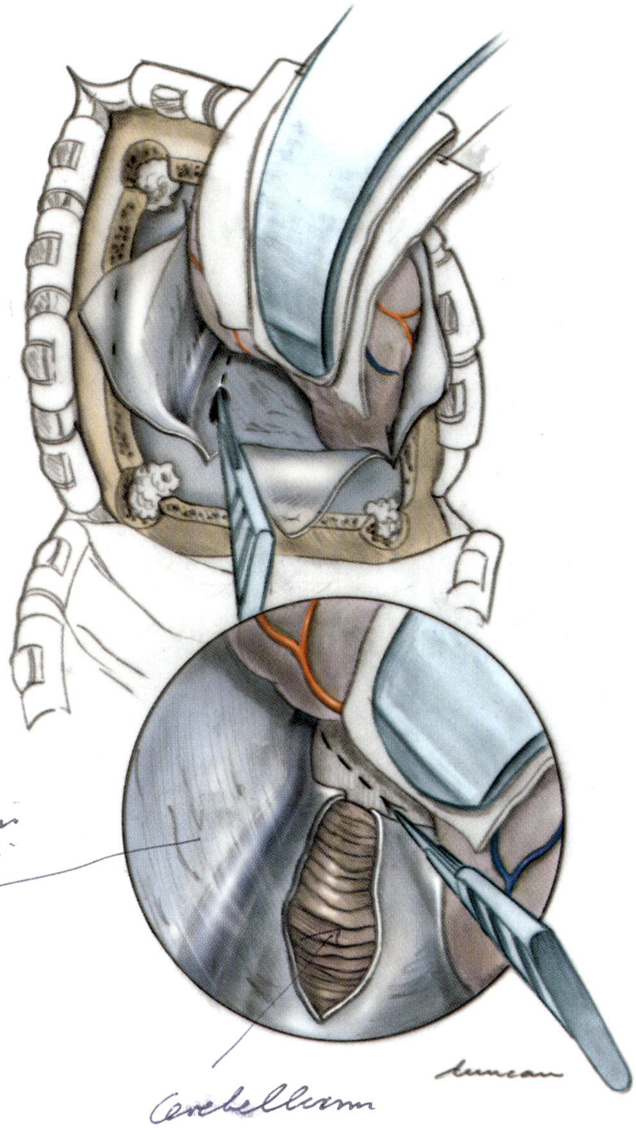

Figure 5–9.

Step 2. The dura mater is tacked to the margins of the bone, and the occipital lobe is lined with hemostatic fabric (Surgicel) and cottonoids and gently retracted. Next, an incision is made in the tentorium cerebelli approximately 5 to 10 mm lateral to the straight sinus. This incision is carried forward to the quadrigeminal cistern. It is important to recognize that the quadrigeminal cistern is dark. Sitting underneath the arachnoid that covers the quadrigeminal cistern is the right basal vein of Rosenthal and the vein of Galen. Accordingly, when initially opening this cistern, the surgeon needs to be careful to avoid inadvertently tearing these veins, which are displaced laterally and posteriorly by the tumor. The best technique is to make a small nick with a sharp #11 blade knife and to use a dissector to extend the opening in the arachnoid.

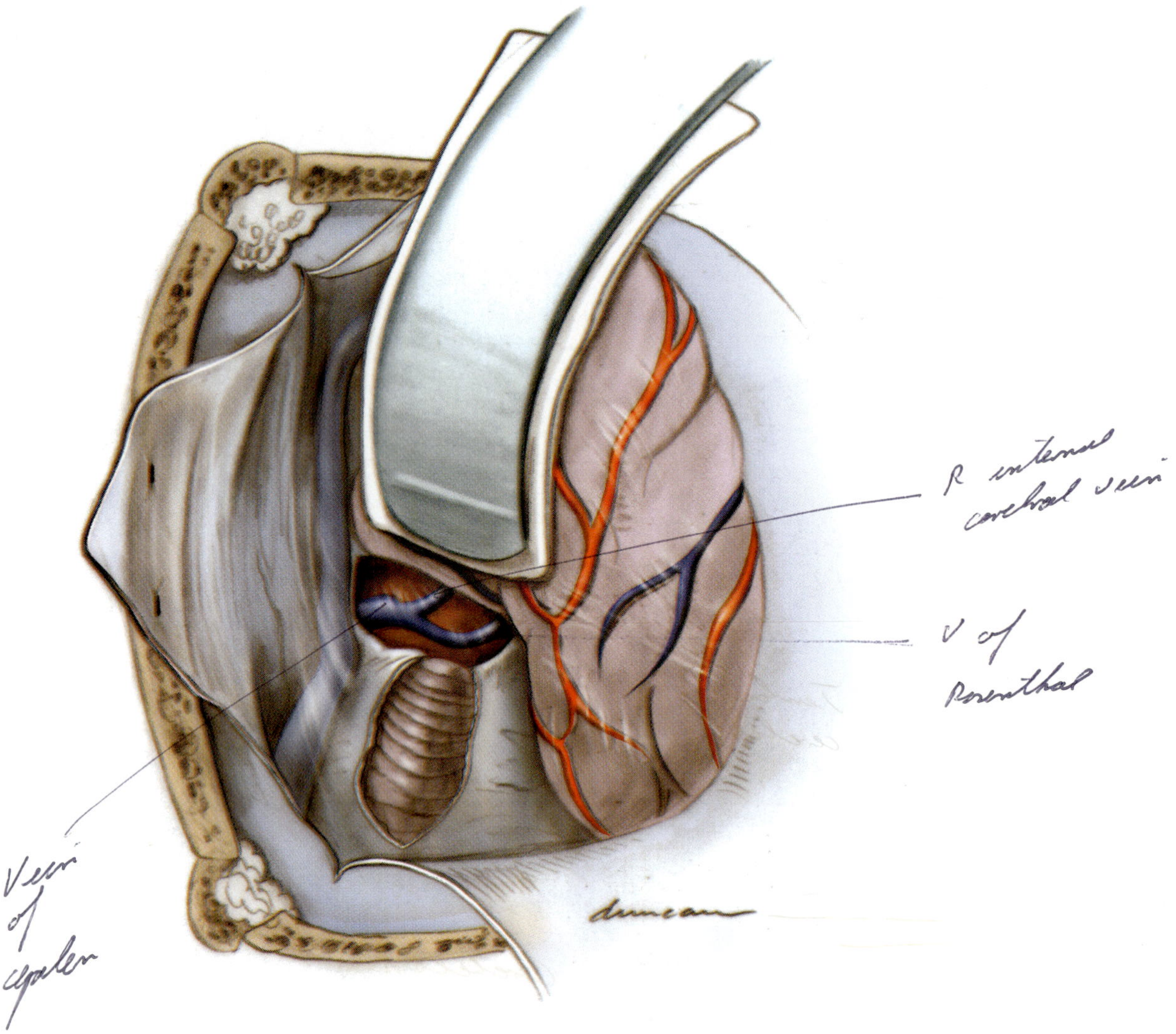

Figure 5–10.

Step 3. After the quadrigeminal cistern has been opened, the splenium of the corpus callosum is retracted gently. This reveals the right basal vein of Rosenthal and, likely, the right internal cerebral vein.

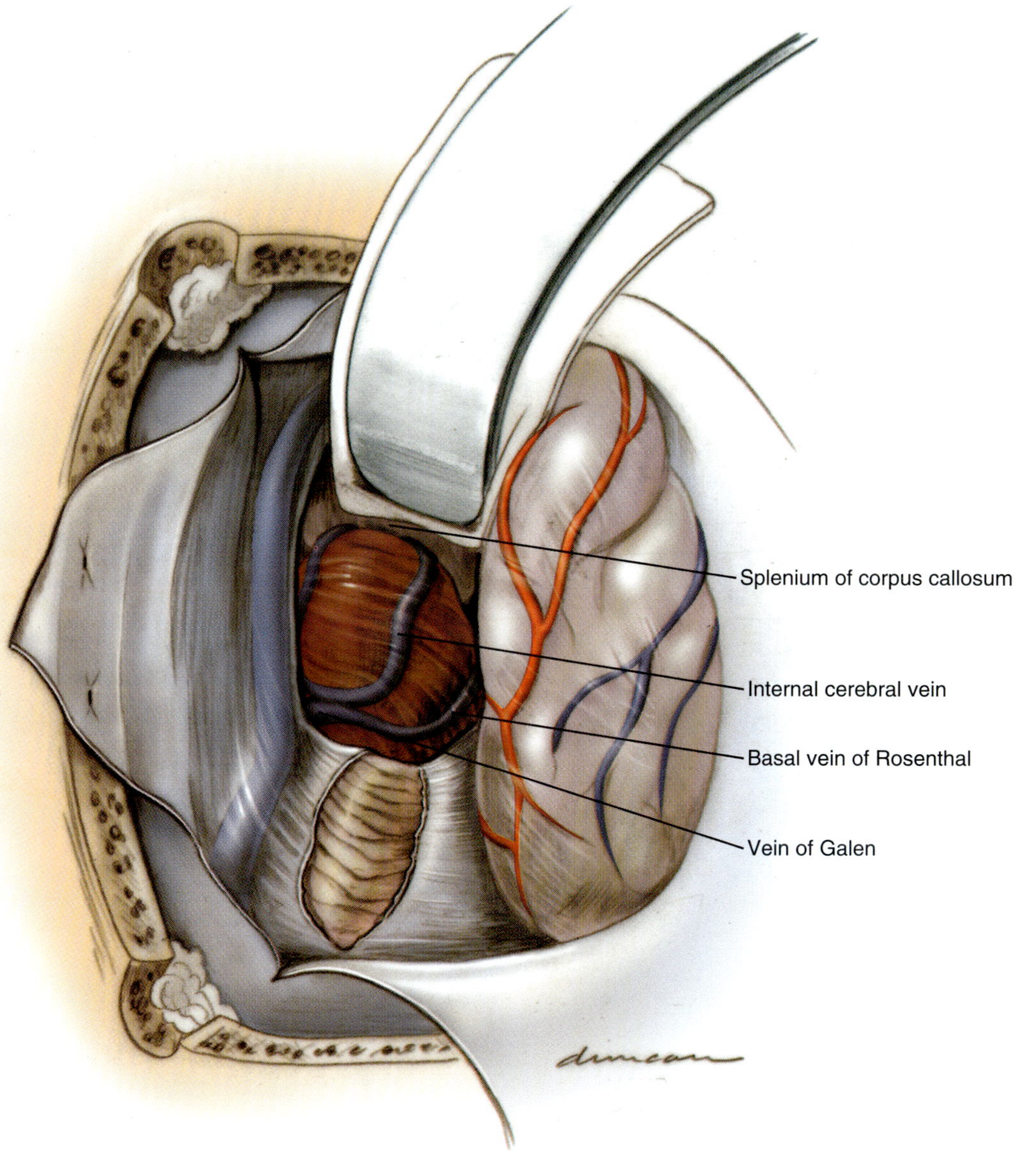

Figure 5–11.

Step 4. The medial occipital lobe and the splenium of the corpus callosum are retracted more vigorously to expose the rostral portion of the tumor. Note that the pertinent veins lie within a layer of arachnoid.

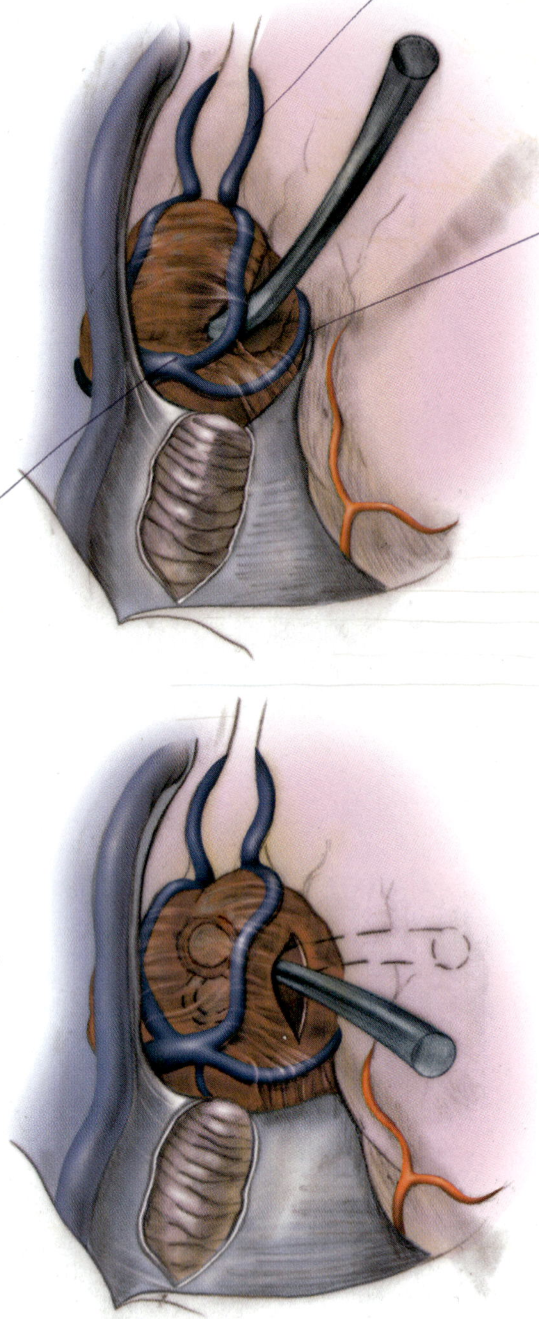

Figure 5–12.

Step 5. The tumor is inspected visually to determine the largest aperture for tumor debulking. This usually occurs between the ipsilateral internal cerebral vein and the basal vein of Rosenthal. The arachnoid and tumor capsule are incised. Small angled curets are used to perform internal debulking of the tumor. A small spatula is used to gently dissect the veins within the ensheathing arachnoid off the tumor capsule. Specifically, the right internal cerebral vein is dissected medially and the basal vein of Rosenthal is dissected laterally and caudally. It is important to perform as vigorous a debulking of the tumor as possible before manipulating the tumor capsule.

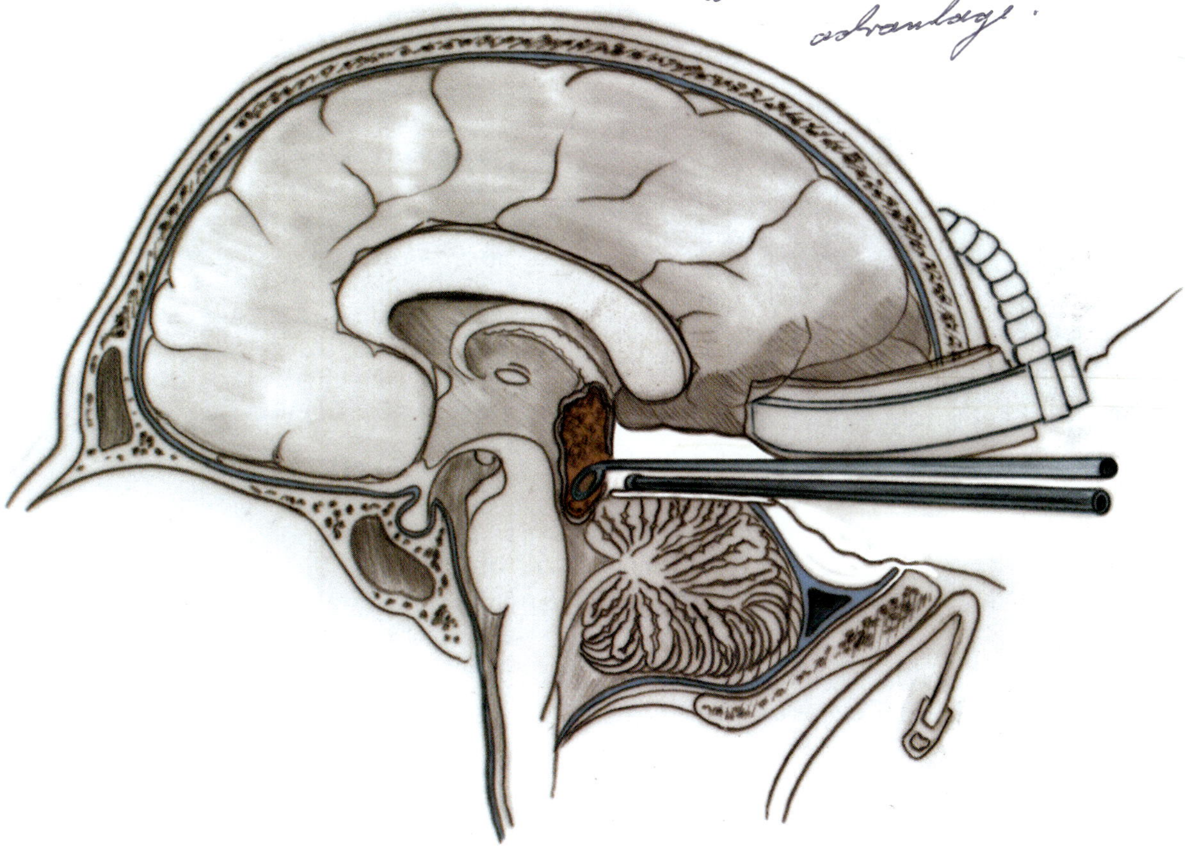

Figure 5–13.

Step 6. This illustration of a midsagittal section of the brain emphasizes why a parietooccipital craniotomy with a transtentorial approach can be useful in removing pineal tumors that have a marked caudal extension. It is difficult to remove the inferior extension of a pineal tumor through a suboccipital approach because of the need for significant retraction of the cerebellum. Alternatively, a transtentorial approach allows a downward line of sight because the occipital lobe is retracted laterally and the surgeon works through the interhemispheric fissure. The cerebellum is protected with a cottonoid and displaced downward with a #5 or #7 straight suction tip. Long angled curettes are used to debulk the tumor. The tumor capsule is worked gently upward into the operative field. The collicular plate is usually caudal and ventral to the tumor.

ARTERIOVENOUS FISTULA OF THE LATERAL AND SIGMOID DURAL SINUSES

Dural arteriovenous fistulas of the lateral and sigmoid sinuses typically present with intractable pulsatile tinnitus and headaches. On neurologic examination, a bruit and, often, papilledema are detected, indicative of increased intracranial pressure. The nidus of the arteriovenous fistula is found at the junction of the transverse and sigmoid sinuses. It has been proposed that these fistulas result from thrombosis or stenosis of the transverse sinus. The blood supply to these lesions is complicated but includes feeding vessels from the external carotid artery, including the occipital artery, the posterior and the middle meningeal arteries, and vascularized petrous bone. There almost always is a blood supply from the internal carotid artery through arterial branches that originate from the meningohypophysial trunk. Occasionally, these fistulas may parasitize cortical arterial branches. The goal of the operation is to disconnect the fistula. The fistula not only causes pulsatile tinnitus, but it can lead to cortical venous hypertension. The presence of cortical venous hypertension with this type of fistula indicates an increased risk of seizures and hemorrhage.

It is important to determine whether the sigmoid sinus on the side of the fistula is patent or thrombosed. If it is patent, it must be preserved. The vein of Labbé likely drains antegradely into it. In this circumstance, the arterial feeding vessels from the dura mater over the occipital lobe and the cerebellum, the tentorium cerebelli, and the petrous bone are disconnected. If the sigmoid sinus is thrombosed, it is easier technically to disconnect the fistula. Specifically, the transverse sinus is ligated approximately 2 cm from the torcular Herophili and rotated outward and used as a handle to expose the inner blood supply coming from the tentorium cerebelli. Next, the transverse sinus is devascularized down to its junction with the sigmoid sinus, and the sigmoid sinus is packed with hemostatic fabric. This leads to additional thrombosis of the sigmoid sinus and obliteration of the fistula at the level of the petrous bone.

In the following example, the sigmoid sinus is patent. Therefore, the goal of the operation is to disconnect the fistula without inducing thrombosis of the sigmoid sinus. Technically, this is more difficult to achieve because it is difficult to visualize the tentorium cerebelli along the inner side of the transverse sinus. The occipital lobe and the cerebellum both are retracted. This allows the tentorium cerebelli to be incised, cauterized, and divided along the inner side of the transverse sinus down to its junction with the sigmoid sinus. Thereafter, the bipolar cautery is used to extensively cauterize the dura mater along the petrous bone, both in the posterior cranial fossa and along the occipital lobe. In effect, this will also cauterize and induce thrombosis of the petrosal sinus, which usually participates in the fistula.

Preoperative embolization is useful for obliterating much of the blood supply from the external carotid artery. This facilitates intraoperative hemostasis. However, embolization or ligation of the external carotid artery in itself does not lead to obliteration of the lesion. In fact, it has an adverse effect by driving the blood supply deeper, making subsequent surgical resection more difficult and dangerous.

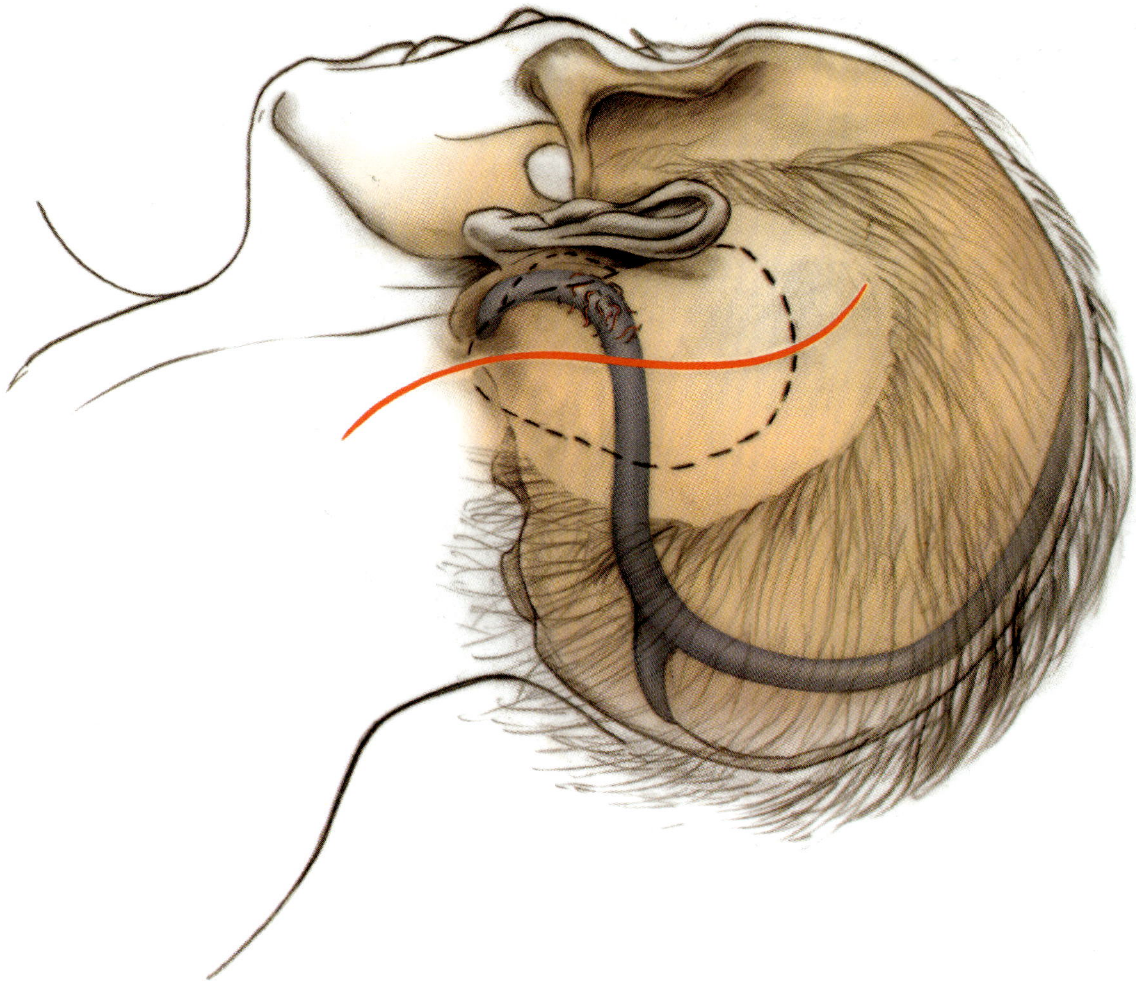

Figure 5–14.

Step 1. The position of the patient's head is similar to that used in a standard suboccipital approach for acoustic neuroma or microvascular decompression surgery. Specifically, the body is supine, with the head rotated parallel to the floor and held in a pinion. It is important not to overrotate the neck, because this causes significant postoperative neck discomfort and might lead to compression of the jugular vein and, subsequently, increased intracranial pressure. Alternatively, the operating table can be rotated laterally. In this operation, it is important to have a lumbar drain in place to facilitate drainage of the cerebrospinal fluid, because the cisterna magna will not be immediately available for drainage after bone removal.

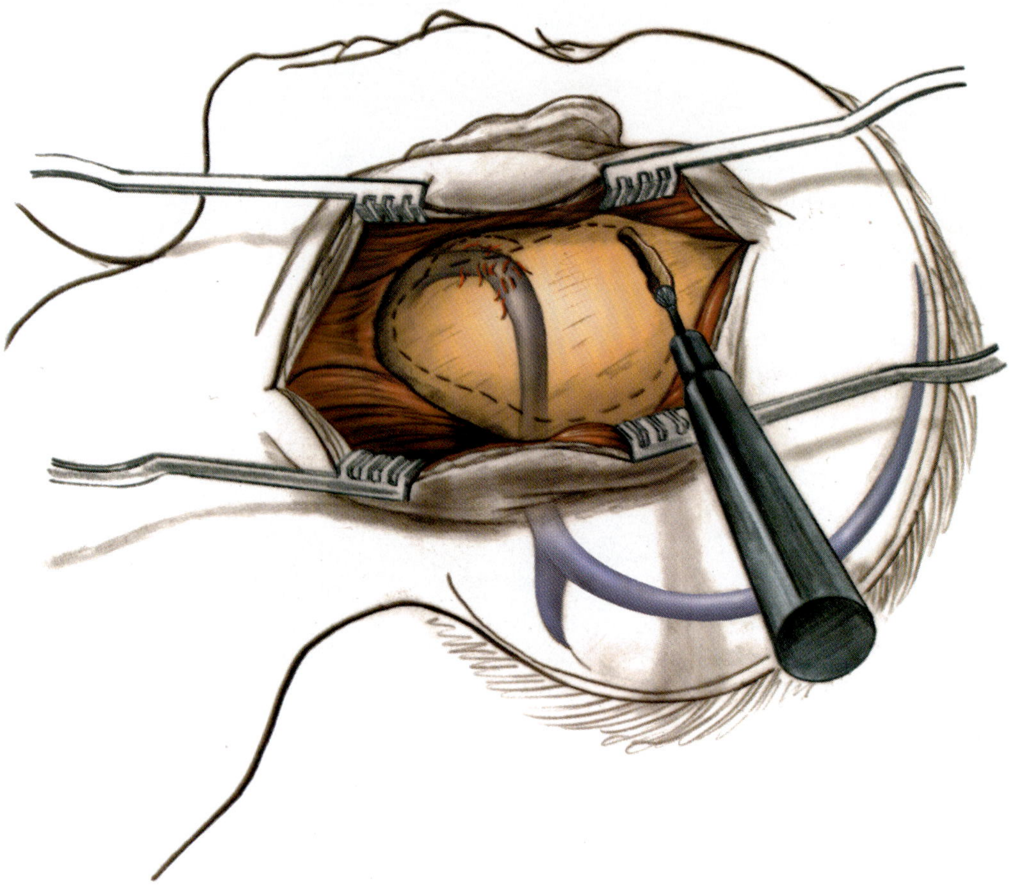

Figure 5–15.

Step 2. The craniotomy is made with a high-speed air drill and a diamond bur. A diamond bur is best because it helps with hemostasis by cauterizing the venous and arterial channels in the bone diploë. The air drill should be held at approximately a 30-degree angle to prevent drilling vertically through the bone. Drilling should proceed uniformly around the craniotomy.

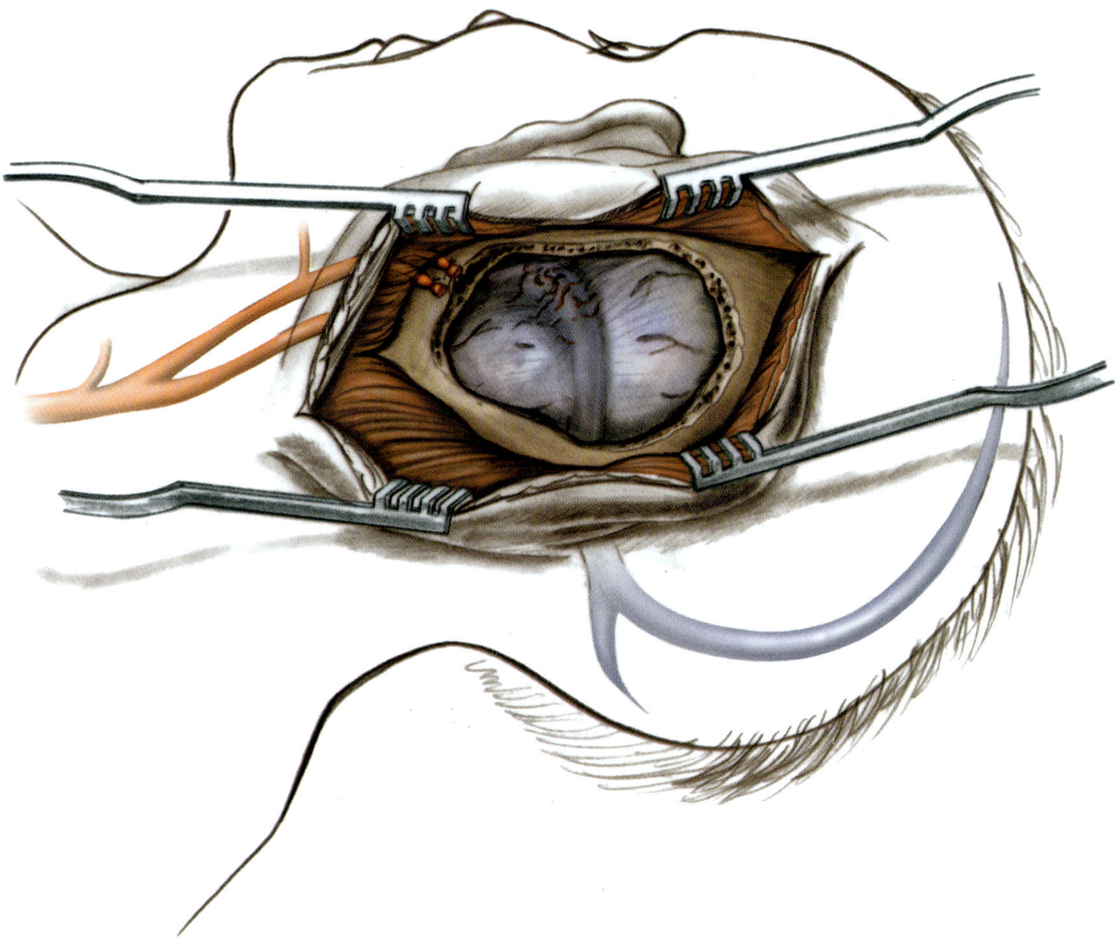

Figure 5–16.

Step 3. After the inner cortical layer has been identified around the circumference of the craniotomy, the bone flap can be removed with a small curved periosteal elevator. As the bone flap is removed, bleeding may occur from the dural arterial and venous vessels. This can be controlled with a large piece of absorbable gelatin sponge. Preoperative embolization decreases the risk of significant hemorrhage during removal of the bone flap.

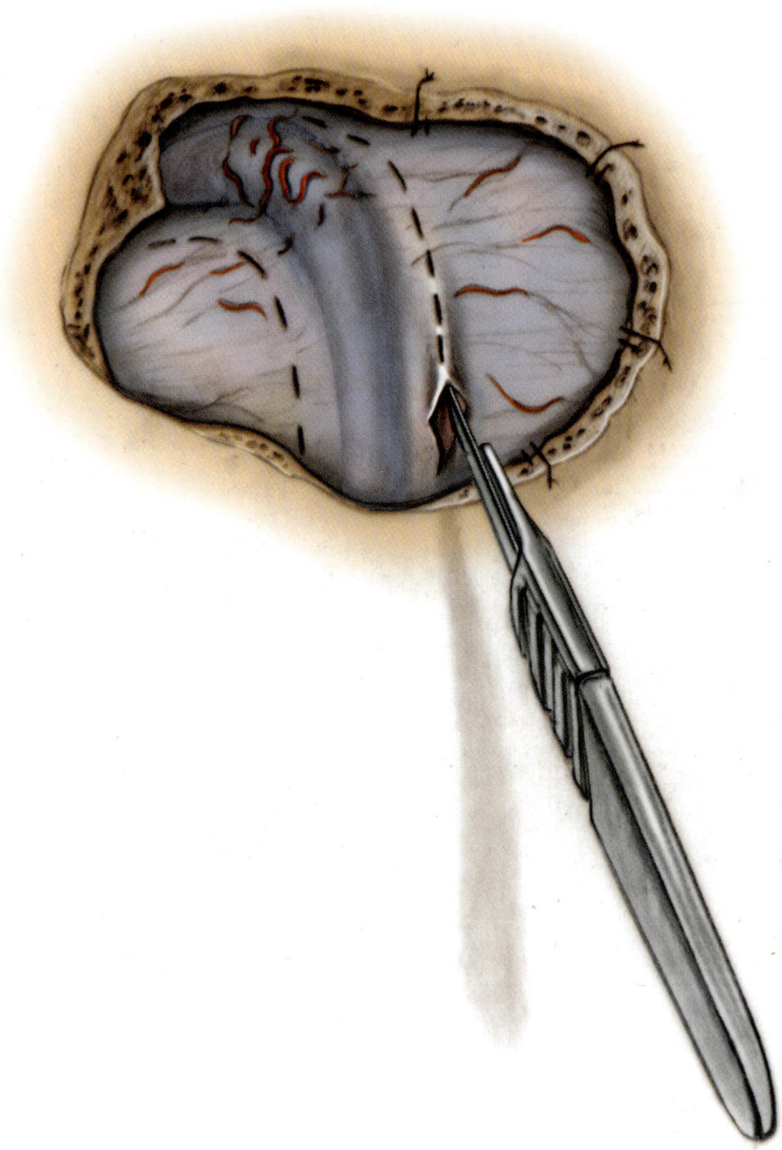

Figure 5–17.

Step 4. A high-speed air drill and a diamond bur are used to unroof the sigmoid sinus by removing the lateral aspect of the mastoid bone. It is unnecessary to remove the mastoid to the point at which the semicircular canals are identified. It is necessary to visualize the dura mater medial to the sigmoid sinus so it can be cauterized. The *dashed lines* on the figure indicate the two parallel incisions that are made above and below the transverse sinus. It is important to ensure that these incisions are approximately 7 to 10 mm lateral to the sinus to allow a good edge for subsequent sewing of the dural grafts. These incisions are made by first cauterizing the dura mater and then incising it with a #11 blade knife. A cottonoid is placed through the incision to protect the underlying parenchyma of the brain. The incisions are extended laterally with a small dissecting scissors or knife. As the junction between the transverse and sigmoid sinuses is approached, the dura mater becomes more vascular.

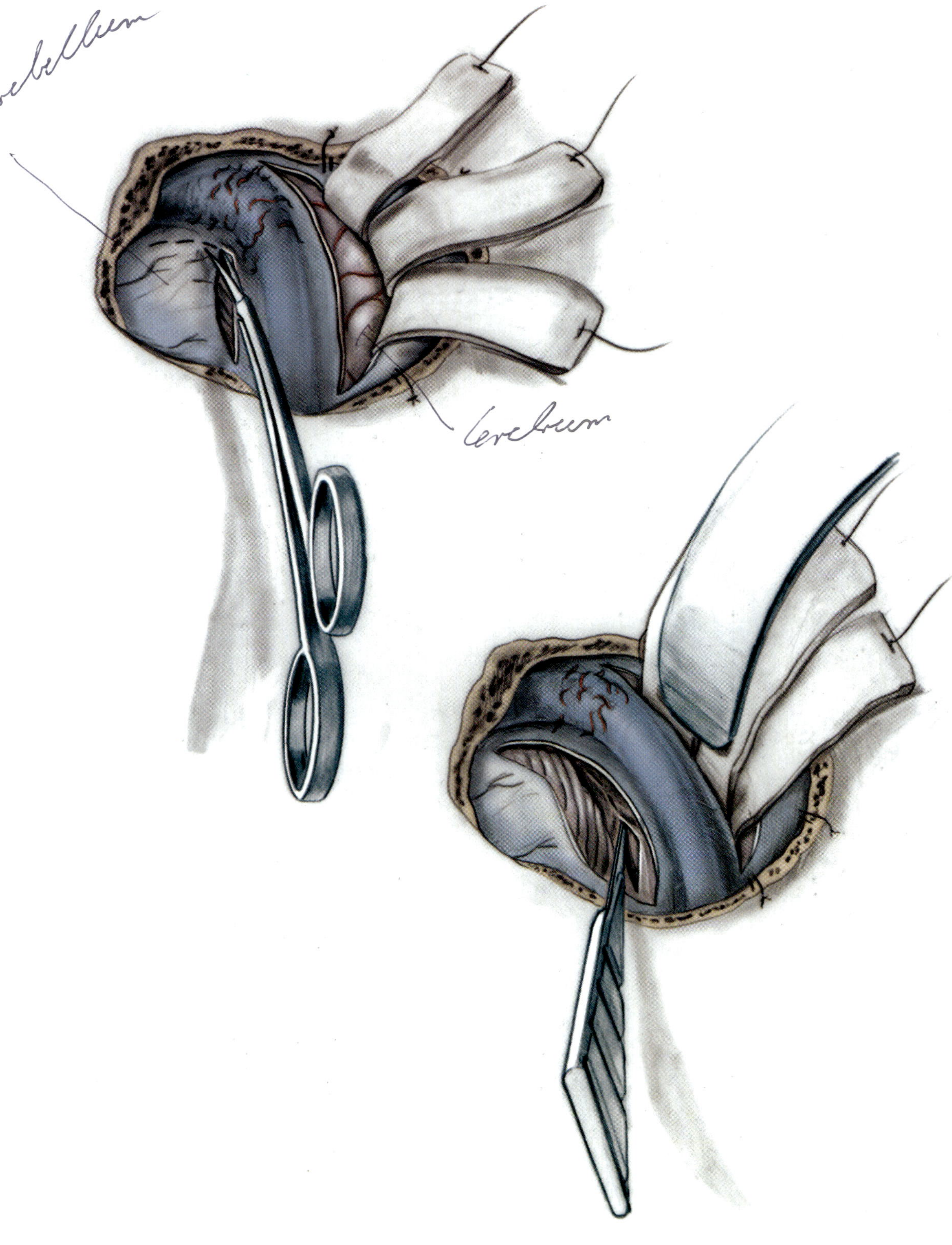

Figure 5–18.

Step 5. The dura mater has been cauterized and divided as far as the junction of the transverse and sigmoid sinuses. Cottonoids have been placed to protect both the cerebellum and the occipital lobe. The next step is to section the medial tentorium cerebelli. This is difficult because the sigmoid sinus is to be preserved and, therefore, cannot be rotated outward as a handle. It is best to use the microscope for good illumination. An incision is made in the tentorium with a #11 blade knife. The underlying brain parenchyma is protected with cottonoids. The incision is carried to the petrous bone using cautery and the #11 blade knife.

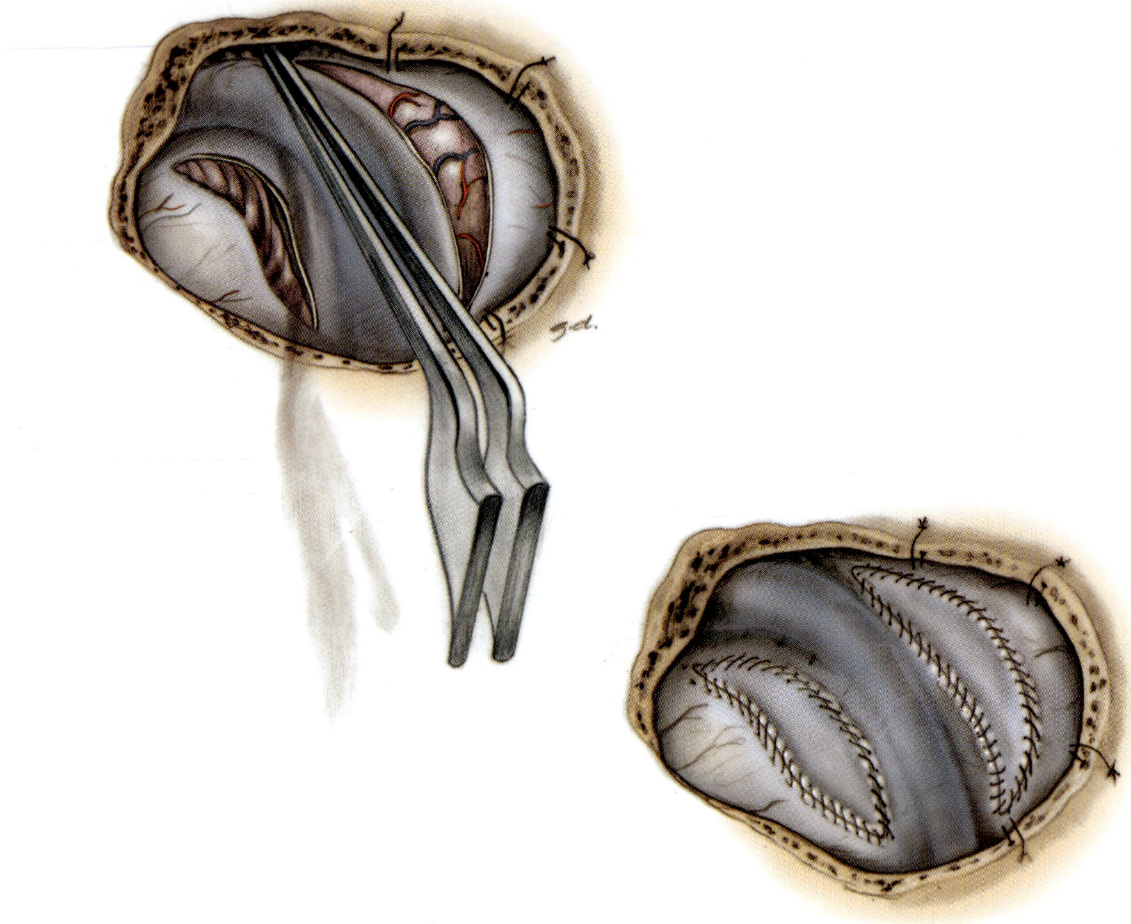

Figure 5–19.

Step 6. At this point, in addition to the occipital and suboccipital dura mater having been sectioned, the tentorium cerebelli has been divided to the petrous apex. The bipolar cautery is used to extensively cauterize the dura mater lying along the inner side of the petrous bone. The dura mater is cauterized from both an occipital and a suboccipital approach. It is important to irrigate the surgical field while cauterizing to prevent burning a hole through this lateral dura mater. If the petrosal sinus is opened inadvertently, it is packed with a small piece of hemostatic fabric. The dura mater lateral to the sigmoid sinus that was revealed by the earlier unroofing of the mastoid sinus is also cauterized. Afterward, the two dural openings are closed with dural grafts.

6

Modified Pterional Approach

Copyright © 1999 Mayo Foundation.

The modified pterional craniotomy, or anterior temporal approach, developed by Sundt provides good access to the upper basilar artery and the basilar caput. One of the major principles of the modified pterional approach is that the temporal lobe is retracted in an anterior-to-posterior direction to allow access to an aneurysm along the floor of the middle cranial fossa. This type of anterior-to-posterior retraction is well tolerated as long as the Sylvian fissure is widely divided. Another advantage of this approach is that it usually is possible to repair the aneurysm without a cutout clip, which sometimes can be difficult to place precisely. Furthermore, it is easier to identify and to dissect the opposite P_1 segment of the posterior cerebral artery through a modified pterional approach than with a subtemporal approach.

When contemplating the approach to a basilar caput aneurysm, two important considerations are the relationship of the neck of the aneurysm to the posterior clinoid process and the projection of the dome of the aneurysm. The modified pterional approach is best suited for aneurysms that are within 1.5 cm in either direction of the posterior clinoid process. For high basilar caput aneurysms, a subtemporal approach through a frontotemporal zygomatic craniotomy may offer a better line of site, with less retraction of the brain. For low basilar caput or basilar trunk aneurysms, a subtemporal transtentorial approach works well.

Approximately one-half of the aneurysms of the basilar caput have a dome that projects posteriorly. Therefore, the back wall of the aneurysm is related intimately to the thalamoperforating arteries that arise from the P_1 segment and the caput. Visualization and dissection of these perforating arteries may be extremely difficult, especially with a large posteriorly projecting dome. In that case, additional surgical maneuvers, including temporary occlusion of the basilar artery or deep hypothermic circulatory arrest, may be necessary to collapse the dome to facilitate the dissection of these perforating arteries off the back wall of the aneurysm.

The second most common projection is straight superior. Larger superiorly projecting aneurysms may present with obstructive hydrocephalus. In smaller superiorly projecting aneurysms, dissecting the thalamoperforating arteries is technically easier than it is for posteriorly projecting domes. The least common projection is anteriorly toward the dorsum sellae. When performing the dissection, a small cottonball can sometimes be placed between the basilar artery and the clivus to facilitate the dissection of the underside of the neck of the aneurysm.

ANATOMY

Perforating arteries originate from the posterior aspect of the basilar artery as it ascends along the pons. Small paramedian perforating arteries can be found within 2 to 3 mm caudal to the basilar bifurcation. One perforating artery may arise from the basilar caput. These basilar perforating vessels enter the interpeduncular cistern along with the posterior thalamoperforating arteries that originate from the P_1 segment of the posterior cerebral artery.

The posterior thalamoperforating arteries, branches of the P_1 segment, are asymmetric and may originate as one or more thalamoperforating trunks that branch within the interpeduncular cistern. The anterior thalamoperforating arteries originate from the posterior communicating artery. Also, branches of the P_2 segment of the posterior cerebral artery are referred to as the "thalamogeniculate" and "peduncular perforating arteries." These perforating arteries perfuse the mammillary bodies, the posterior thalamus, the hypothalamus, the subthalamus, the substantia nigra, the oculomotor and trochlear nuclei, the red nucleus, the mesencephalic reticular formation, the pretectum, the rostral medial floor of the fourth ventricle, and part of the posterior limb of the internal capsule. Injury to these perforating vessels leads to devastating neurologic outcomes.

The short and the long lateral circumflex arteries originate from the medial aspect of the P_1 and P_2 segments. They wrap around the midbrain in parallel with the posterior cerebral artery to perfuse the geniculate bodies, the collicular plate, and the cerebral peduncles.

As emphasized by Sundt, in superiorly projecting aneurysms, the P_1 segments are frequently adherent to the base of the aneurysm, especially when the bifurcation is low. If the P_1 segments are densely adherent to the neck and cannot be sharply dissected free, Drake cutout clips are necessary to obliterate the aneurysm, with the thalamoperforating arteries passing through the aperture of the cutout clip.

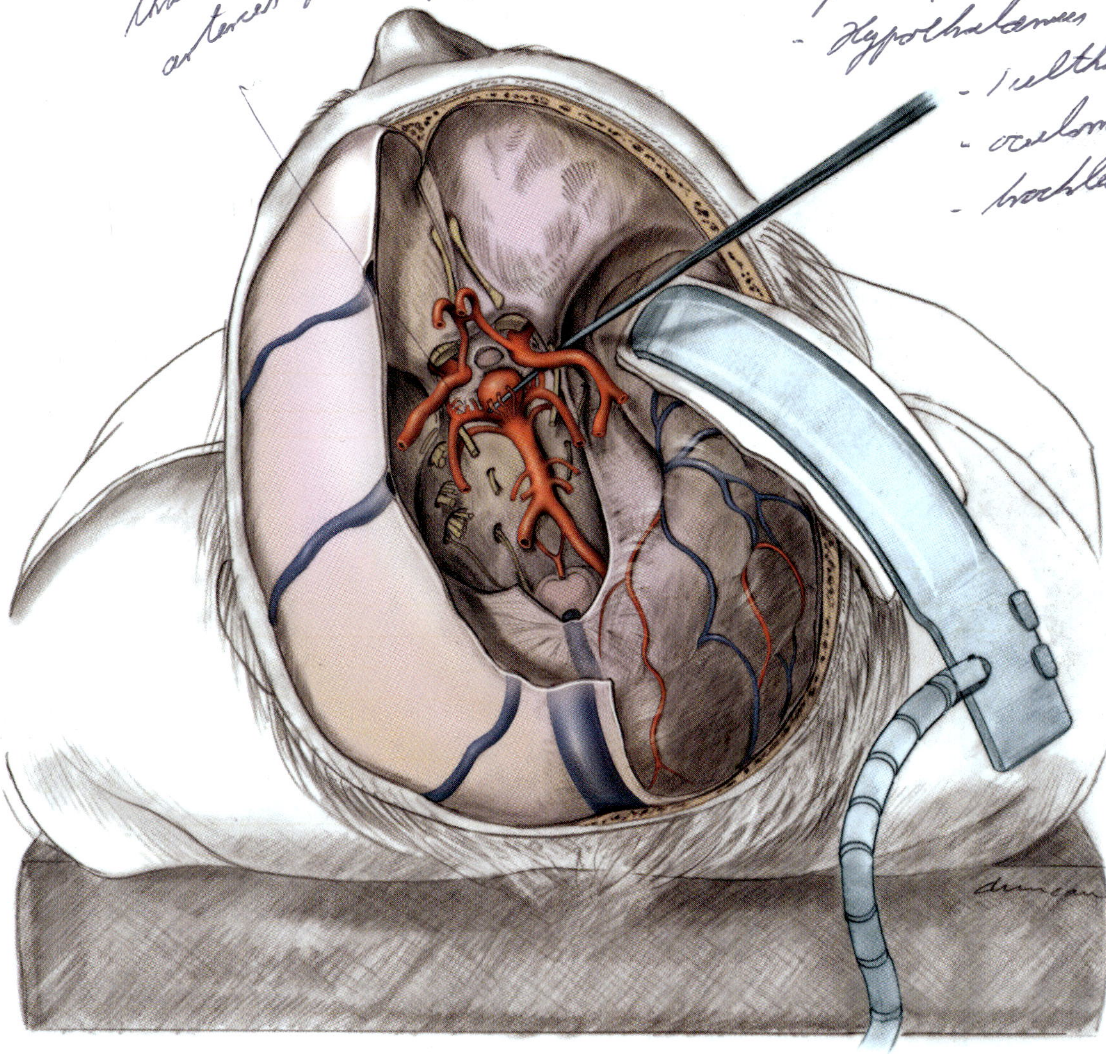

Figure 6–1.

With the modified pterional approach, the patient's head is rotated 15 to 20 degrees and slightly flexed, approximately 15 degrees. Therefore, there is no head extension compared to a standard pterional craniotomy. Flexion of the head rotates the posterior clinoid process forward and brings the basilar caput into the line of sight through a middle cranial fossa trajectory. With this approach, it is necessary to retract the temporal lobe in an anterior-to-posterior direction. The posterior communicating artery may clutter the microoperative field. If so, it often can be ligated safely at its junction with the posterior cerebral artery as long as its origin from the internal carotid artery appears to be sufficiently large and there is no fetal-type circulation. The posterior communicating artery and its perforating branches are then swept forward.

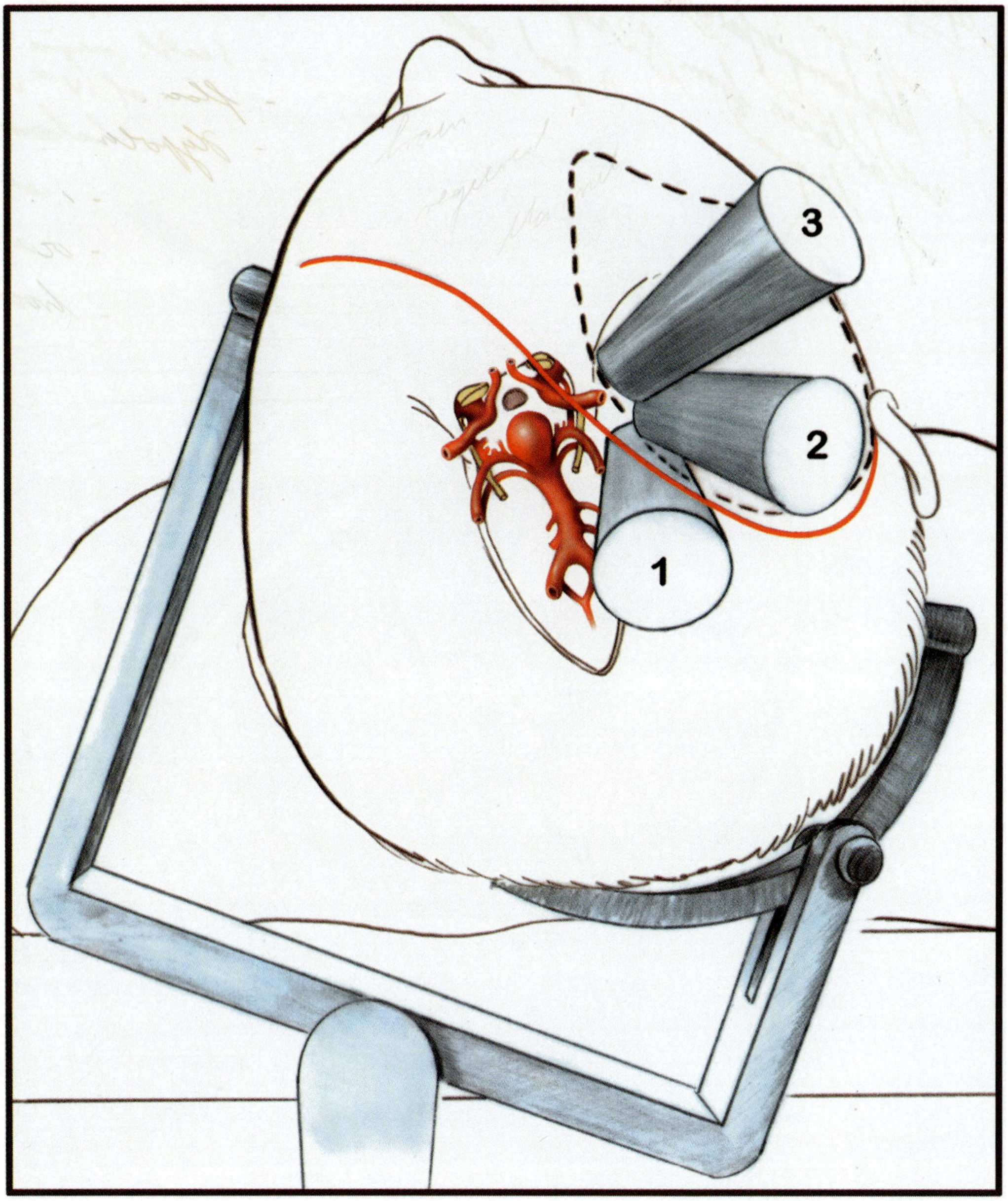

Figure 6–2.

This approach uses a craniotomy that exposes more of the floor of the middle cranial fossa than a standard pterional approach does. Therefore, the skin incision must curve posteriorly above the ear. The temporalis muscle is reflected anteriorly with the skin flap. The lower edge of the craniotomy is made with a high-speed air drill to remove the inferior portion of the temporal squamous bone, thereby allowing a middle cranial fossa approach. As the operation progresses, the angle of view progresses laterally. One, initially, the view is along the Sylvian fissure, to aid in its dissection. Two, after the temporal lobe has been retracted posteriorly, the arachnoid along the edge of the tentorium cerebelli and the oculomotor nerve is dissected free. Three, after this is accomplished, the head of the operating microscope is shifted more laterally as the surgeon works across the middle cranial fossa to approach the basilar caput. Because of this shifting line of sight, it is important that the scrub nurse and the overlying brain table be sufficiently caudal so that the space along the patient's shoulder is open and free. In this way, the surgeon can sit comfortably with his or her arm resting on the patient's shoulder, with adequate room for the microscope head. A standard frontotemporal craniotomy is used for the exposure.

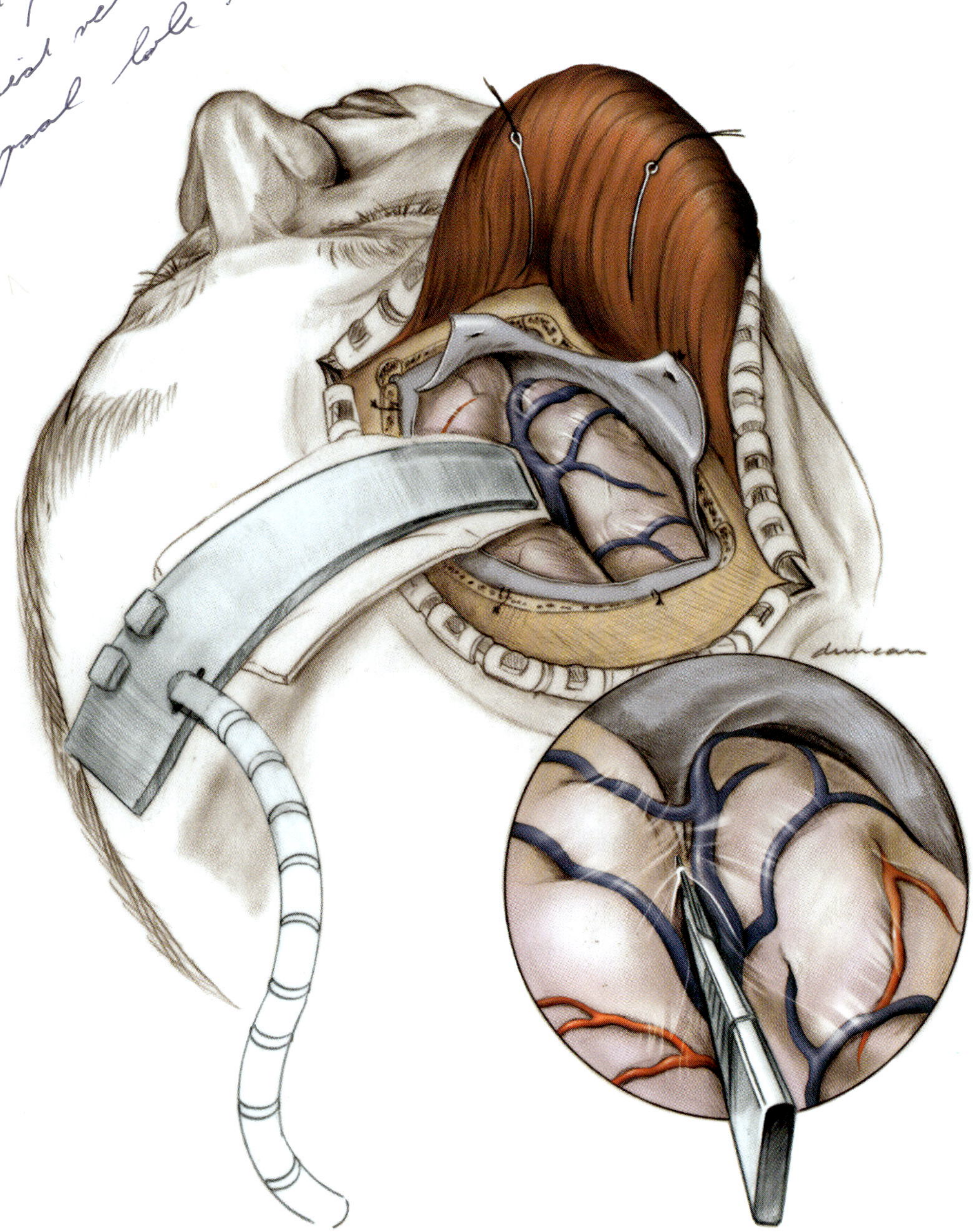

Figure 6–3.

Step 1. After the frontotemporal craniotomy has been performed, the dura mater is opened and tacked to the margins of the bone. Under the operating microscope, the Sylvian fissure is widely divided. The more completely the bridging arachnoid is divided, the less traction there will be on the frontal lobe as the temporal lobe is displaced posteriorly.

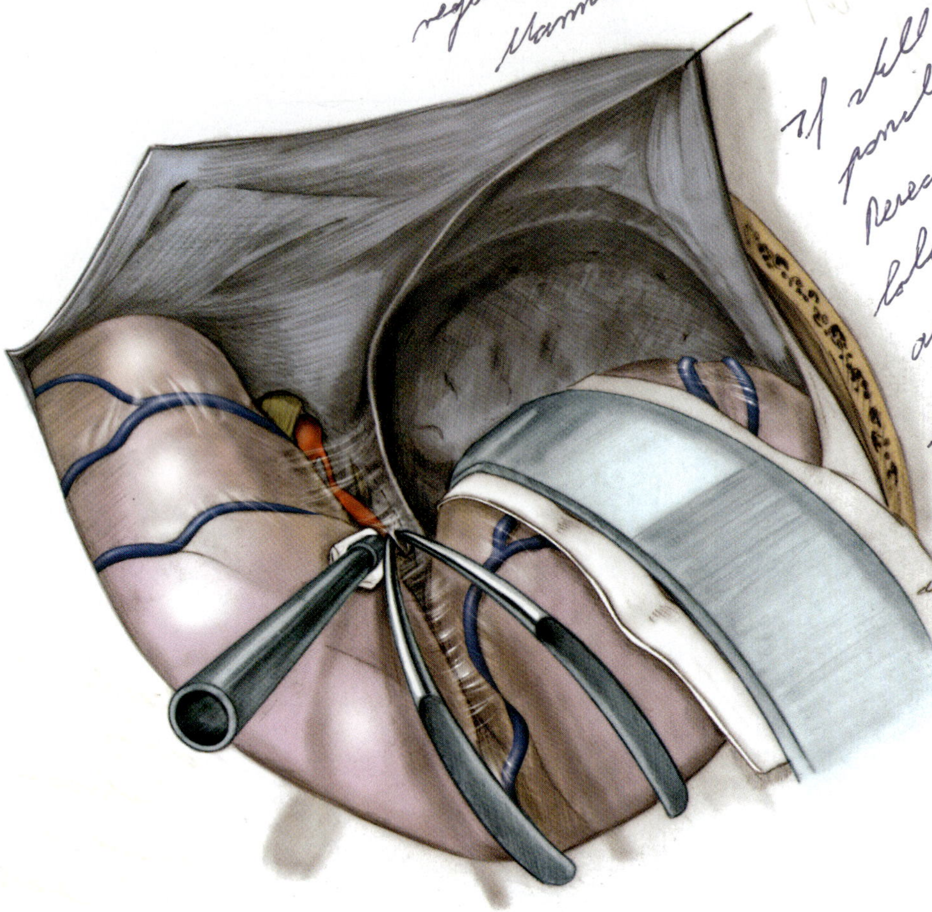

Figure 6–4.

Step 2. The tip of the temporal lobe is lined with hemostatic fabric (Surgicel) and cottonoids (Americot) and gently retracted in a posterior direction. Typically, bridging veins come off the tip of the temporal lobe and must be cauterized and divided. After the temporal lobe has been retracted posteriorly, any bridging arachnoid deep along the edge of the tentorium cerebelli between the frontal and temporal lobes must be separated. As the temporal lobe is retracted, brain relaxation is required. Draining cerebrospinal fluid through a lumbar needle and administering mannitol intravenously help facilitate brain relaxation. In rare circumstances, the brain may still be tight and the surgeon will not be able to obtain good access along the edge of the tentorium cerebelli. In this case, the tip of the temporal lobe and uncus, which contains the amygdala, can be removed. The risk of memory impairment with removal of the nondominant medial temporal lobe is minimal.

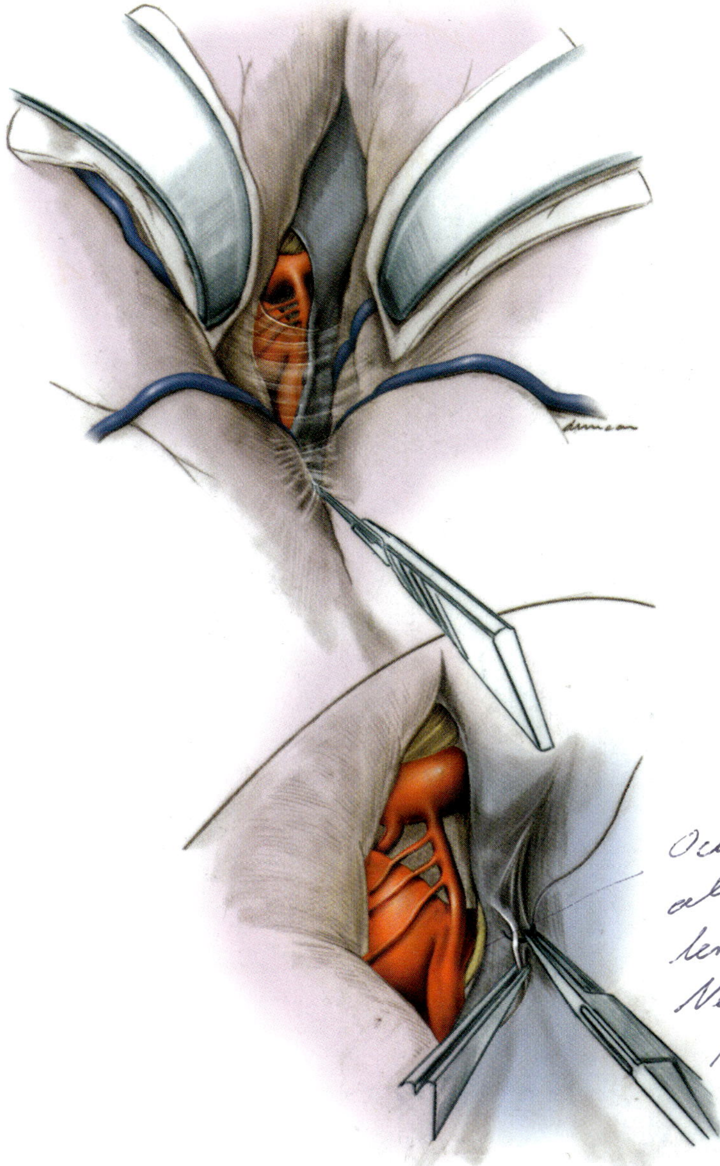

Figure 6–5.

Step 3. Under high magnification, the edge of the tentorium cerebelli is identified. The arachnoid overlying it is incised and separated with a fine dissecting spatula. It may be necessary to place a small retractor along the underside of the frontal lobe, which will displace the internal carotid artery medially. Along the edge of the tentorium cerebelli, the most important landmark is the oculomotor nerve. Overlying this nerve is the posterior cerebral artery, which the surgeon follows to the basilar caput. After the oculomotor nerve has been identified, the edge of the tentorium cerebelli is retracted laterally by placing a tacking suture into the temporal dura mater. When placing the suture, it is important to avoid the trochlear nerve and to make sure that the suture is as tight as possible to provide maximal retraction of the edge of the tentorium cerebelli. The best way to tie the suture is to throw the first two knots in the same direction. This allows cinching the knot downward. The third throw is done in reverse to lock the knot.

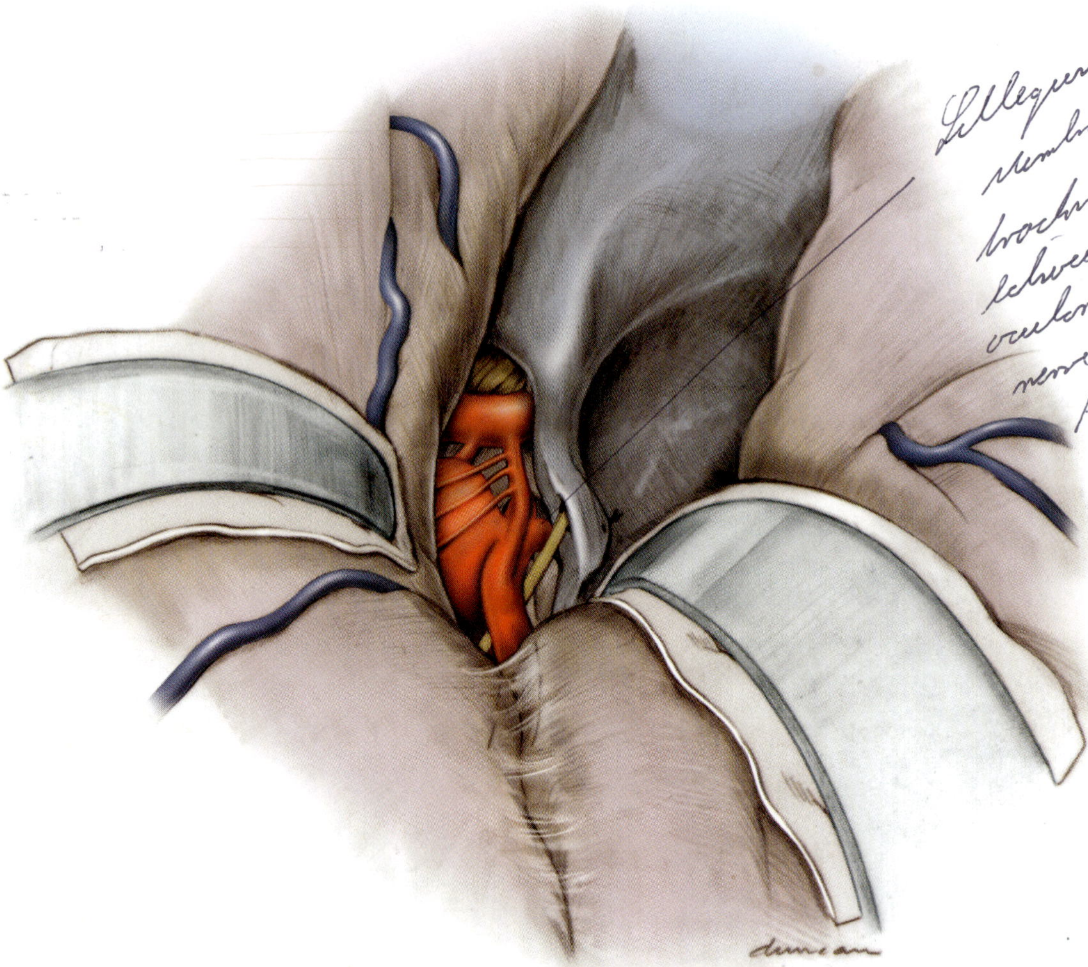

Figure 6–6.

Step 4. The medial temporal lobe, including the uncus, is retracted to better identify the edge of the tentorium cerebelli. The oculomotor nerve is identified, and the posterior cerebral artery is followed medially to the basilar caput. It is necessary to dissect the arachnoid (Liliequist's membrane) between the oculomotor nerve and the posterior cerebral artery to provide access to the basilar trunk. With low-lying bifurcations, access to the basilar trunk is provided between the oculomotor nerve and the tentorium cerebelli. Before dissecting out the aneurysm, it is best to ensure that the basilar artery is visualized and free in case a temporary clip must be placed. In fact, it is best to have the scrub nurse load the clip and the surgeon practice placing it to make sure that an aneurysm clip of correct length has been chosen. It also is important to have two suction tips available: a smaller #5 or #7 suction tip is used for the dissection and a large #15-French suction tip is hooked to the wall suction and is immediately available should the aneurysm rupture prematurely.

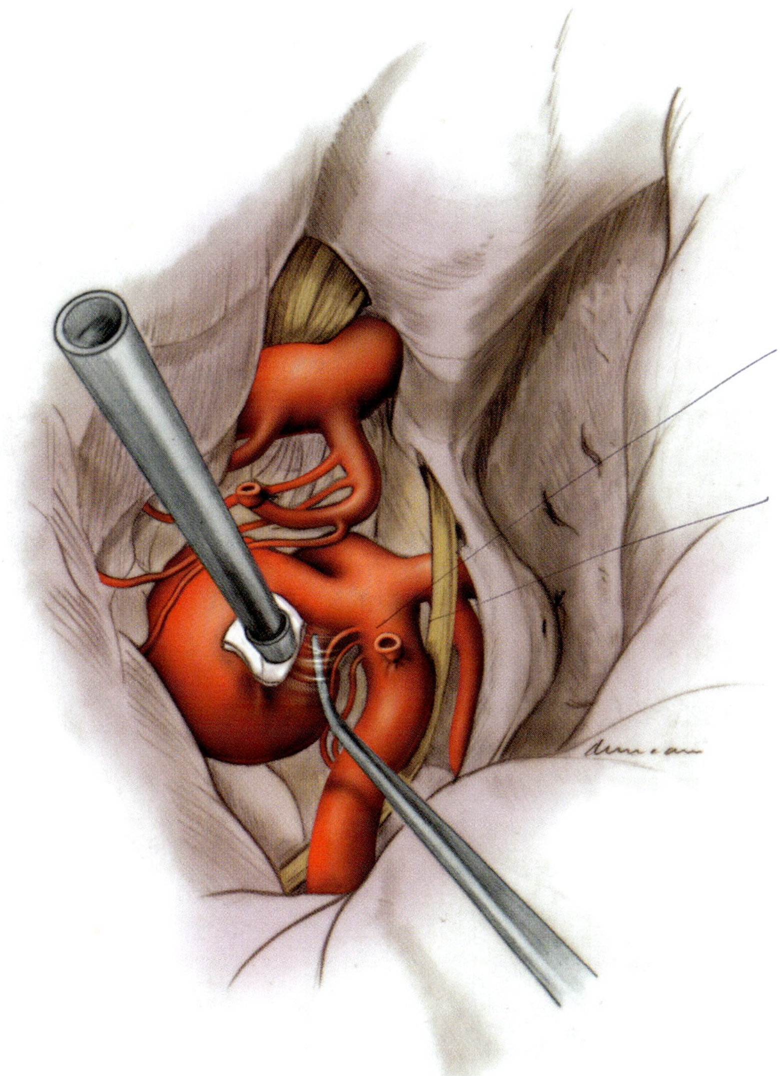

Figure 6–7.

Step 5. The posterior communicating artery is often in the line of sight. It usually can be ligated close to the posterior cerebral artery and, along with its perforating arteries, be swept forward in its own arachnoid sheath out of harm's way. Although small wire clips can be used to ligate the posterior communicating artery, these clips occasionally can be in the way. Therefore, ligation with an 8-0 or 9-0 monofilament suture is best. Dissection of the aneurysm starts along the proximal posterior cerebral artery to identify the thalamostriate arteries that originate from the P_1 segment and their relationship to the neck of the aneurysm. These perforating arteries can be swept off as a sheet in continuity with the perforating arteries along the basilar caput on the back side of the neck of the aneurysm, because they are ensheathed in a thin layer of arachnoid. Therefore, first identifying the correct plane along the proximal P_1 segment will aid in dissection of the small perforating arteries along the back side of the aneurysm.

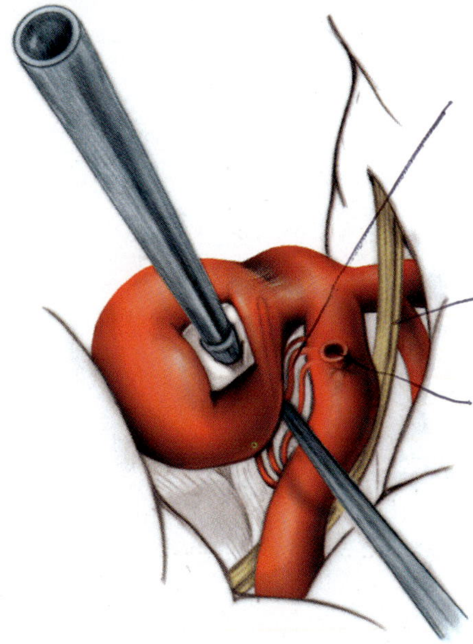

Figure 6–8.

Step 6. After the thalamogeniculate perforating arteries have been dissected off the ipsilateral posterior cerebral artery and basilar caput, a piece of absorbable gelatin sponge (Gelfoam) is placed between them and the neck of the aneurysm. This keeps these small vessels out of harm's way when the aneurysm clip is placed.

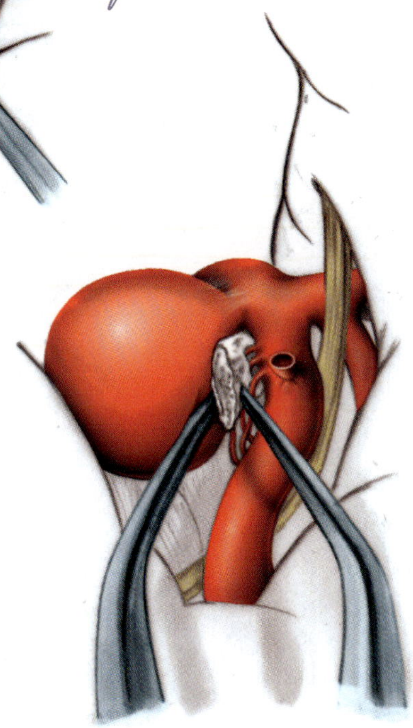

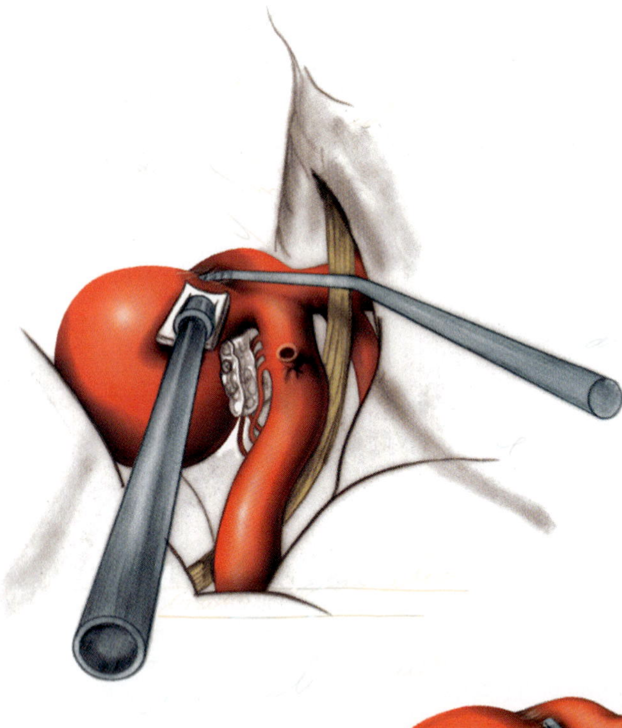

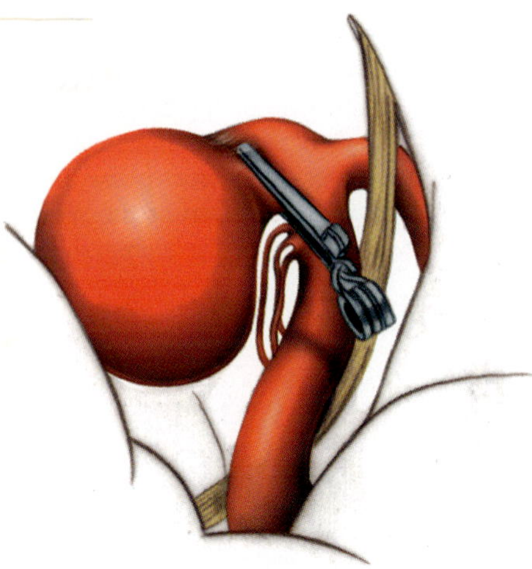

Figure 6–9.

Step 7. The contralateral P_1 segment is dissected off the neck of the aneurysm to identify the thalamogeniculate trunk that originates from that P_1 segment. A small ball-tip dissector or angled spatula works best. The dome of the aneurysm is manipulated gently with a #5 or #7 suction tip and a cottonoid. If the surgeon is concerned about rupturing the aneurysm, there are several options to consider. One, the patient's systolic blood pressure can be decreased to 80 to 90 mm Hg to soften the dome. Two, the basilar artery can be occluded temporarily just above or below the oculomotor nerve. Depending on the position of the basilar caput, placement of a temporary aneurysm clip can be difficult and may clutter the operative field. After the contralateral P_1 segment has been dissected off the neck of the aneurysm, a small piece of absorbable gelatin sponge is placed if a major thalamogeniculate trunk has been identified. An aneurysm clip is then placed across the neck of the aneurysm, parallel to the posterior cerebral arteries. The absorbable gelatin sponge is removed, and the dome of the aneurysm is aspirated. It is mandatory to make sure—absolutely sure—that no perforating vessels are caught within the aneurysm clip.

Figure 6–10.

A, In the sequence illustrated here, the aneurysm ruptured prematurely during dissection. The best strategy is to change immediately to a larger suction tip and to capture the dome. The neck can quickly be dissected free and the aneurysm clip placed. *B*, Alternatively, a temporary aneurysm clip can be placed on the basilar artery between the posterior cerebral artery and the superior cerebellar artery. Depending on the degree of collateral blood flow through the posterior communicating arteries, there may be a surprising amount of back bleeding through the aneurysm despite temporary occlusion of the basilar artery. After the aneurysm has been clipped, the temporary clip is removed to restore blood flow. Thereafter, the dome of the aneurysm is manipulated to ensure that all the perforating vessels are free. If prolonged temporary occlusion is anticipated, it is best to have the anesthesiologist normalize blood pressure and to administer a cerebral protective agent such as thiopental (2 to 3 mg/kg). Increasing the patient's blood pressure increases potential collateral blood flow, and the cerebral protective agent decreases metabolic demand.

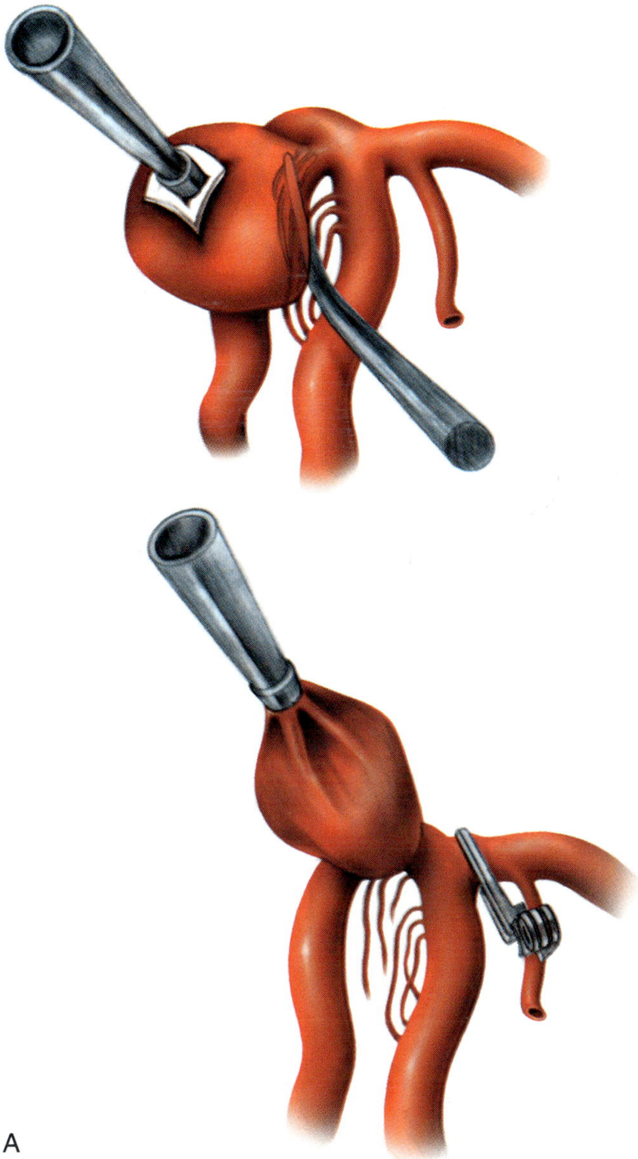

A

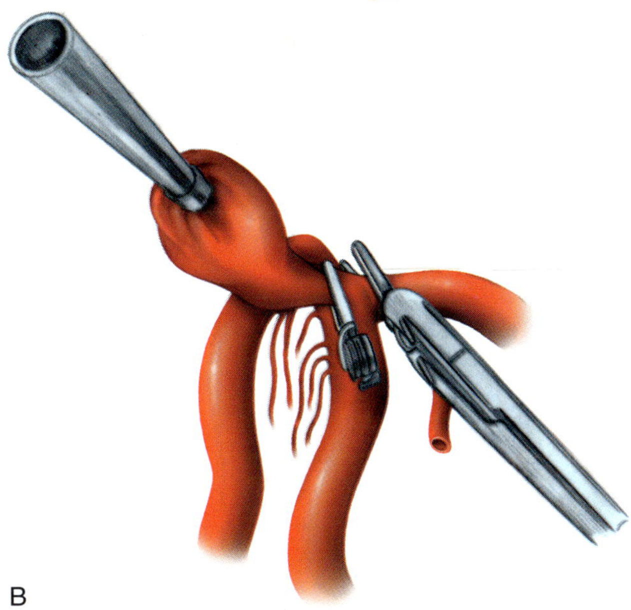

B

7

Temporal Approach

Copyright © 1999 Mayo Foundation.

A temporal craniotomy necessary for a subtemporal approach is useful to access aneurysms of the basilar caput at or below the level of the posterior clinoid process and those involving the upper one-third of the basilar trunk. This approach also provides good exposure for neoplasms, cysts, and vascular malformations that involve the tentorial notch, the medial temporal lobe, or the lateral aspect of the mesencephalon.

Regardless of the lesion, several principles should be adhered to in using the subtemporal approach. One, it is important to optimize the position of the patient's head so that it is nearly horizontal and extended approximately 10 degrees. Maintaining the head in a horizontal position aids in surgical orientation, and extending the head lessens the need for retraction of the temporal lobe. Two, it is important to remove residual temporal bone with rongeurs until the floor of the middle cranial fossa is reached. Three, it is necessary to protect the vein of Labbé, which nearly always is visualized along the posterior margins of the craniotomy. The vein of Labbé can be buttressed with absorbable gelatin sponge (Gelfoam) and cottonoids (Americot). Four, it usually is necessary to enhance brain relaxation with the use of lumbar spinal drainage and mannitol. Fifth, because medial temporal lobe structures are retracted, the perioperative use of anticonvulsants is prudent. Sixth, some mastoid air cells often are exposed when the temporal squamous bone is removed with rongeurs. A watertight dural closure decreases the risk of postoperative otorrhea.

BASILAR CAPUT ANEURYSM

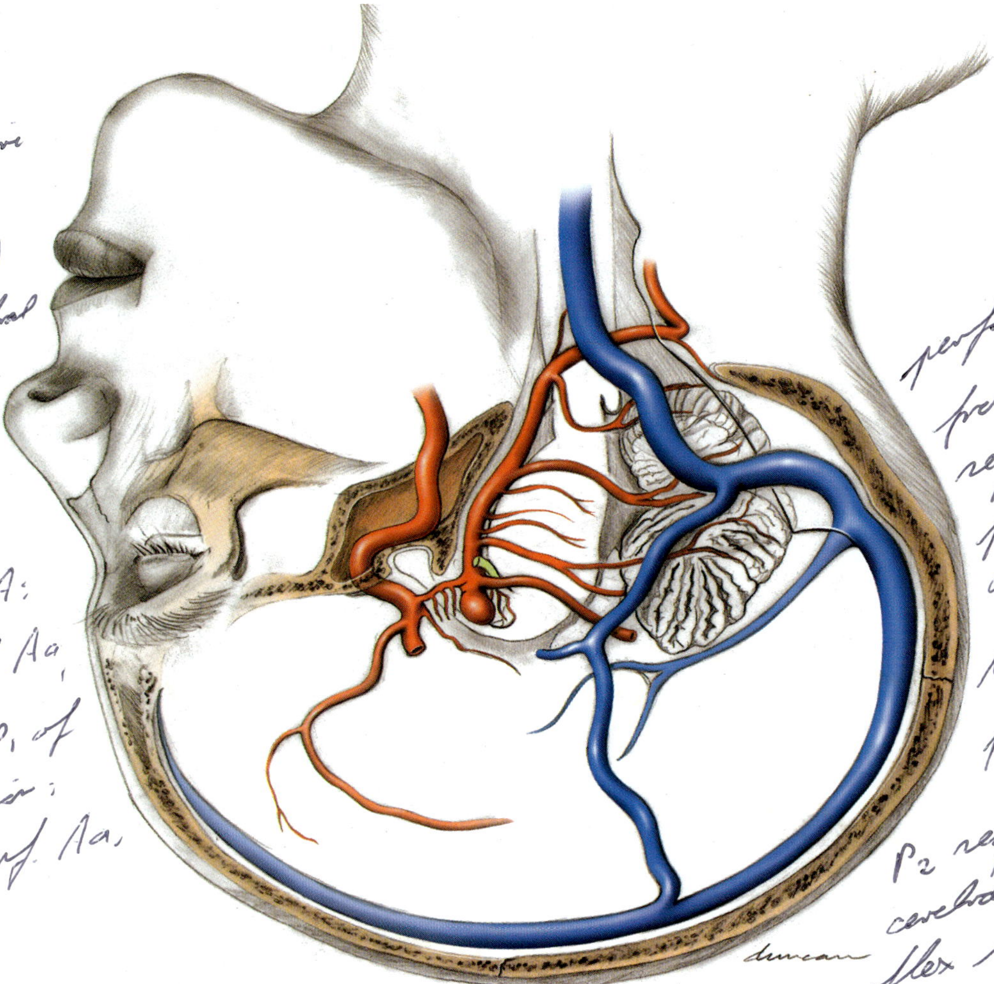

Figure 7–1.

In most cases, the upper basilar artery and caput should be approached from the right side in patients who have a dominant left hemisphere. This decreases the risk of injury to the dominant temporal lobe, medial temporal lobe structures, and vein of Labbé. However, in a patient with a P_1-P_2 aneurysm on the left side, a left subtemporal approach is required. Illustrated here is the vascular anatomy visualized through a subtemporal approach. The basilar caput is at the level of the dorsum sellae in approximately 50 percent of patients, superior to the dorsum sellae in 30 percent, and inferior in 20 percent. Approximately 80 percent of all aneurysms of the basilar caput are within 1.0 cm of the dorsum sellae. In tall persons, the bifurcation of the basilar artery tends to be at a lower level, below the level of the posterior clinoid process. Often, the P_1 segments are attached to the neck of the aneurysm, requiring the use of a fenestrated or cutout clip. It has been suggested that with increasing age, the basilar artery becomes progressively more tortuous and the level of its bifurcation becomes progressively more inferior.

The perforating arteries include ones that originate from the posterior communicating artery, the posterior aspect of the basilar bifurcation, and the P_1 segment of the posterior cerebral artery. The perforating arteries from the posterior communicating artery are termed the "anterior thalamoperforating arteries," and those from the P_1 segment are called the "posterior thalamoperforating arteries." Perforating branches from the P_2 segment of the posterior cerebral artery are termed the "thalamogeniculate" and "peduncular perforating arteries." Some of the thalamoperforating arteries supply the mammillary bodies, and the rest go through the interpeduncular fossa to supply the posterior thalamus, hypothalamus, subthalamus, substantia nigra, red nucleus, oculomotor and trochlear nuclei, mesencephalic reticular formation, pretectum, rostral medial floor of the fourth ventricle, and part of the posterior limb of the internal capsule.

Circumflex arteries also originate from the distal P_1 and P_2 segments and encircle the midbrain, running parallel and medial to the posterior cerebral artery. The short circumflex arteries primarily perfuse the geniculate bodies, and the long circumflex arteries supply the superior and inferior colliculi, the geniculate bodies, part of the cerebral peduncle, and part of the mesencephalic tegmentum. With the subtemporal approach, the primary vein at risk is the vein of Labbé, which runs along the posterior aspect of the craniotomy.

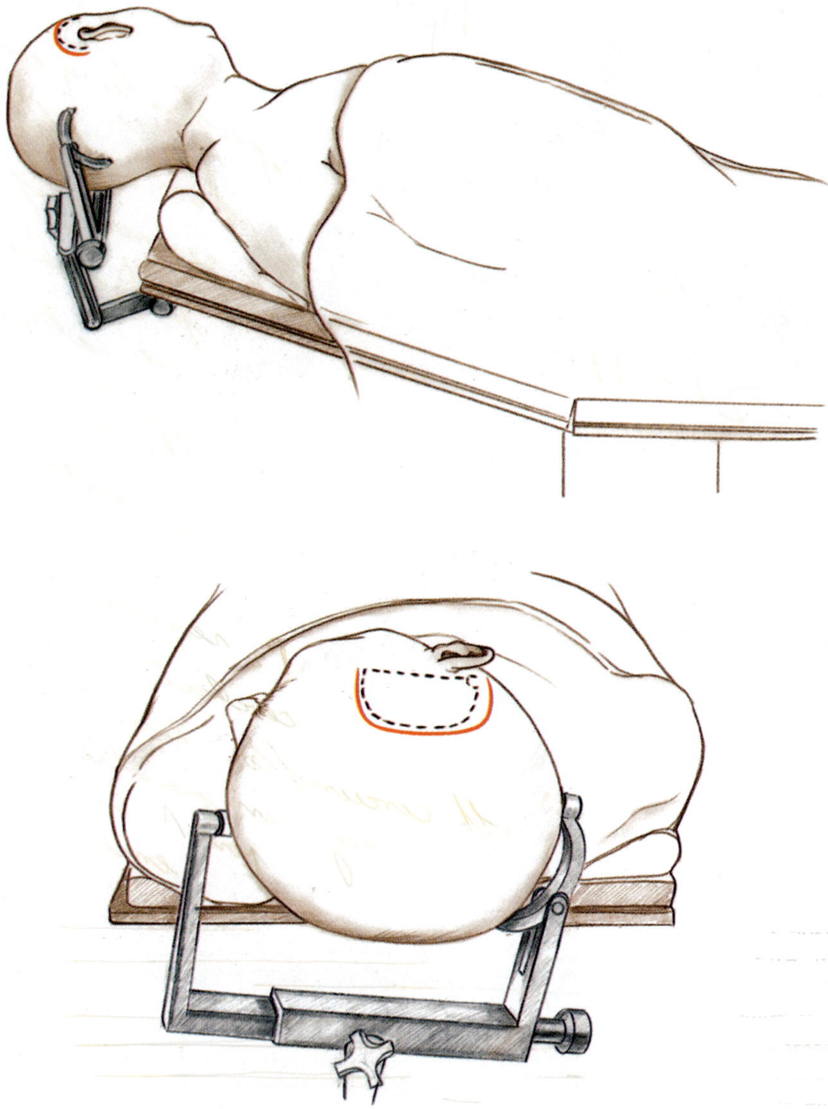

Figure 7–2.

Step 1. The patient's head is positioned nearly horizontal at 10 to 15 degrees and extended approximately 15 degrees. The U-shaped incision is centered over the ear. To avoid injury to the facial nerve, it is important to make sure that the anterior limb of the incision ends approximately 1.0 cm above the midportion of the zygoma.

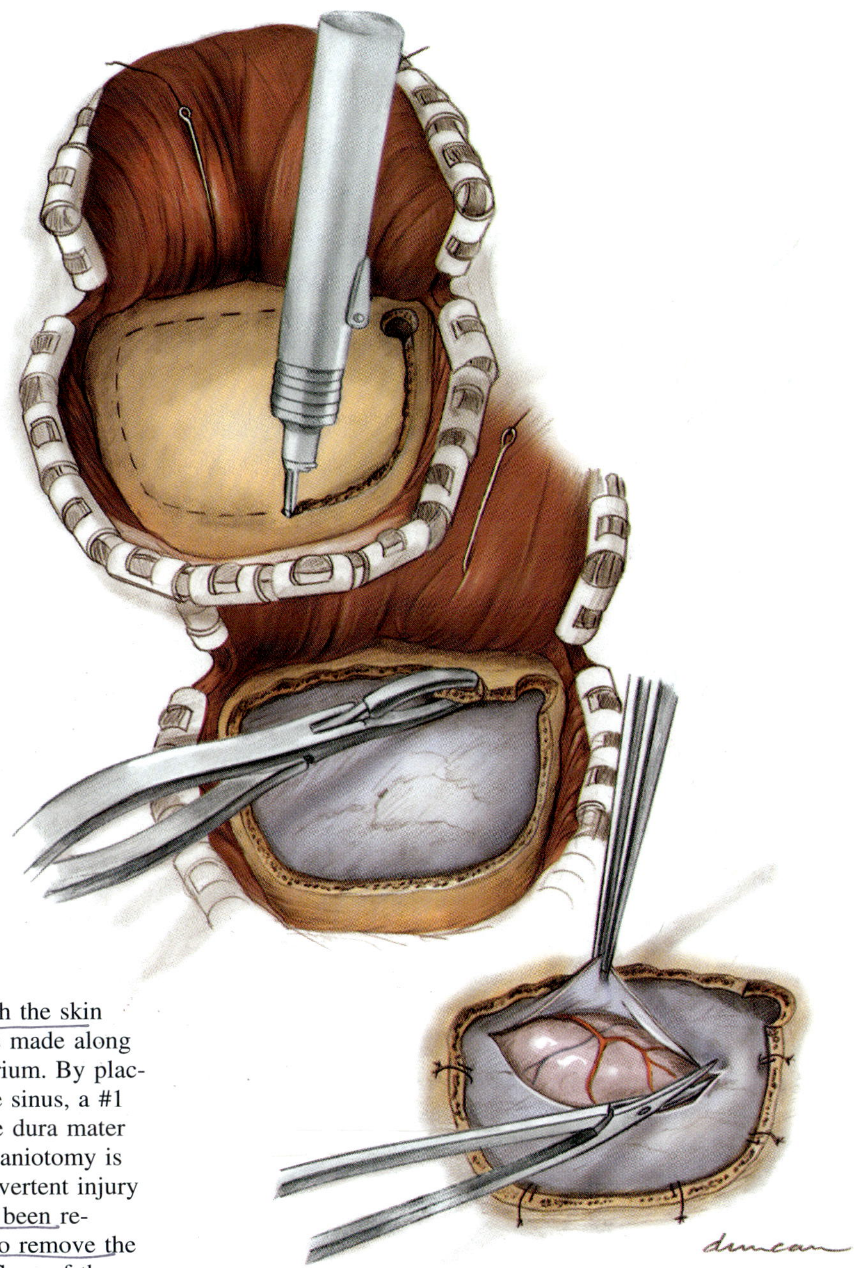

Figure 7–3.

Step 2. The temporalis muscle is turned with the skin flap and retracted with fishhooks. A bur hole is made along the posteroinferior aspect of the exposed calvarium. By placing this bur hole in the region of the transverse sinus, a #1 or #3 Penfield dissector can be used to peel the dura mater off the underside of the bone flap before the craniotomy is performed, thereby minimizing the risk of inadvertent injury to the transverse sinus. After the bone flap has been removed, it is important to use Adson rongeurs to remove the inferior temporal squamous bone down to the floor of the middle cranial fossa. The more bone that is removed, the better the angle of view along the temporal floor, with less retraction on the brain. Thereafter, the dura mater is tacked to the margins of the bone and then opened in a U-shaped fashion. Next, the dura mater is retracted by repositioning the fishhooks previously used to hold the temporalis muscle.

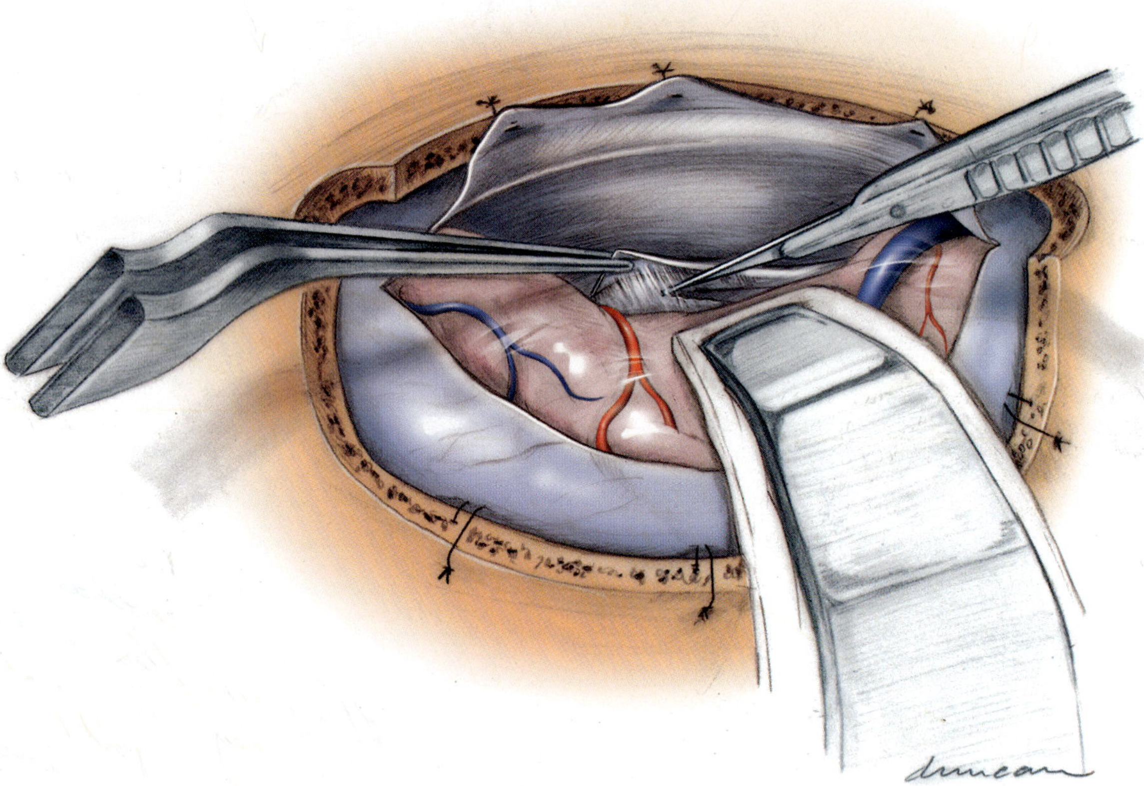

Figure 7–4.

Step 3. The vein of Labbé is protected with absorbable gelatin sponge and cottonoids. The mid-temporal lobe is retracted with a Yasargil self-retaining retractor. During this retraction, the temporal lobe is elevated approximately 1.5 to 2.0 cm. Brain retraction is facilitated with the use of lumbar spinal drainage and mannitol. The edge of the tentorium cerebelli is retracted with a toothed pickup, and the arachnoid is incised and opened with a #11 blade knife. During this incision and dissection, it is important to identify both the oculomotor and the trochlear nerves to ensure that they are not inadvertently injured.

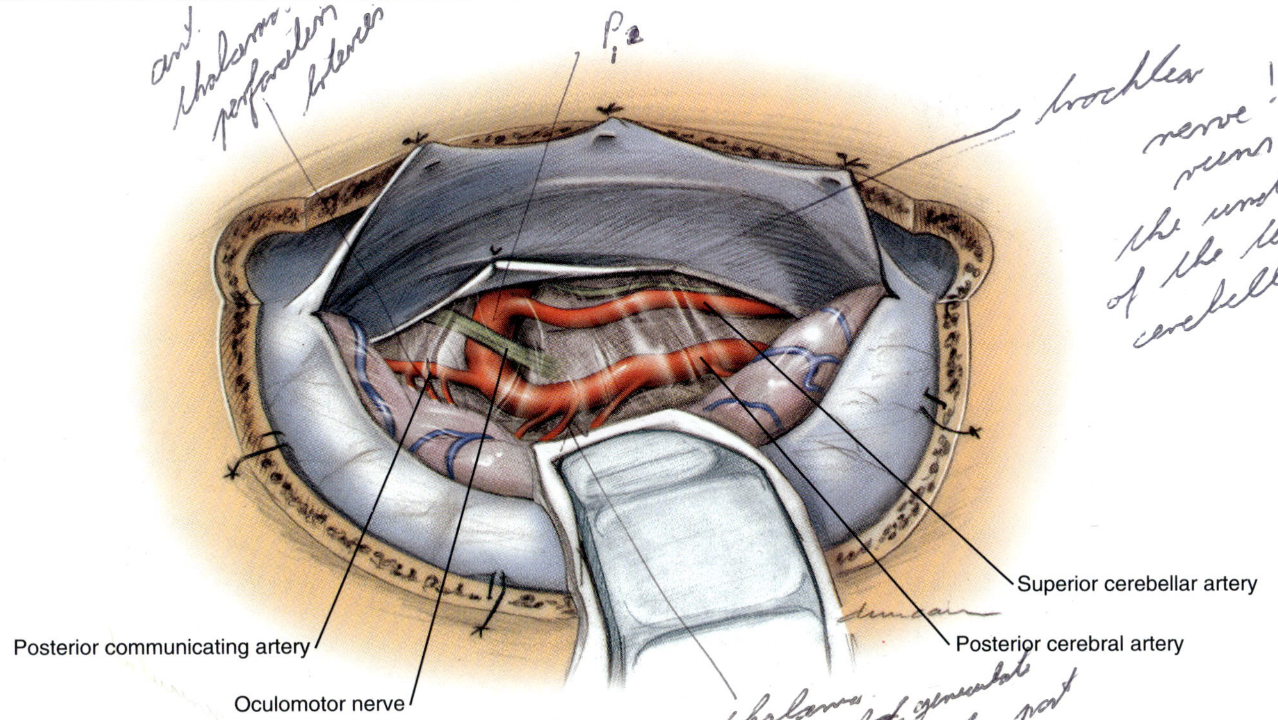

Figure 7–5.

Step 4. The edge of the tentorium cerebelli is tacked lateral to the floor of the middle cranial fossa with an interrupted suture. The stitch is placed anterior to the trochlear nerve, which runs along the underside of the tentorium cerebelli. The oculomotor nerve is the landmark for orientation.

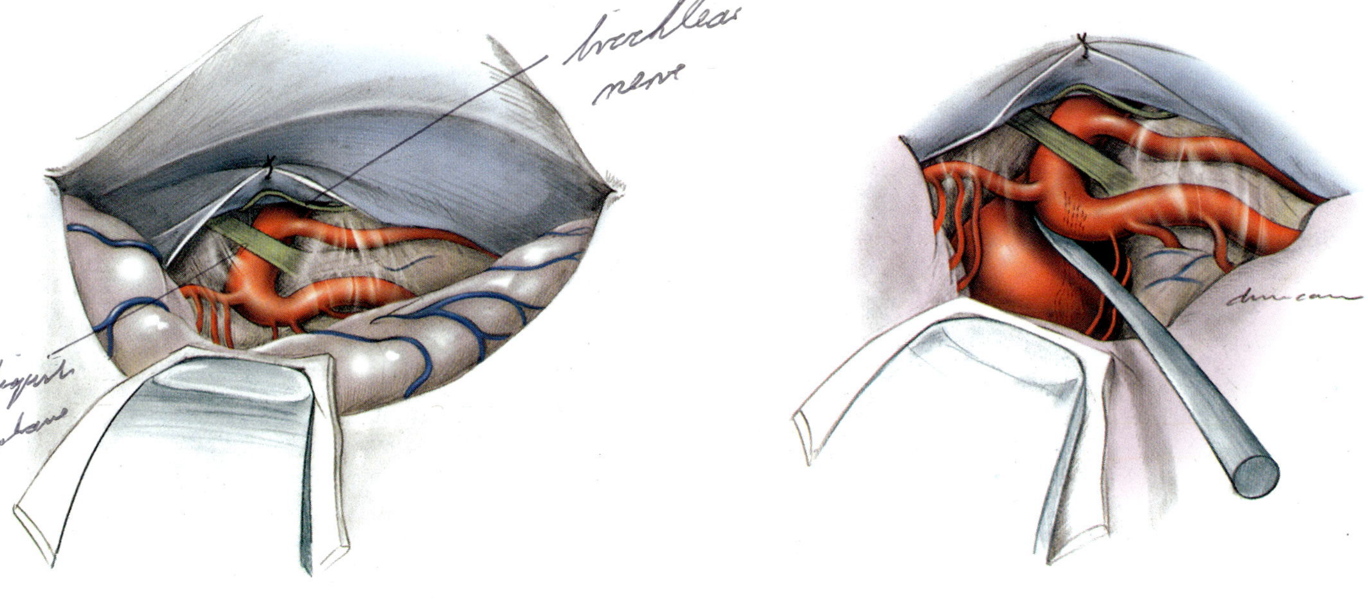

Figure 7–6.

Step 5. The Yasargil retractor is placed deeper to elevate the uncus. The oculomotor nerve is followed medially to identify the basilar trunk and the posterior cerebral artery. If a subarachnoid hemorrhage has occurred, the blood clot is removed gently with controlled suction and irrigation. The arachnoid lateral to the oculomotor nerve is incised to allow identification of the superior cerebellar artery. Next, Liliequist's membrane is divided to remove the blood clot from the prepontine cistern. If the bifurcation of the basilar artery is low, it usually is not necessary to divide the arachnoid along the underside of the oculomotor nerve. After the basilar trunk has been identified, a small spatula is used to dissect the basilar trunk free should a temporary clip have to be placed. The proximal ipsilateral posterior cerebral artery is then identified. The neck of the aneurysm is retracted posteriorly with a #7 suction tip and a cottonoid to allow the contralateral P_1 segment to be identified.

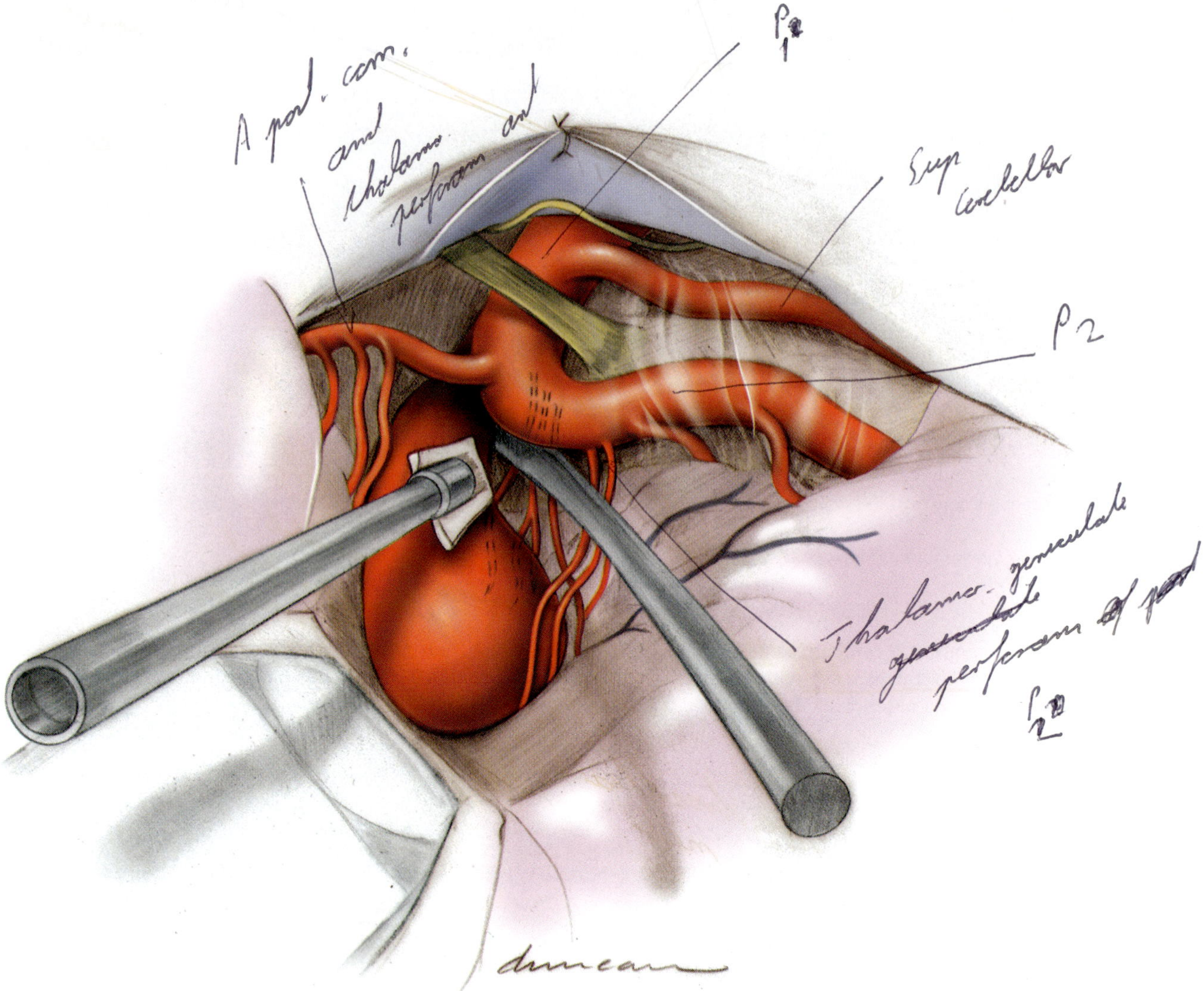

Figure 7–7.

Step 6. A plane of dissection is created starting with the perforating arteries that originate from the ipsilateral P_1 segment and working along the posterior wall of the aneurysm toward the contralateral P_1 segment. This typically requires retraction of the neck of the aneurysm anteriorly, using a small suction tip and cottonoid. Deliberately maintaining systolic blood pressure at 70 to 80 mm Hg softens the neck. Alternatively, the basilar trunk can be occluded temporarily. If temporary occlusion is chosen, hypotension should be avoided. Maintaining reasonable perfusion through the perforating vessels makes their identification and subsequent dissection easier. Note that the combination of occlusion of the proximal basilar trunk and hypotension may increase the risk of ischemic injury.

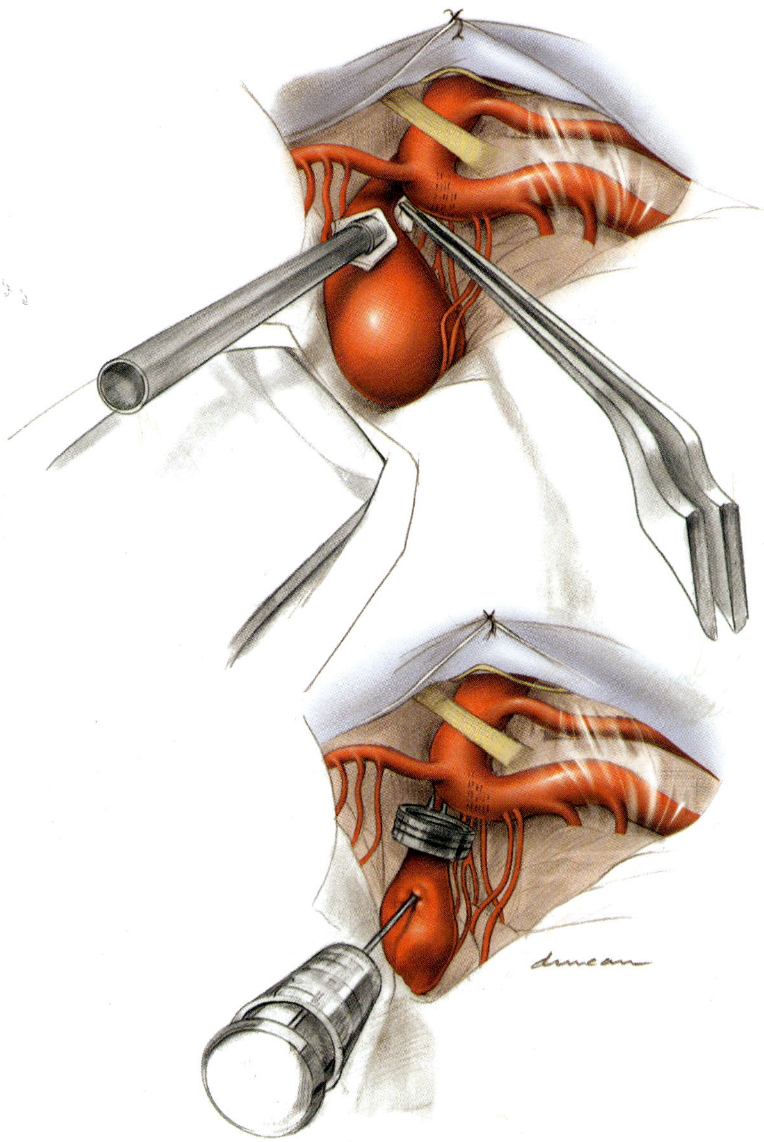

Figure 7–8.

Step 7. The plane of dissection that starts along the ipsilateral P_1 segment is carried along the back wall of the aneurysm. Generally, the perforating arteries that come off both the P_1 segments and the basilar caput can be dissected off the neck of the aneurysm as a sheet because they usually are attached to arachnoid. The vessels at greatest risk from this exposure are the perforating arteries that originate from the contralateral P_1 segment. Accordingly, it is mandatory to dissect the neck of the aneurysm free from the left P_1 segment and to make sure there are no thalamoperforating vessels. After this dissection has been completed, a piece of absorbable gelatin sponge can be used to displace these vessels. Before the aneurysm clip is placed, the back wall of the neck of the aneurysm is retracted anteriorly and the sheath of perforating arteries is reinspected, including identifying of the piece of absorbable gelatin sponge sitting between the neck of the aneurysm and the contralateral P_1 segment. After this has been identified, the aneurysm clip is placed. If the proximal P_1 segment has been dissected off the neck of the aneurysm, a straight aneurysm clip can be used. However, if this proximal ipsilateral P_1 segment cannot be dissected off the neck of the aneurysm, a fenestrated clip must be placed to preserve the posterior cerebral artery and its perforating arteries. In this case, some of the perforating arteries may run through the fenestration of the clip. Thus, it is technically more difficult to place a fenestrated clip. After the aneurysm has been secured, the dome is aspirated with a small needle to ensure that complete obliteration has been achieved. After the dome has been collapsed, the back wall of the neck of the aneurysm and aneurysm clip are reinspected to make sure that no perforating arteries have been entrapped.

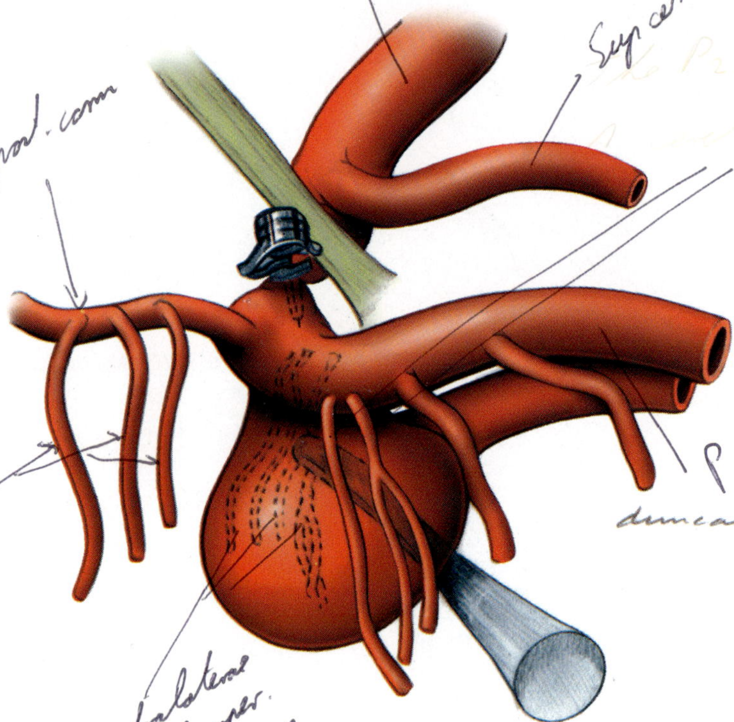

Figure 7–9.

Illustrated here is the use of a temporary basilar clip during intraoperative rupture of an aneurysm. Under ideal circumstances, the best clip placement is between the posterior cerebral artery and the superior cerebellar artery. Placement of a temporary clip can in itself be difficult depending on the relationship of the basilar artery to the tentorium cerebelli. Specifically, placement of a small clip is desirable because it is less likely to be in the way during subsequent dissection. However, depending on the degree of exposure, it is possible that only a very long straight clip can be used to occlude temporarily the basilar artery. Thus, before beginning dissection on the aneurysm, the surgeon should choose several potential aneurysm clips to be used to occlude temporarily the basilar artery and to practice placing them on the basilar trunk to determine which clip will work and will not be in the way of the dissection. After the appropriate temporary clip has been chosen, it should be loaded on the aneurysm clip applier for quick use.

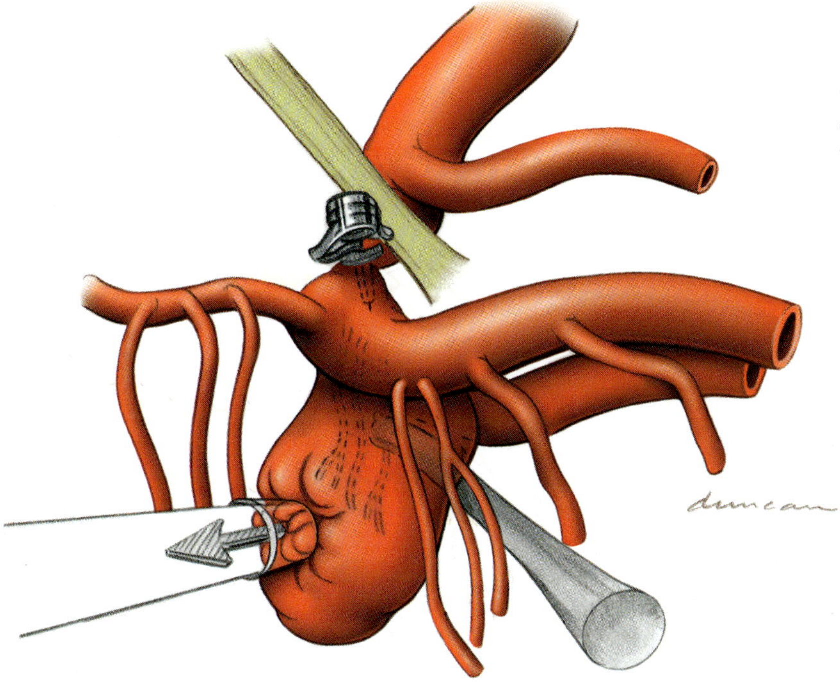

Figure 7–10.

If the aneurysm ruptures, the suction tip is used to aspirate the dome. The surgeon can then quickly maneuver the dome with the suction tip while dissecting off the perforating vessels.

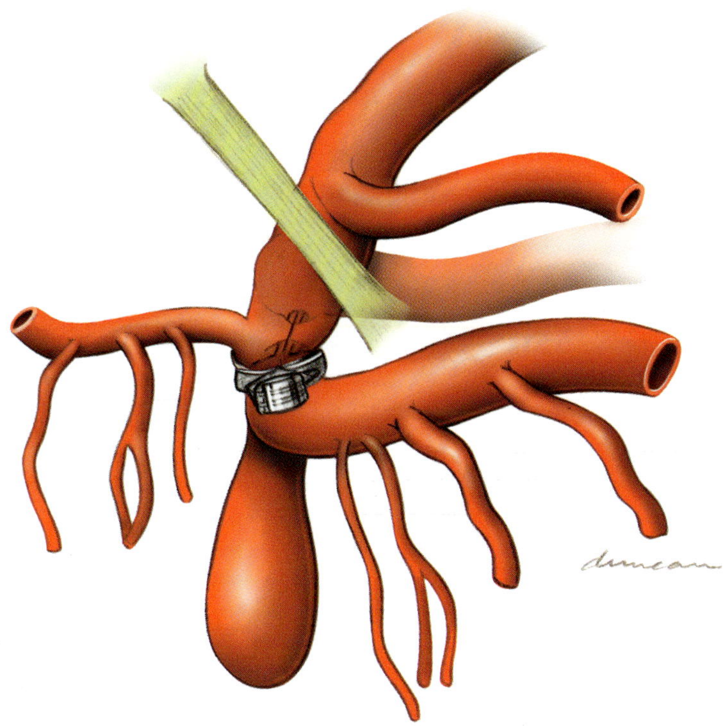

Figure 7–11.

Illustrated here is the typical use of a Drake-type or fenestrated aneurysm clip that encircles the proximal P_1 segment. When placing this clip, it is important to make sure not only that the opposite P_1 segment is patent but that the perforating arteries that come off the ipsilateral P_1 segment have not been entrapped. In attempting to preserve the opposite P_1 segment, it often is necessary to leave a small remnant of the neck of the aneurysm to prevent encroachment.

POSTERIOR CEREBRAL ARTERY ANEURYSM

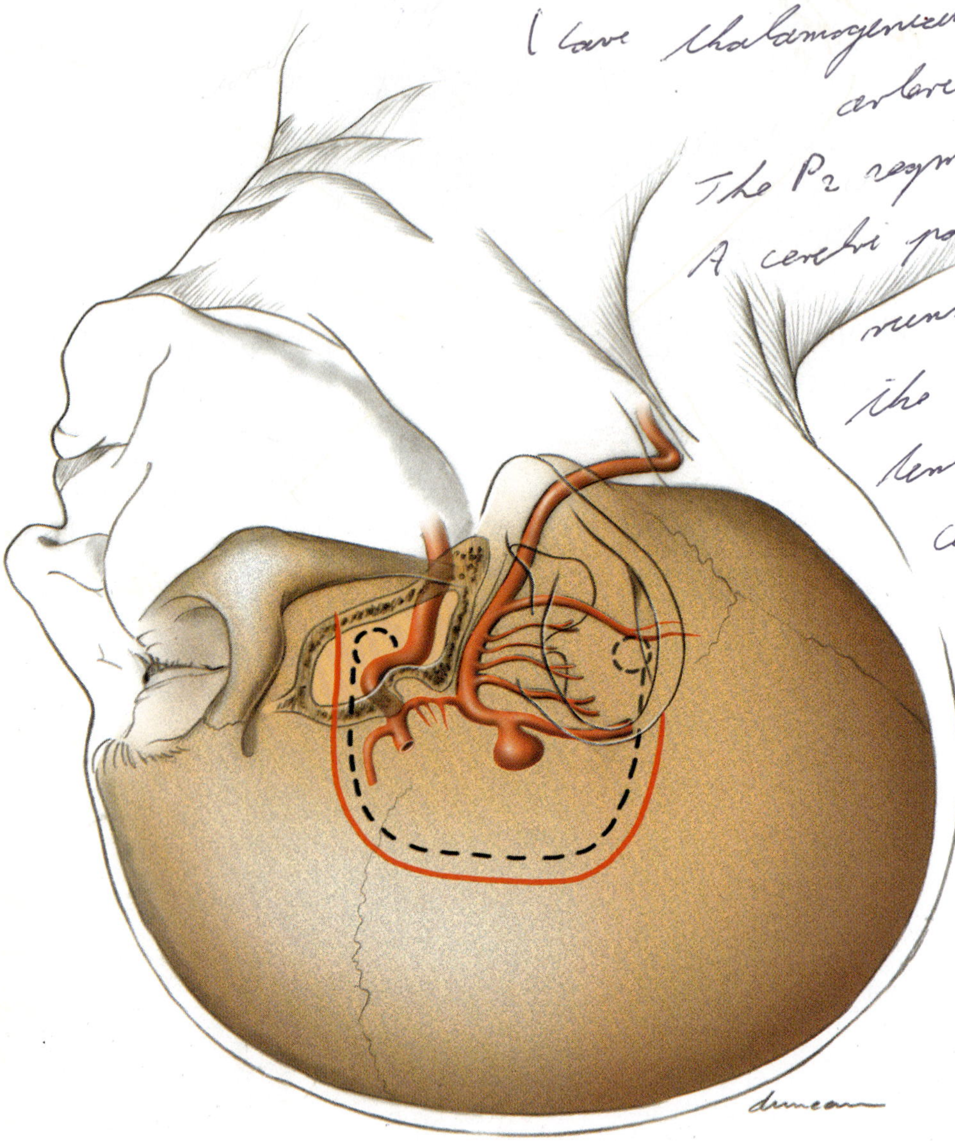

Figure 7–12.

Most aneurysms of the proximal posterior cerebral artery tend to occur along the P_2 segment, as the artery runs adjacent to the tentorium cerebelli. Perhaps trauma to the posterior cerebral artery by compression against the tentorium cerebelli promotes the development of aneurysms in this location. In addition to the posterior cerebral artery, the vessels at risk include the thalamogeniculate arteries that may originate from the P_2 segment. It is important to emphasize that the temporal lobe must be retracted carefully when using a subtemporal approach to aneurysms in this location. Excessive retraction along the temporal lobe may tear the dome of the aneurysm, which usually is attached to or embedded in the uncus.

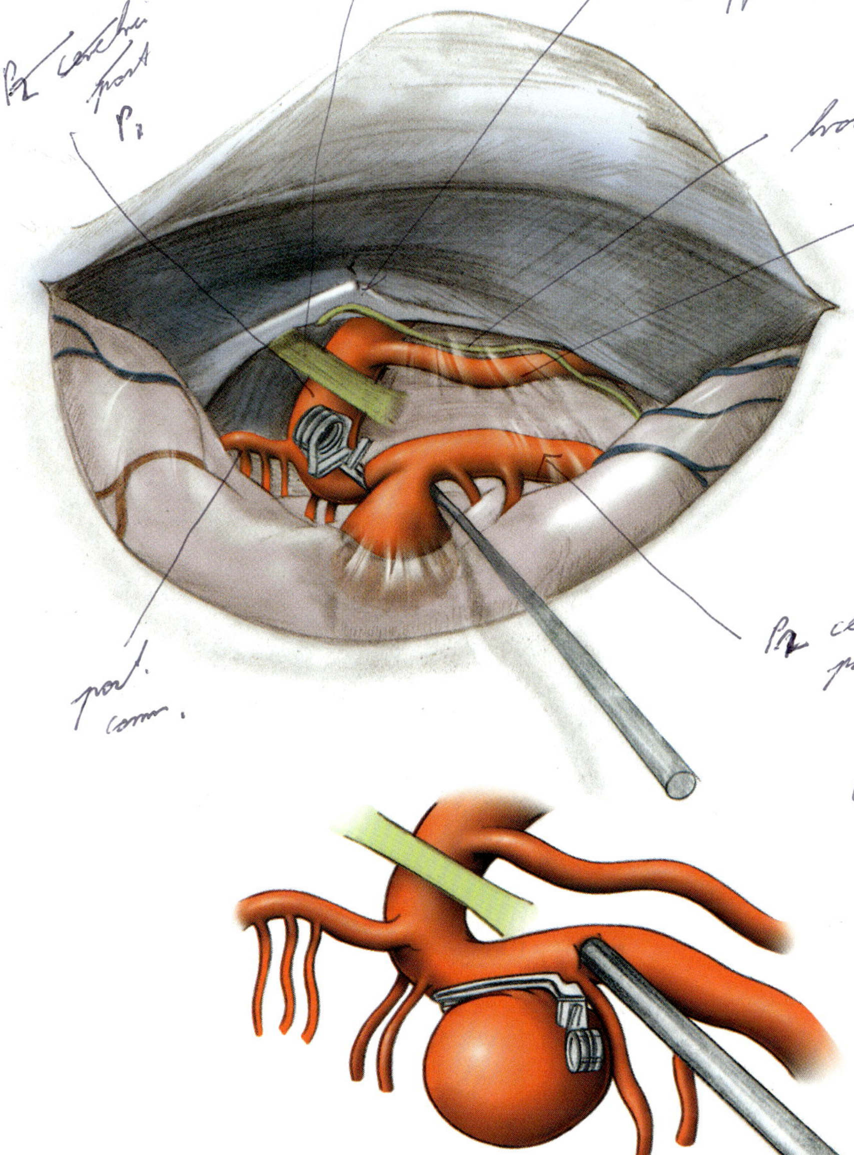

Figure 7–13.

The exposure is identical to that used for an aneurysm of the basilar caput. It is reasonable to place a small temporary clip along the posterior cerebral artery just distal to the posterior communicating artery if space permits. The neck of the aneurysm is dissected free from the posterior cerebral artery. It is not necessary to work the dome of the aneurysm out from the temporal lobe. Either a right angled clip placed parallel to the posterior cerebral artery or a straight clip placed perpendicularly can be used. The angled clip is superior in preserving patency of the posterior cerebral artery. After the aneurysm clip has been placed, it is important to make sure that the distal posterior cerebral artery is patent. A small micro Doppler probe is useful in determining whether the artery is patent.

SUPERIOR CEREBELLAR ARTERY ANEURYSM

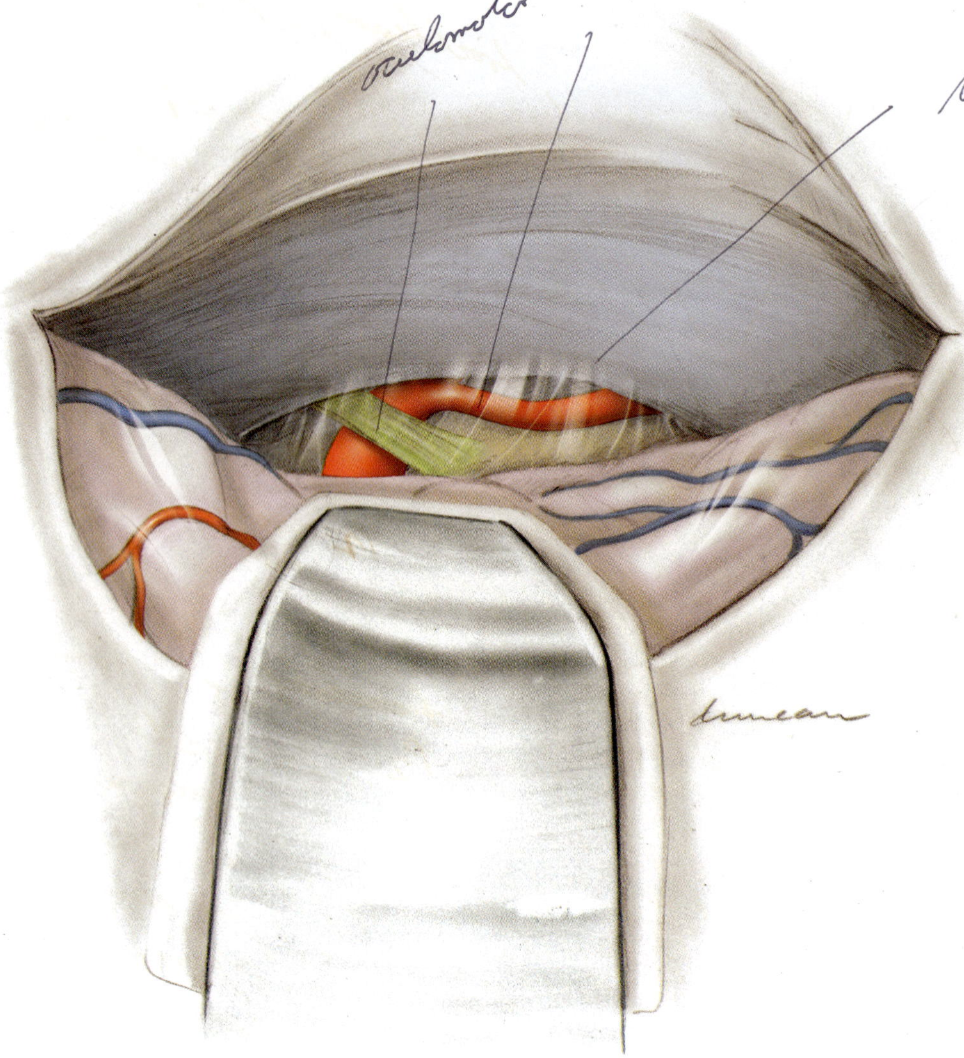

Figure 7–14.

Step 1. The subtemporal approach to an aneurysm of the superior cerebellar artery is identical to that used for an aneurysm of either the basilar caput or the proximal posterior cerebral artery. After the appropriate craniotomy has been completed, the vein of Labbé is protected and the temporal lobe is gently retracted.

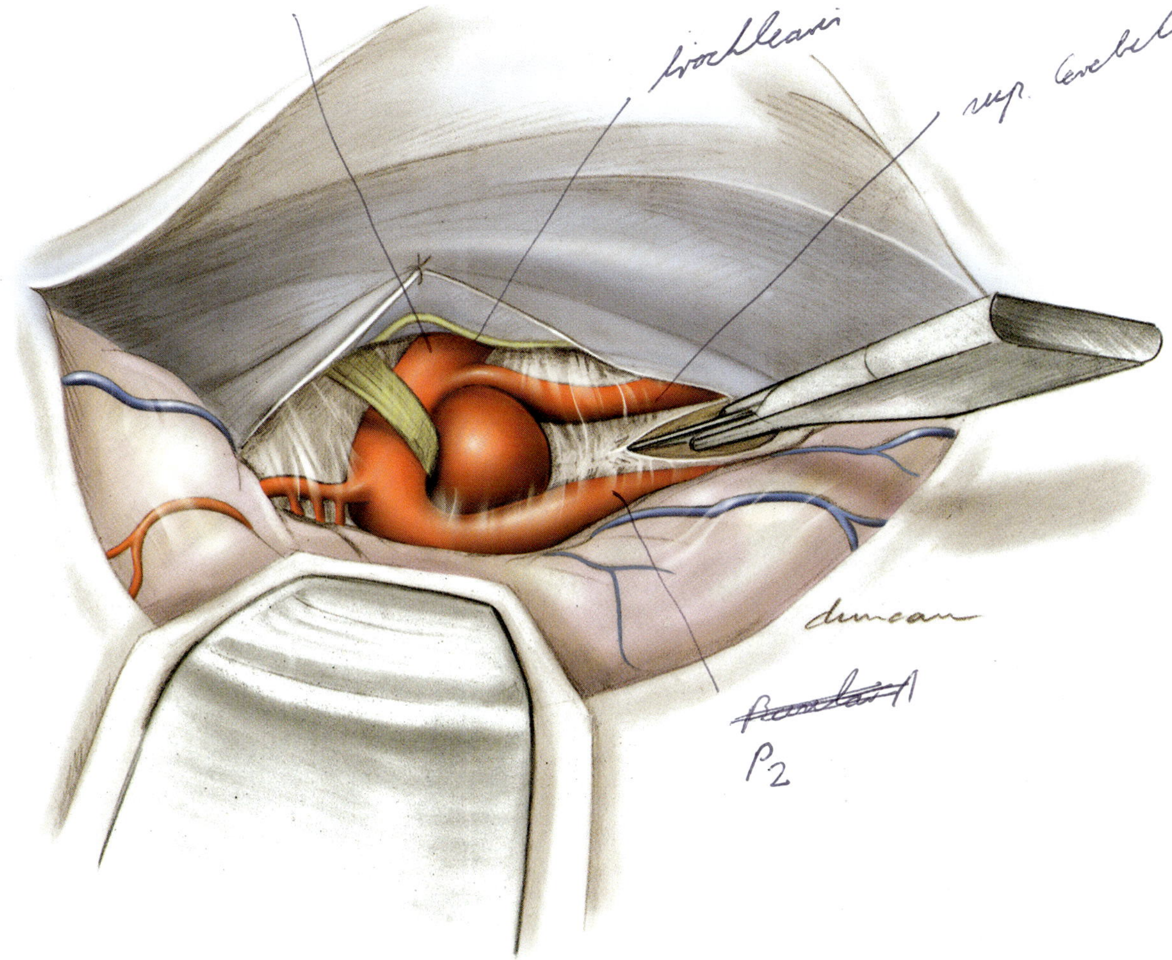

Figure 7–15.

Step 2. The arachnoid between the posterior cerebral artery and the superior cerebellar artery is incised after the location of the trochlear nerve has been identified. A #11 blade knife is used to incise the arachnoid. A small ball-tip dissector can be used to peel the arachnoid anteriorly toward the basilar trunk. If space permits, it is best first to identify the basilar trunk proximal to the superior cerebellar artery in case a temporary clip has to be applied.

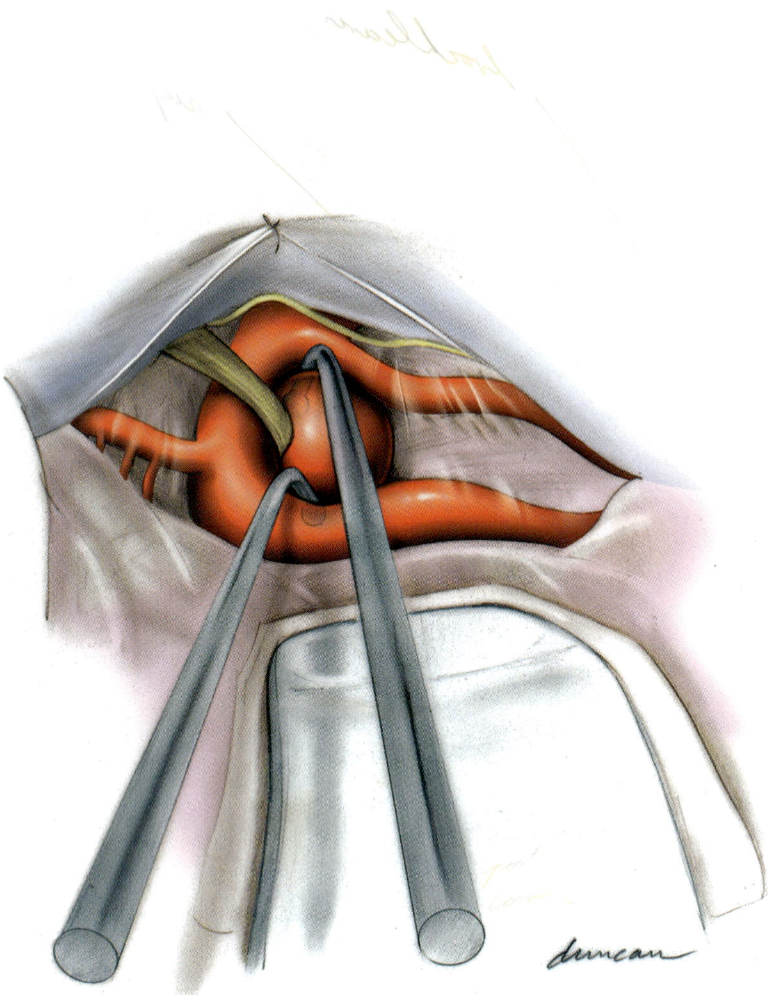

Figure 7–16.

Step 3. A small angled ball-tip dissector works well for dissecting the neck of the aneurysm off both the posterior cerebral artery and the superior cerebellar artery.

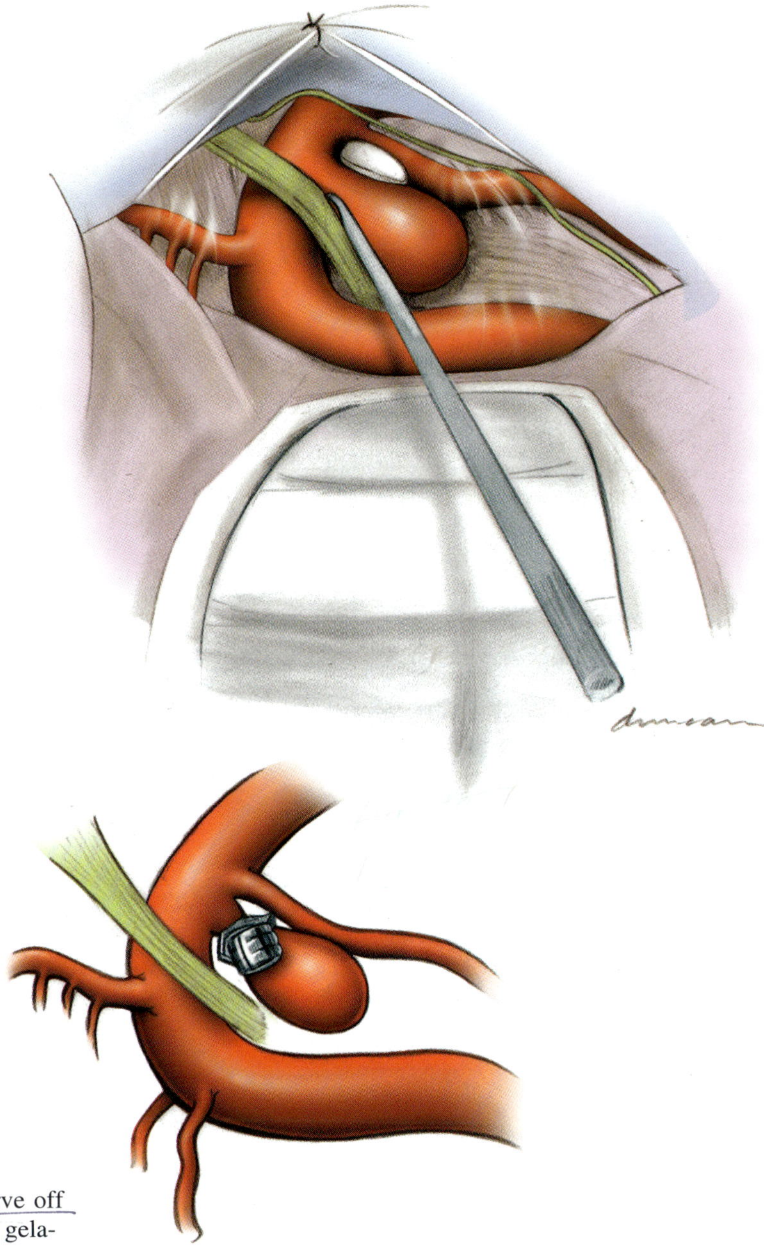

Figure 7–17.

Step 4. It is important to dissect the oculomotor nerve off the neck of the aneurysm. A small piece of absorbable gelatin sponge can be placed between the neck of the aneurysm and the oculomotor nerve and the superior cerebellar artery to keep these structures safe. A straight aneurysm clip is used to obliterate the neck of the aneurysm. As in all aneurysm repairs, it is important to aspirate the dome of the aneurysm to make sure that complete occlusion has occurred.

BASILAR TRUNK ANEURYSM

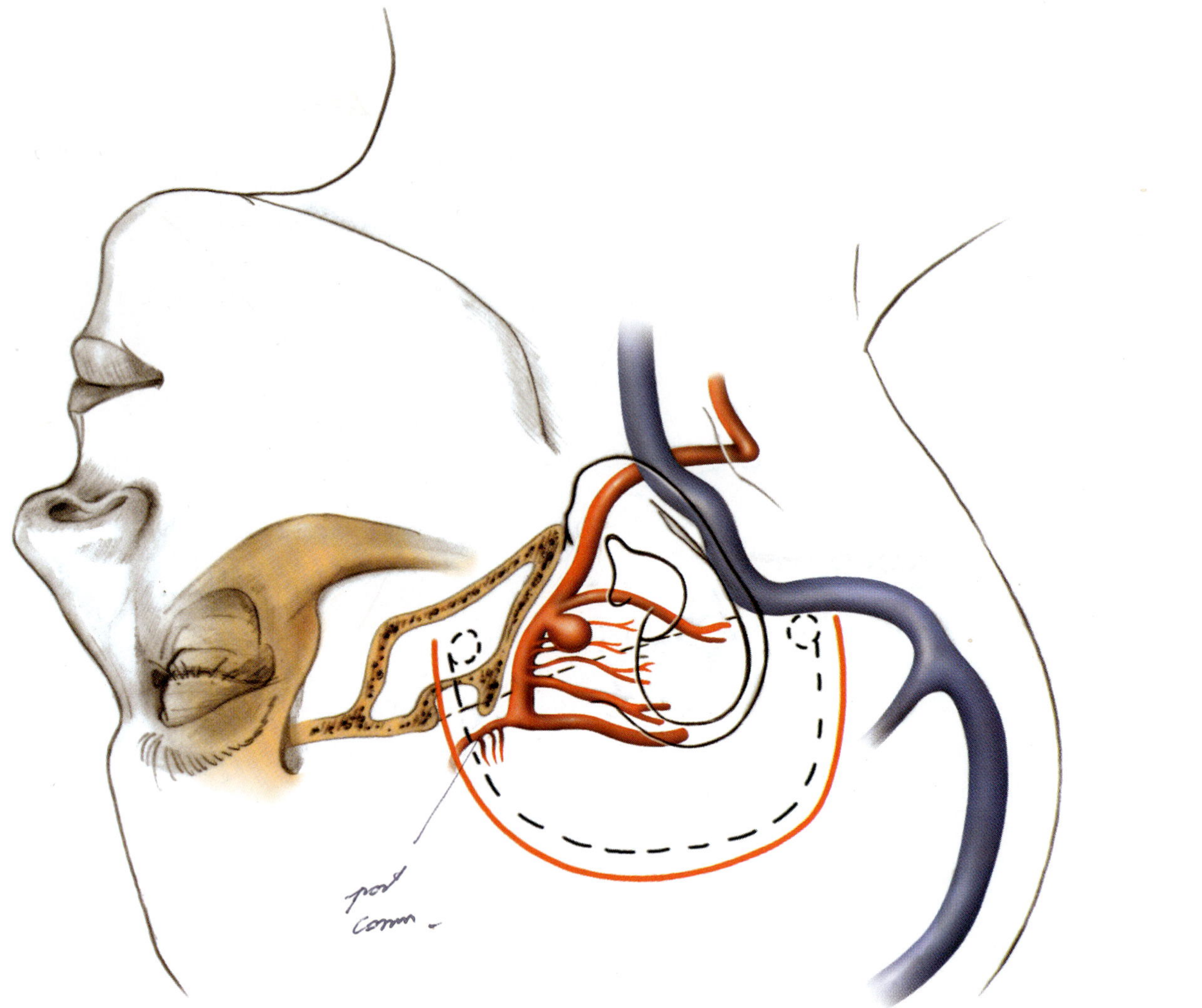

Figure 7–18.

The aneurysm of the basilar trunk illustrated here occurs close to the origin of the anterior inferior cerebellar artery. Through a subtemporal approach, it will be necessary to incise the tentorium cerebelli to obtain exposure of the posterior cranial fossa. The variation in the basilar artery and its perforating arteries is great. In addition to the major branches, many paramedian and short and long circumflex pontine arteries arise from the basilar trunk. The paramedian arteries originate from the dorsal aspect of the basilar artery and supply the pons. Occlusion of these paramedian arteries can produce significant dysfunction, including hemiplegia, quadriplegia, and disconjugate eye movements. Occlusion of one of the circumferential vessels will also likely produce cerebellar dysfunction.

Vital branches from the basilar A → long and short pontine circumflex arteries

→ lesion of these
hemiplegia
Quadriplegia
dysconjugate eye movements
cerebellar dysfunction

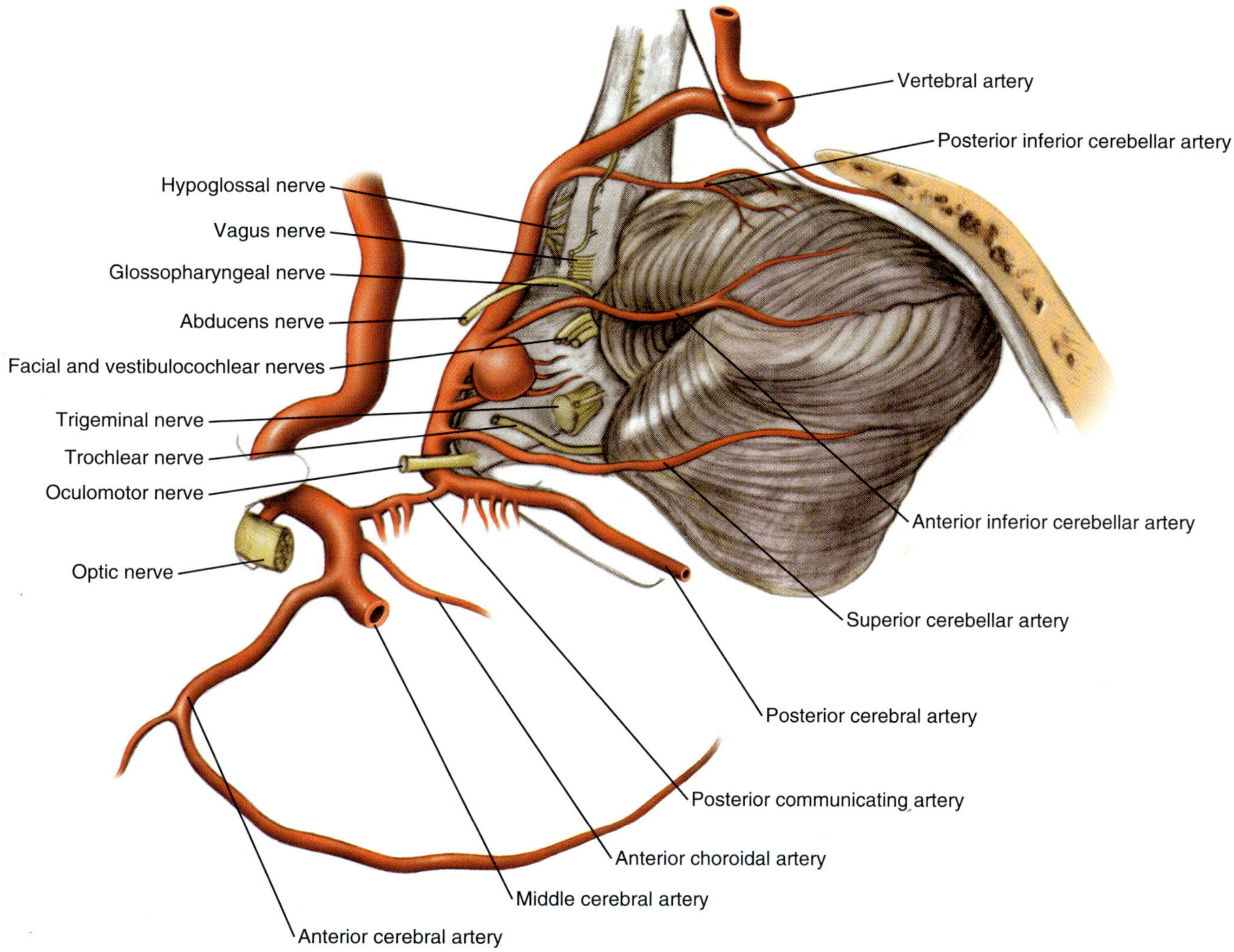

Figure 7–19.

Illustrated here are the neurovascular relationships along the basilar trunk that need to be considered when repairing aneurysms of the basilar trunk.

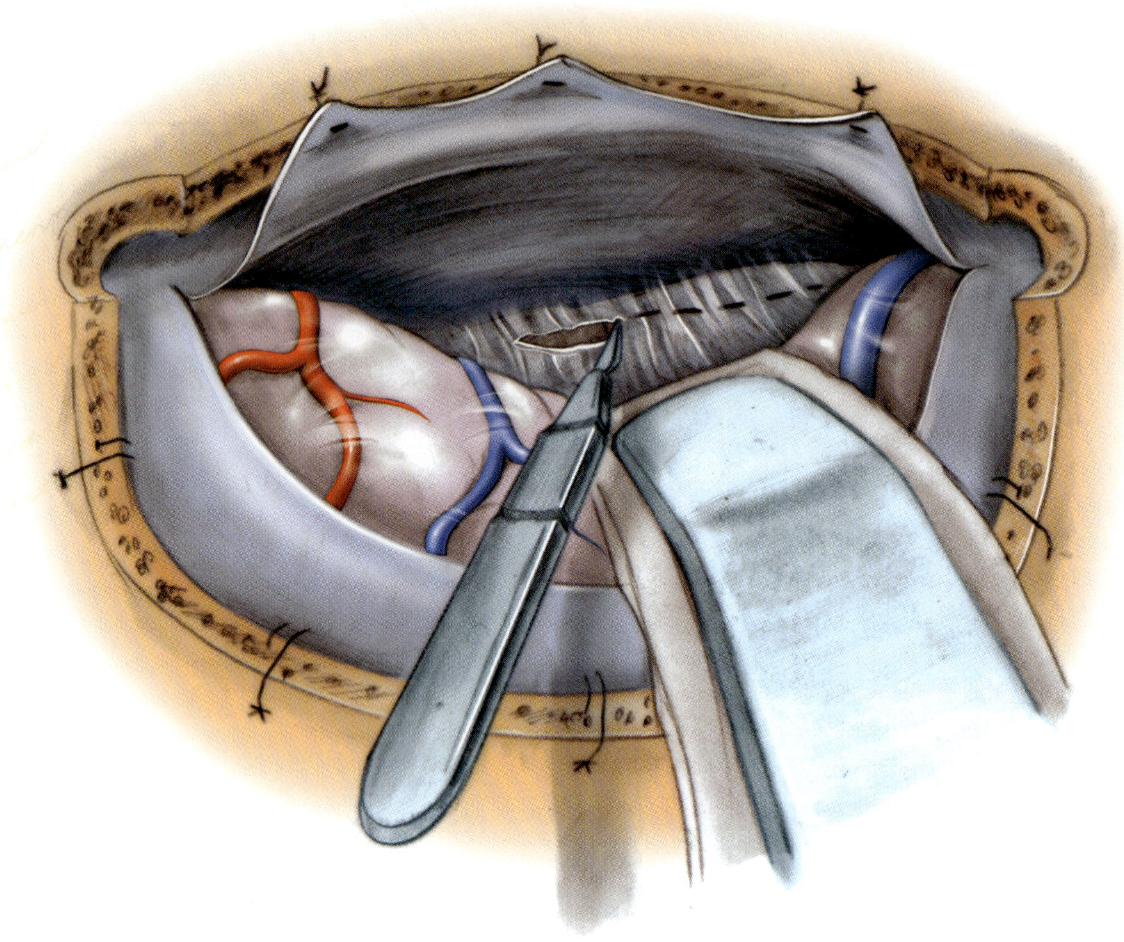

Figure 7–20.

Step 1. A standard subtemporal craniotomy is performed. The vein of Labbé is protected. The mid-temporal lobe is retracted gently to identify the edge of the tentorium cerebelli adjacent to the cerebral peduncles. The trochlear nerve is identified beneath the arachnoid. Next, the tentorium cerebelli is incised posterior to the trochlear nerve, approximately 1.5 cm behind the petrous ridge, for a distance of approximately 2.0 cm. The anterior leaf of the incision is cauterized, folded forward, and tacked to the floor of the middle cranial fossa. The incision in the tentorium cerebelli is carried up to, but not through, the petrosal vein.

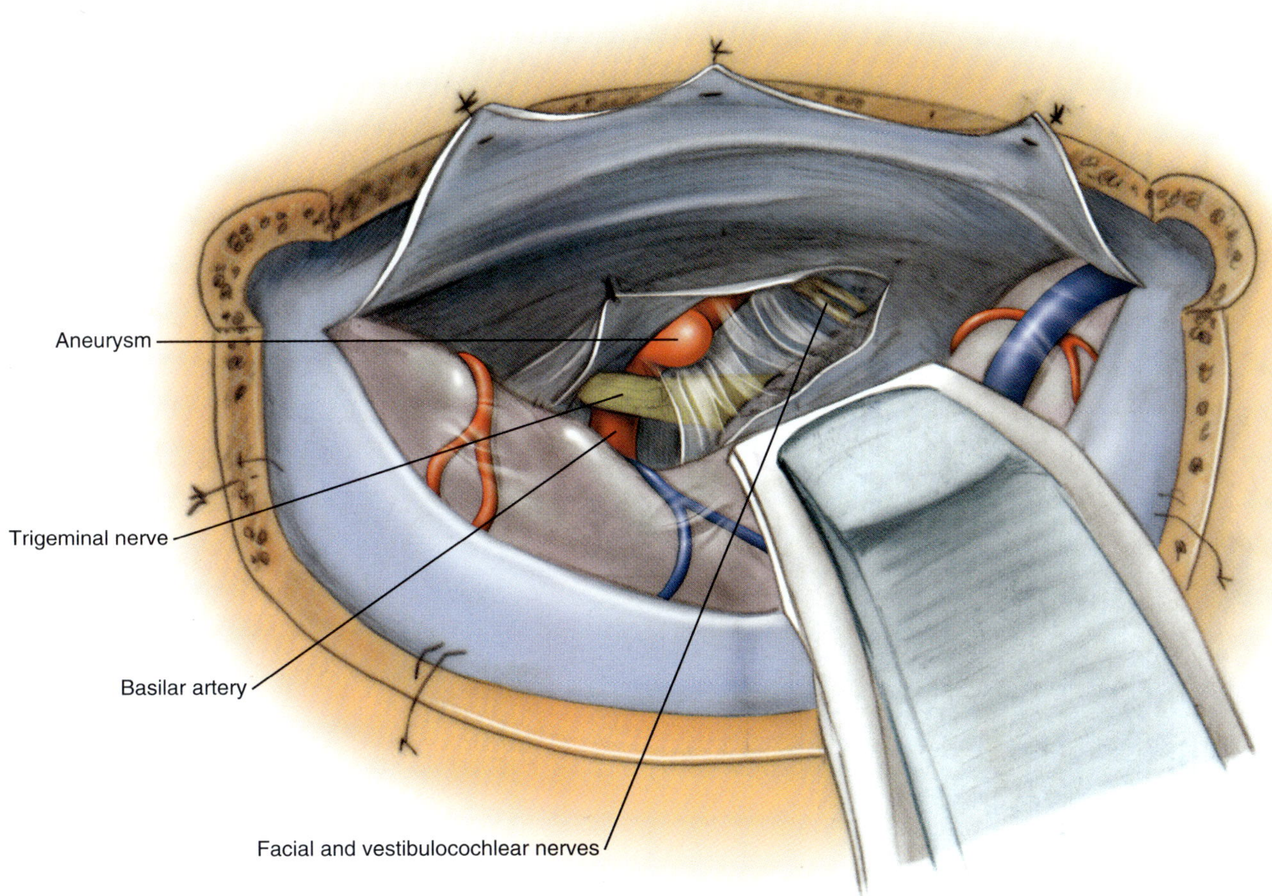

Figure 7–21.

Step 2. The arachnoid underneath the tentorium cerebelli is opened with a #11 blade knife. The trigeminal nerve is medial, and the facial nerve and the vestibulocochlear nerve are lateral in this exposure. After the petrosal vein has been visualized, it should be cauterized and divided. It may be necessary to extend the incision in the tentorium cerebelli laterally after the petrosal vein has been divided.

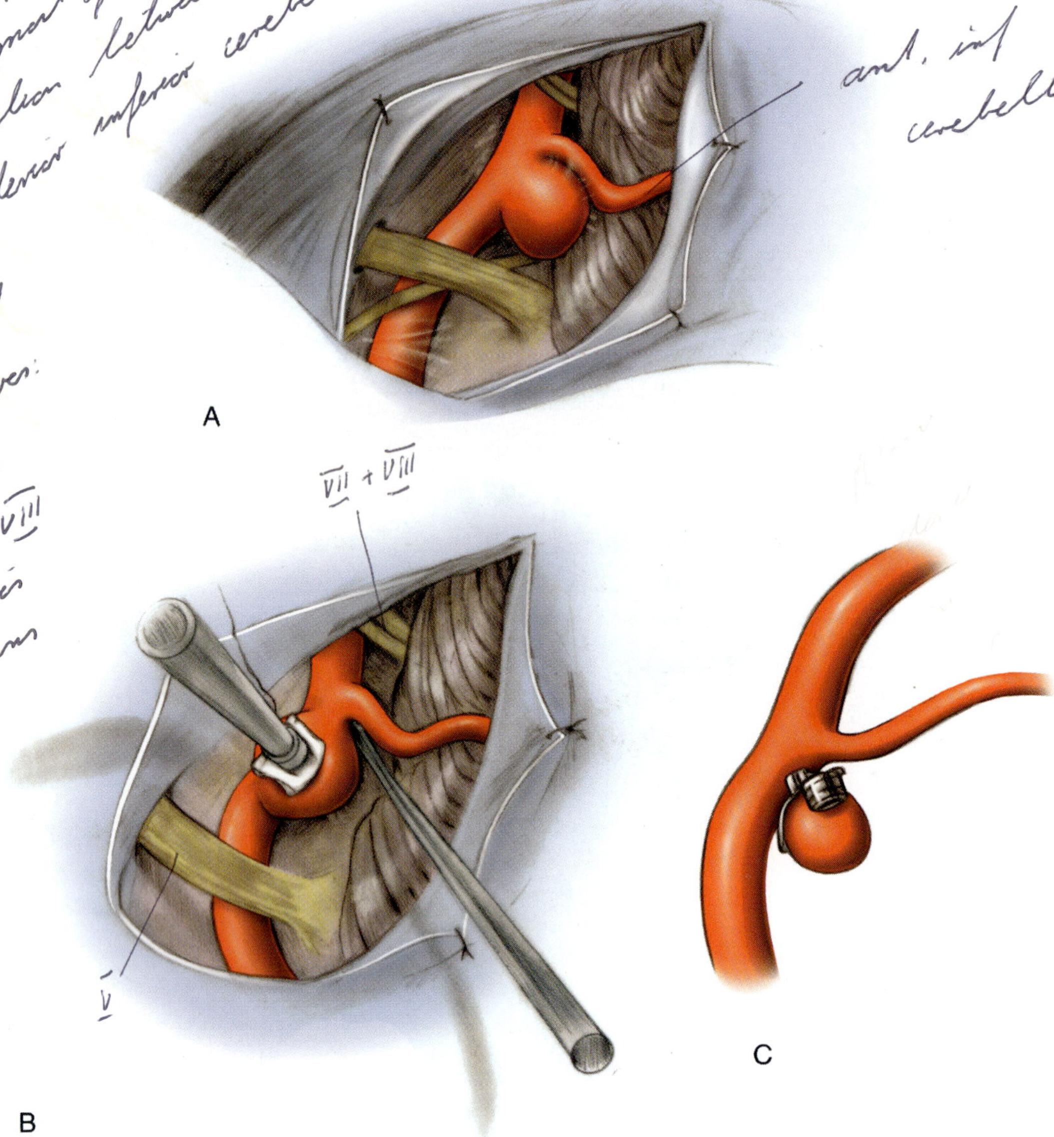

Figure 7–22.

Step 3. *A*, A small retractor is placed between the trigeminal nerve medially and the facial and vestibulocochlear nerves laterally. If the aneurysm has hemorrhaged, blood can be removed gently with suction and irrigation. **Step 4**. The anterior inferior cerebellar artery is identified laterally and followed to the basilar artery.

Step 5. *B*, Aneurysms in this location typically arise at the junction of the anterior inferior cerebellar artery and the basilar trunk. Although they usually project laterally, the configuration of the aneurysm with the anterior inferior cerebellar artery can be complicated. The dome of the aneurysm is retracted gently with a #5 or #7 suction tip and cottonoid, and a spatula is used to dissect the neck of the aneurysm free.

C, A small straight or curved clip works well in this location. However, depending on the degree of exposure, a long straight clip may be needed to obliterate the neck of the aneurysm.

TENTORIUM MENINGIOMA

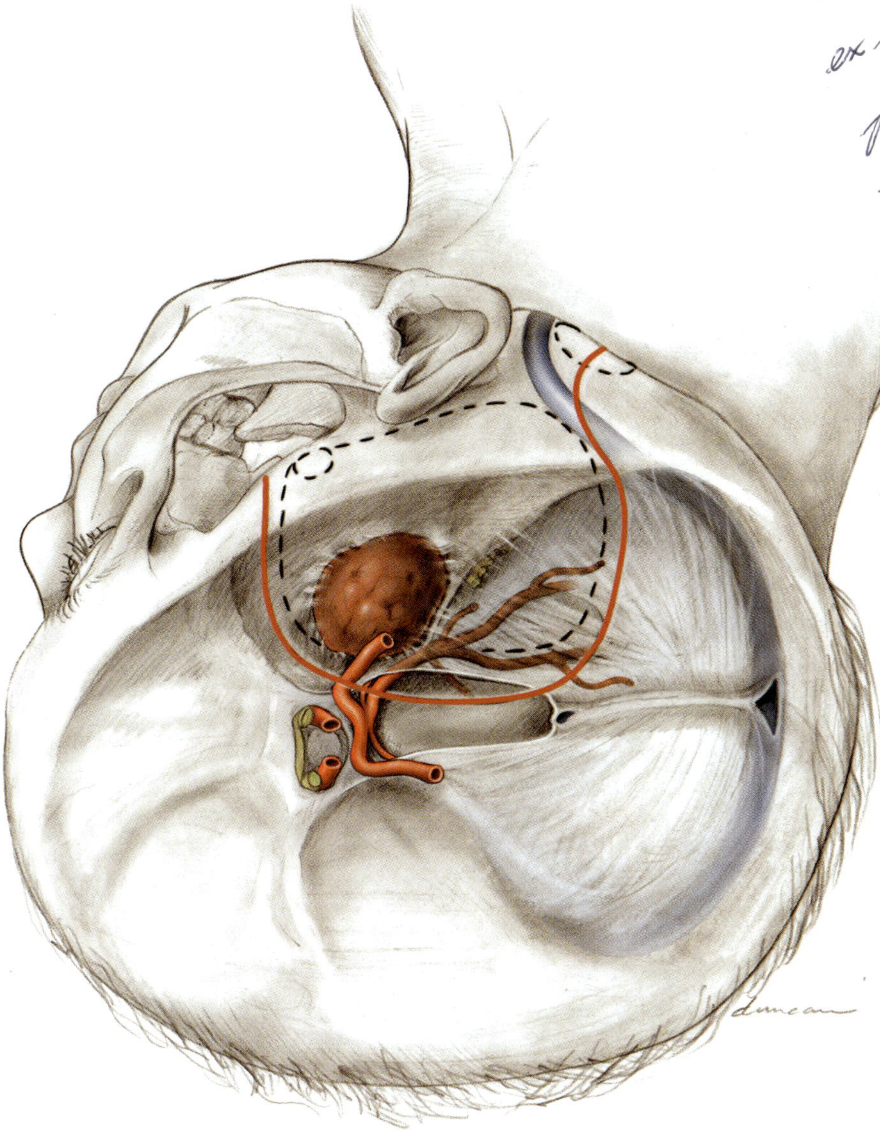

Figure 7–23.

Tumors such as meningiomas along the edge of the tentorium cerebelli typically have extensions into both the middle and the posterior cranial fossae. Smaller tumors can be approached directly through a subtemporal approach, with sectioning of the tentorium cerebelli. However, for large tumors that have a significant extension into the posterior cranial fossa, a subtemporal approach may need to be combined with a suboccipital approach. Accordingly, it is necessary to plan an incision that allows the surgeon access to both the middle and posterior cranial fossae. The position of the patient's head is similar to that described for an aneurysm of the basilar trunk, in which the head is 10 to 15 degrees to the horizontal and extended approximately 15 degrees. A question-mark incision behind the ear can be extended down if a suboccipital craniotomy is necessary.

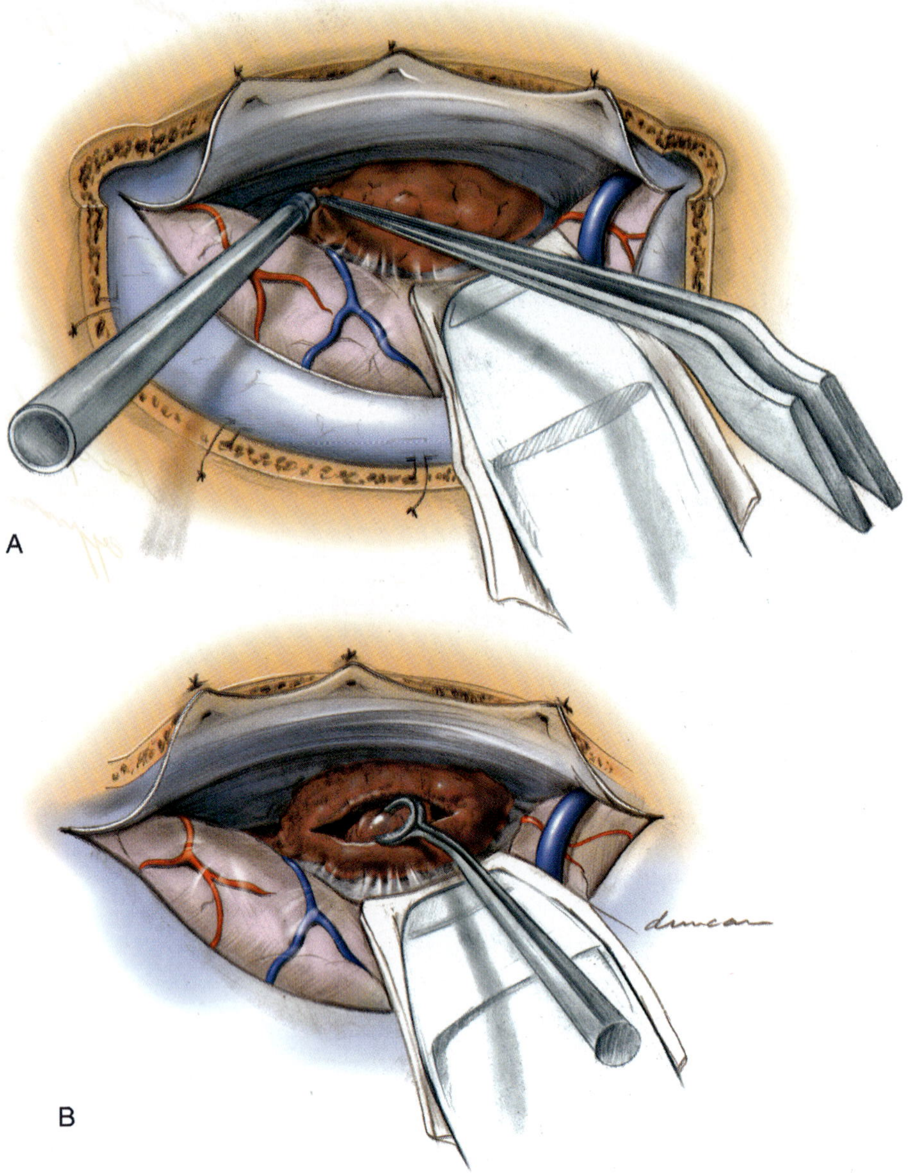

Figure 7–24.

Step 1. *A*, A subtemporal approach is used in the series of illustrations shown here. After the vein of Labbé has been protected, a Yasargil retractor is used to elevate the temporal lobe gently to identify the tumor along the tentorium cerebelli. These tumors are vascular, deriving their blood supply from the dura mater of the middle and posterior cranial fossa. Accordingly, before the tumor is debulked, it is best to attack this blood supply by vigorously cauterizing its dural attachment using a bipolar cautery.

Step 2. *B*, After the blood supply of the tumor has been cauterized, the tumor is debulked with curets, an ultrasonic aspirator, or a laser.

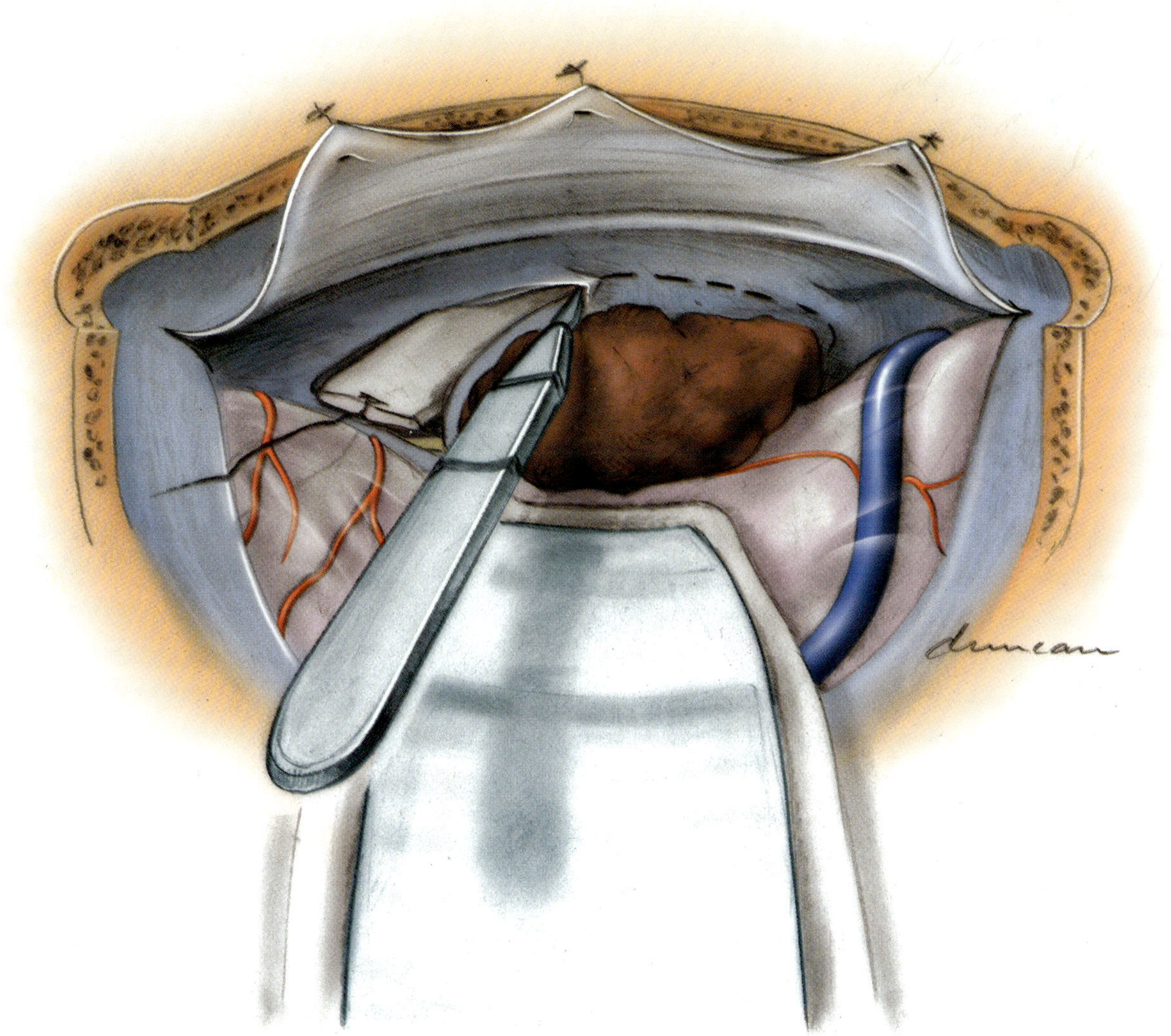

Figure 7–25.

Step 3. After some of the tumor has been debulked, the tentorium cerebelli is incised posterior to the petrous ridge. A cottonoid can be placed along the underside of the edge of the tentorium cerebelli to prevent inadvertent injury to the trigeminal nerve and petrosal vein.

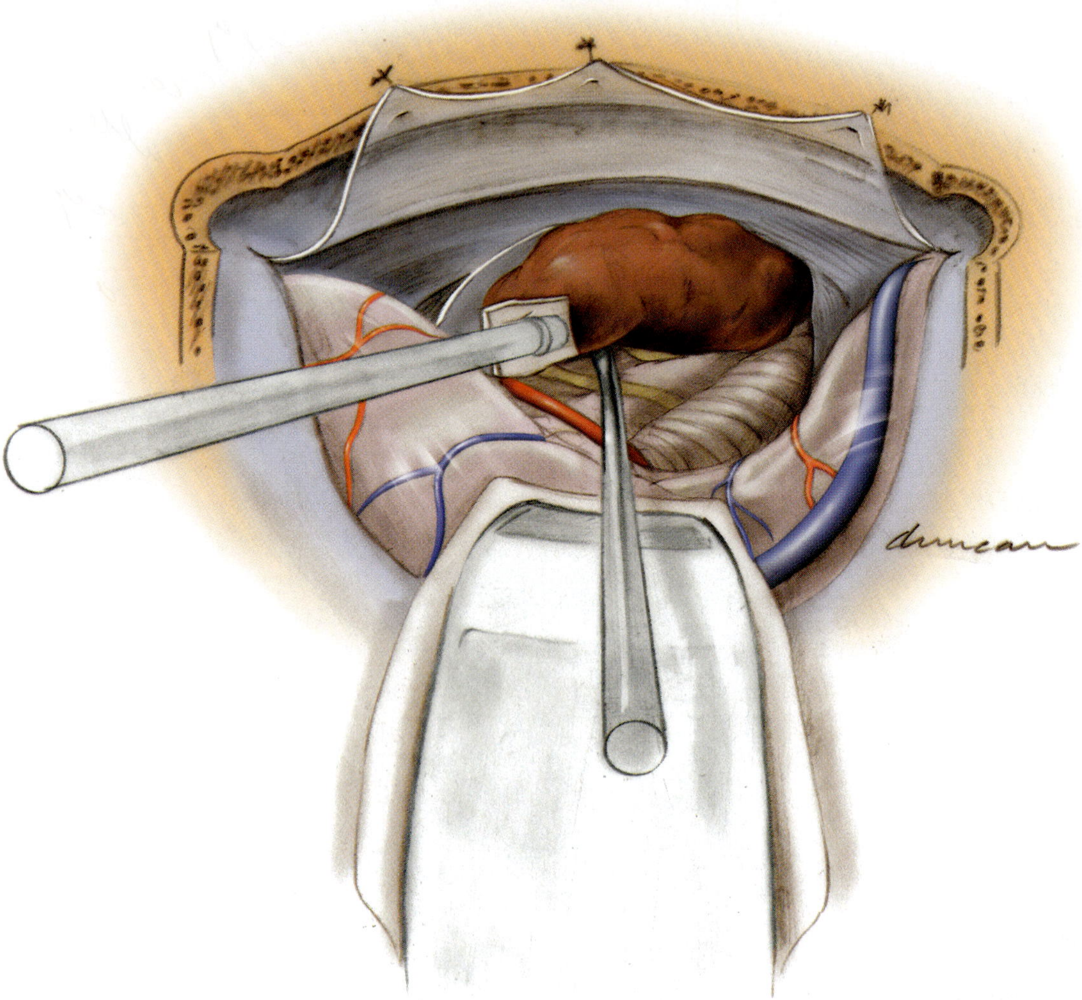

Figure 7–26.

Step 4. After the tentorium cerebelli has been incised, the medial edge of the tentorium and the tumor are retracted laterally to dissect the underside of the tumor off the arachnoid that overlies the trigeminal nerve, the pons, the facial nerve, and the vestibulocochlear nerve. The petrosal vein is often seen running into the underside of the tumor, close to the trigeminal nerve, and must be cauterized and divided.

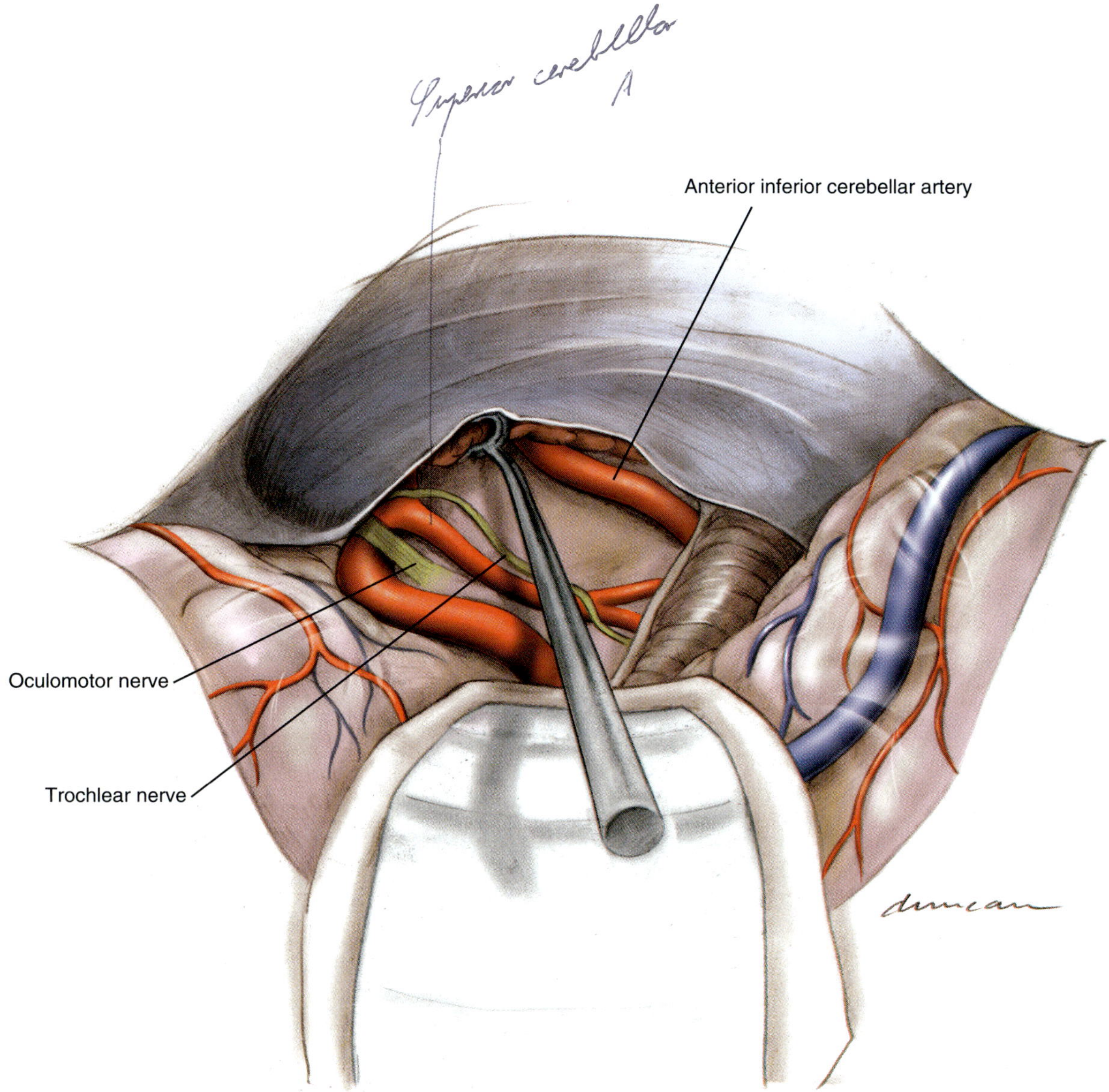

Figure 7–27.

Step 5. After most of the tumor has been debulked and removed, the extension of the tumor along the underside of the tentorium cerebelli in the posterior cranial fossa is visualized. Ring curets usually can be used to scrape the tumor off the dura mater. If the tumor has a large extension into the cerebellopontine angle, a suboccipital craniotomy should be performed to allow better access to this extension into the posterior cranial fossa. Because of the relationship of the tumor to the cranial nerves, intraoperative electromyographic monitoring of the trigeminal, facial, and vestibulocochlear nerves is necessary. Respecting the arachnoid layer will protect these cranial nerves and the adjacent vascular structures.

8

Lateral Suboccipital Approach

Copyright © 1999 Mayo Foundation.

ARTERIAL SUPPLY

The arterial supply of the posterior fossa consists of the vertebral and basilar arteries and their branches. The pertinent anatomic features of the arterial and venous systems are illustrated in Figures 8–1 to 8–3.

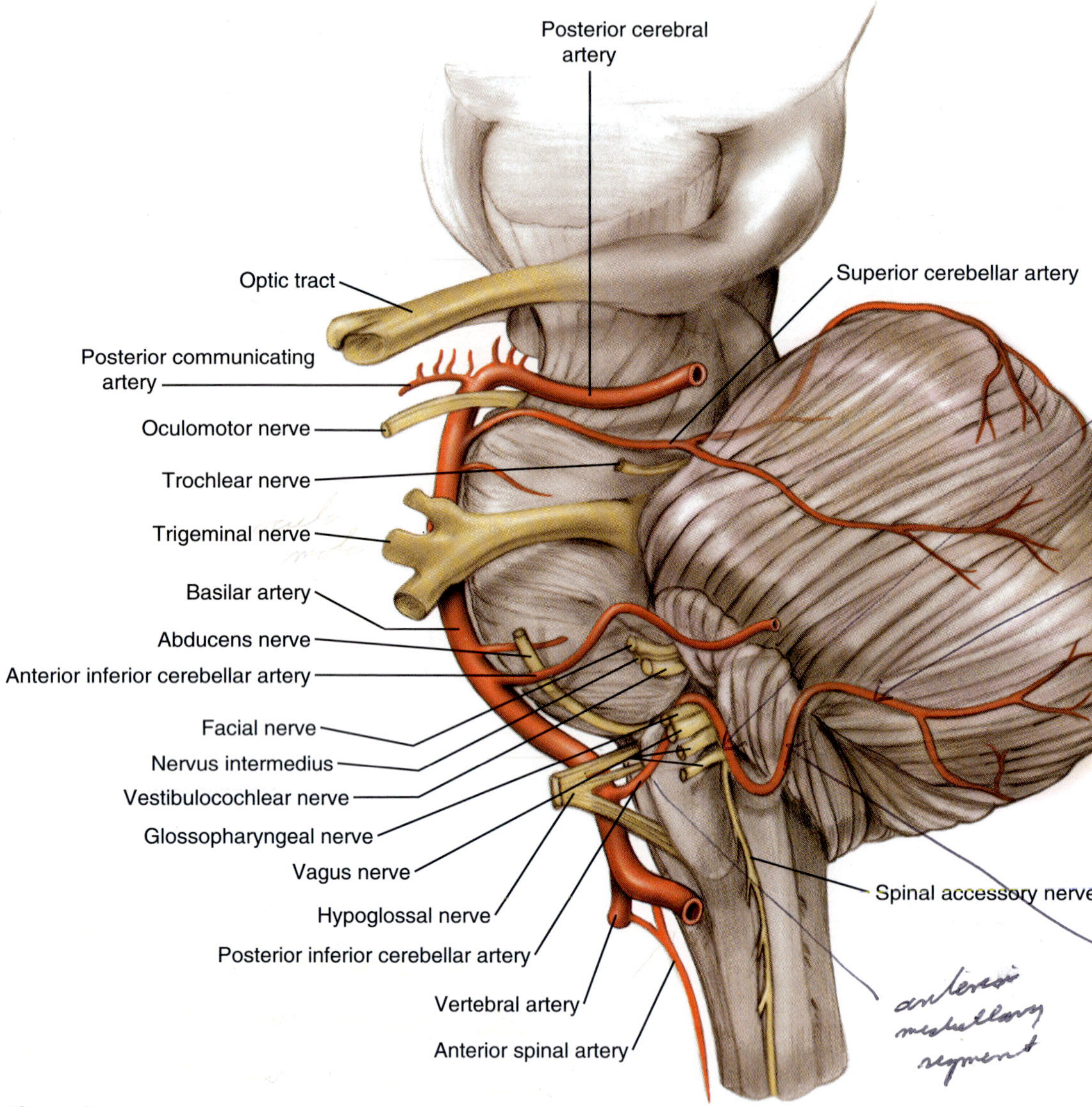

Figure 8–1.

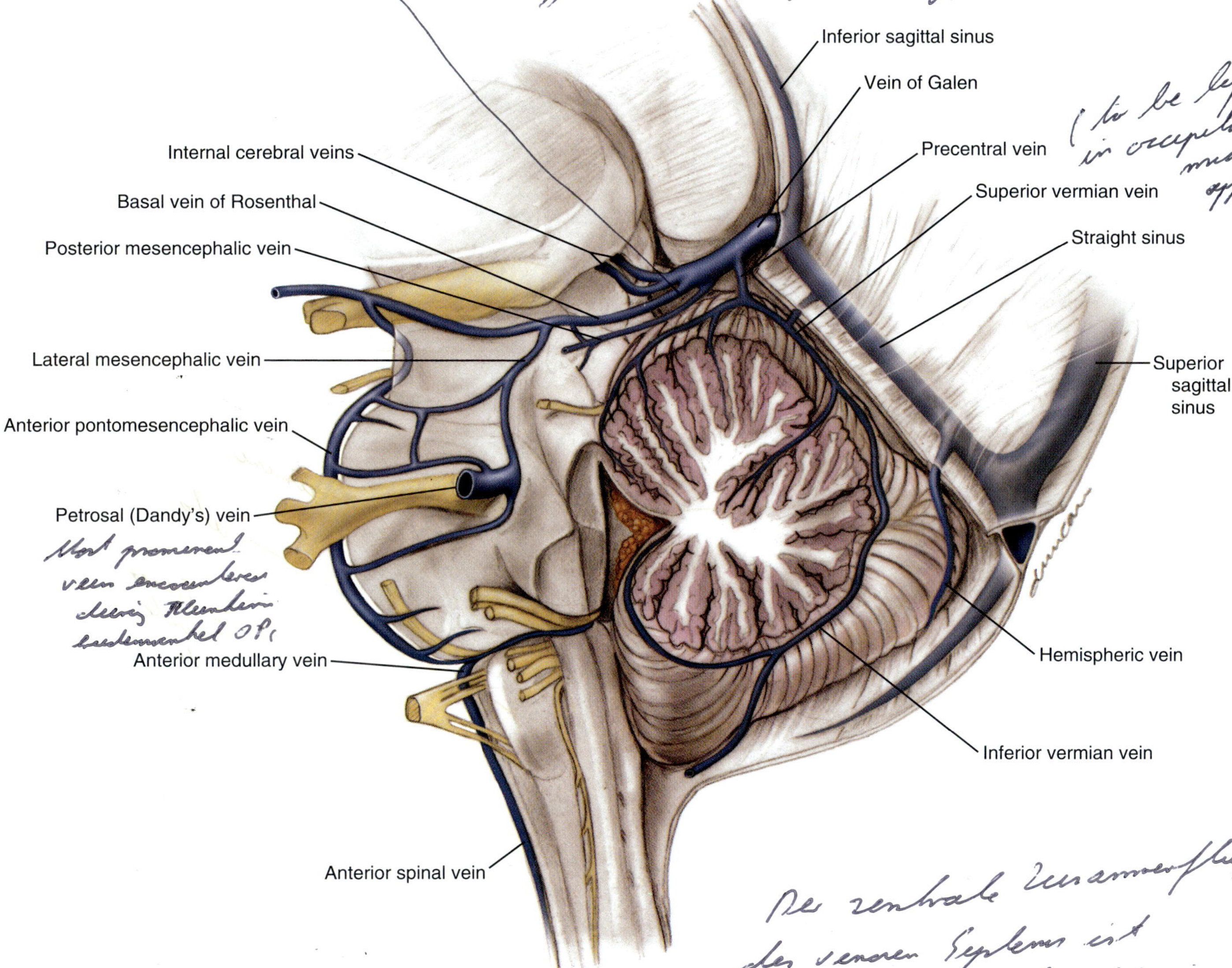
Inferior sagittal sinus
Vein of Galen
Internal cerebral veins
Precentral vein
Superior vermian vein
Basal vein of Rosenthal
Straight sinus
Posterior mesencephalic vein
Lateral mesencephalic vein
Superior sagittal sinus
Anterior pontomesencephalic vein
Petrosal (Dandy's) vein
Hemispheric vein
Anterior medullary vein
Inferior vermian vein
Anterior spinal vein

Figure 8–2.

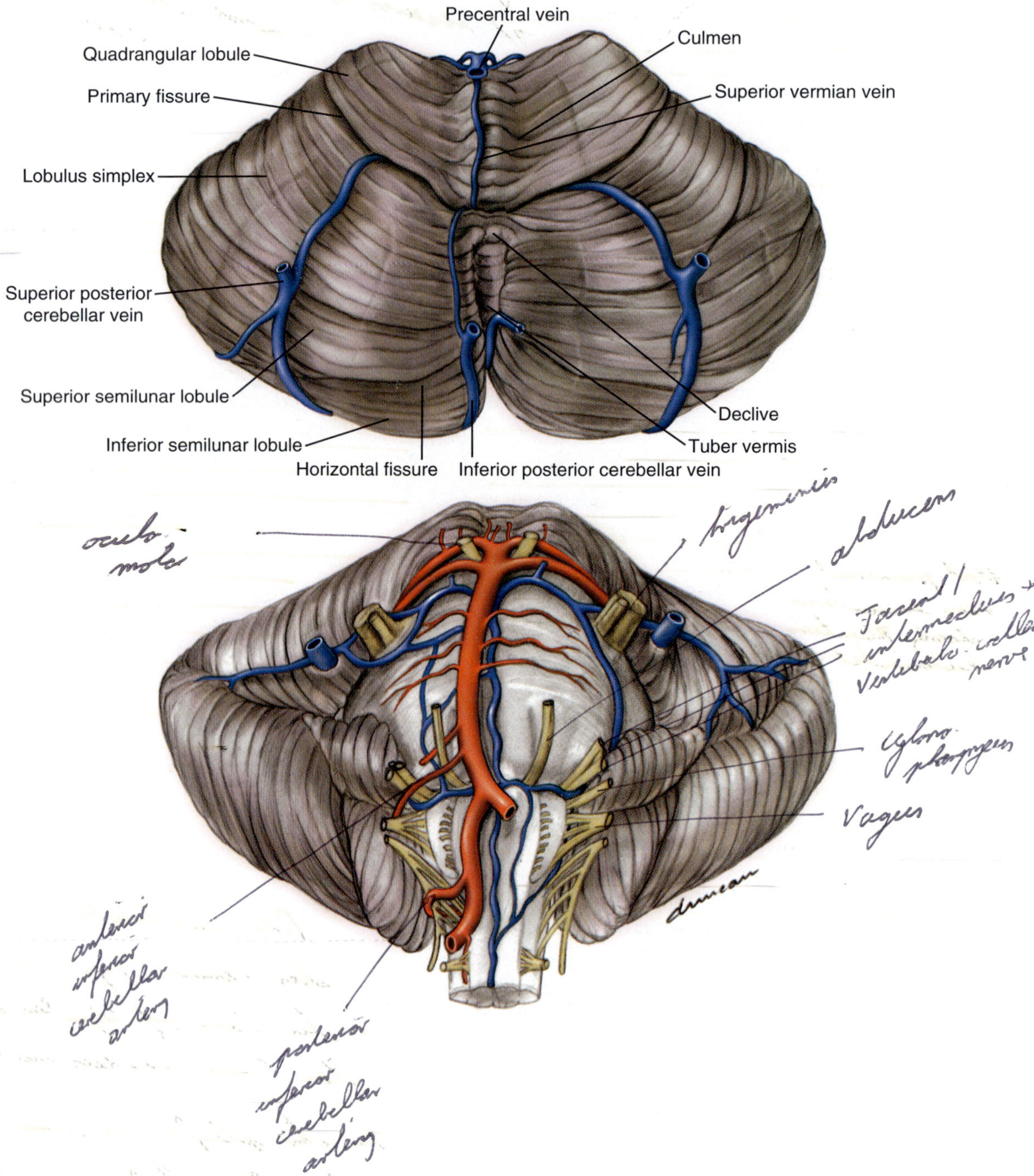
Precentral vein
Culmen
Quadrangular lobule
Primary fissure
Superior vermian vein
Lobulus simplex
Superior posterior
cerebellar vein
Superior semilunar lobule
Declive
Inferior semilunar lobule
Tuber vermis
Horizontal fissure
Inferior posterior cerebellar vein

Figure 8–3.

Vertebral Artery

The vertebral artery originates as the first branch of the subclavian artery and enters the transverse foramen of C-6. At C-3, the artery turns laterally and enters the foramen of C-2. After exiting through the foramen of C-1, it curves behind the atlantooccipital joint to lie horizontally along the posterior arch of C-1. This horizontal segment is called the "pars atlantica." As the vertebral artery courses medially, it curves rostrally and passes through the foramen magnum. Along the transverse segment of the vertebral artery, there are usually muscular branches that anastomose with branches of the external carotid artery. The posterior meningeal branch often originates from the middle portion of this segment. It also has been reported that the posterior inferior cerebellar artery originates from the pars atlantica in approximately 5 percent of patients.

After the vertebral artery penetrates the dura mater, it goes laterally and then ventrally or anteriorly to join the contralateral vertebral artery to form the basilar artery. In approximately two-thirds of patients, this union occurs at or just below the inferior pontine sulcus. In approximately 15 percent of patients, one vertebral artery is dominant, and in 5 to 10 percent a nondominant vertebral artery ends as the posterior inferior cerebellar artery and does not join the contralateral vertebral artery.

Branches of the vertebral artery include the posterior inferior cerebellar artery, direct perforating branches to the medulla, the anterior spinal artery, small meningeal branches, and, occasionally, a posterior spinal artery.

Posterior Inferior Cerebellar Artery

The posterior inferior cerebellar artery is quite variable. In approximately 50 percent of patients, it originates from the proximal third of the intracisternal portion of the vertebral artery. In 5 to 10 percent of patients, one posterior inferior cerebellar artery is absent. In these patients, the ipsilateral anterior inferior cerebellar artery is hypertrophic or dominant and perfuses the area normally supplied by the posterior inferior cerebellar artery. Occasionally, both posterior inferior cerebellar arteries may be absent; alternatively, there can be duplications of the vessels.

The first segment of the posterior inferior cerebellar artery goes laterally around the medulla and is called the "anterior medullary segment." The artery then curves caudally to form a loop along the lateral aspect of the medulla; this is called the "lateral medullary segment." This segment typically courses between the rootlets of the spinal accessory nerve. At the posterior margin of the medulla, the posterior inferior cerebellar artery turns superiorly to complete the caudal loop. The portion of the artery that passes superiorly to form a cranial loop is called the "posterior medullary segment." Branches that originate from the apex of the cranial loop go to the choroid plexus of the fourth ventricle and the cerebellar tonsil. Distal to the origin of these branches, the posterior inferior cerebellar artery crosses the cerebellar tonsil to form the "supratonsillar segment." Originating from the supratonsillar segment are medial branches that supply the vermis and lateral branches that supply the cerebellar hemisphere.

Basilar Artery

In approximately 80 percent of patients, the left and right vertebral arteries join to form the basilar artery. This occurs along the anterior surface of the medulla, close to the pontomedullary junction. With increasing age, the basilar artery tends to become more curved and, sometimes, ectatic. If the vertebral artery is large on one side, the basilar artery is usually deviated to the opposite side. It also may have fenestrations. The basilar artery extends rostrally along the ventral surface of the pons and terminates in the interpeduncular cistern by dividing into the left and right posterior cerebral arteries. In approximately one-half of patients, the basilar caput is at the level of the posterior clinoid process. Branches of the basilar artery include the anterior spinal, pontine, labyrinthine, anterior inferior cerebellar, superior cerebellar, mesencephalic, and posterior cerebral arteries. The internal auditory or labyrinthine artery originates from the anterior inferior cerebellar artery in approximately 85 percent of patients. In the other 15 percent, it originates from the trunk of the basilar artery. The labyrinthine artery joins the vestibulocochlear nerve. Medial and lateral pontine branches originate from the trunk of the basilar artery. Other pontine branches originate from both the anterior inferior cerebellar and superior cerebellar arteries. These pontine branches perfuse the pons and medulla.

Anterior Inferior Cerebellar Artery

The anterior inferior cerebellar artery originates, in most patients, from the proximal two-thirds of the basilar artery. Typically, the left and right anterior inferior cerebellar arteries originate at the same level. Duplication of one of these arteries occurs in approximately 10 to 15 percent of patients. The artery courses laterally and inferiorly over the anterior surface of the pons. The artery often has a second loop adjacent to the internal acoustic meatus. At its origin in about 80 percent of patients, the anterior inferior cerebellar artery is anterior to the origin of the abducens nerve. As mentioned above, the labyrinthine artery is a branch of the anterior inferior cerebellar artery. Branches of the anterior inferior cerebellar artery perfuse the pons, middle cerebellar peduncle, flocculus, tegmentum, and cerebellar hemisphere.

Superior Cerebellar Artery

In 85 percent of patients, the left and right superior cerebellar arteries arise from the basilar artery as a single trunk. Variations include two smaller branches of the superior cerebellar artery, one of which runs medially and the other laterally; origin from the posterior cerebral artery; and dual trunks that unite to form a single superior cerebellar artery. At its origin, the superior cerebellar artery is separated from the posterior cerebral artery by the oculomotor nerve. The segments of the superior cerebellar artery include the mesencephalic segment below the oculomotor nerve, the lateral pontine mesencephalic segment below the trochlear nerve and separated from the posterior cerebral artery by the edge of the tentorium cerebelli, the cerebellar mesencephalic segment located between the cerebellum and midbrain, and the cortical segment. The lateral branch of the superior cerebellar artery supplies the superior aspect of the cerebellar hemispheres, the superior cerebellar peduncle, the dentate nucleus, and a portion of the middle cerebellar peduncle. The medial branch perfuses the rostral surface of the cerebellar hemisphere and the vermis.

VENOUS DRAINAGE

The venous drainage of the posterior fossa can be divided into three systems: the Galenic system, anterior petrosal system, and posterior (or tentorial) system.

Galenic System

The Galenic system includes the precentral cerebellar vein, the superior vermian vein, the anterior pontomesencephalic vein, and the posterior and lateral mesencephalic veins.

The precentral cerebellar vein is located in the midline in the fissure between the lingula and the central lobule of the vermis. It is formed by the union of veins from the brachium pontis and vermis. It sits posterior to the collicular plate and precentral lobule of the vermis to enter the vein of Galen. It is an important landmark during supracerebellar approaches to the pineal and tectal plate region.

The superior vermian vein curves along the anterior surface of the culmen and receives tributaries from the vermis. It also enters the vein of Galen, either with or just adjacent to the precentral cerebellar vein. The posterior mesencephalic vein originates from the outer aspect of the cerebral peduncle and curves around the brain stem in the ambient cistern. Often, it is adjacent to the basal vein of Rosenthal. One of the main tributaries to the posterior mesencephalic vein is the lateral mesencephalic vein, which is an important landmark for identifying the junction of the tegmentum and the cerebral peduncle. The anterior pontomesencephalic vein is a complex of small veins that runs along the ventral and rostral surfaces of the pons and mesencephalon. This vein curves along the interpeduncular fossa below or caudal to the cerebral peduncle to drain into either the basal vein of Rosenthal or the posterior mesencephalic vein.

Petrosal System

The petrosal system of veins receives multiple tributaries from the cerebellum, pons, and medulla. They unite to form the petrosal vein. The petrosal vein, or "Dandy's vein," is the most important cisternal bridging vein encountered during cerebellopontine angle operations. It drains laterally, adjacent to the trigeminal nerve, into the superior petrosal sinus. It collects venous blood from the middle and superior cerebellar peduncles, ventral cerebellum, pons, flocculus, medulla, and lateral region of the fourth ventricle. These tributary veins collect close to the dorsal root entry zone of the trigeminal nerve and form the bridging petrosal vein. Despite the relatively large drainage territory of the petrosal vein, it can be cauterized and divided, with low risk of venous infarction.

Posterior System

The posterior system of veins drains directly posterolaterally into the torcular Herophili. The inferior vermian vein curves posterosuperiorly along the inferior surface of the vermis and receives blood from the hemispheric veins of the cerebellar tonsils and caudal cerebellum.

The inferior petrosal sinus originates in the posterior region of the cavernous sinus. It travels along the apex of the petrous ridge, where it is crossed by the abducens nerve in Dorello's canal, and then runs down along the clivus to enter the jugular foramen. The left and inferior petrosal sinuses communicate with each other through the basilar plexus, which is located along the ventral aspect of the clivus. Also, some small veins from the hypoglossal canal, condyle region, and foramen magnum enter the inferior petrosal sinus. When a far lateral suboccipital approach is used, with removal of the occipital condyle, these veins can be the source of considerable nuisance bleeding.

ACOUSTIC NEURILEMOMA

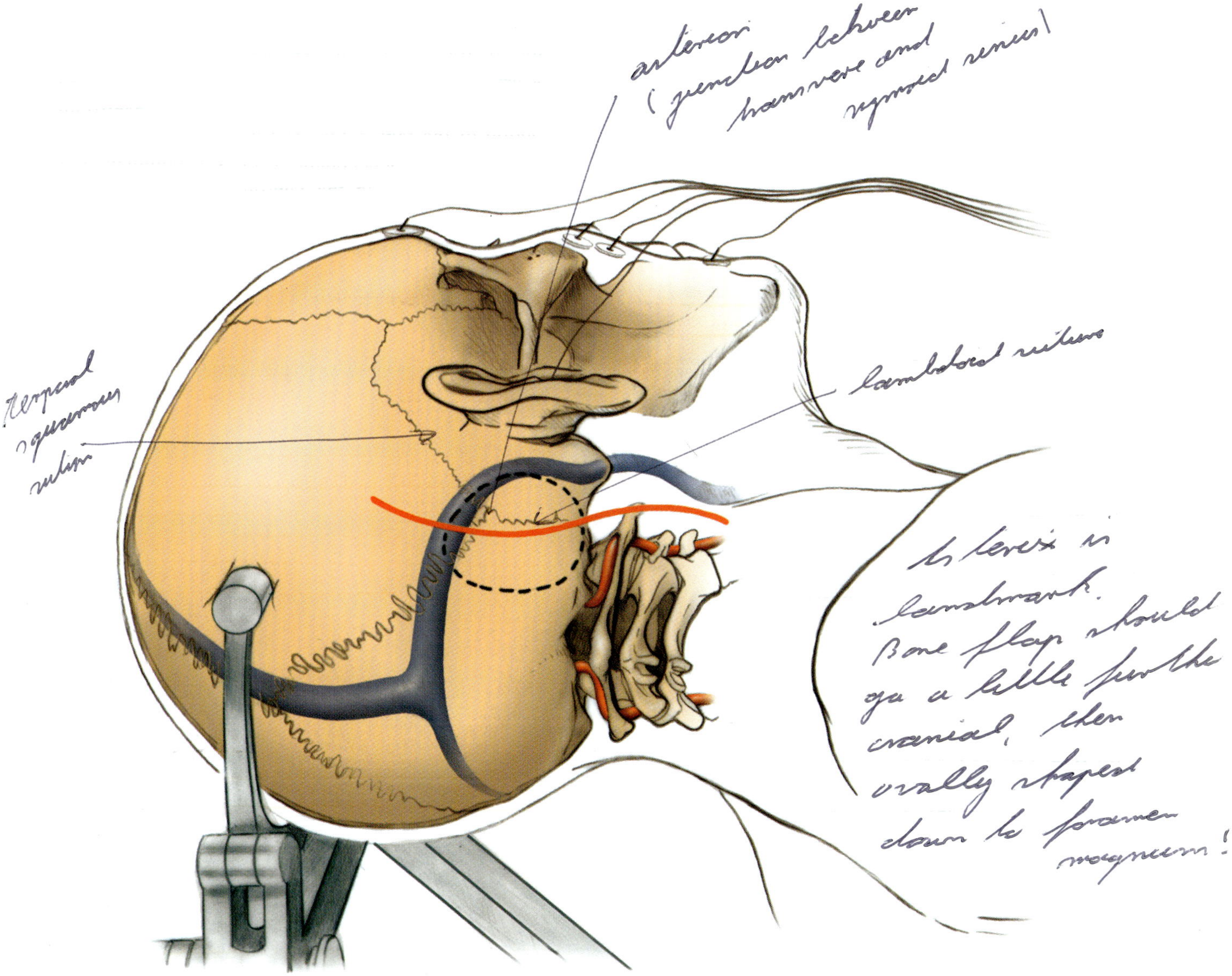

Figure 8–4.

A gentle S-shaped incision provides access to the cerebellopontine angle. The extent of bony removal, through either a craniotomy or craniectomy, depends on the type of lesion and surgical approach. For most lesions, it is best to identify the junction of the transverse and sigmoid sinuses. This visual identification facilitates the surgeon's orientation. The asterion, which is formed by the junction of the lambdoid suture and the temporal squamous suture, lies over this junction and is a useful landmark when planning bony removal. Also, there may be a mastoid emissary vein that originates from the proximal part of the sigmoid sinus. For resection of an acoustic neurilemoma, bony removal should extend down to the foramen magnum. Electromyographic monitoring of the cranial nerves is essential when resecting an acoustic neurilemoma.

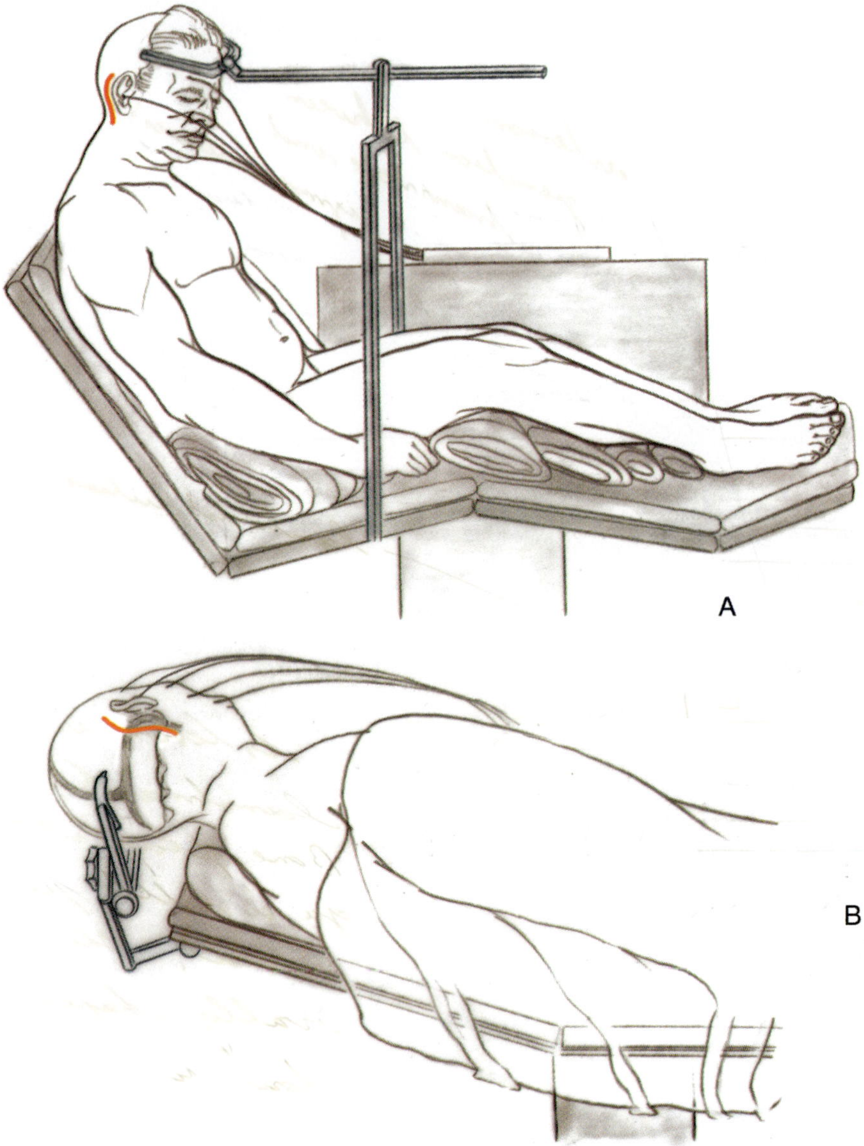

Figure 8–5.

Two patient positions can be used for resecting acoustic neurilemomas. *A*, If the sitting position is chosen, the head should be slightly flexed and rotated toward the surgeon by 15 to 20 degrees. This rotation helps decrease the need for cerebellar retraction and shortens the distance between the tumor and the surgeon. In this way, the surgeon's arms are less extended, and they can be placed more comfortably on an armrest.

B, If the supine position is chosen, it is important not to overrotate or overextend the patient's head, because this may cause compression of the contralateral jugular vein and possibly an increase in intracranial pressure. Propping up the patient's ipsilateral shoulder decreases the degree of neck rotation. However, it is important that this "propped up" shoulder not protrude too high, otherwise it will interfere with the surgeon comfortably resting his or her arm on the patient's shoulder while resecting the tumor.

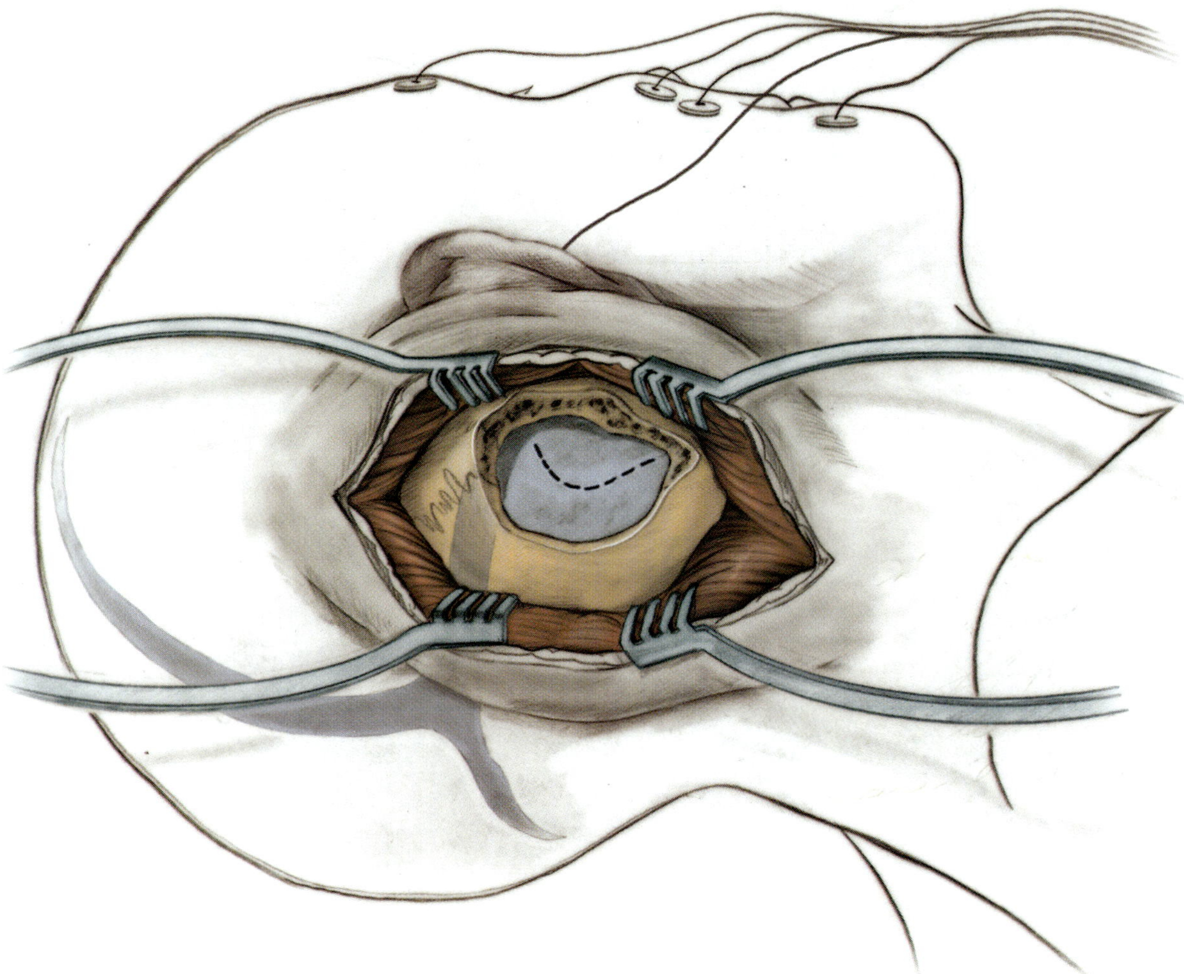

Figure 8–6.

Step 1. The asterion is identified, and a bur hole is placed. The craniectomy is performed with Adson rongeurs. A small angled Kerrison rongeur can be used to undermine and to remove bone to identify the junction of the transverse sinus and the sigmoid sinus. However, when placing the foot plate of the Kerrison rongeur underneath the bone, the surgeon must be careful, especially in young children, not to tear the sigmoid sinus, which may interdigitate with the overlying bone. An alternative is to use a high-speed air drill and diamond bur. Removing sufficient bone laterally to identify the first 4 to 6 mm of the edge of the sigmoid sinus decreases the degree of retraction on the cerebellum. The mastoid air cells are waxed. After the dura mater is closed, a piece of muscle is harvested and placed against the mastoid air cells for reinforcement.

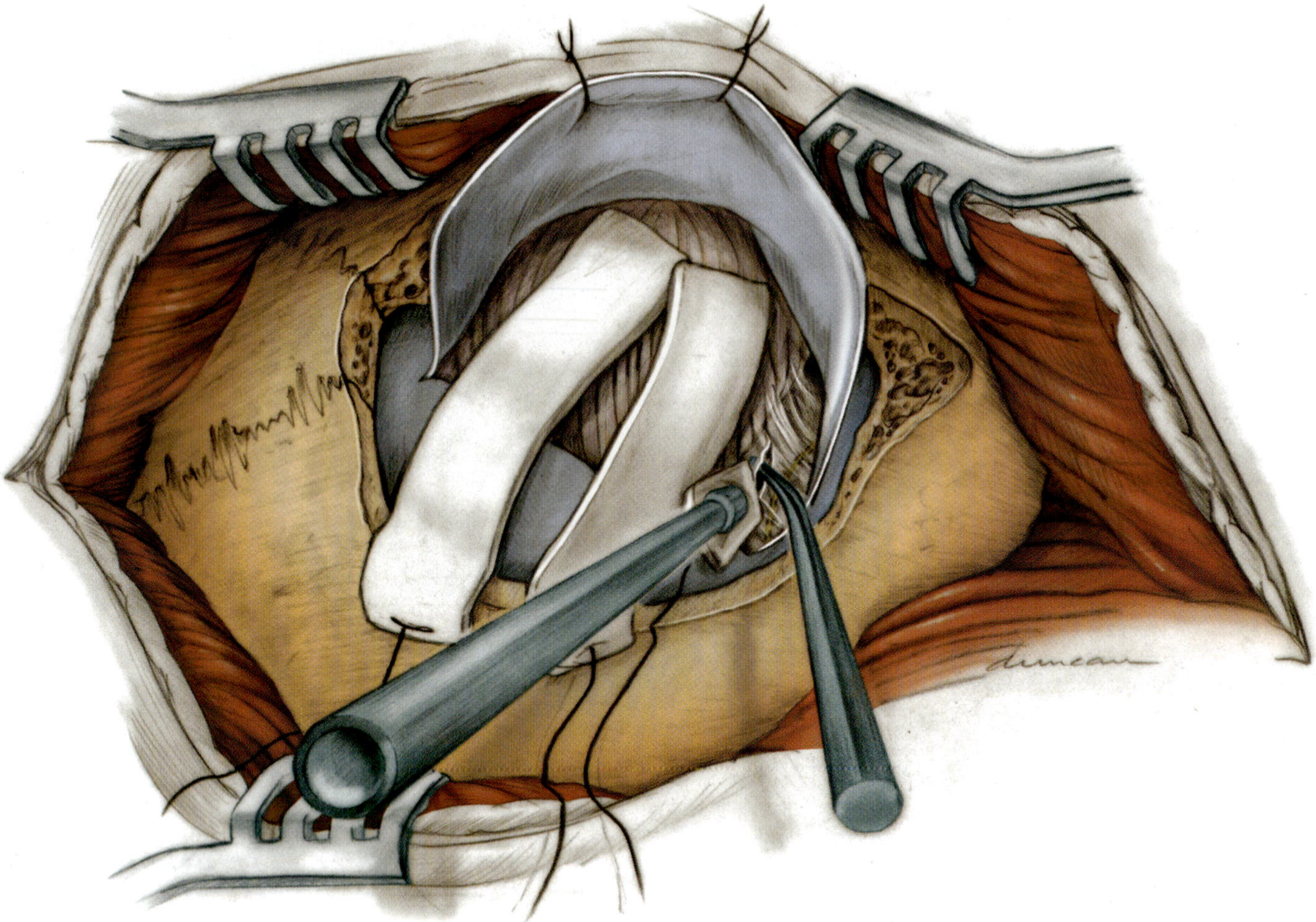

Figure 8–7.

Step 2. The dura mater is opened and tacked to the margins of the muscle. When approaching large tumors of the cerebellopontine angle, a useful maneuver is to incise the arachnoid over the cisterna magna. This provides immediate release of cerebrospinal fluid and considerably enhances the ease of exposure. It is best to incise the arachnoid closest to the cerebellum. In this way, the arachnoid will drape over and protect the lower cranial nerves during the operation. Rarely with massive tumors, it may be necessary to partially resect the lateral 1.0 cm of the cerebellar hemisphere to gain exposure.

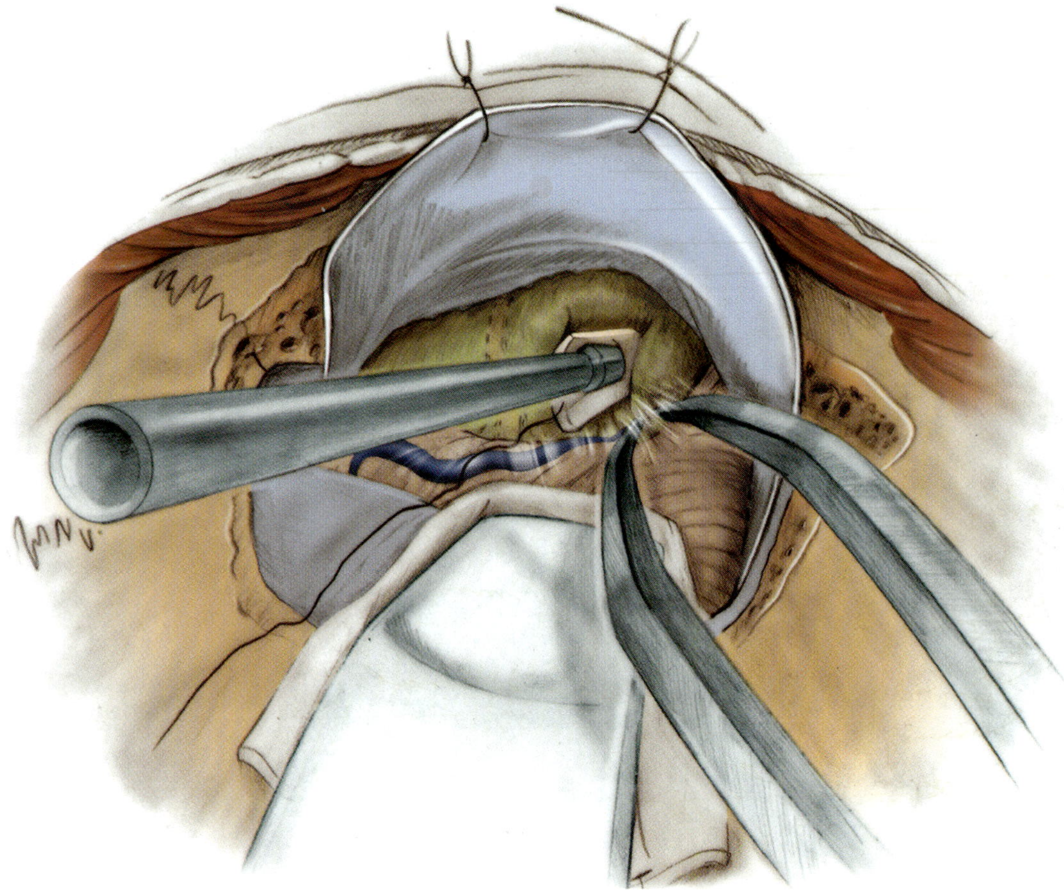

Figure 8–8.

Step 3. The exposed cerebellum is lined with hemostatic fabric (Surgicel), after which a cottonoid (Americot) is placed. The hemostatic fabric prevents the cottonoid from being stuck to the cerebellum at the end of the operation. Next, the cerebellum is gently retracted with a #7 suction tip. When first gaining access to the cerebellopontine angle, rotation of the operating table improves the angle of microscopic view. Arachnoid adhesions occur between the cerebellum and tumor capsule. These adhesions should be peeled back toward the cerebellum with a bipolar forceps or a small flat dissector. Several tributaries of the petrosal vein usually lie on the cerebellum and pons. These veins are extremely useful in identifying the pial surface and, thus, the junction between the pons and the tumor capsule. It is important to keep these veins and arachnoid adhesions with the cerebellum and pons. This pial layer merges with the thin layer of arachnoid that separates the facial and vestibulocochlear nerve complex from the tumor capsule. If the pial plane becomes obscure during the dissection, the surgeon should dissect another aspect of the tumor and work back toward the area of difficulty.

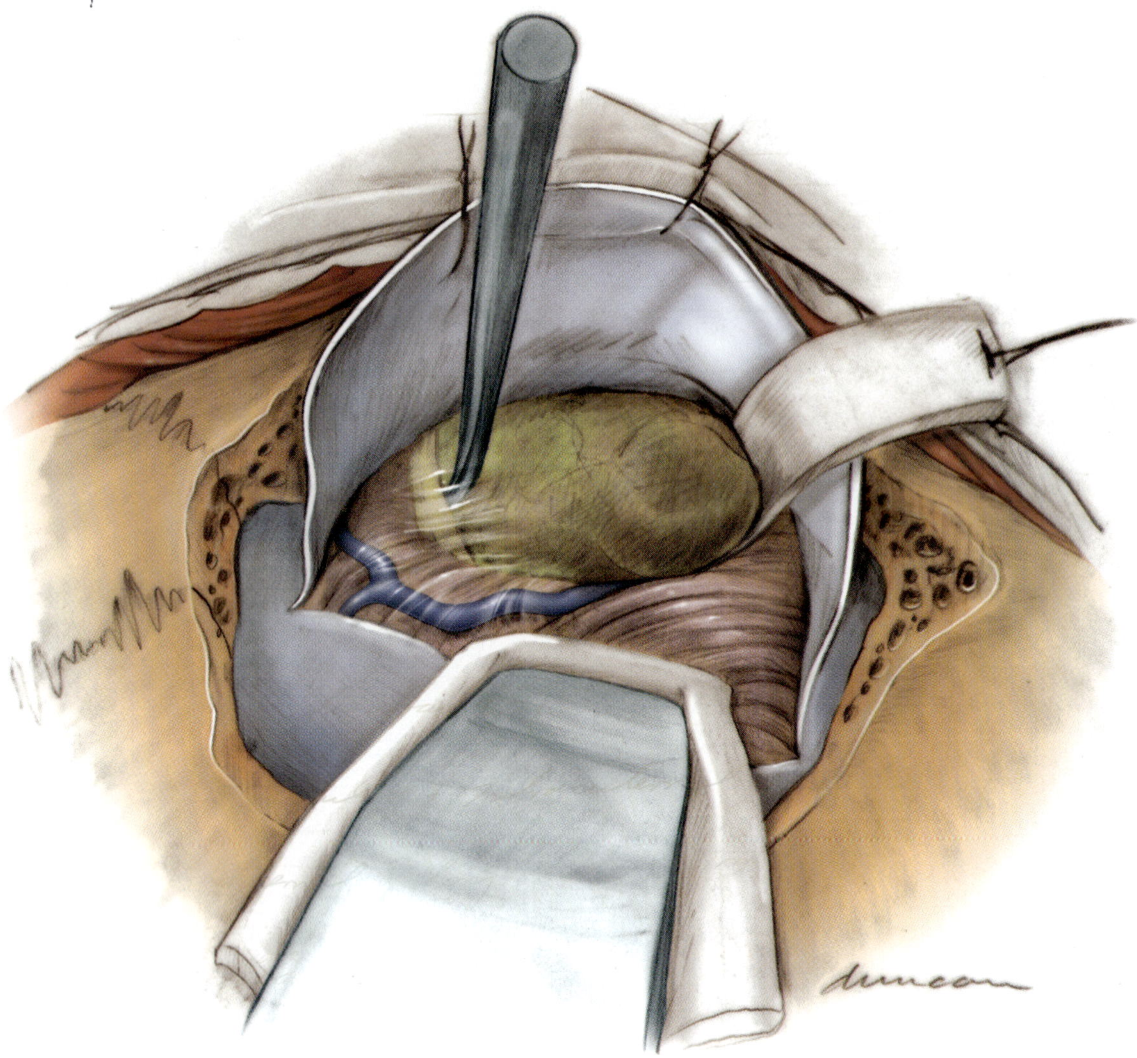

Figure 8–9.

Step 4. Typically, the trigeminal nerve is displaced rostrally and sometimes ventrally. An arachnoid layer separates the trigeminal nerve from the tumor capsule. This arachnoid is continuous with the arachnoid overlying the facial and vestibulocochlear nerve complex. It also is continuous with the pial layer of the pons. Therefore, the trigeminal nerve is dissected off the tumor capsule with its arachnoid intact. Similarly, the arachnoid overlying the lower cranial nerves is preserved. The arachnoid over the glossopharyngeal and vagus nerves is continuous with the arachnoid overlying the facial and vestibulocochlear nerve complex. It also is continuous with the pial layer of the lower pons.

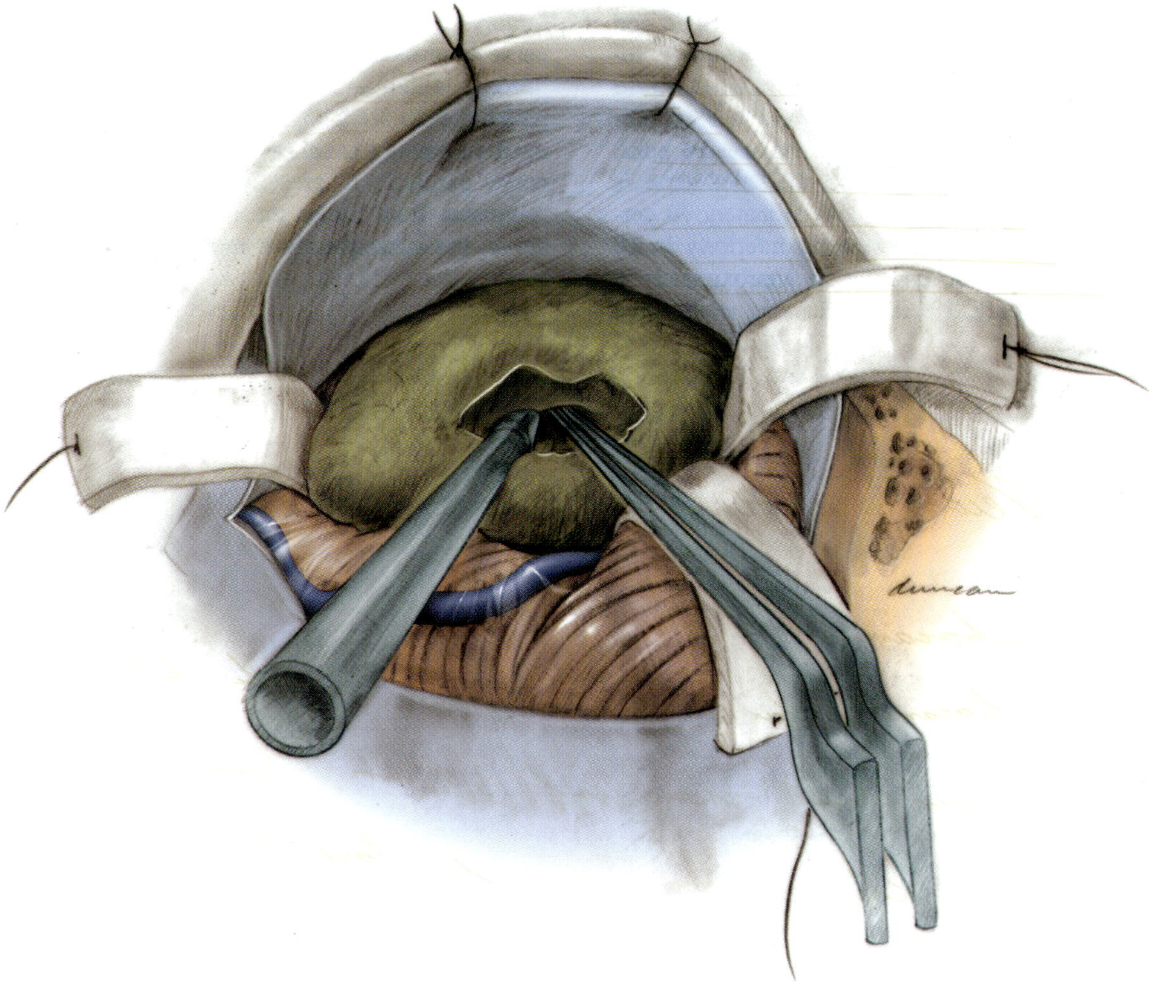

Figure 8–10.

Step 5. Tumor debulking is done with a bipolar cautery or an ultrasonic aspirator. It is important not to be overly aggressive along the ventral aspect of the tumor when debulking the center. Otherwise, the surgeon may inadvertently punch through the capsule or the deep side of the tumor and injure the facial and vestibulocochlear nerve complex. It is important to recognize that an ultrasonic aspirator can cause vibratory injury to the facial nerve. Moreover, aggressive bipolar cautery without irrigation can cause heat injury.

Acoustic neurilemomas are divided into four grades, depending on size. The relevance of the grading system is related to the prognosis regarding preservation of the facial nerve. Grade 1 tumors are intracanalicular in location and have a longitudinal diameter of 1 to 10 mm. Grade 2 tumors are both intracanalicular and intracisternal and have a longitudinal diameter up to 20 mm. Grade 3 tumors are intracisternal, have a longitudinal diameter of 30 mm, and abut the pons. Grade 4 tumors have a longitudinal diameter greater than 30 mm and displace the pons. In grade 3 or 4 acoustic neurilemomas, the facial nerve is displaced anteriorly or ventrally in approximately 70 percent of patients, rostrally in 10 percent, inferiorly in 10 percent, and posteriorly or dorsally in approximately 5 percent. Most commonly, the facial nerve is ventral and slightly rostral along the tumor capsule, but near the internal acoustic meatus, the nerve tends to be more posterior or dorsal. Therefore, when initially debulking the tumor, it is important to stay away from the porus acoustica. In approximately two-thirds of patients with acoustic tumors not related to Recklinghausen's disease, the facial nerve is preserved as a thin bundle, and in the other one-third, it is thin and splayed against the tumor capsule. In patients with Recklinghausen's disease, the facial nerve most commonly is splayed and thin, and the risk of facial nerve paralysis is greater. In most patients, the tumor originates from either the inferior or superior vestibular nerve, but subsequently it may involve the cochlear division.

Neurinoma Grading:

1) Intracanalicular 1-10 mm
2) Intracanalicular + Intracisternal up to 20 mm
3) Intracisternal long. ext 30 mm, touch the pons
4) Longer than 30 mm and displace the pons

In Grade 3+4 Neurinomas:

Facial nerve displaced: anteriorly 70% (then deep to tumour)
rostrally 10% (with trigeminus)
Inferior 10% (with vagus + glosso)
dorsally 5% (then on capsule)

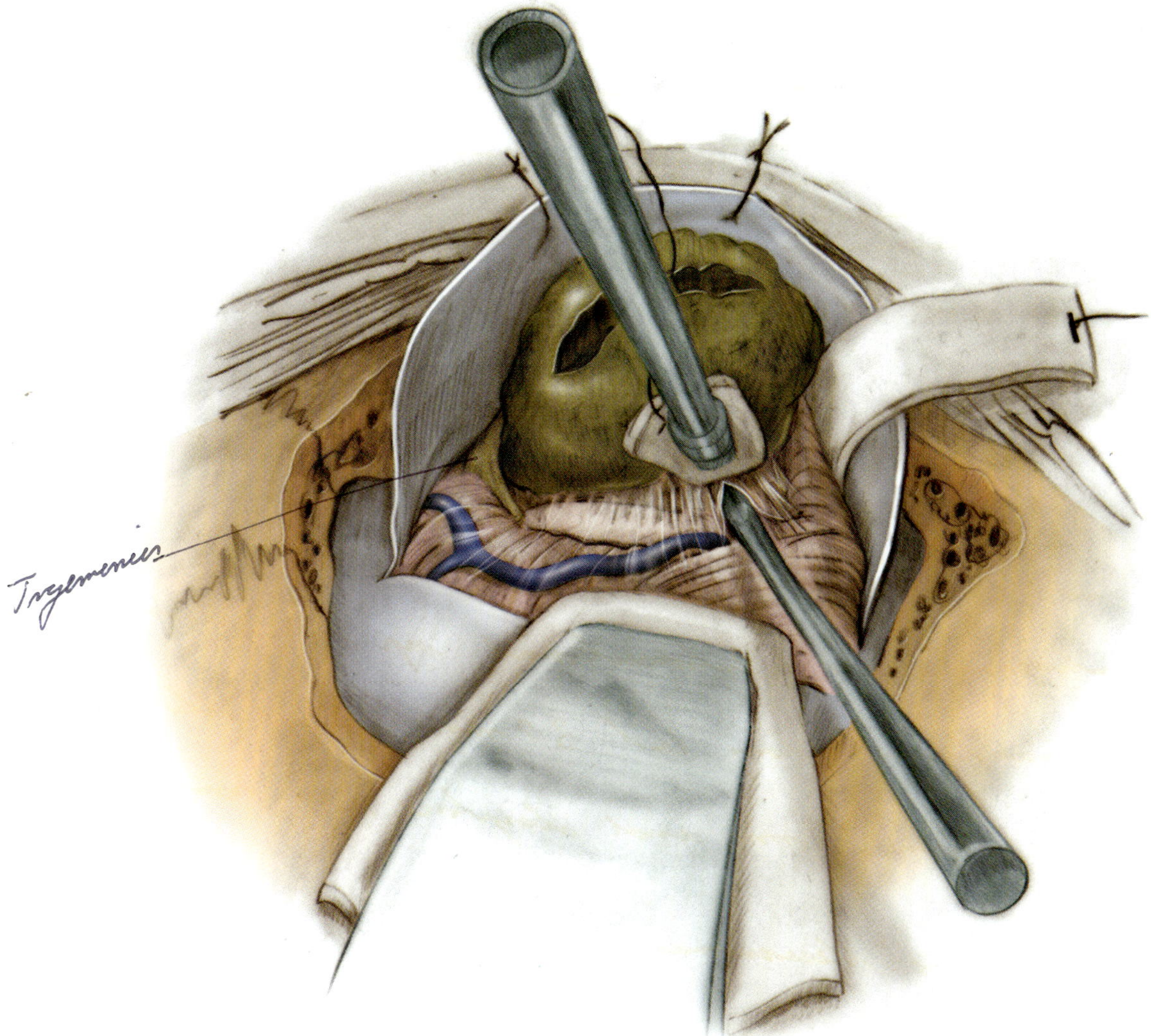

Figure 8–11.

Step 6. After the tumor has been debulked, the suction tip with a small cottonoid is used to gently rotate and lift the tumor away from the pons. However, before this maneuver is performed, it is important to identify the arachnoid over the trigeminal nerve and lower cranial nerves and the place where it merges with the pial surface of the pons is identified. Often, the thin facial nerve is translucent. However, a very thin layer of arachnoid usually separates the facial and cochlear nerves from the tumor capsule. As the tumor is retracted laterally, a small spatula is used to push the thin arachnoid away from the tumor capsule, and an attempt is made to maintain the integrity of this layer, with the more clearly defined arachnoid along the underside of the trigeminal nerve and the arachnoid lying along the upper aspect of the lower cranial nerves.

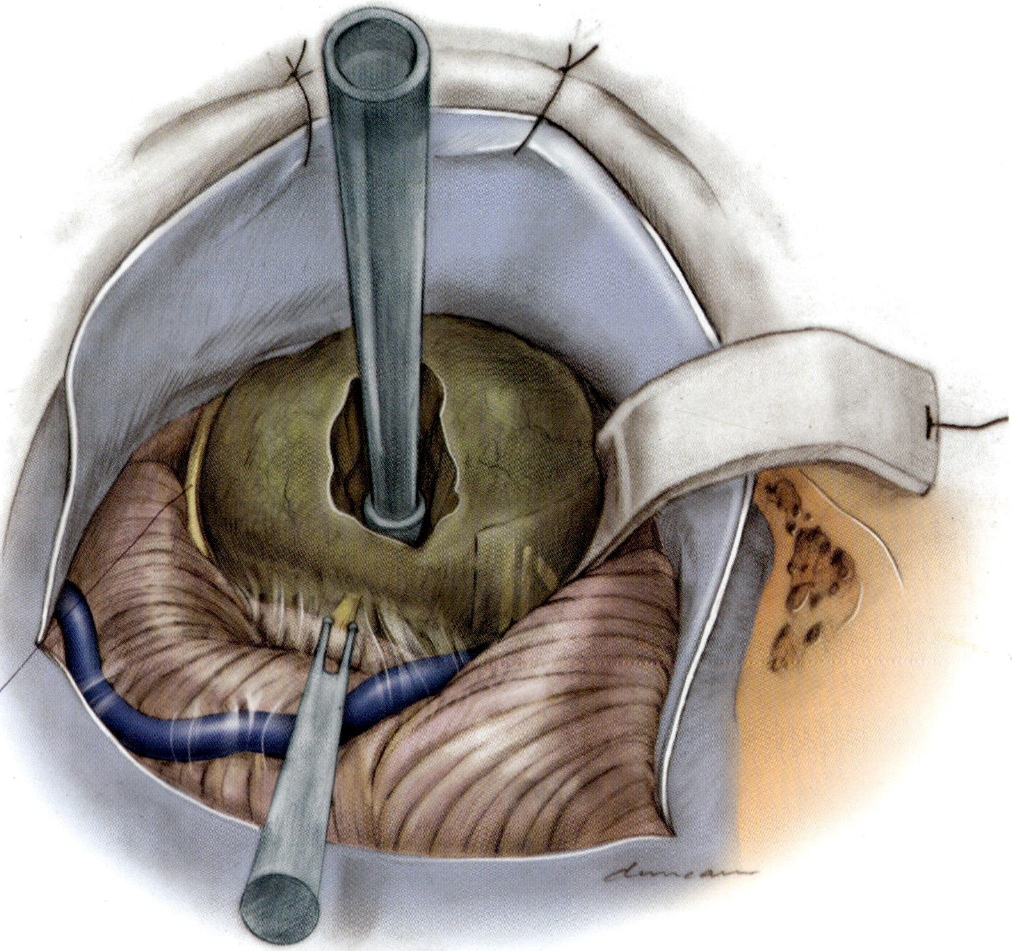

Figure 8–12.

Step 7. At the junction of the pons with the tumor capsule, bipolar stimulation in combination with electromyographic monitoring is used to identify the facial nerve. With a spatula or forceps, the arachnoid adhesions are dissected or peeled with the facial nerve. These adhesions are never sharply dissected off the tumor capsule.

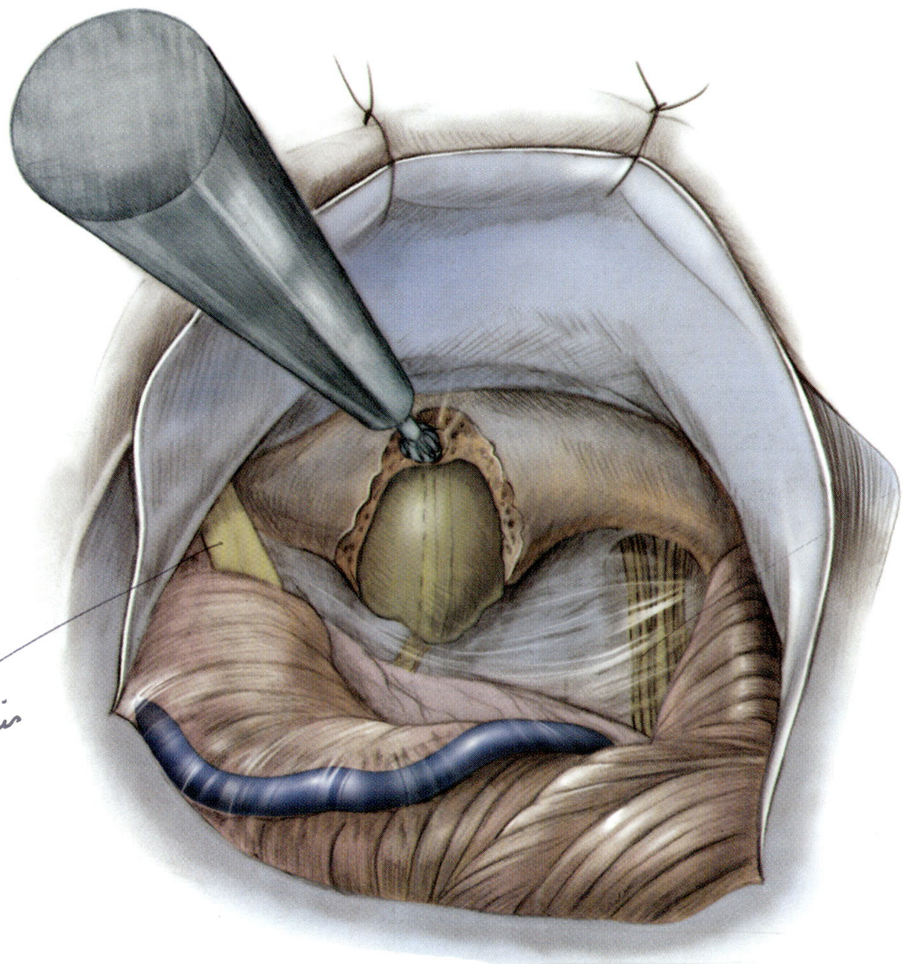

Figure 8–13.

Step 8. By step 8, the majority of tumor has been removed. The tumor within the internal acoustic meatus is exposed with careful drilling of the porus acoustica. If it is difficult to identify the facial nerve along the tumor capsule during the initial dissection, the porus acoustica should be removed earlier. The facial and cochlear nerves then can be identified and followed medially into the cerebellopontine angle.

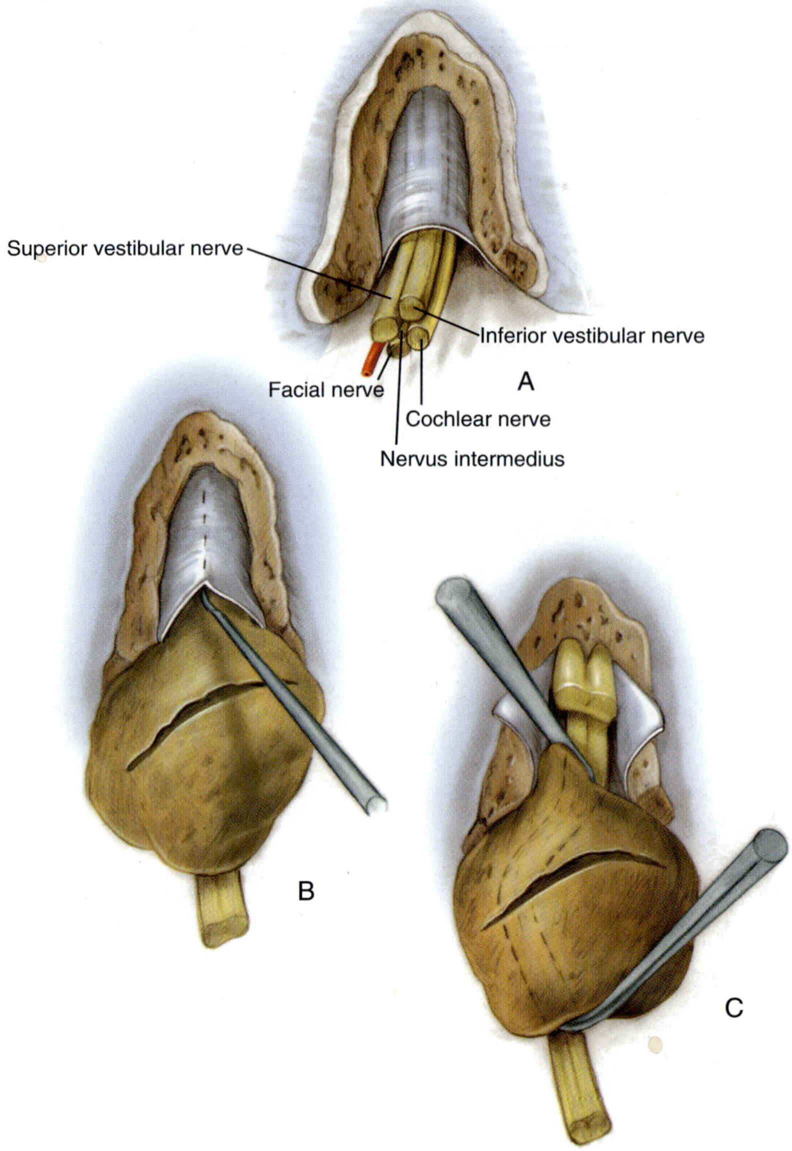

Figure 8–14.

A, The normal anatomy within the internal acoustic meatus. The internal acoustic meatus is covered by a thin layer of dura mater. Within it are the facial and vestibulocochlear nerves, including the nervus intermedius. Typically, there is at least one small labyrinthine artery, and in approximately one-half of patients, a lateral loop of the anterior inferior cerebellar artery enters the proximal portion of the internal acoustic meatus. The facial nerve is against the anterosuperior aspect of the internal acoustic meatus, and the cochlear nerve is against the anteroinferior aspect. The superior and inferior vestibular nerves are posterior to the facial and cochlear nerves. The superior and inferior vestibular nerves are separated by the transverse crest. The small nervus intermedius is intimately related to the facial nerve and usually posterior to it, adjacent to the cochlear nerve.

B, After the porus acoustica has been removed with a high-speed air drill, the thin dura mater is incised with a sickle knife.

C, Next, normal-appearing superior and inferior vestibular nerves are identified and sectioned at their junction with the tumor, and then the facial and cochlear nerves are identified in the internal acoustic canal. The tumor is gently dissected off these nerves with a small spatula. As the facial nerve exits from the internal acoustic meatus to enter the subarachnoid space, it usually is quite thin and compressed against the opening or rim. The surgeon works back and forth from both a brain stem and internal acoustic meatus perspective until the tumor is dissected off the arachnoid that overlies the thin facial nerve. After the tumor has been resected, the facial nerve is stimulated at its origin from the brain stem to assess residual conduction. Some mild bleeding usually occurs along the facial nerve. This is treated best with small bits of hemostatic agent, such as absorbable gelatin sponge (Gelfoam) or hemostatic fabric, followed by irrigation, instead of bipolar cautery. After immaculate hemostasis has been achieved, the surface of the cerebellum is inspected to ensure that there are no retraction hemorrhages. Next, the dura mater is closed with a graft in a watertight fashion, and the mastoid air cells are rewaxed. If a craniotomy was performed, the bone flap is reapproximated with small titanium plates, wires, or monofilament sutures. If a craniectomy was performed, a new bone plate can be fashioned with either acrylate or newer bone matrix materials. According to anecdotal experience with removal of acoustic neurilemoma, replacement of a bone flap decreases postoperative headache. Before suturing, the muscle is injected with 0.25 percent bupivacaine to decrease postoperative neck pain.

CEREBELLOPONTINE ANGLE MENINGIOMA

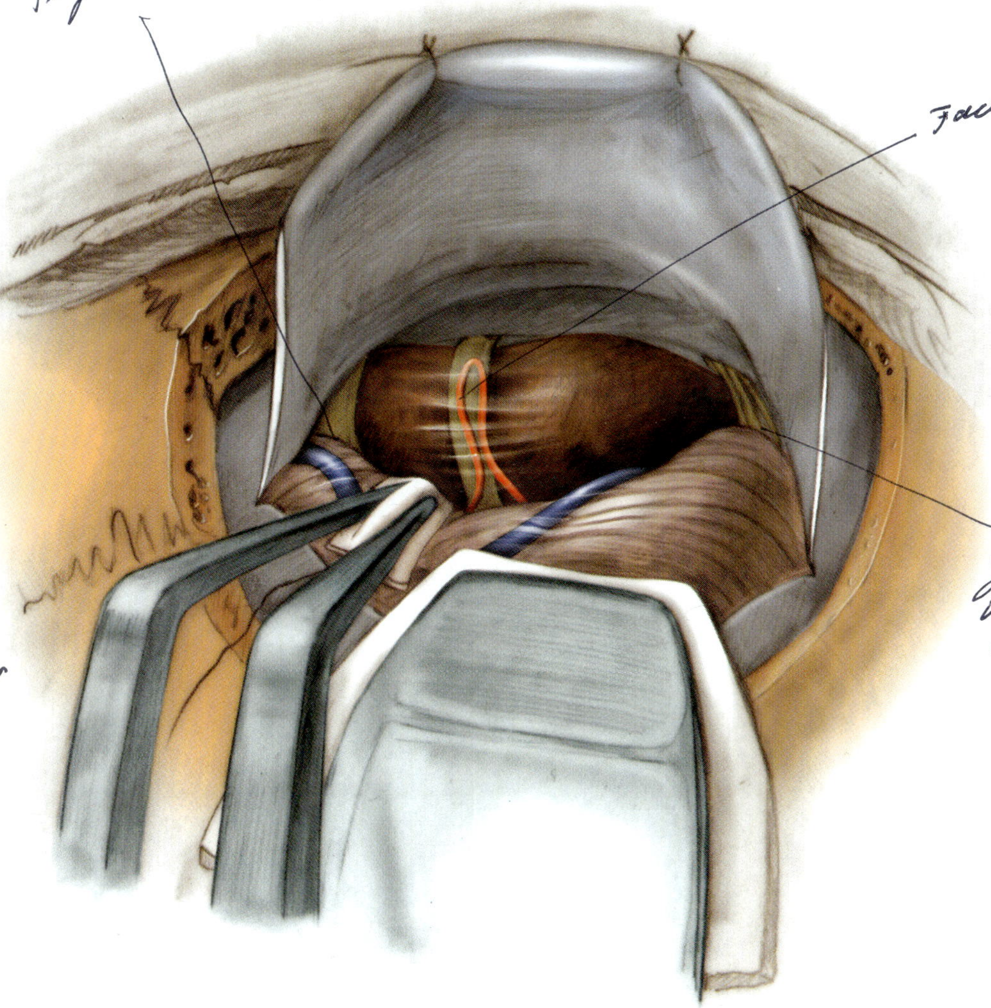

Figure 8–15.

Step 1. The patient position is similar to that for resection of an acoustic neurilemoma. Specifically, a supine, park bench, or sitting position can be used. The craniectomy or craniotomy is identical to that used for an acoustic neurilemoma: the junction between the transverse sinus and the sigmoid sinus is identified, and the bone is removed as far as the foramen magnum. Approximately 2 cm medially from the transverse sinus and sigmoid sinus, the dura mater is opened and tacked to the margins of the muscle. The rest of the dura mater is left intact to protect the cerebellum, keeping it out of harm's way. The cerebellum is lined with hemostatic fabric and cottonoids and gently retracted. Lateral rotation of the operating room table facilitates entry into the cerebellopontine angle, with less retraction on the cerebellum. Typically, the trigeminal nerve is displaced rostrally at the margins of the exposure adjacent to the petrosal vein. The facial and vestibulocochlear nerves are usually displaced dorsally and encountered during the initial retraction of the cerebellum. The lower cranial nerves are displaced caudally.

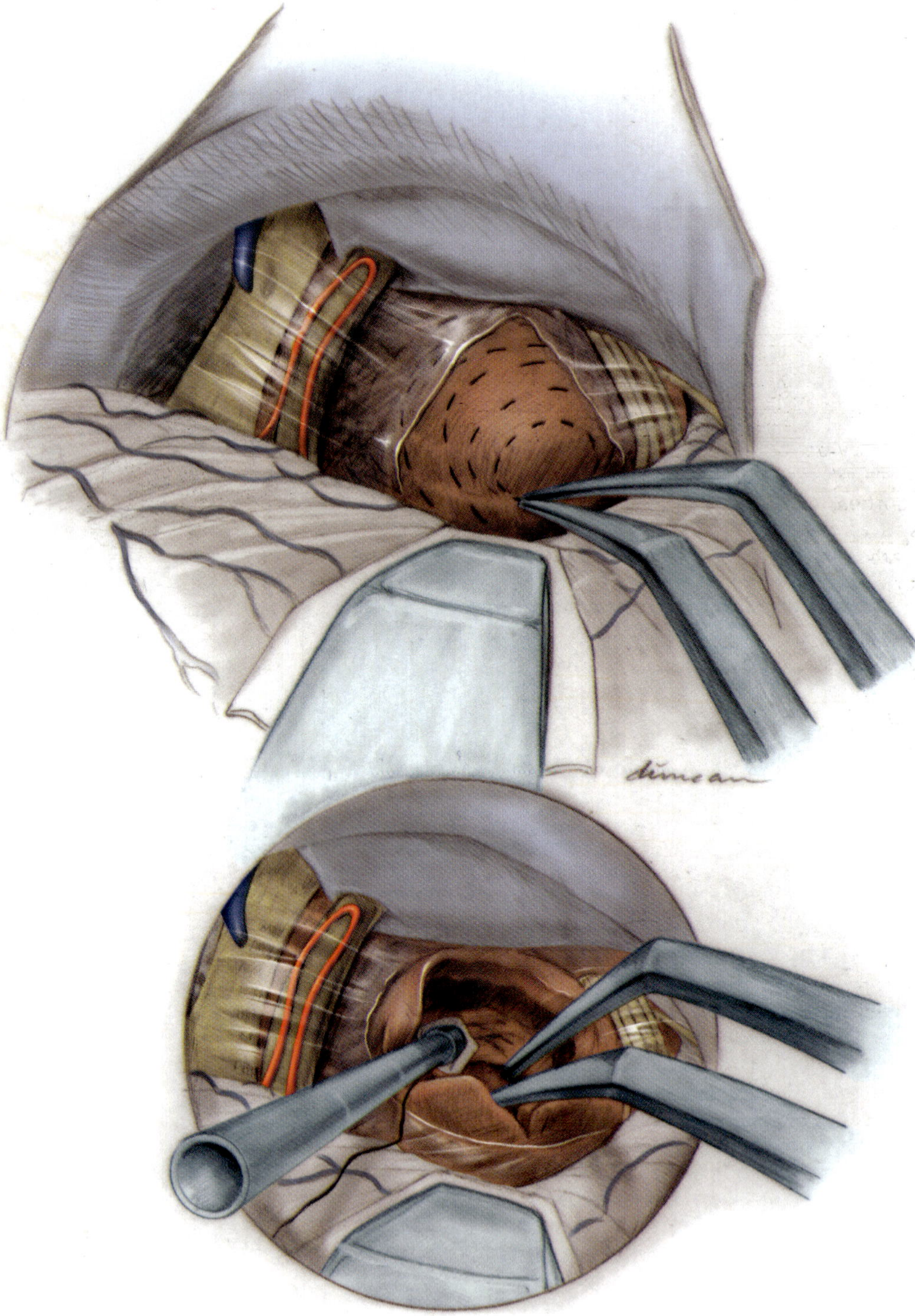

A

B

Figure 8–16.

Step 2. *A*, The trajectory or approach for resecting the tumor depends on the way the cranial nerves have been displaced. In this illustration, the facial and vestibulocochlear nerves have been displaced rostrally. Therefore, the tumor will initially be approached caudally, below the facial and vestibulocochlear nerves. If during the initial exposure the facial nerve has been displaced caudally, the tumor is approached between the trigeminal and the facial and vestibulocochlear nerves. Regardless of the approach, it is valuable to preserve the arachnoid that overlies the facial and vestibulocochlear nerves. This arachnoid layer helps to protect these nerves and their vascular supply from injury. During the operation, brain stem auditory evoked potentials are a valuable tool in helping to preserve audition. For example, an increasing latency in wave 5 during the resection suggests that cerebellar retraction is excessive. In this case, the retractor blade should be loosened. Constant monitoring of the facial nerve during the dissection prevents excessive manipulation. During any exposure of the cerebellopontine angle, it is important to watch the petrosal vein. Often, it is best to cauterize "Dandy's vein" if it appears to be under tension or it obscures exposure. When cauterizing this vein, it is important to cauterize it completely and to cut it only partially with a microscissors, after which the vein is again cauterized and then severed. Bleeding or oozing may occur from the petrosal vein at its junction with the transverse sinus. It is better to treat this with absorbable gelatin sponge packing instead of attempting cauterization. Occasionally, bleeding may occur from the top of the cerebellum because of tearing of small bridging veins. These veins usually cannot be visualized directly. Packing with absorbable gelatin sponge is also useful in this situation. Following the resection, it is important to remove the absorbable gelatin sponge from the top of the cerebellum and to irrigate to ensure that no hematoma has been trapped.

B, After the arachnoid has been dissected off the tumor capsule, an incision is made in the midportion of the meningioma, and a bipolar cautery, laser, or ultrasonic aspirator is used to core out the tumor.

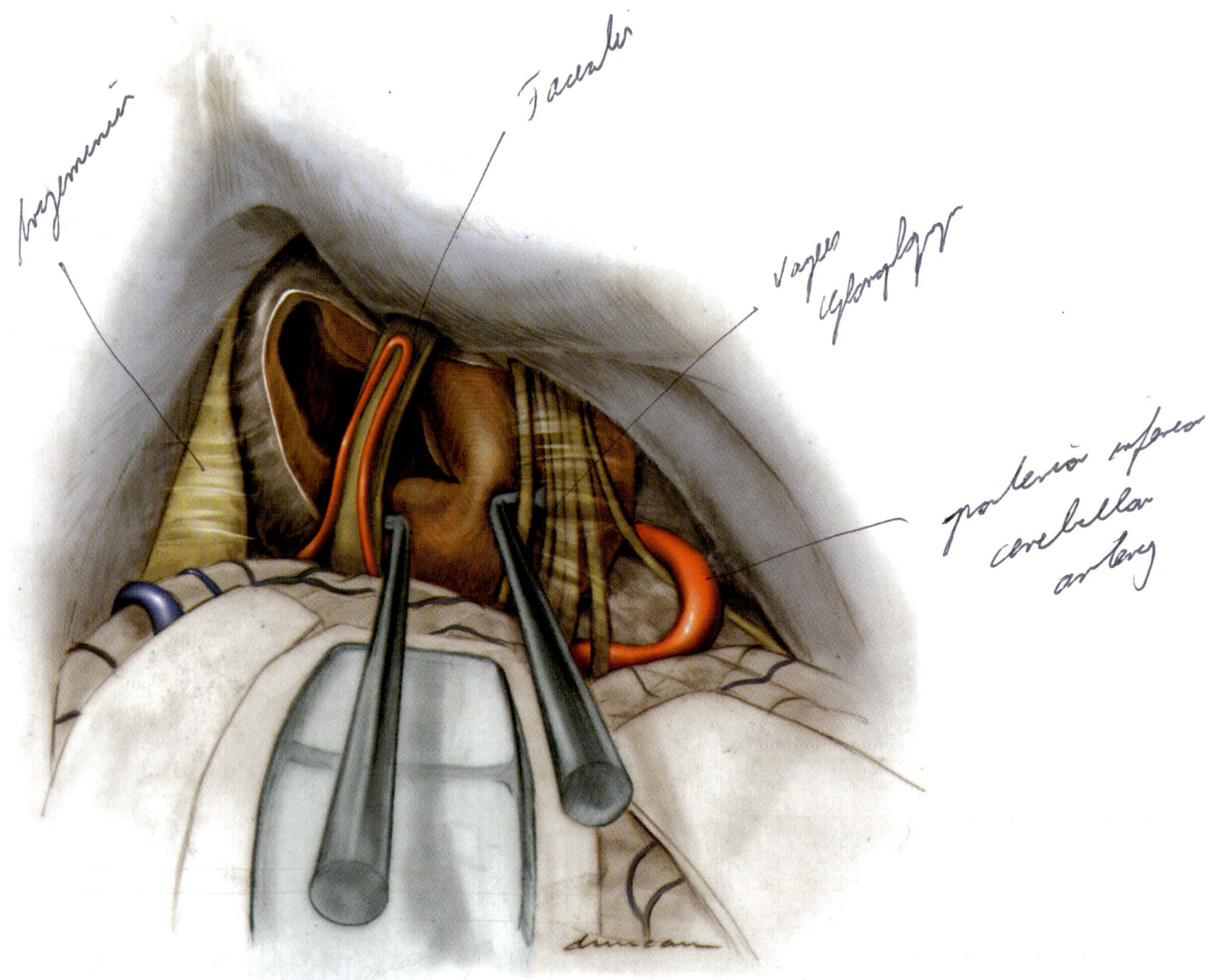

Figure 8–17.

Step 3. After the tumor has been debulked, a small ball tip or similar dissector is used to dissect the cranial nerves off the tumor capsule. The lower cranial nerves usually can be swept off in a sheath of arachnoid. Dissecting the facial and vestibulocochlear nerves off the tumor capsule must be done with care. During this dissection, it is important to press against the tumor capsule instead of against the nerves.

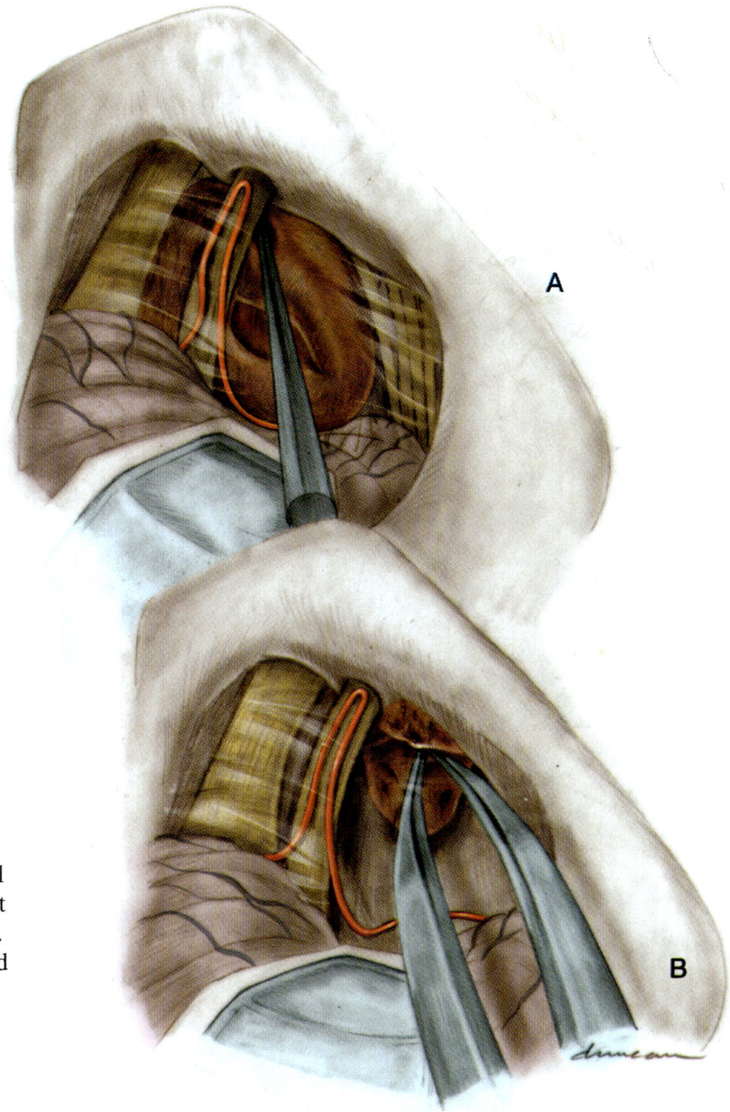

Figure 8–18.

Step 4. *A*, After the tumor has been dissected off the cranial nerves, additional debulking is performed. Next, a small spatula is used to dissect the tumor off the trigeminal nerve. Also, a spatula or ball-tip dissector is used to dissect the tumor off the distal facial and vestibulocochlear nerves. Remember that preserving the arachnoid over the facial and vestibulocochlear nerves helps to protect these structures. The tumor usually flattens these nerves against the internal acoustic meatus.

Step 5. *B*, The residual nubbin of tumor along the petrous ridge is cauterized with a bipolar cautery and then removed. Small curets can be useful in removing less well visualized tumor from around corners. After the tumor has been resected, it is important to meticulously cauterize the dural attachment of the tumor in a wide fashion to decrease recurrence.

MICROVASCULAR DECOMPRESSION FOR TRIGEMINAL NEURALGIA

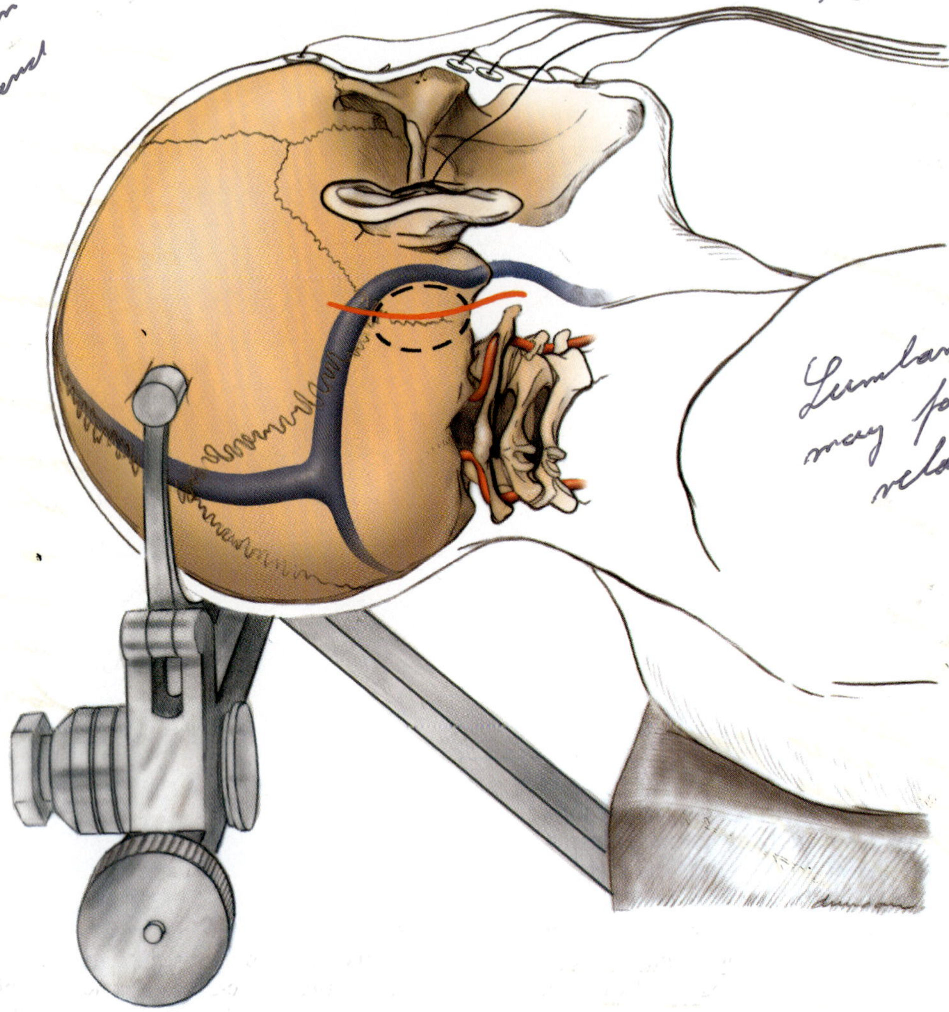

Figure 8–19.

Step 1. A straight or gentle curve incision is used in this exposure. The craniectomy must identify the junction between the transverse sinus and the sigmoid sinus. It does not need to extend down to the foramen magnum. The first bur hole is placed at the asterion. An Adson rongeur is used to bite bone laterally until the junction of the transverse and sigmoid sinuses is identified. Although electromyographic monitoring is not mandatory, it provides a degree of security in protecting the cranial nerves. Placement of a lumbar needle can be helpful in younger patients. Specifically, withdrawal of approximately 10 to 20 mL of cerebrospinal fluid through the lumbar needle facilitates cerebellar displacement. Often, a retractor is not necessary. One disadvantage of the lumbar needle is the risk of postoperative low-pressure headaches. After the craniectomy, the dura mater is opened in a curved fashion. The cerebellum is lined with hemostatic fabric and a cottonoid and gently retracted with a #7 suction tip. The arachnoid bulging over the trigeminal nerve is incised. The immediate drainage of cerebrospinal fluid provides adequate relaxation of the cerebellum. The surgeon's view and approach to the trigeminal nerve can be improved by rotating the operating room table from side to side.

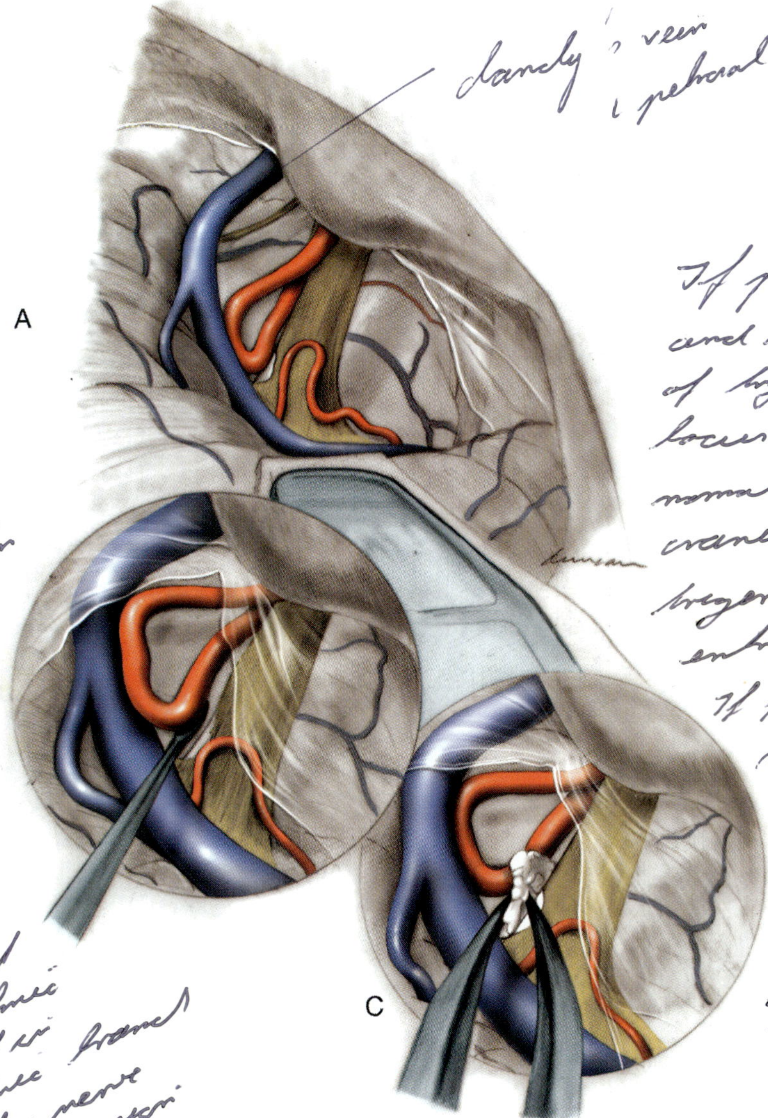

Figure 8–20.

Step 2. *A*, With gentle retraction of the cerebellum, the petrosal vein is encountered. If the petrosal vein is under tension or is at risk of being injured during the dissection, it should be cauterized, partially divided, recauterized, and then completely severed. From this operative approach, the facial and vestibulocochlear nerves are visualized at the caudal end of the exposure. The arachnoid over these structures should be left intact.

Step 3. *B*, It is mandatory to clearly identify and expose the dorsal root entry zone of the trigeminal nerve. For patients with pain in the ophthalmic or maxillary distribution, the site of vascular compression is usually along the rostral side of the dorsal entry zone; however, if the pain is in the mandibular distribution, the site of compression is located caudally. A focal area of discoloration or demyelination is often present at the site of vascular compression. A small dissector or spatula is used to gently dissect the tethering arachnoid and to lift off the vascular loop.

Step 4. *C*, Before permanently displacing the vascular loop, it is important to examine the circumference of the dorsal root entry zone to ensure there are no other sites of vascular compression. Next, a small piece of polytef (Teflon) is used to displace the vascular compression off the dorsal root entry zone. Some surgeons use cotton or another type of packing material, including muscle, and others place a suture in the underside of the tentorium cerebelli and create a sling around the artery.

If a site of vascular compression cannot be identified, a difficult decision must be made about what the next step should be. There are several alternatives. First, the nerve can be compressed three to five times with a bipolar forceps. Such traumatic compression often is successful in alleviating the pain. Second, the trigeminal nerve can be partially sectioned. If the patient has pain in the maxillary or mandibular distribution, the lower one-half to two-thirds of the nerve can be sectioned. However, if the pain is in the ophthalmic distribution, it is better to compress the nerve instead of performing a rhizotomy, which may result in corneal anesthesia dolorosa. Before either nerve compression or rhizotomy is considered, the surgeon must be absolutely certain that there is no arterial or venous compression. The possibility of not finding any arterial or venous compression and the alternatives to this should be discussed thoroughly with the patient before the operation.

MICROVASCULAR DECOMPRESSION FOR HEMIFACIAL SPASM

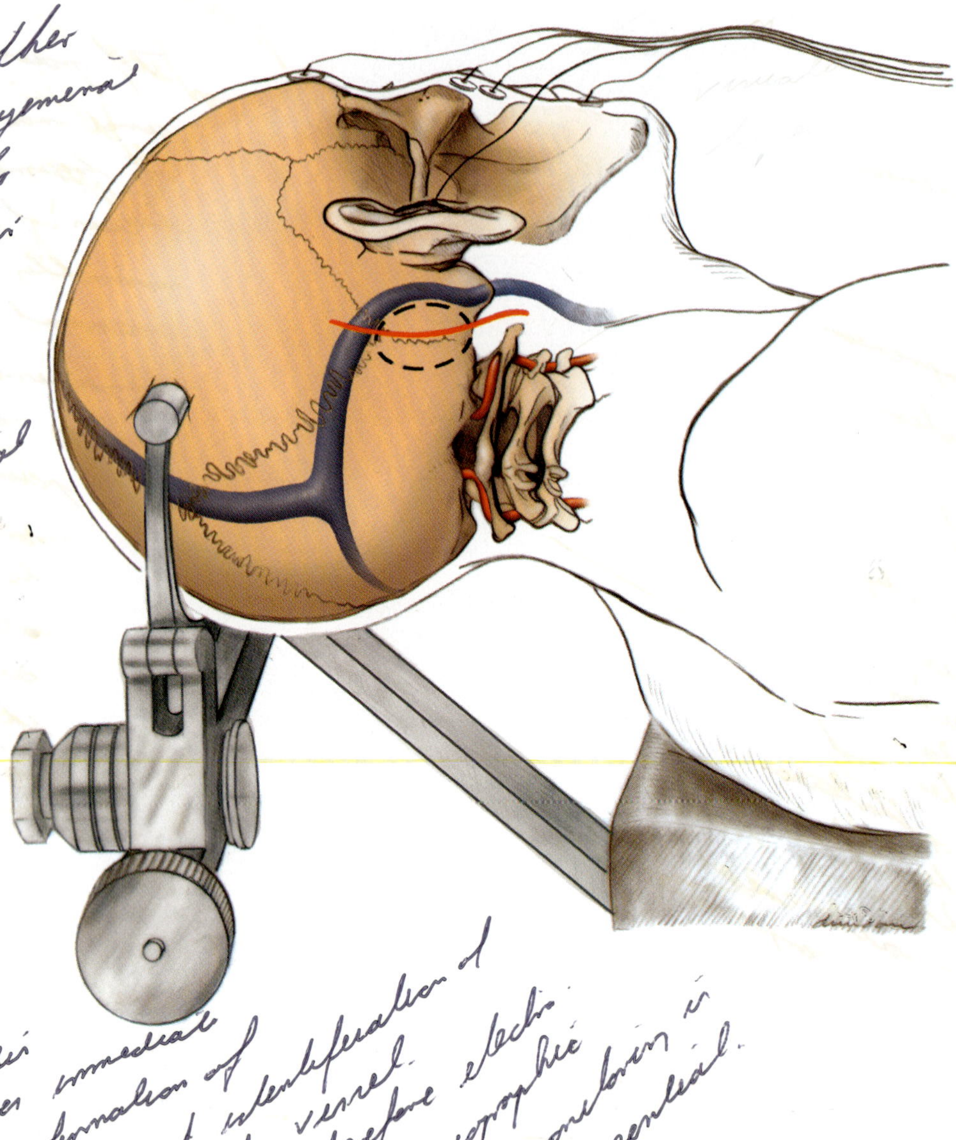

Figure 8–21.

Step 1. Bone removal for treatment of hemifacial spasm should extend lower than that typically used for surgical treatment of trigeminal neuralgia. It is valuable to outline the junction of the transverse sinus and sigmoid sinus at the upper end of the craniectomy. The rationale for having more inferior exposure of bone is that the facial nerve should be approached from a caudal direction, between it and the glossopharyngeal nerve. This is contrary to approaching the facial nerve directly laterally or rostrally below the trigeminal nerve. The latter two approaches have an increased risk of causing hearing loss. Electromyographic monitoring for hemifacial spasm is required for several reasons. First, it helps preserve cochlear nerve function. Second, patients with hemifacial spasm have an abnormal electromyographic lateral spread reflex. Lifting off the arterial compression leads immediately to the loss of the lateral spread reflex. Thus, the surgeon immediately has intraoperative confirmation that the correct vascular compression has been identified. This is in contrast to microvascular decompression for trigeminal neuralgia, in which there is no direct confirmation that successful decompression has been achieved.

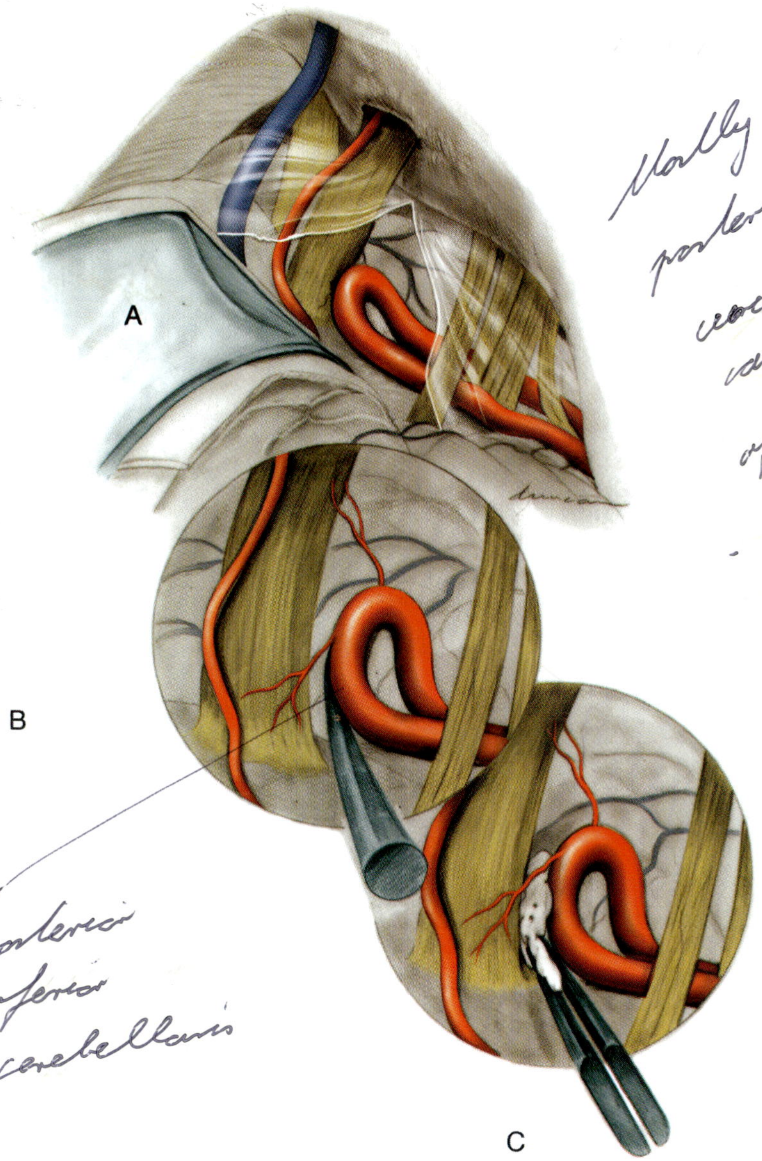

Figure 8–22.

Step 2. *A*, The dura mater is opened in a curved fashion and tacked to the margin of the muscle. The cerebellum is lined with hemostatic fabric and a cottonoid and gently retracted. As mentioned above, the facial nerve is approached from a more caudal or inferior approach, above the glossopharyngeal nerve. A lumbar needle can be placed to drain cerebrospinal fluid to enhance the ease of exposure. Alternatively, the cisterna magna can be opened during the initial retraction of the cerebellum for cerebrospinal fluid drainage. After gentle retraction of the cerebellum, the arachnoid below the facial and vestibulocochlear nerves is incised.

Step 3. *B*, In most circumstances, the vascular compression is due to a loop of the posterior inferior cerebellar artery. The vascular loop is gently lifted off the dorsal root entry zone of the facial nerve with a small dissector. There typically are a few small branches of the posterior inferior cerebellar artery that supply the facial nerve; these must be preserved. After the vascular loop has been dissected and lifted off the facial nerve, electromyographic monitoring should show an immediate loss of the lateral spread reflex. The surgeon can let the vascular loop fall back onto the facial nerve to determine whether the lateral spread reflex returns. This is additional confirmation that the correct vascular compression has been identified.

Step 4. *C*, The vascular loop is displaced from the dorsal root entry zone by packing the space with polytef. During this packing, it is important for the technician to continue to monitor electromyographically the lateral spread reflex. The return of this reflex during the packing is a strong indication that the vascular loop had slipped back onto the facial nerve.

PONTINE CAVERNOUS HEMANGIOMA

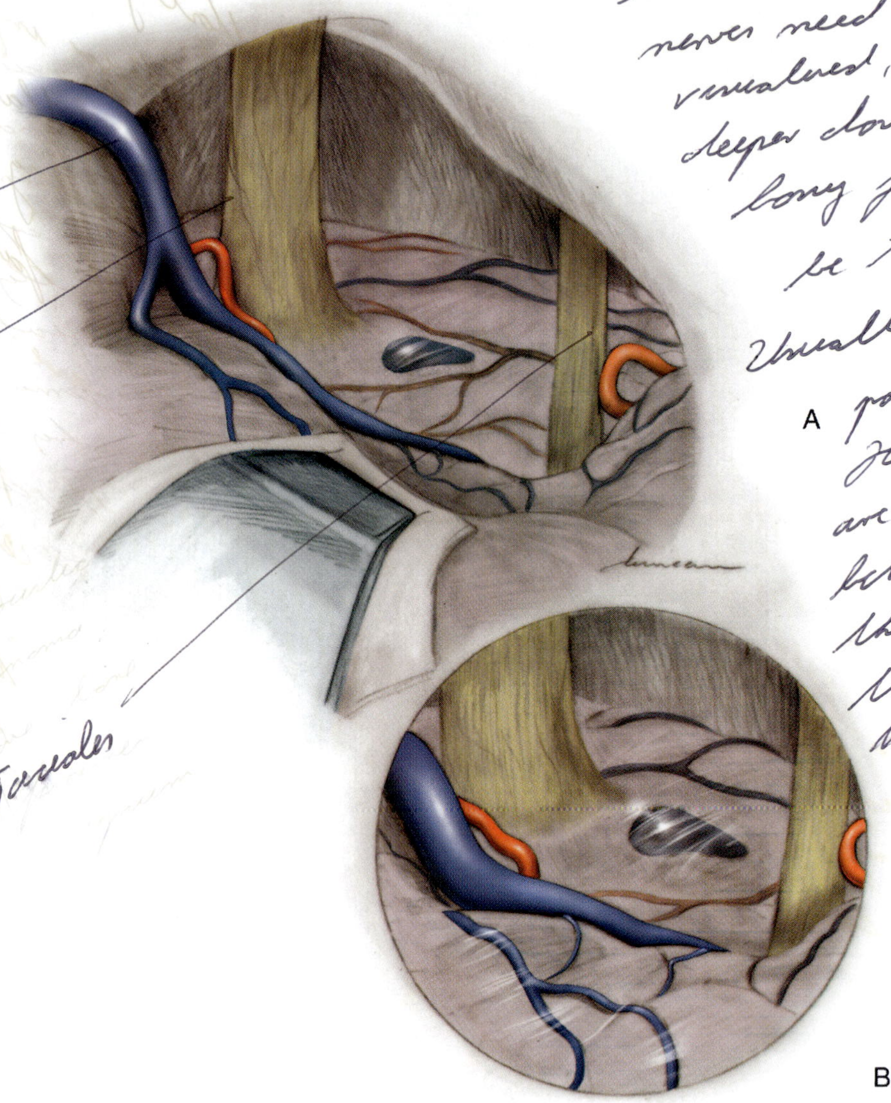

Figure 8–23.

Step 1. *A*, The craniotomy or craniectomy for exposure of a pontine cavernous hemangioma is similar to that for microvascular decompression of the facial nerve. Specifically, the bony exposure must identify the junction between the transverse sinus and the sigmoid sinus for orientation. It also should extend sufficiently inferiorly or caudally that the surgeon can identify the glossopharyngeal and vagus nerves. After the dura mater has been opened, the cerebellum is lined with hemostatic fabric and cottonoids and gently displaced with a small tapered retractor. With most pontine cavernous hemangiomas, some hemosiderin or bluish discoloration of the pial surface is apparent under high magnification.

B, The best place to enter the cavity of the pontine hematoma is between the trigeminal and facial nerves in an avascular portion of the pons. Although a large area of the pial surface may be stained with hemosiderin, it is best to enter at the point of bluish discoloration that indicates the location of the hematoma cavity.

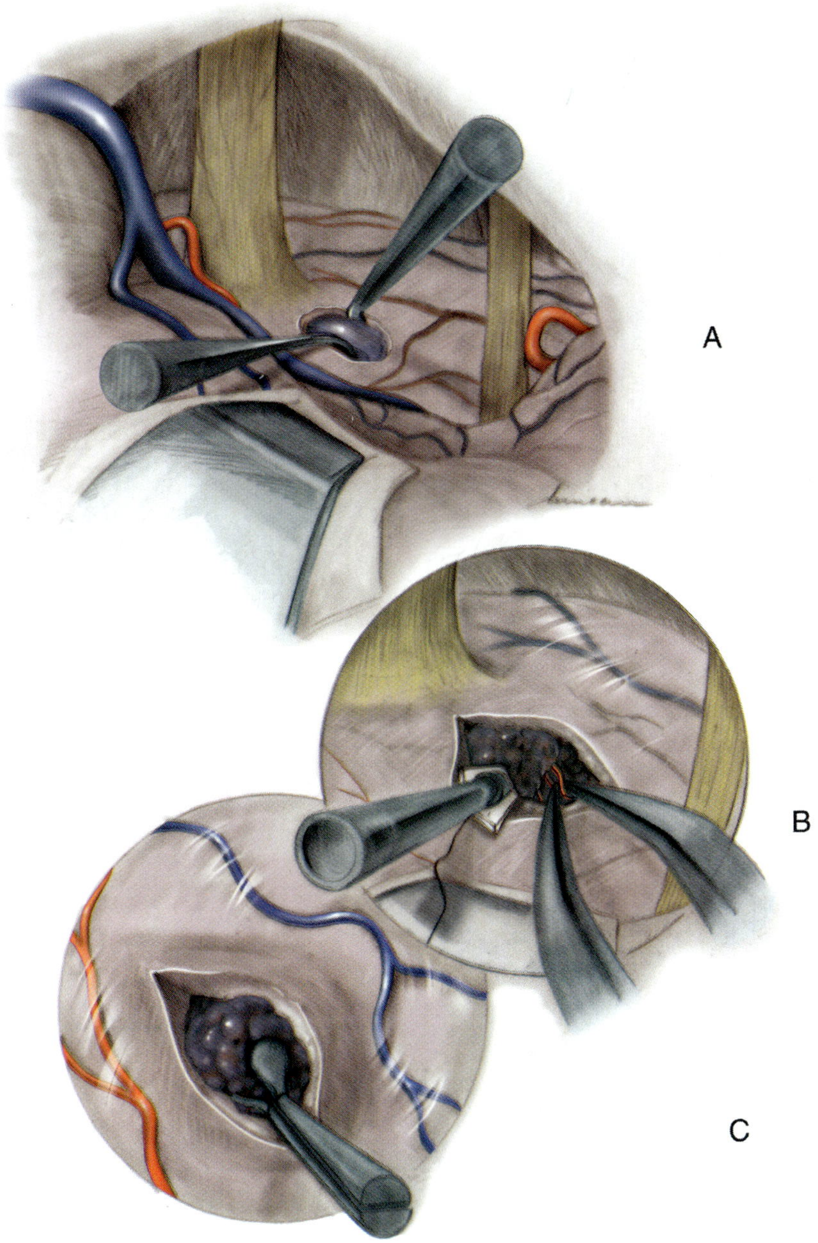

Figure 8–24.

Step 2. *A*, The pial surface of the pons is cauterized and incised vertically over a length of approximately 6 to 7 mm. Two small spatulas are moved in a back and forth manner to deepen the incision until the hematoma capsule is identified.

Step 3. *B*, The hematoma cavity is entered and the clot removed. Within the clot, the cavernous hemangioma is identified as a purplish-reddish mulberry lesion that usually is small, approximately 4 to 5 mm. Generally, three to five small arterial feeding vessels supply the cavernous hemangiomas, which should be cauterized individually and divided with a microscissors.

Step 4. *C*, After the cavernous hemangioma has been isolated, it is removed with a small cup forceps.

ANEURYSMS OF THE POSTERIOR INFERIOR CEREBELLAR ARTERY

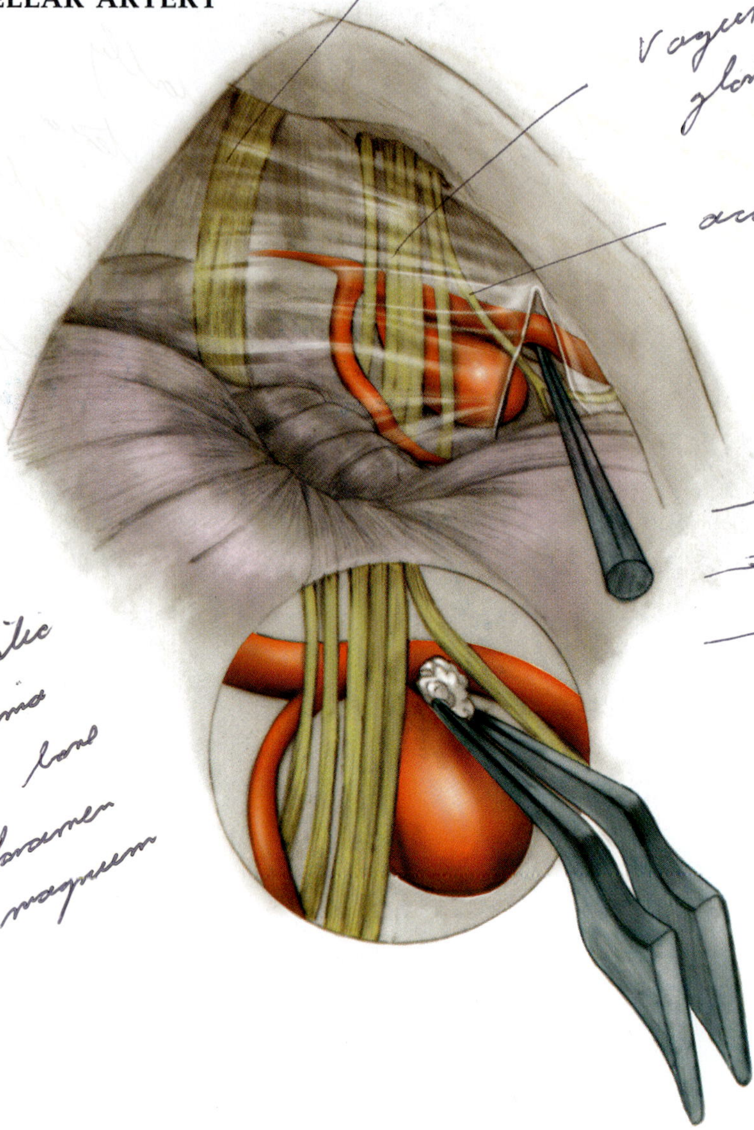

Figure 8–25.

Step 1. *A*, The position of the patient is the same as that used for removing an acoustic neurilemoma. Either a sitting or supine position can be used. A supine or park bench position is used most often; however, for lower lying aneurysms of the posterior inferior cerebellar artery, a sitting position actually works better. One of the risks of this surgical procedure is injury to the vagus nerve. With low-lying aneurysms approached through a sitting position, the cerebellar tonsil is lifted up and the aneurysm is approached behind the vagus nerve instead of going through the nerve, which often is necessary when the patient is supine or in the park bench position. Regardless of the position of the patient, the craniectomy or craniotomy must be similar to that for an acoustic neurilemoma. It is best to identify the junction between the transverse sinus and the sigmoid sinus for surgeon orientation. Also, it is mandatory to remove bone down to the foramen magnum. After the dura mater has been opened, the cerebellum is gently retracted and the lower cranial nerves are identified. It is best to open up the arachnoid caudally, below the spinal accessory nerve. This allows early identification and isolation of the vertebral artery.

Step 2. *B*, The dissection is carried distally along the vertebral artery until the aneurysm is identified. In almost all circumstances, the glossopharyngeal, vagus, and spinal accessory nerves lie over the aneurysm to some extent. Ideally, it is best to work either below or above the vagus nerve instead of working through its rootlets. When working from a more rostral approach, the glossopharyngeal nerve will serve as a buffer and protect the vagus nerve. After the proximal neck of the aneurysm has been identified, a small piece of absorbable gelatin sponge can be placed to preserve the separation of the neck from the vertebral artery.

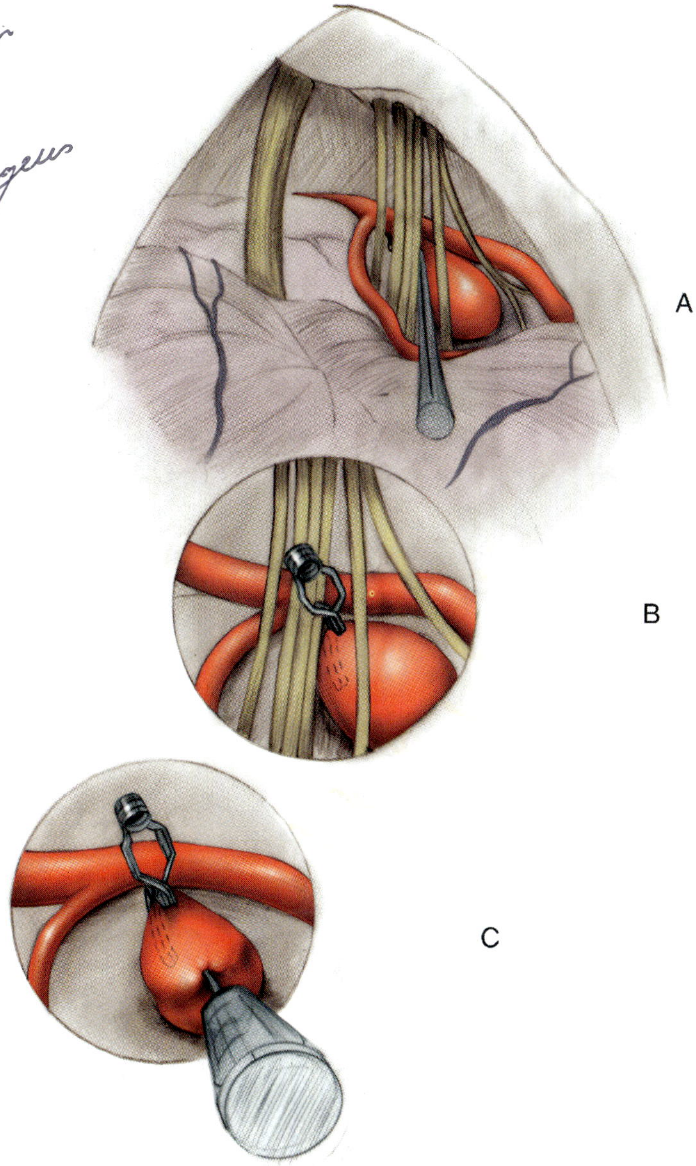

Figure 8–26.

Step 3. *A*, The distal neck of the aneurysm must be identified. Nearly always, it is intimately associated with the origin of the posterior inferior cerebellar artery. As illustrated here, the vagus nerve lies over the neck; therefore, the surgeon must work through the rootlets of the nerve.

Step 4. *B*, After the neck has been identified, the aneurysm is repaired, usually with a small curved or bayonet clip.

Step 5. *C*, The dome of the aneurysm is aspirated and the origin of the posterior inferior cerebellar artery is inspected. A small Doppler probe is valuable in confirming patency and flow through both the posterior inferior cerebellar and vertebral arteries. During the immediate postoperative convalescence, the patient should be observed for potential airway obstruction or aspiration from possible injury to the vagus nerve.

ANEURYSMS OF THE VERTEBROBASILAR JUNCTION

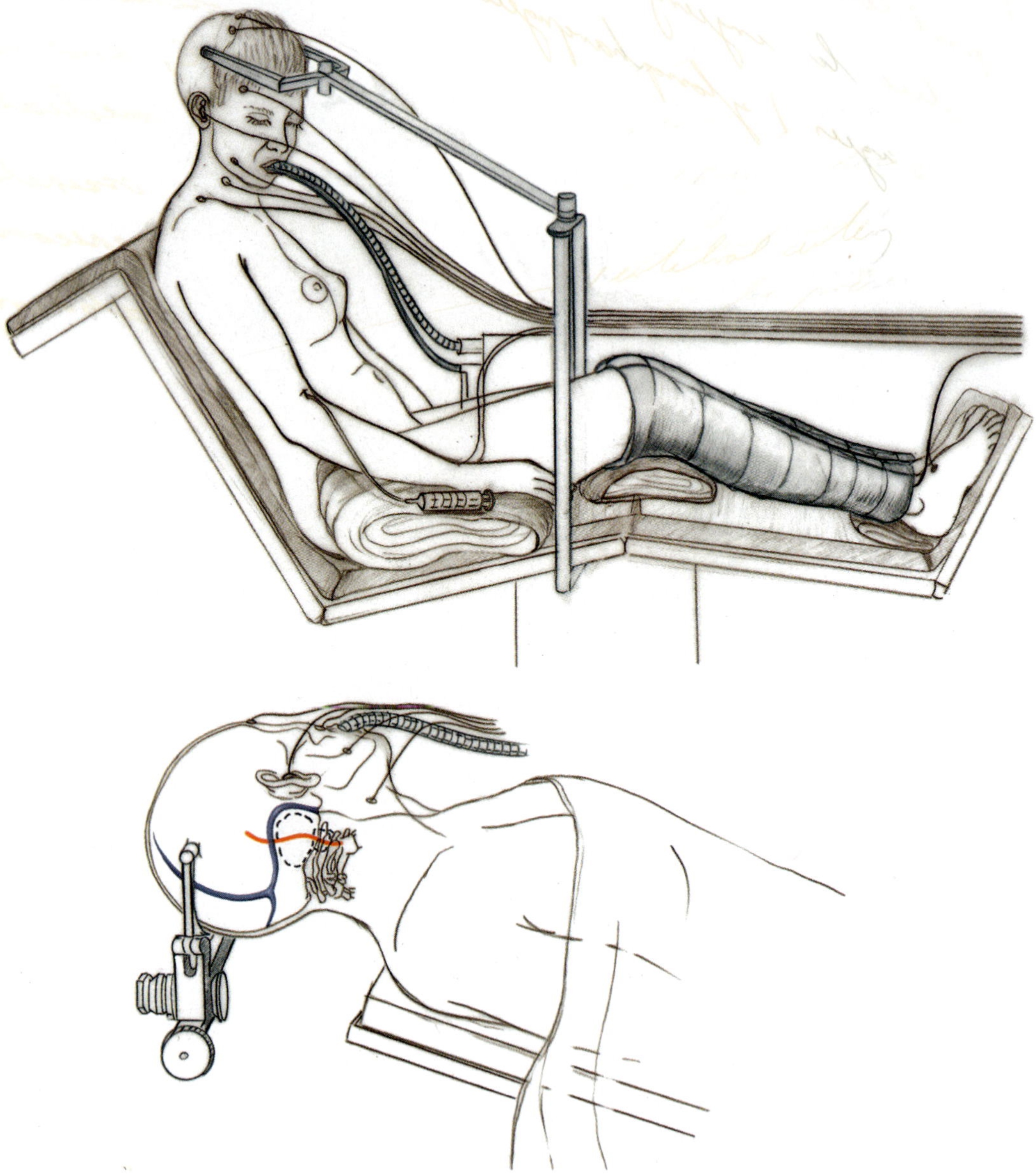

Figure 8–27.

Illustrated are the two patient positions used for exposure of an aneurysm of either the posterior inferior cerebellar artery or the vertebrobasilar trunk.

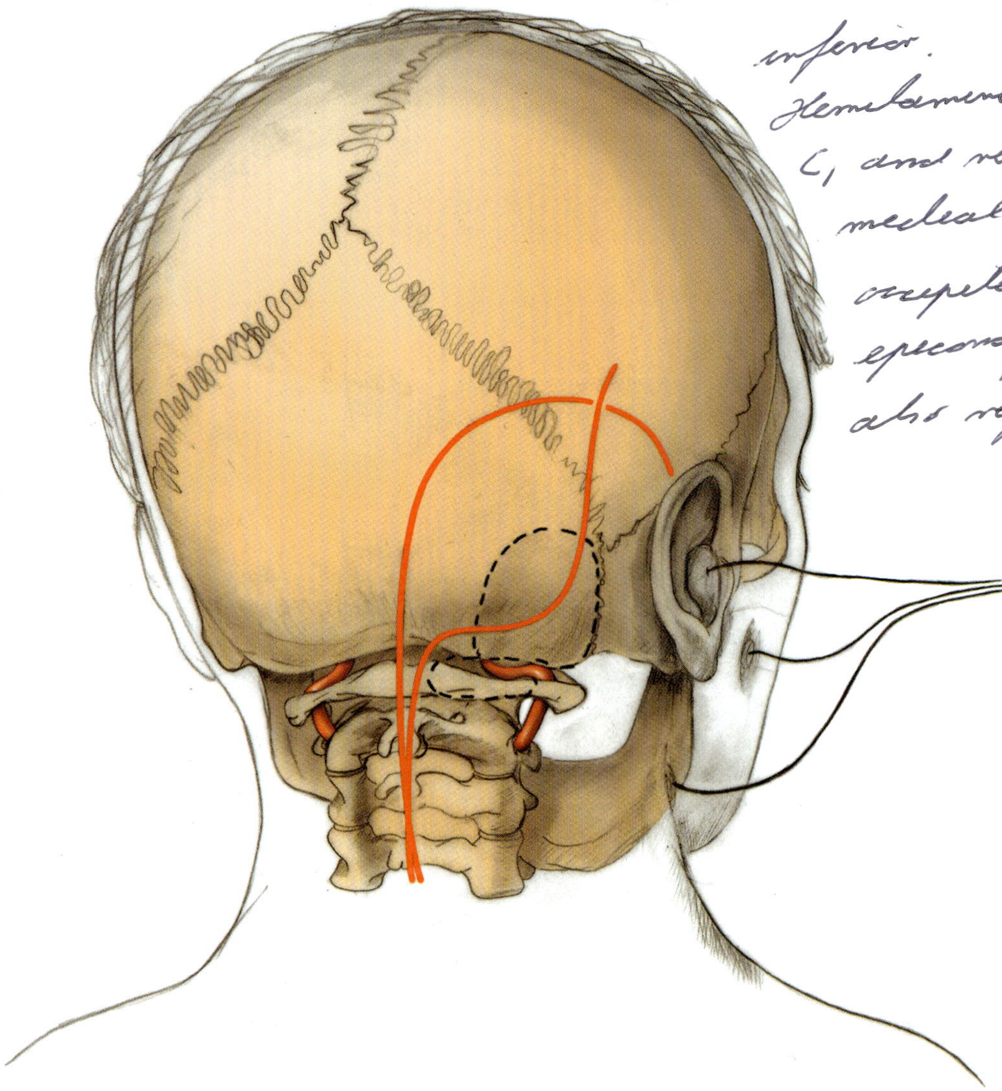

Figure 8–28.

Step 1. Two different incisions can be used for exposure of an aneurysm of the vertebrobasilar junction. Bone removal must extend from the junction of the transverse and sigmoid sinuses down to the foramen magnum. Furthermore, it usually is best to remove the medial third of the occipital condyle. A hemilaminectomy of C-1 must also be performed. It is easier to expose the foramen magnum and the occipital condyle through the inverted S-shaped incision. Note that in the sitting position, the head is rotated approximately 20 to 25 degrees. For a large or giant aneurysm of the vertebrobasilar junction or basilar trunk, deep hypothermic circulatory bypass is usually required to provide the degree of brain relaxation and protection necessary for repair of these difficult aneurysms. If this is the case, the supine or park bench position is required.

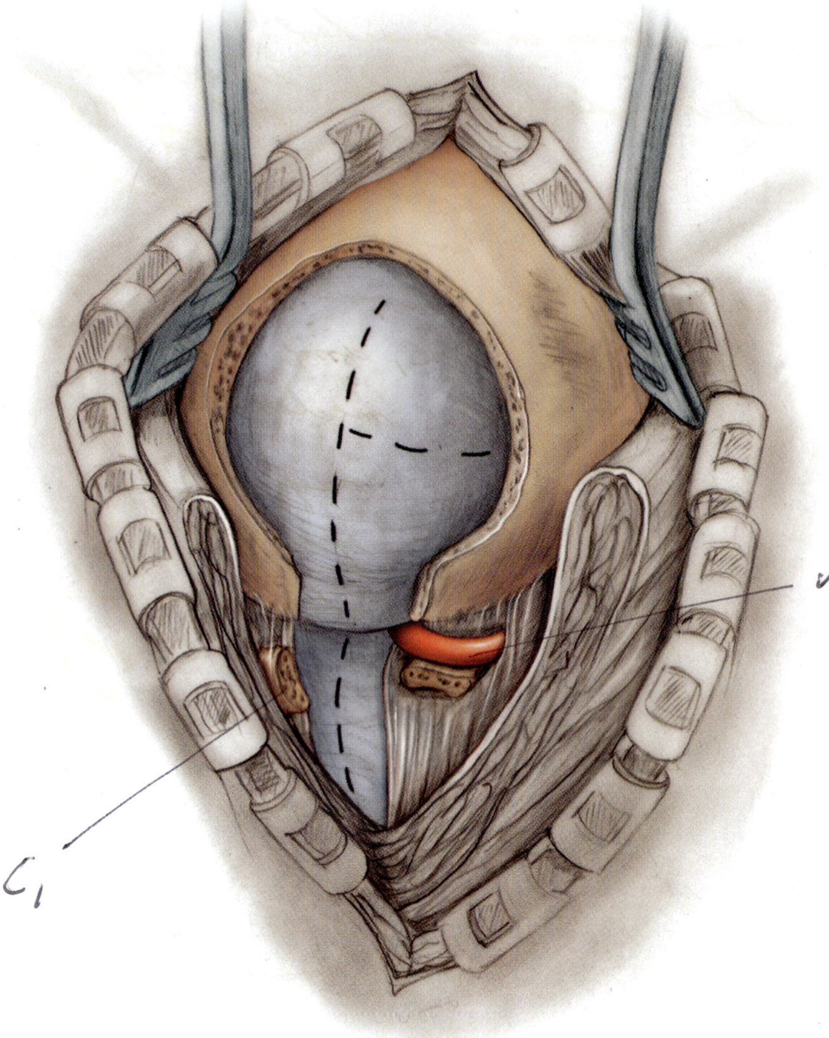

Figure 8–29.

Step 2. Following the hemilaminectomy of the arch of C-1, the vertebral artery is identified, and the medial one-third of the occipital condyle is removed with a high-speed air drill and diamond bur. Next, the dura mater is opened, as shown here.

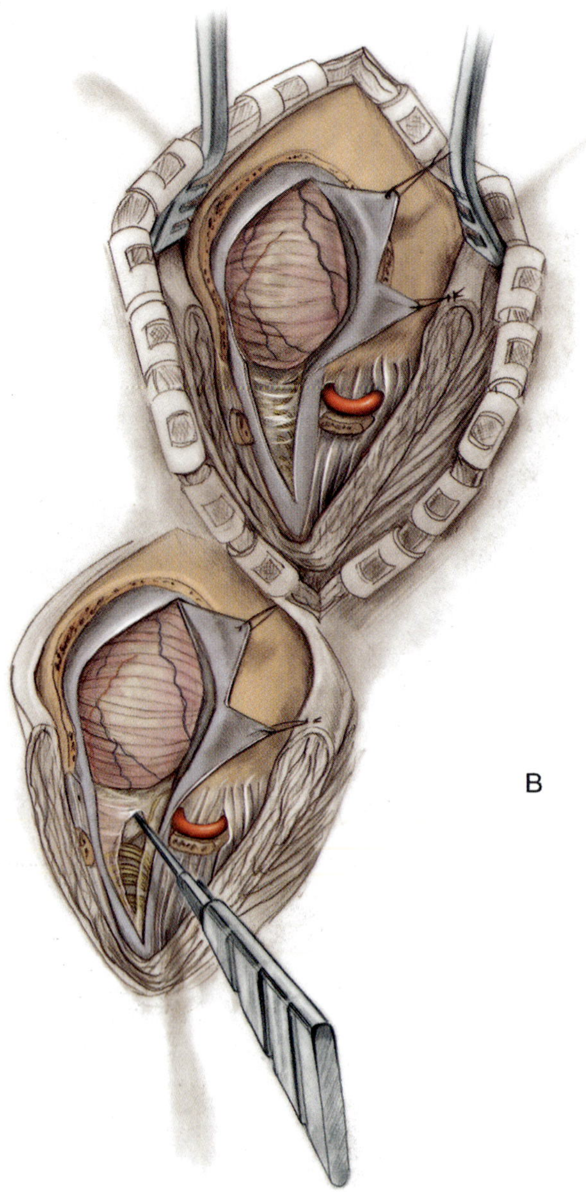

Figure 8–30.

Step 3. *A*, Note that lateral bone removal allows direct access to the cerebellopontine angle. If the lateral exposure is not sufficient to identify the vertebrobasilar junction after the cerebellum has been retracted, the surgeon must consider a presigmoid sinus approach. This requires additional removal of bone over the sigmoid sinus, with a partial mastoidectomy.

Step 4. *B*, The arachnoid is incised over the cisterna magna to drain cerebrospinal fluid to aid cerebellar relaxation.

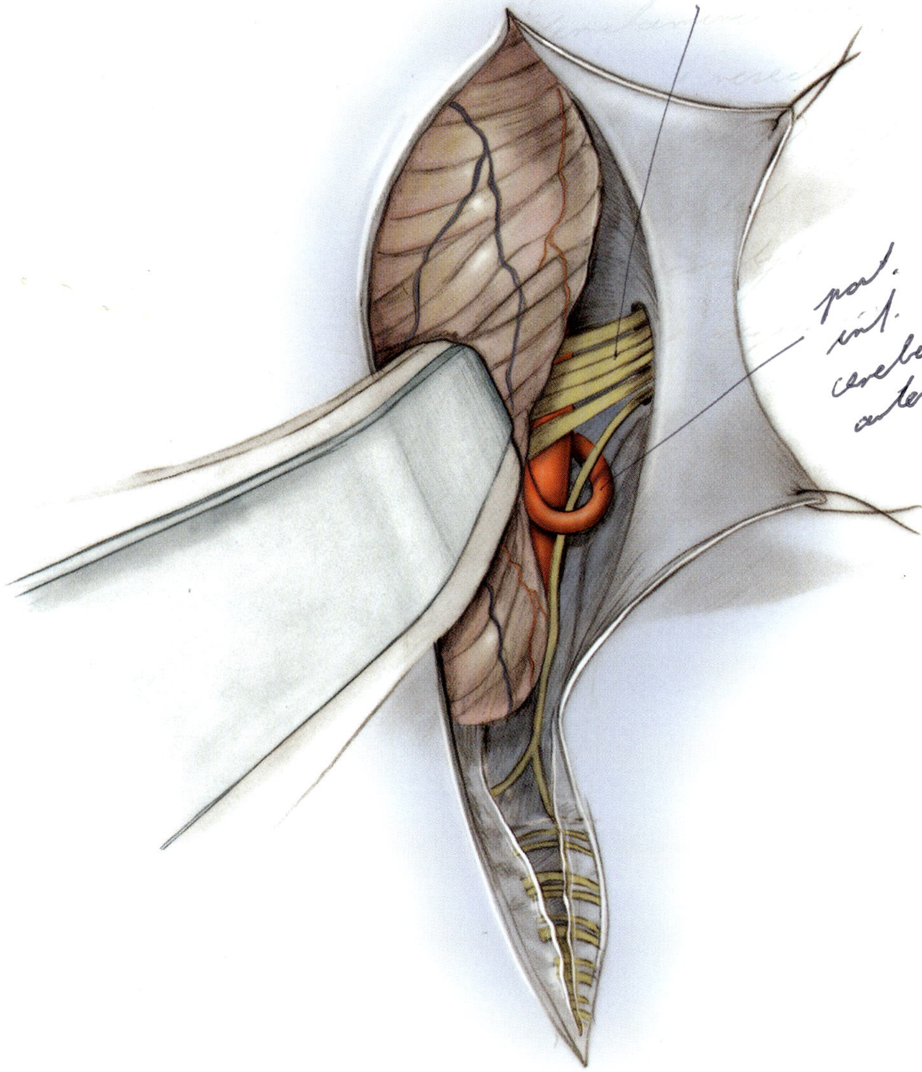

Figure 8–31.

Step 5. The cerebellum is retracted medially and upward. The lower cranial nerves are identified. The posterior inferior cerebellar artery is followed proximally to the vertebral artery.

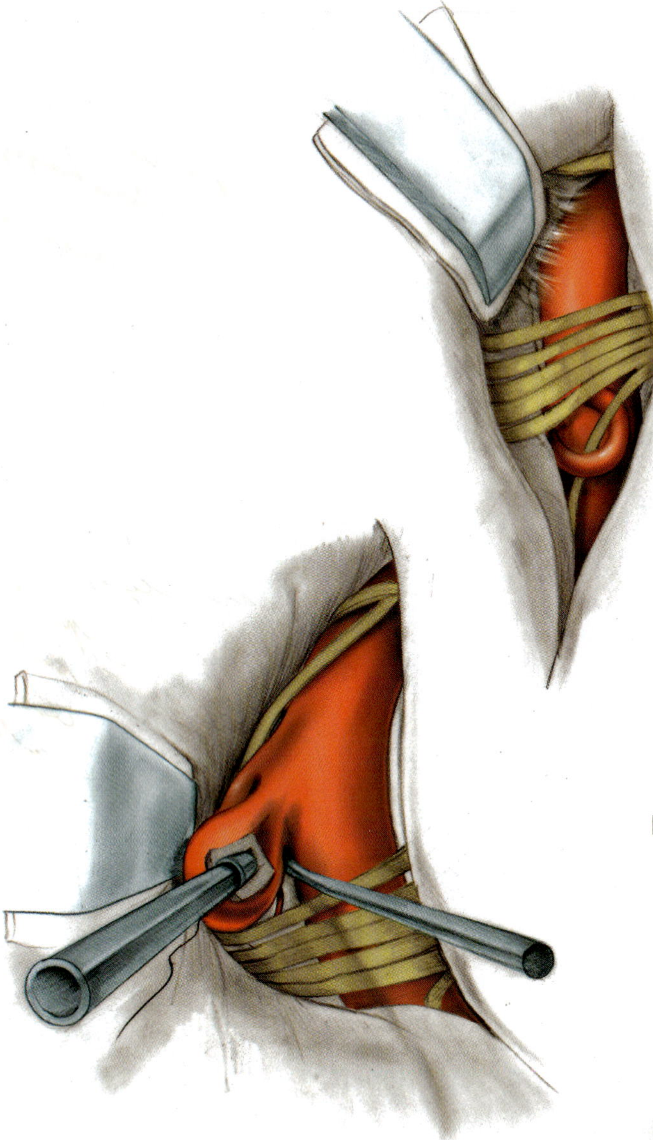

Figure 8–32.

Step 6. *A*, The cerebellum is retracted more aggressively. The vertebral artery is followed distally to identify the vertebrobasilar junction.

Step 7. *B*, The cerebellum is further retracted. It is usually necessary to gently retract the lower pons to better identify the vertebrobasilar junction. Aneurysms in this location generally point caudally. The aneurysm is manipulated gently with a #5 or #7 suction tip and cottonoid. A small spatula is used to dissect the neck of the aneurysm and to identify the anterior spinal artery, which likely is present.

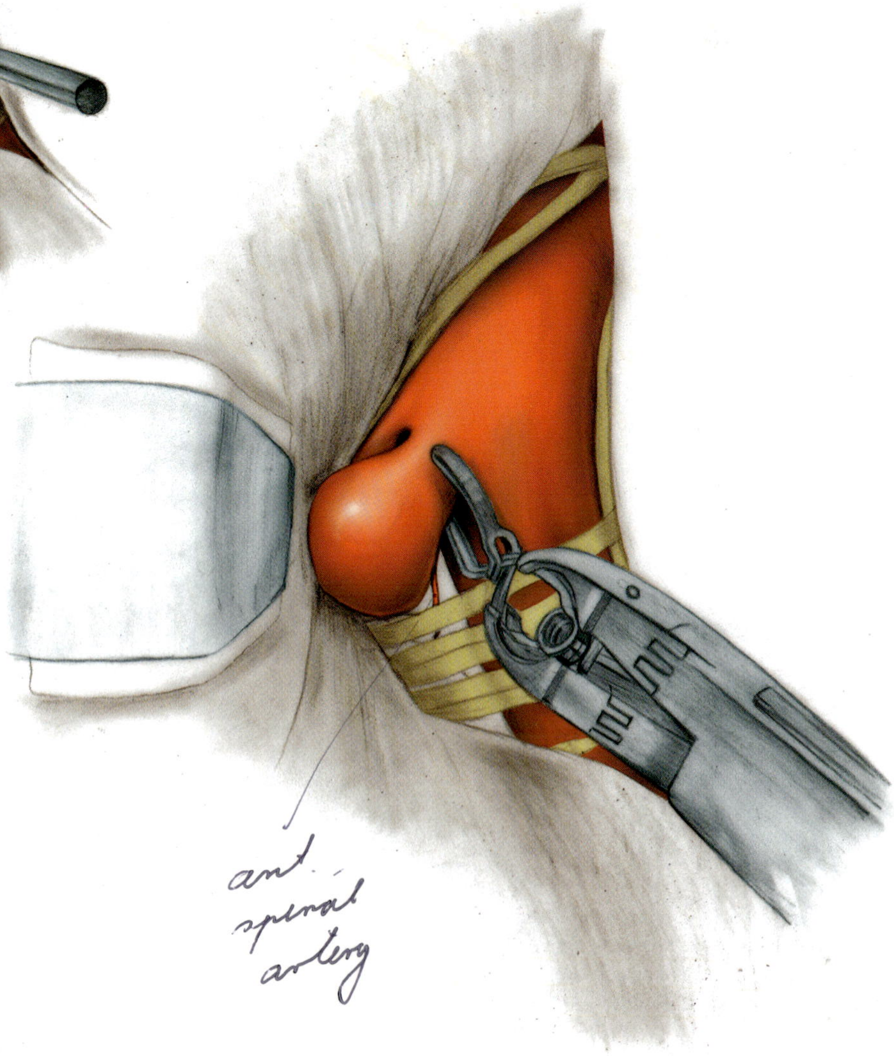

Figure 8–33.

Step 8. After the aneurysm has been dissected, a small straight or slightly curved aneurysm clip is used to obliterate the neck, and the dome of the aneurysm is aspirated to ensure that successful clipping has been achieved. The anterior spinal artery is inspected to make sure that its origin has not been compromised.

JUVENILE CEREBELLAR ASTROCYTOMA

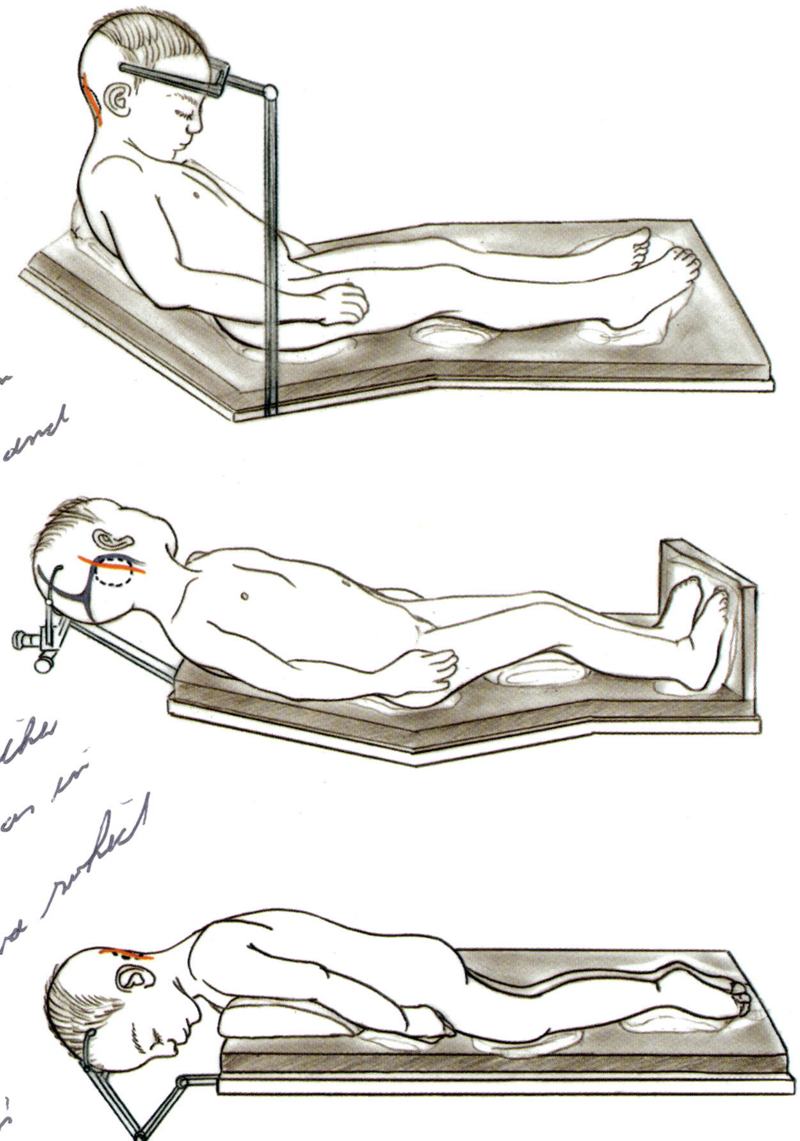

Figure 8–34.

Step 1. Juvenile cerebellar astrocytomas can be approached through several positions, such as those illustrated here. Bony removal should expose most of the involved cerebellar hemisphere and, thus, extend from the sigmoid sinus to the midline and down to the foramen magnum.

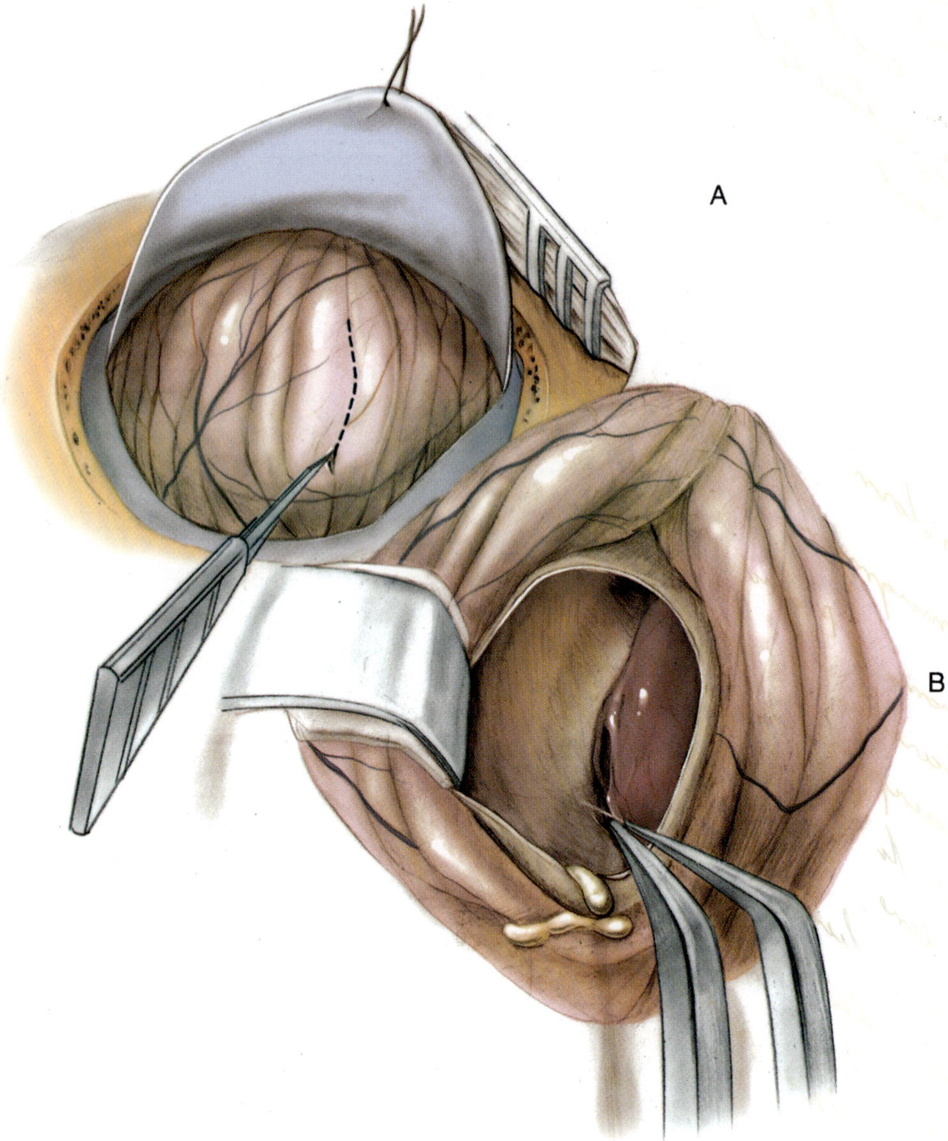

Figure 8–35.

Step 2. *A*, After the dura mater has been opened, the folia of the cerebellum are inspected. With cystic cerebellar astrocytomas, the folia overlying the cyst cavity are usually expanded and enlarged. An incision is made parallel to the folia.

Step 3. *B*, The cyst wall is identified and entered. Drainage of the xanthochromic fluid leads to immediate relaxation of the cerebellum. A small retractor can be used to keep the cyst cavity open for inspection.

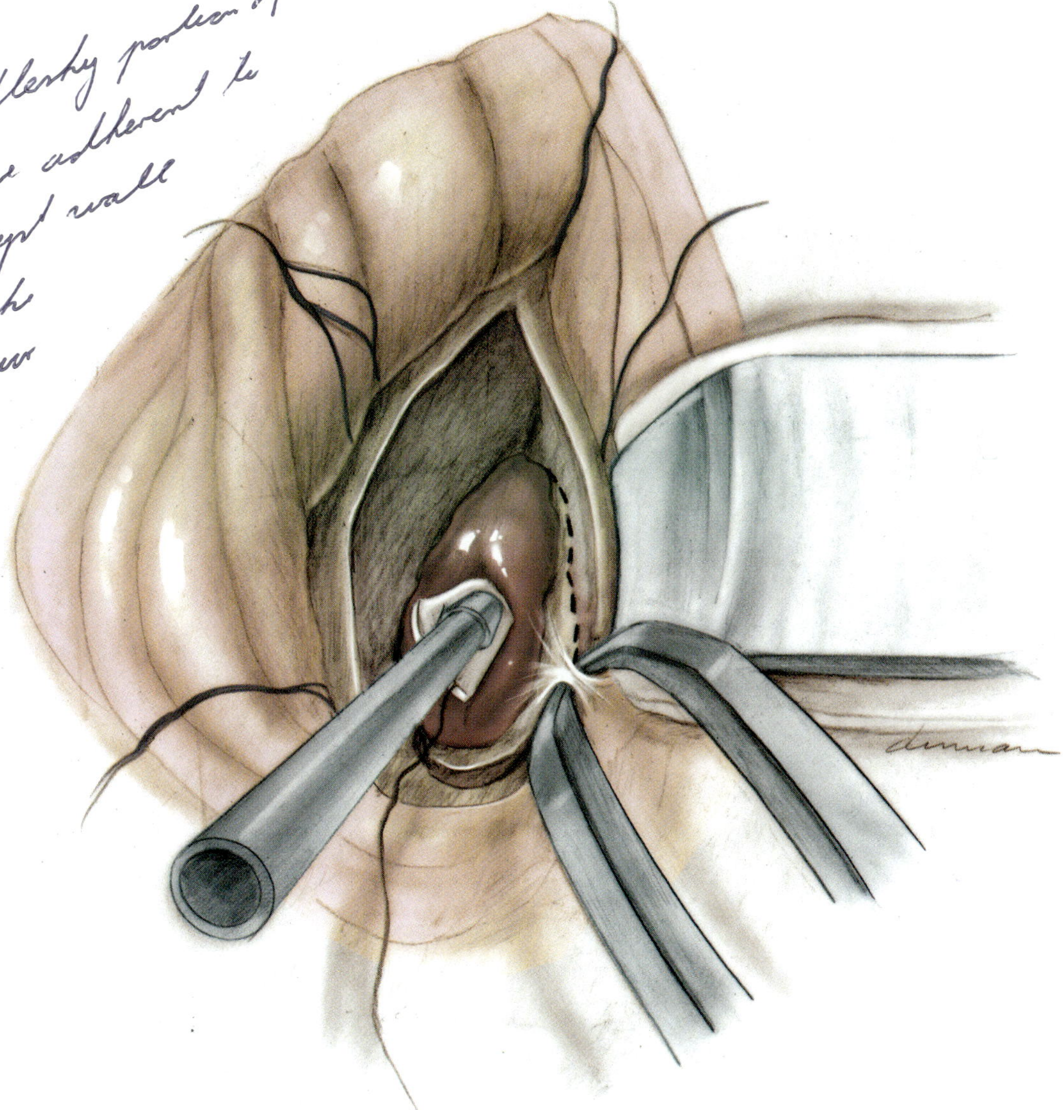

Figure 8–36.

Step 4. With juvenile astrocytomas, the neoplastic portion is a fleshy nodular-appearing mass along one wall of the cyst. It is distinct from the compressed gliotic cerebellar tissue. Surgical cure is achieved by resecting the neoplastic mass. It is not necessary to resect the entire cyst wall. However, a healthy margin of approximately 0.5 cm from the edge of the fleshy neoplastic mass should be used during resection to ensure complete removal of the tumor.

CEREBELLAR HEMANGIOBLASTOMA

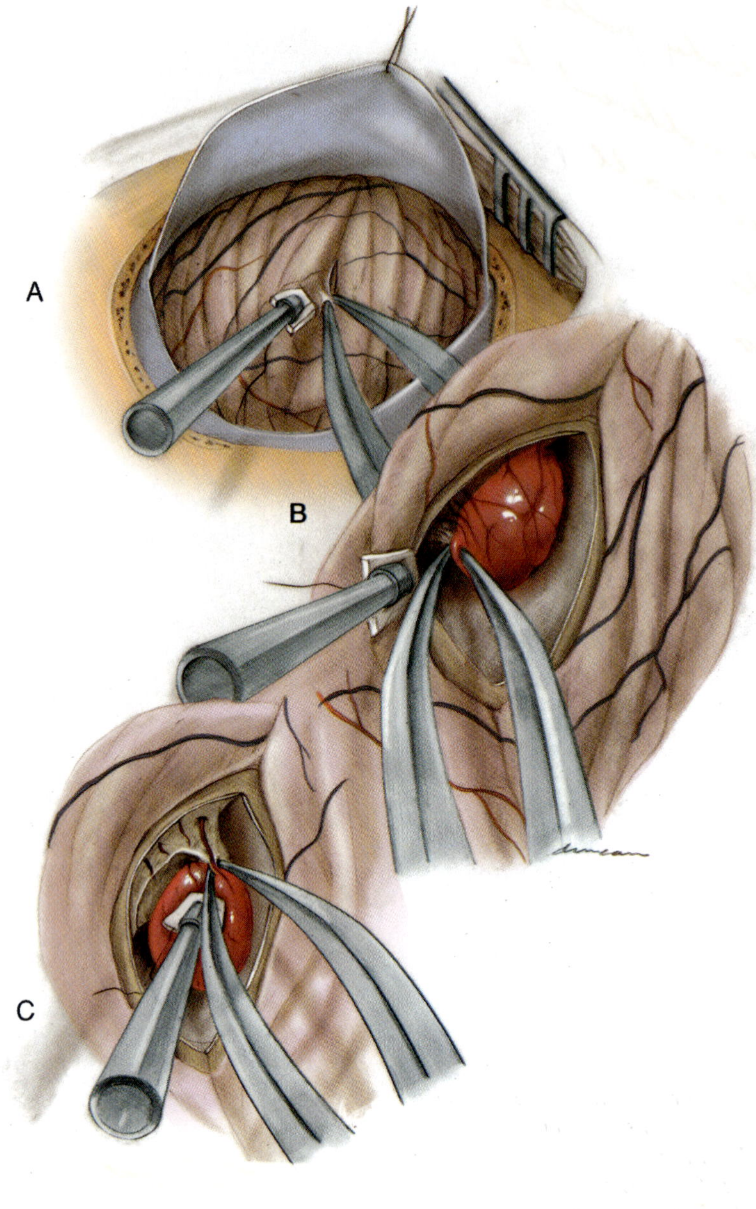

Figure 8–37.

Step 1. The extent of bony removal for a cerebellar hemangioblastoma is similar to that for resection of other hemispheric lesions, such as juvenile astrocytoma and metastatic tumor. Specifically, much of the bone over the involved cerebellar hemisphere should be removed, extending laterally from near the midline to the sigmoid sinus.

Step 2. *A*, After the dura mater has been opened, the cerebellum is inspected. Most hemangioblastomas are associated with a large cyst. Therefore, the folia are often enlarged and expanded over the epicenter of the cyst. An incision is made in an expanded folium and in parallel with the folium.

Step 3. *B*, The cyst is encountered and entered. Drainage of the xanthochromic fluid provides immediate relaxation of the cerebellum. Occasionally, it is necessary to use a small brain spatula to keep the incision open within the cyst after the cerebellum collapses. The interior of the cyst is inspected until the reddish mulberry hemangioblastoma is identified.

Step 4. *C*, After the hemangioblastoma has been identified, the small feeding arteries are cauterized and divided. The hemangioblastoma is gently retracted with a #7 suction tip and cottonoid, and the bipolar cautery is used to separate the tumor from the surrounding cerebellar cyst cavity.

CEREBELLAR METASTASIS

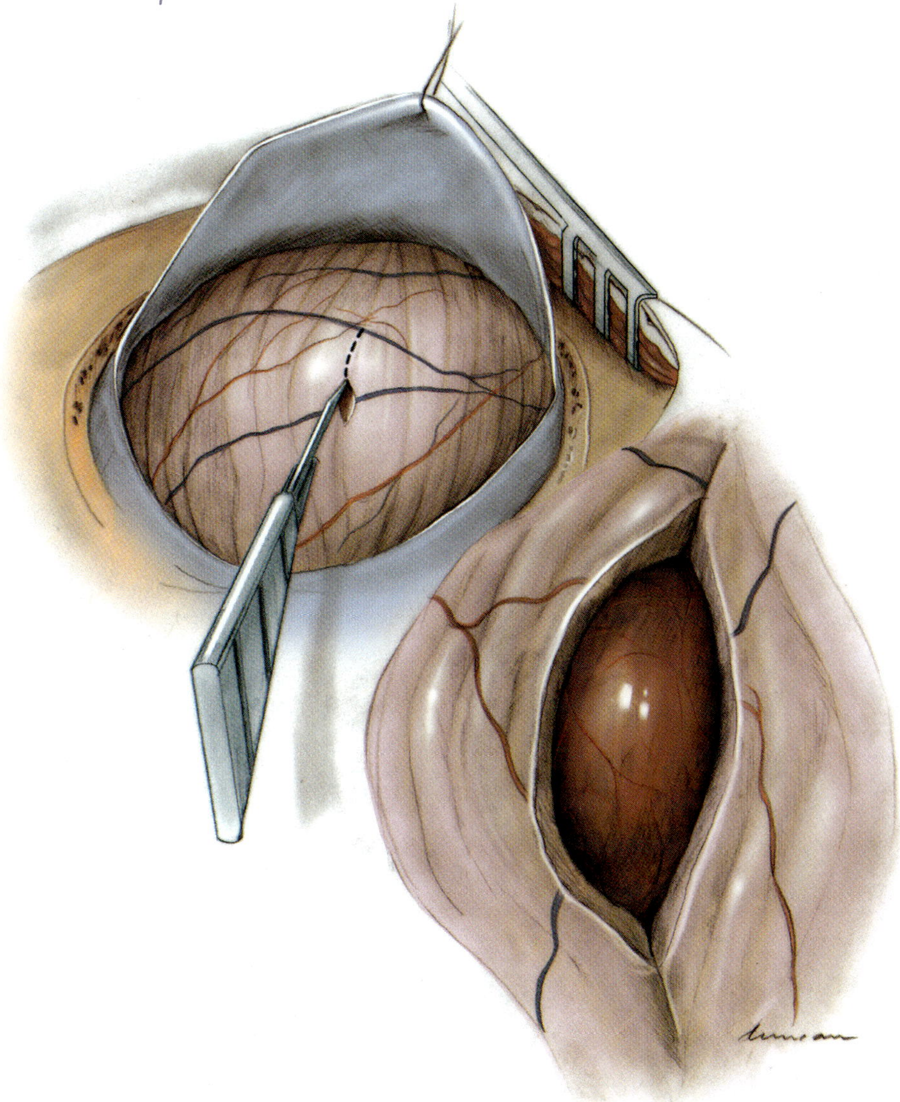

Figure 8–38.

Step 1. A metastasis to the cerebellar hemisphere can be approached with the patient in either a sitting or a supine position. Either a midline or lateral incision over the involved hemisphere can be used. Bone removal should be generous, extending laterally from close to the midline to almost the transverse and sigmoid sinuses. It also should extend down close to the foramen magnum. This large bony removal will afford some decompression of the edematous cerebellum. For a metastasis in the vermis, a midline incision with a bilateral suboccipital craniectomy should be performed. **Step 2**. The dura mater is opened in a curved fashion and tacked to the margins of the muscle. Often, inspection of the cerebellar surface is not revealing about the location of the metastatic tumor. If available, ultrasonography or stereotaxis can be useful in pinpointing the location of the tumor and minimizing the incision in the cerebellum. The incision in the cerebellum should be parallel with the folia and approximately 1 to 1.5 cm long. Most metastatic lesions are encountered within 1.0 cm of the pial surface.

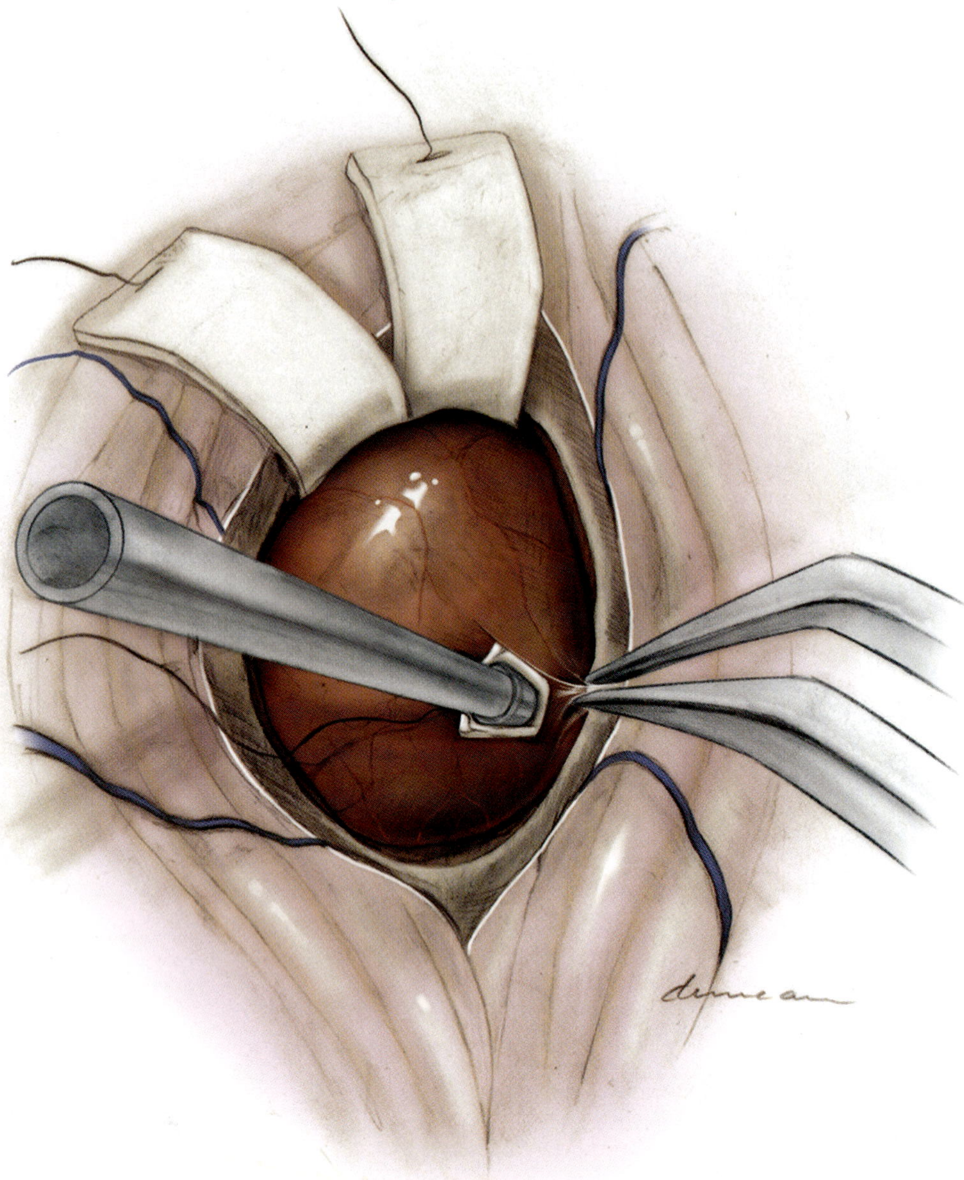

Figure 8–39.

Step 3. After the tumor has been located, a bipolar cautery and #5 or #7 suction tip are used to separate the tumor from the surrounding cerebellar tissue. If necessary, small brain spatulas can be used to gently retract the cerebellum. Some metastatic tumors, such as renal cell carcinoma, can be extremely vascular. The best way to control bleeding is to not enter the tumor but to stay on its periphery, quickly separating it from the surrounding cerebellum.

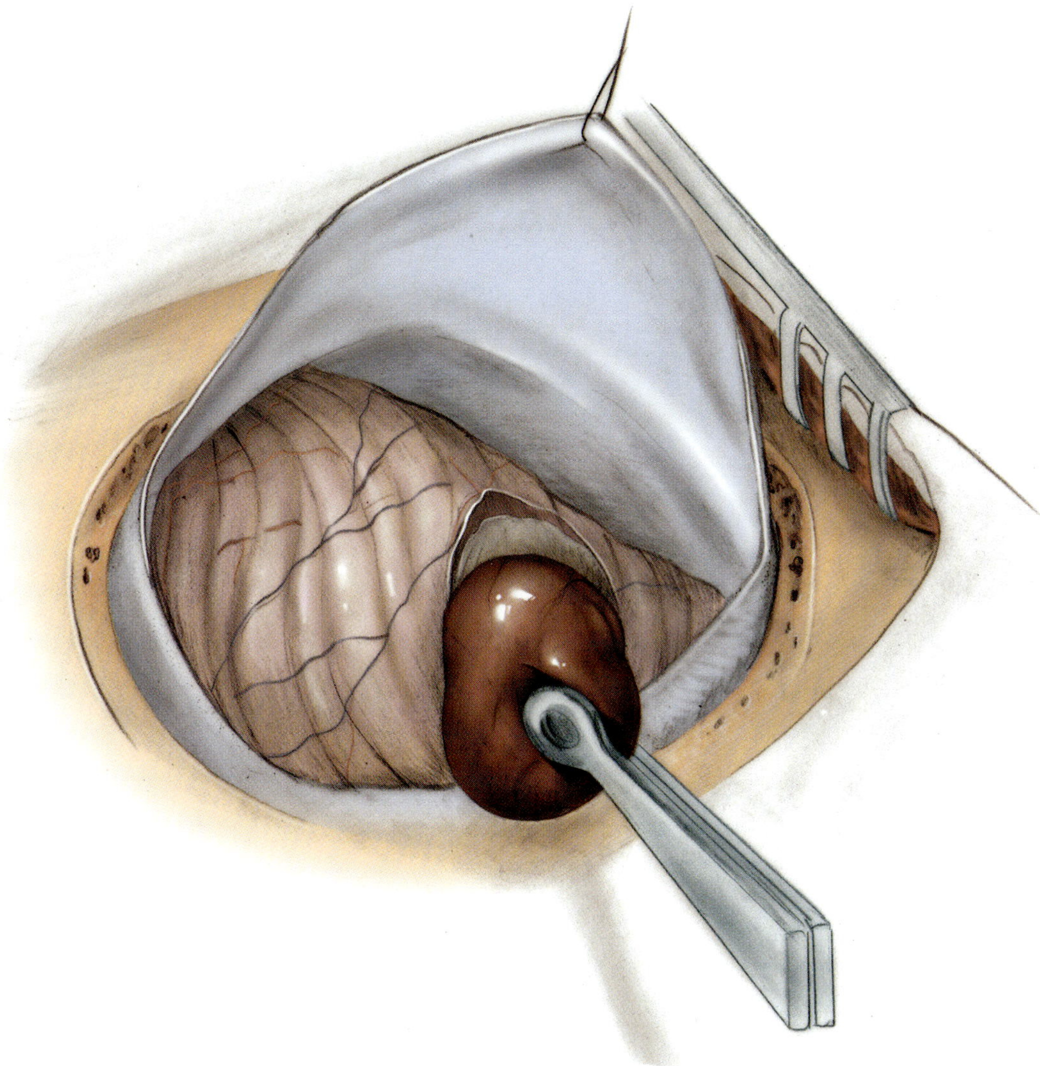

Figure 8–40.

Step 4. After the tumor has been extracted, the resection bed is examined for hemostasis. Secondary closure of the dura mater with pericranium, muscle, or graft is effective treatment if the cerebellum looks edematous.

9

Midline Suboccipital Approach

Copyright © 1999 Mayo Foundation.

ANATOMY

The pertinent neurosurgical anatomy for midline suboccipital approaches is illustrated in Figures 9–1 to 9–3.

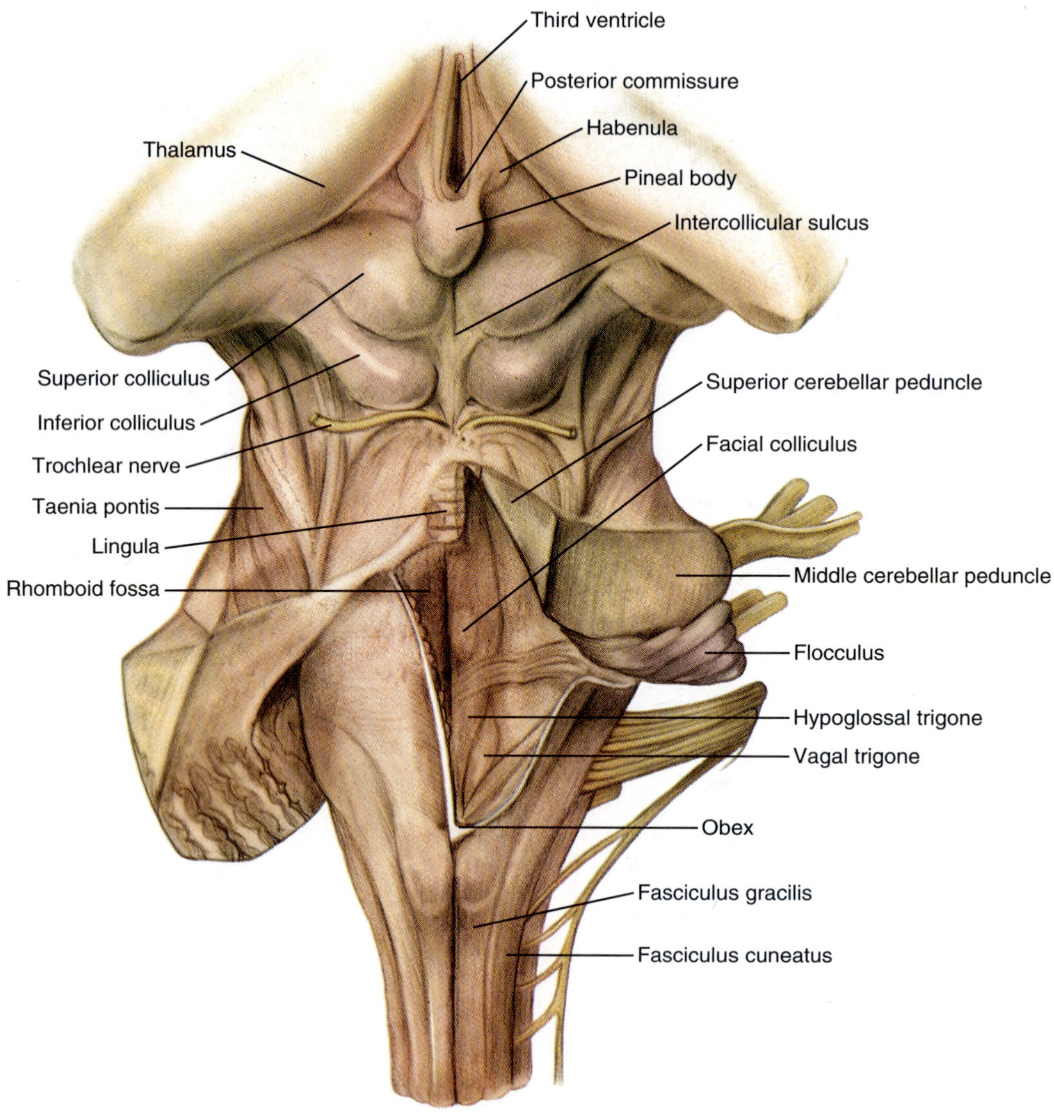

Figure 9–1.

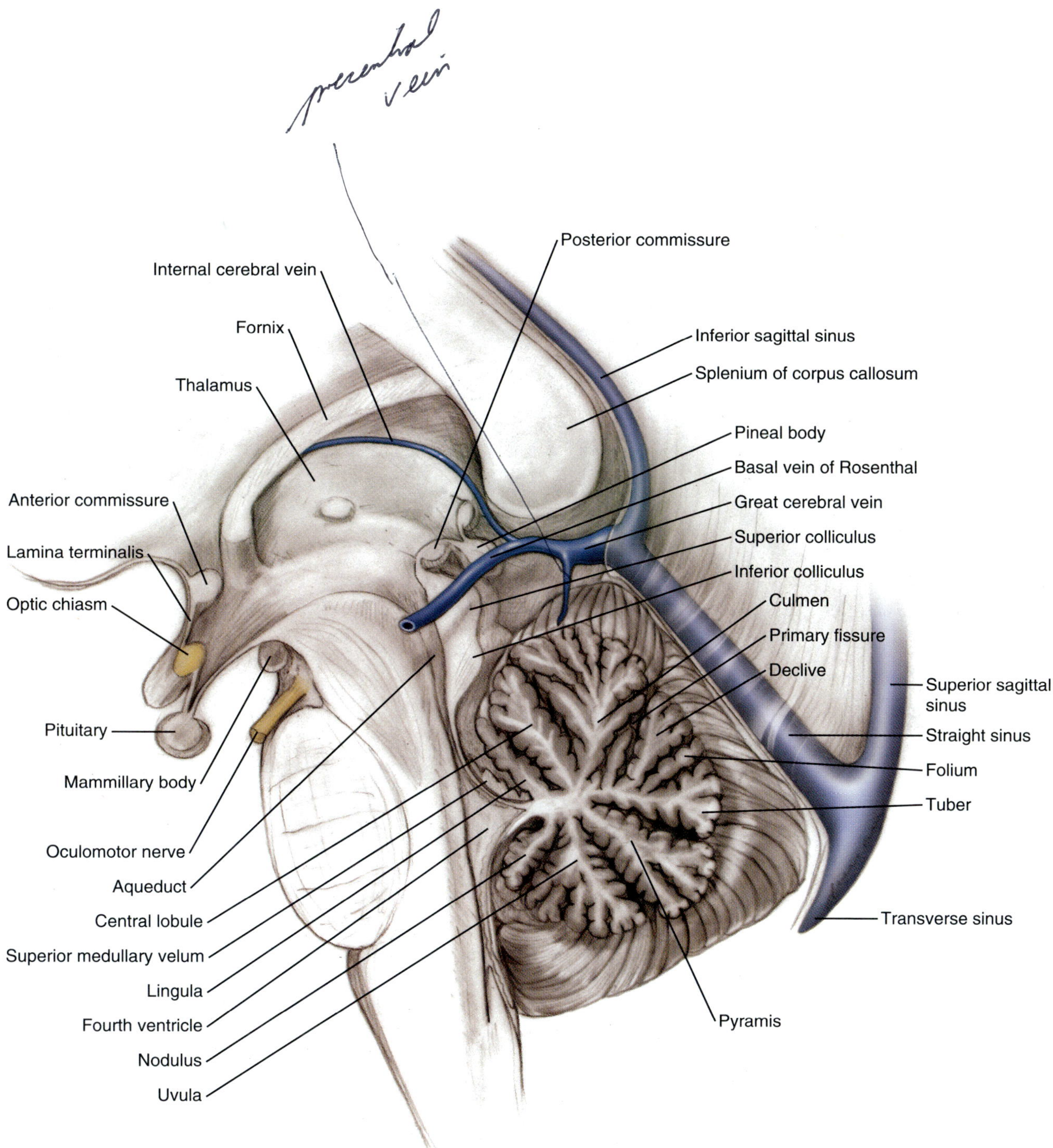
precentral vein
Posterior commissure
Internal cerebral vein
Fornix
Thalamus
Inferior sagittal sinus
Splenium of corpus callosum
Pineal body
Basal vein of Rosenthal
Anterior commissure
Great cerebral vein
Superior colliculus
Lamina terminalis
Inferior colliculus
Optic chiasm
Culmen
Primary fissure
Declive
Superior sagittal sinus
Pituitary
Straight sinus
Folium
Mammillary body
Tuber
Oculomotor nerve
Aqueduct
Transverse sinus
Central lobule
Superior medullary velum
Lingula
Fourth ventricle
Pyramis
Nodulus
Uvula

Figure 9–2.

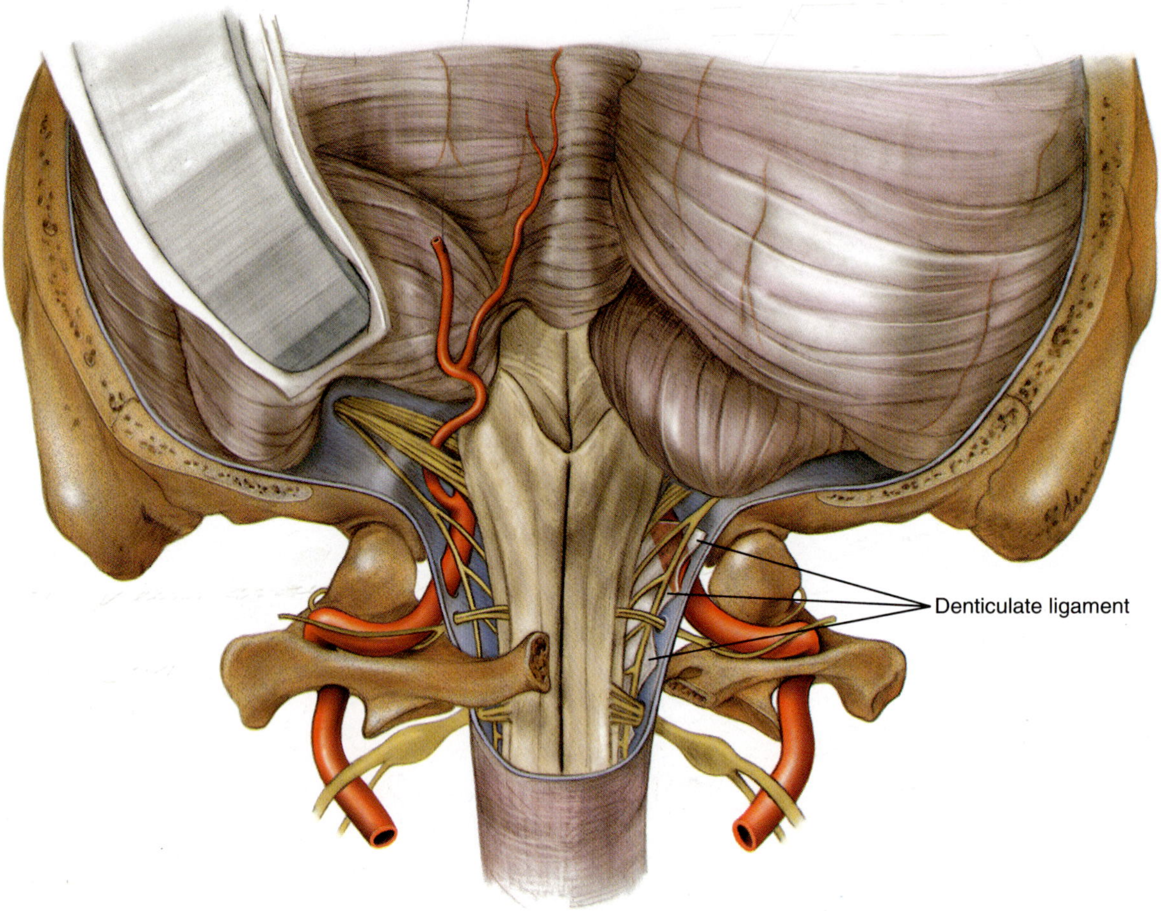

Figure 9–3.

CHIARI MALFORMATION

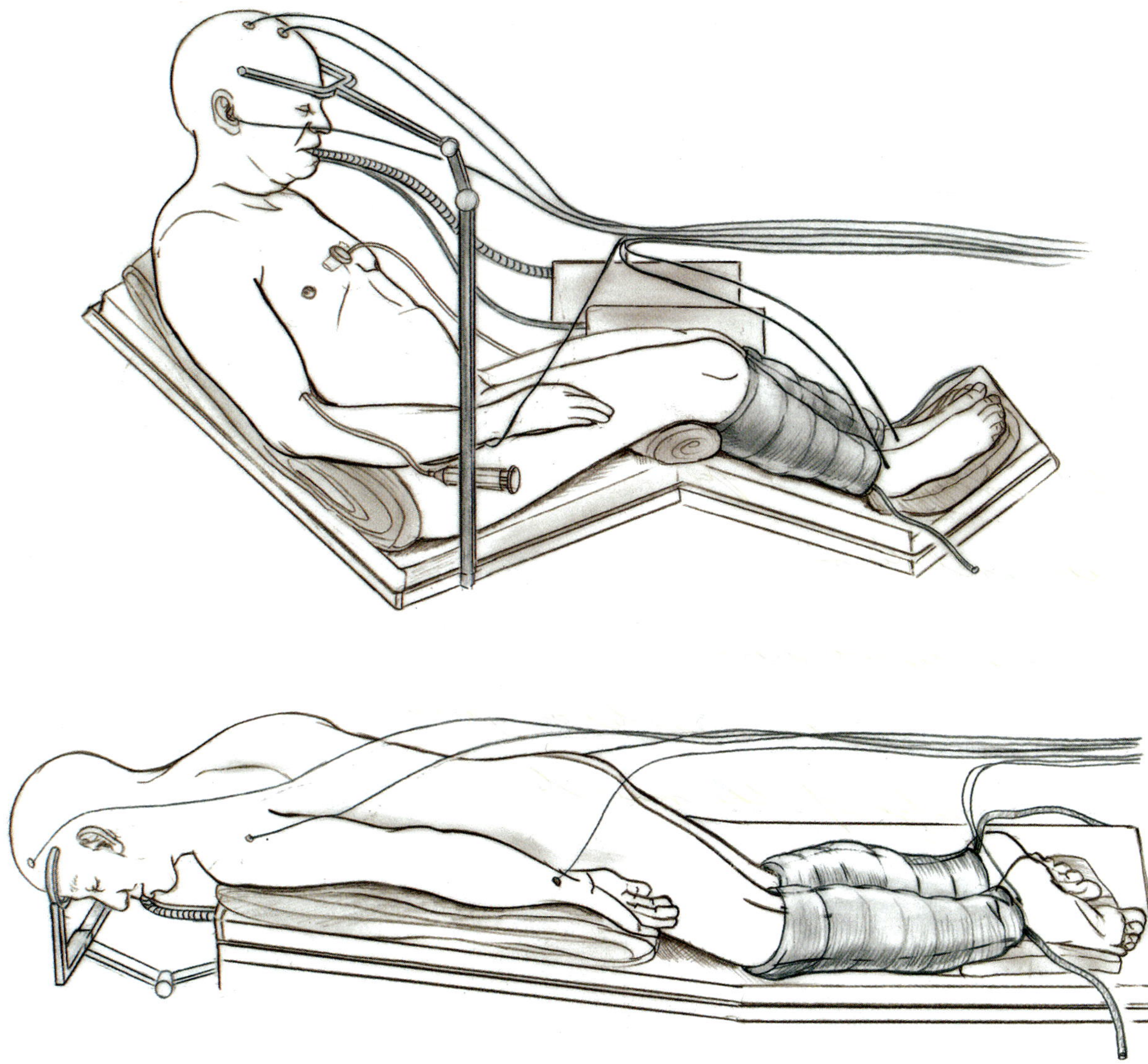

Figure 9–4.

Illustrated are two of the most common patient positions used for midline suboccipital approaches. *A*, The sitting position works well for several reasons. First, compared with the prone position, there is less intrathoracic pressure and, thus, better venous return. Accordingly, brain relaxation is excellent. Second, for less experienced surgeons, the sitting position facilitates surgeon orientation. Third, in the sitting position, blood drains out from the lower end of the incision, but in the prone position blood coming from the cut edge of muscle tends to run into the operative field. Disadvantages of the sitting position include the increased risk of air embolus, pneumocephalus, and brain collapse, resulting in subdural hygroma or hematoma.

B, If the prone position is used, it is important to make sure that the chest rolls are optimally placed to prevent an increase in intrathoracic pressure. Before the patient's head is flexed, it is necessary to confirm that the endotracheal tube is adequately secured. An advantage of the prone position is that the surgeon's assistant can be involved more actively in the operation instead of standing to the side, which occurs if the patient is in the sitting position.

With the sitting position, a central venous catheter, transthoracic Doppler, and transesophageal echocardiography (TEE) are used. If there is Doppler or TEE evidence of a venous air embolus, the anesthesiologist should attempt to

Legend continued on following page

Figure 9–4 *Continued*

aspirate the air through the central venous catheter. At the same time, the surgeon should immediately inspect the operative field to determine the source of the air embolus. The most common sites for air absorption into the venous circulation are through bone diploë, veins located laterally along the craniovertebral junction and between vertebrae C-1 and C-2, and the cut edge of muscle. Accordingly, the surgeon should rewax the bone edges, place absorbable gelatin sponge (Gelfoam) in the epidural space between vertebrae C-1 and C-2 laterally and at the craniovertebral junction, and press wet gauze against the edge of the muscle. If nitrous oxide is used as an anesthetic, it is discontinued. If the above surgical maneuvers do not stop the source of air absorption, jugular vein compression should be performed to facilitate identification of the air leak by causing bleeding from the site that is the source of entry of air into the systemic circulation. Simultaneously, the surgical bed is rotated into a more Trendelenburg position, which lowers the head in relationship to the heart but still allows the surgeon to visualize the wound. If TEE continues to show air absorption, if end-expired carbon dioxide decreases, if end-expired nitrogen increases, if arterial blood pressure begins to decrease, or if TEE shows paradoxical air embolus in the left ventricle, the surgeon must consider rapid closure of the surgical wound. In practice, the need to close a wound because of air embolus with the patient in the sitting position is rare.

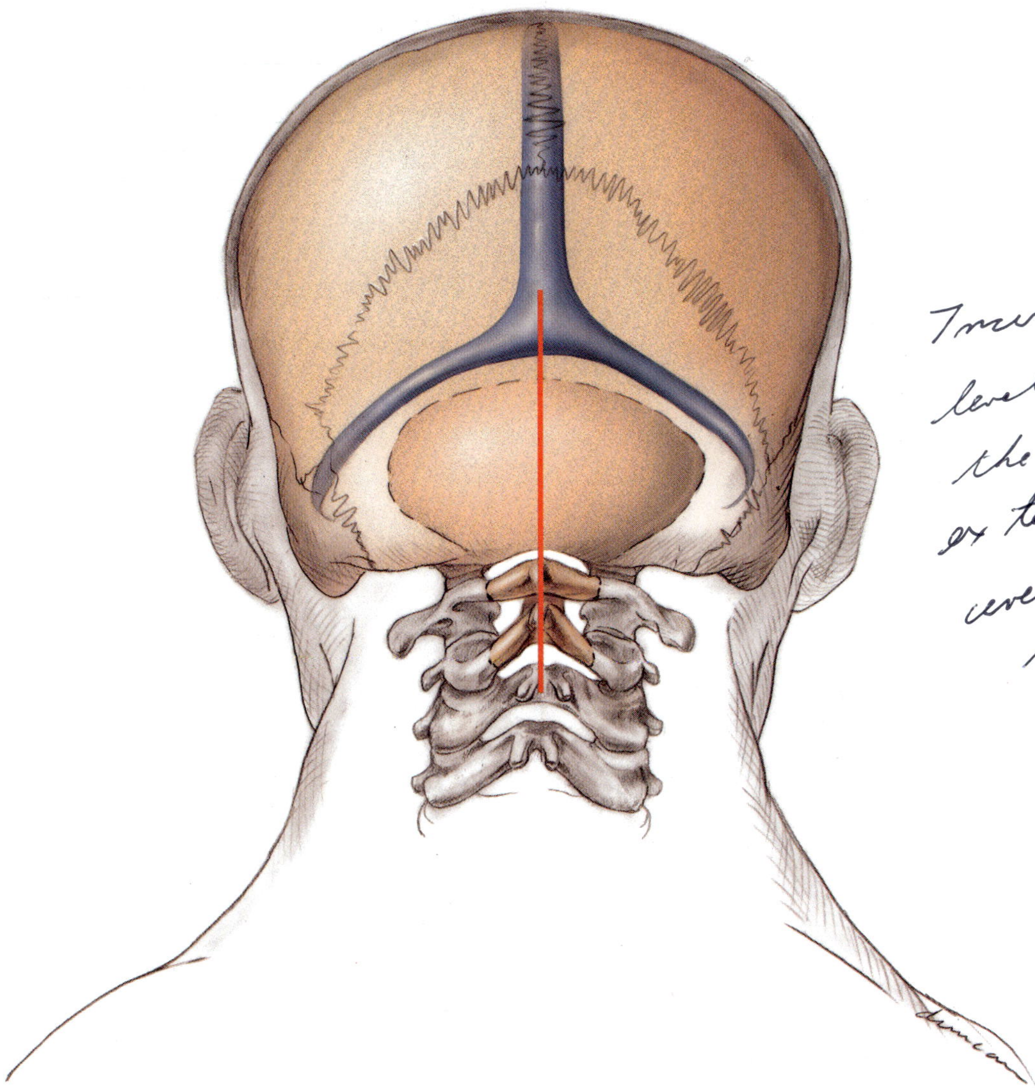

Figure 9–5.

Step 1. In the case of a Chiari malformation, the main goal of the operation is decompression of the posterior fossa. A midline incision is made from the inion down to the cervical lamina one level below the lowest extent of the cerebellar tonsils, as identified on preoperative imaging. It is uncommon for the incision to extend below the level of vertebra C-3. The craniectomy should extend rostrally approximately 1 to 2 cm below the torcular and transverse sinus and laterally approximately 1.0 to 1.5 cm from the sigmoid sinus. At the foramen magnum, bone removal should be carried lateral to the occipital condyles. A laminectomy of C-1 is also performed. Depending on the extent of the tonsillar herniation, it may be necessary to perform additional cervical laminectomies.

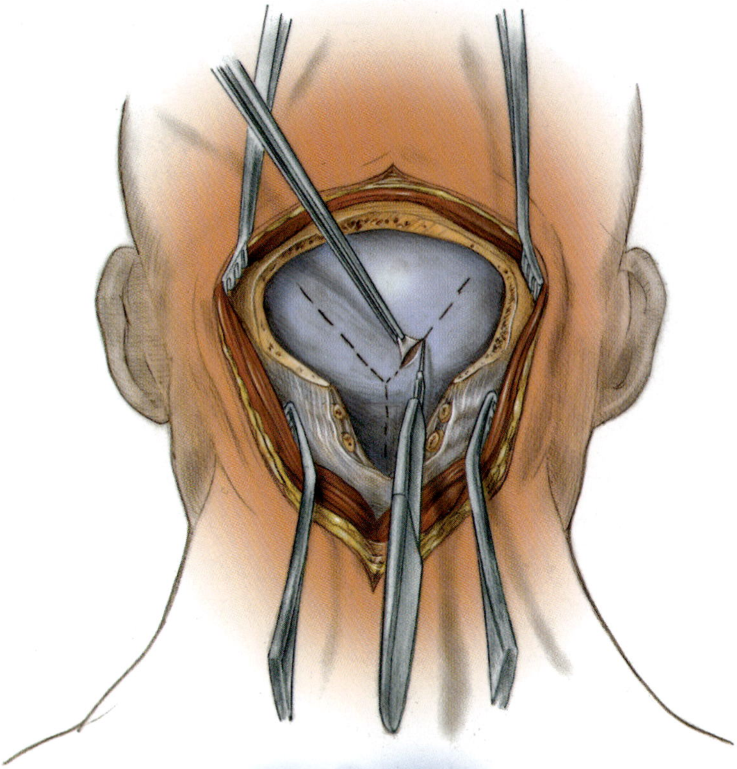

Figure 9–6.

Step 2. Note that in the process of exposing the calvarium, a triangular pedicle of muscle and fascia is left attached to the external occipital protuberance. This will facilitate muscle closure at the end of the operation. In the example shown here, a laminectomy of both C-1 and C-2 has been performed. The dura mater is opened in the standard Y-shaped fashion, which is used in almost all midline approaches to the posterior fossa. Some patients have a midline occipital sinus that can be the source of bleeding when the dura mater is opened. In this case, it is best to open the dura mater over each cerebellar hemisphere first before crossing the midline. After the dura mater has been opened, the dural leaves are tacked to the margins of the muscle. If there is oozing from the torcular, a piece of absorbable gelatin sponge or muscle can be packed against it before the upper dural fold is tacked.

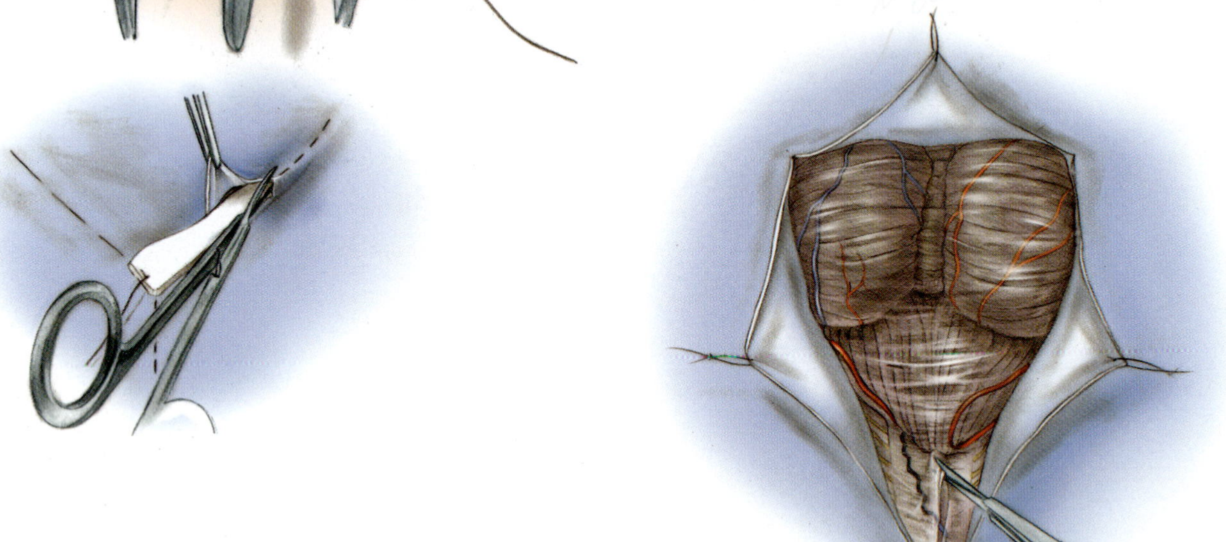

A

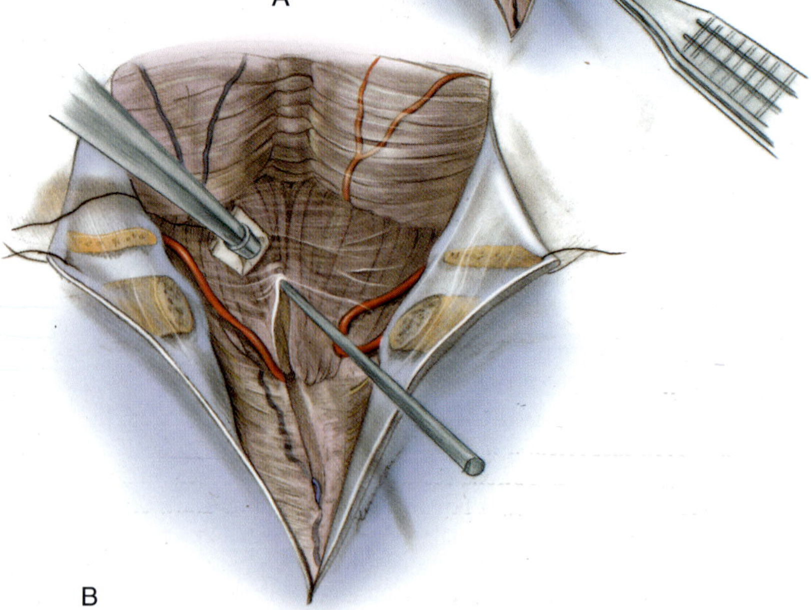

B

Figure 9–7.

Step 3. *A*, In Chiari malformations, the arachnoid is often thickened, and it acts like tethering bands against the cerebellar tonsils at the foramen magnum. Therefore, it is necessary to incise the arachnoid. A small jeweler's forceps can be used to hold the arachnoid while a sharp #11-blade knife or microscissors is used to cut the arachnoid. After a hole has been made in the arachnoid, cerebrospinal fluid immediately drains through it.

B, The rest of the arachnoid can easily be opened with a small ball-tip dissector or knife. Sometimes, arachnoid adhesions tether the posterior inferior cerebellar artery to the dura mater, requiring sharp dissection.

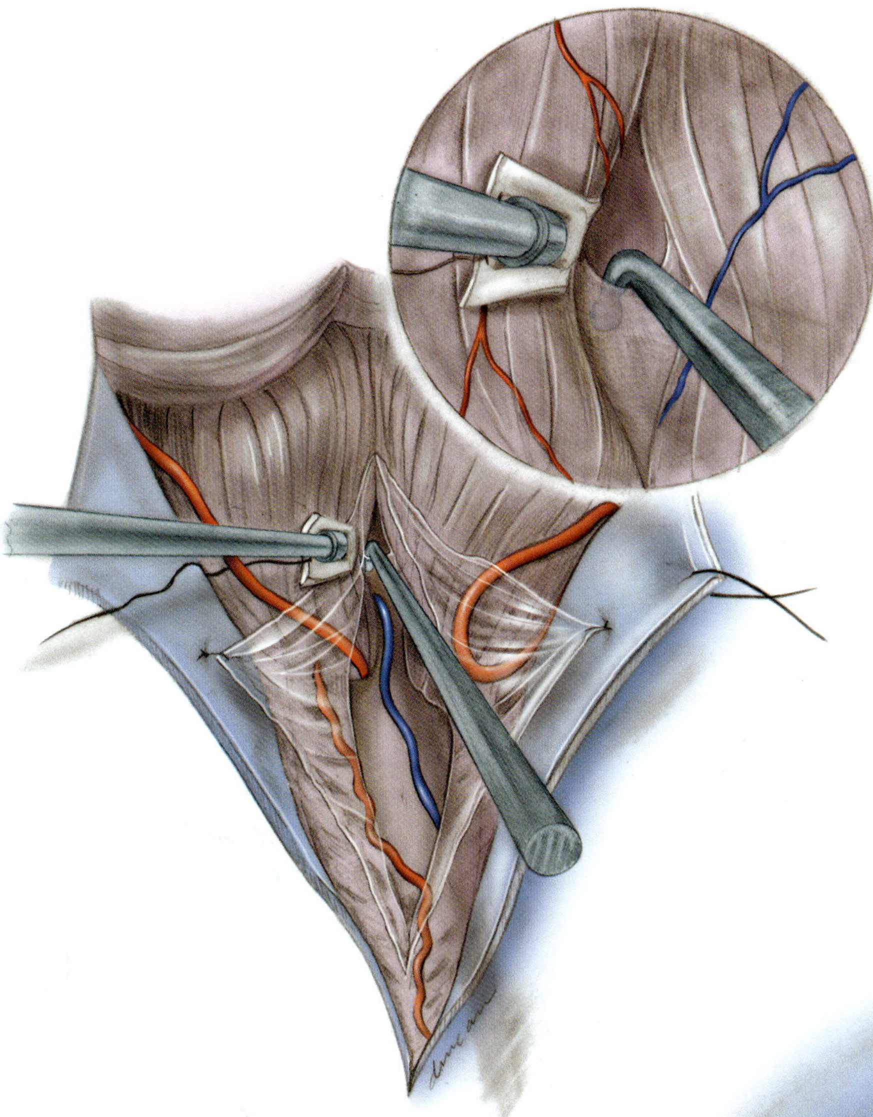

Figure 9–8.

Step 4. After the arachnoid has been opened, some surgeons tack it to the dura mater. An alternative is to excise the arachnoid over the cerebellar tonsils. Thereafter, the fourth ventricle should be inspected to make sure there are no arachnoid adhesions that prevent communication of the fourth ventricle with the cisterna magna. In patients with an associated syrinx, a small ball-tip dissector can be used to identify the obex and to make sure that adhesions do not prevent the flow of cerebrospinal fluid out of the syrinx into the subarachnoid space.

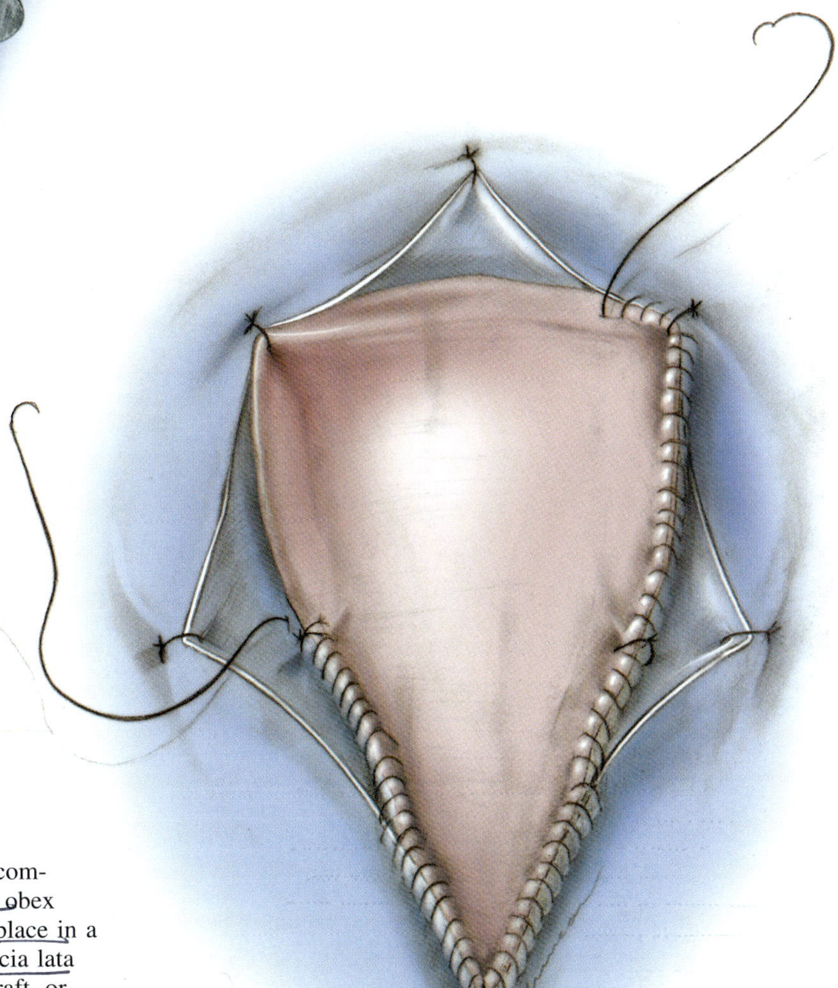

Figure 9–9.

Step 5. After the cerebellar tonsils have been decompressed and the floor of the fourth ventricle and the obex have been inspected, a loose dural graft is sewn in place in a watertight fashion. Options for this graft include fascia lata harvested from the leg, a bovine or cadaver dural graft, or possibly pericranium. It usually is difficult to obtain a piece of pericranium large enough to cover the dural opening for this particular operation, using a midline incision.

SUBOCCIPITAL SUPRACEREBELLAR APPROACH TO PINEAL REGION TUMORS

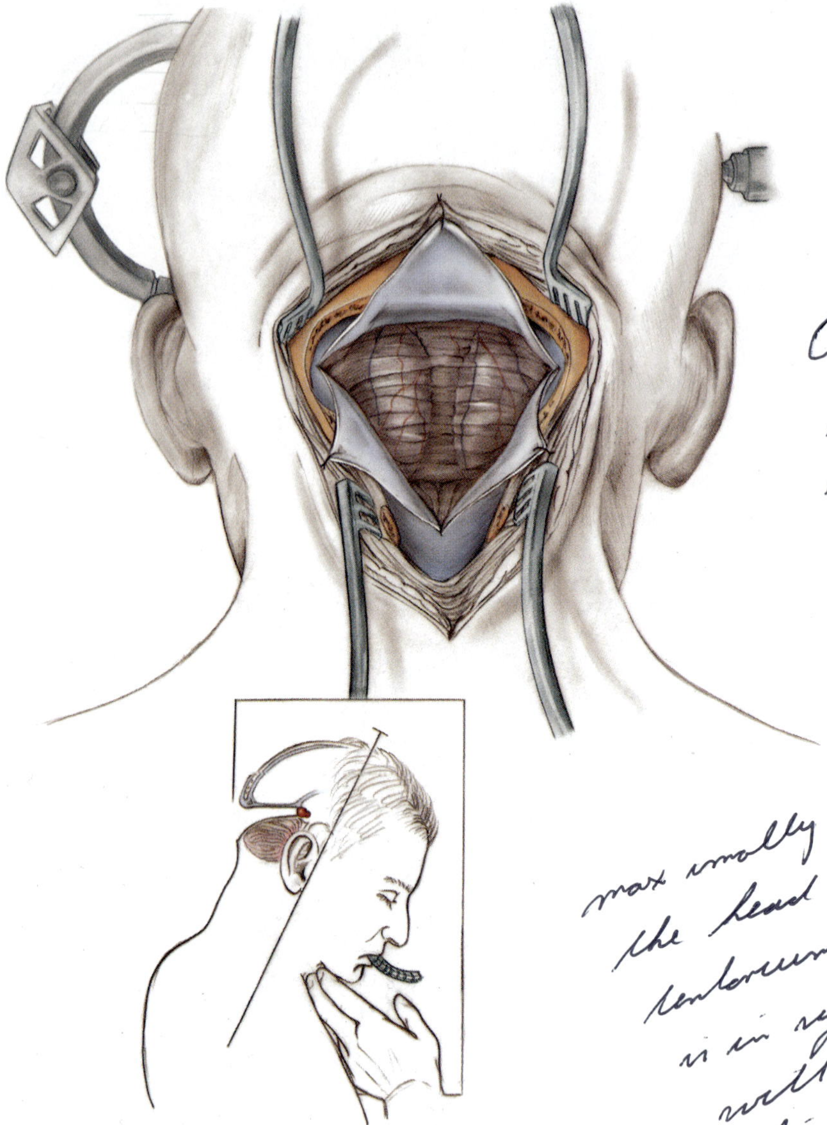

Figure 9–10.

Step 1. This operation can be performed with the patient in either a sitting or prone position. However, the sitting position offers an easier approach to tumors in this region. Regardless of body position, it is essential to make sure that the head is maximally flexed so that the tentorium cerebelli is parallel with the surgeon's line of sight. This will lessen the need for downward retraction of the cerebellum. When positioning the patient's head, the anesthesiologist typically places two fingers underneath the chin to prevent overflexion. Excessive flexion of the head leads to kinking and compression of the jugular veins, which can increase intracranial venous distention and intracranial pressure. A midline incision is used, similar to the one described above for treating a Chiari malformation. However, bone removal is extended more rostrally to expose approximately 5 mm of the torcular and transverse sinus. It also is advantageous to perform a laminectomy of C-1 to decompress the foramen magnum. The arachnoid over the cisterna magna should be opened for drainage of cerebrospinal fluid to provide relaxation of the cerebellum.

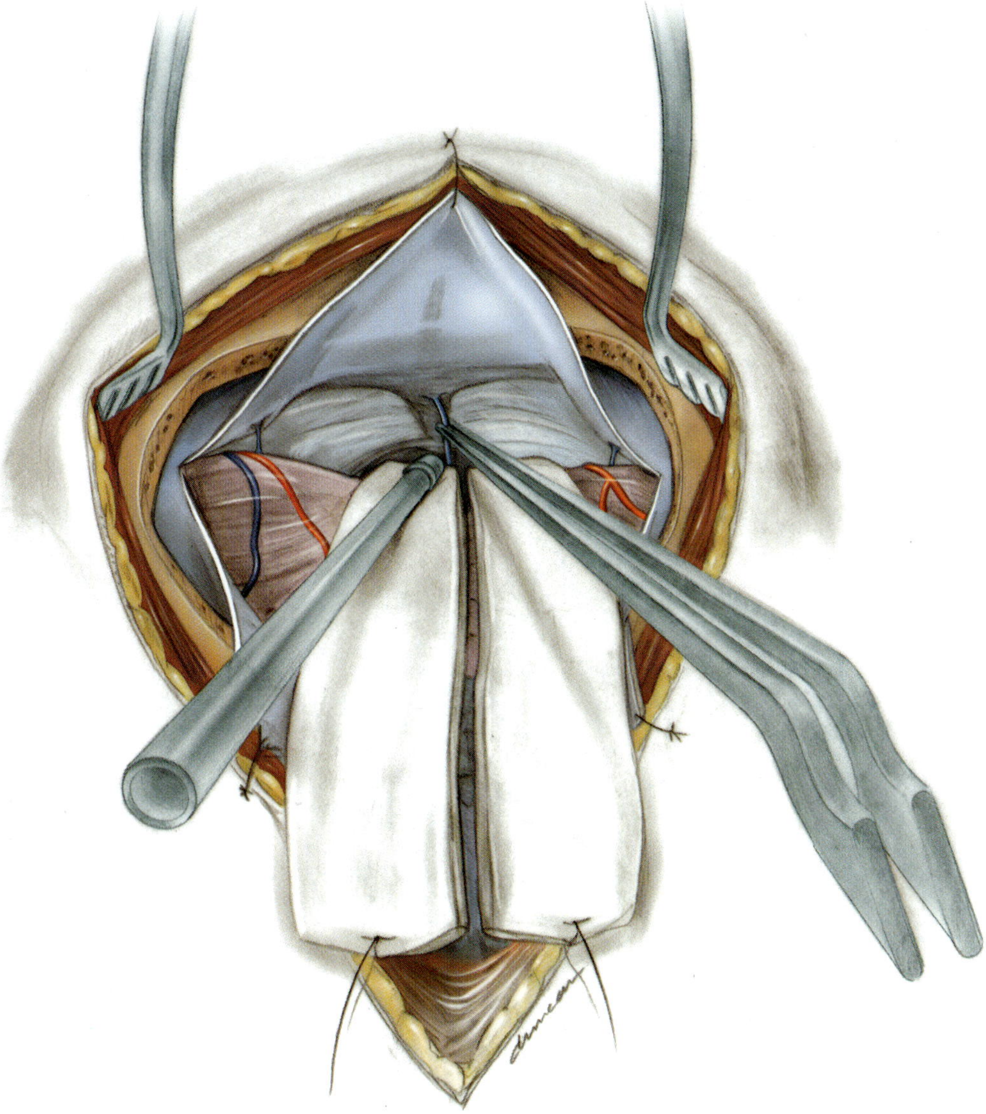

Figure 9–11.

Step 2. After the arachnoid over the cisterna magna has been opened, the cerebellum will sag caudally. The top of the cerebellum is lined with hemostatic fabric (Surgicel) and cottonoids and gently retracted with a #5 or #7 suction tip and bipolar cautery. It is important to limit the number of cottonoids used, otherwise they will narrow the exposure. Several small veins usually come off the top of the cerebellum and run to the underside of the tentorium cerebelli; they should be cauterized and divided. Note how the torcular and transverse sinus are retracted upward by tacking the dura mater, thereby providing an additional 3 to 4 mm of exposure.

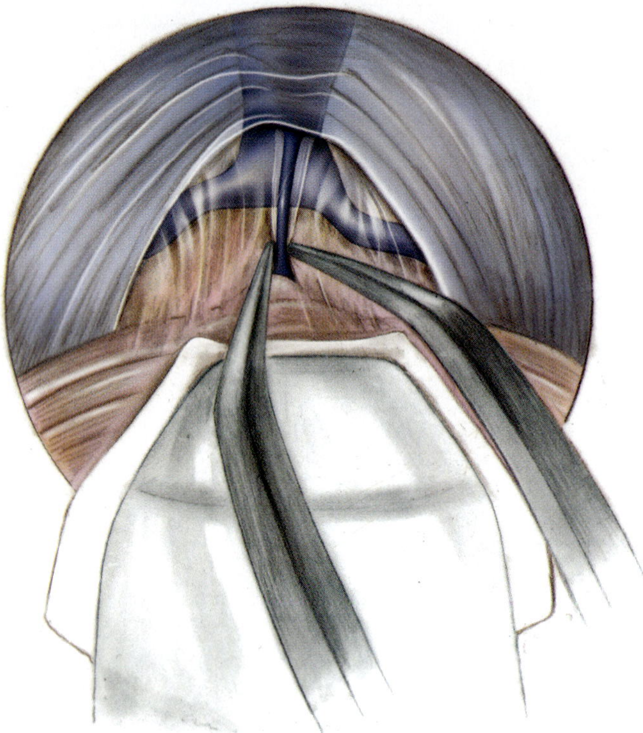

Figure 9–12.

Step 3. Under higher magnification, the surgeon extends the dissection deeper toward the precentral vein. If necessary, a single retractor blade can be placed over the roof of the cerebellum. The precentral vein is ensheathed by arachnoid and extends to the vein of Galen. The precentral vein may have several tributaries. This vein should be completely cauterized and divided.

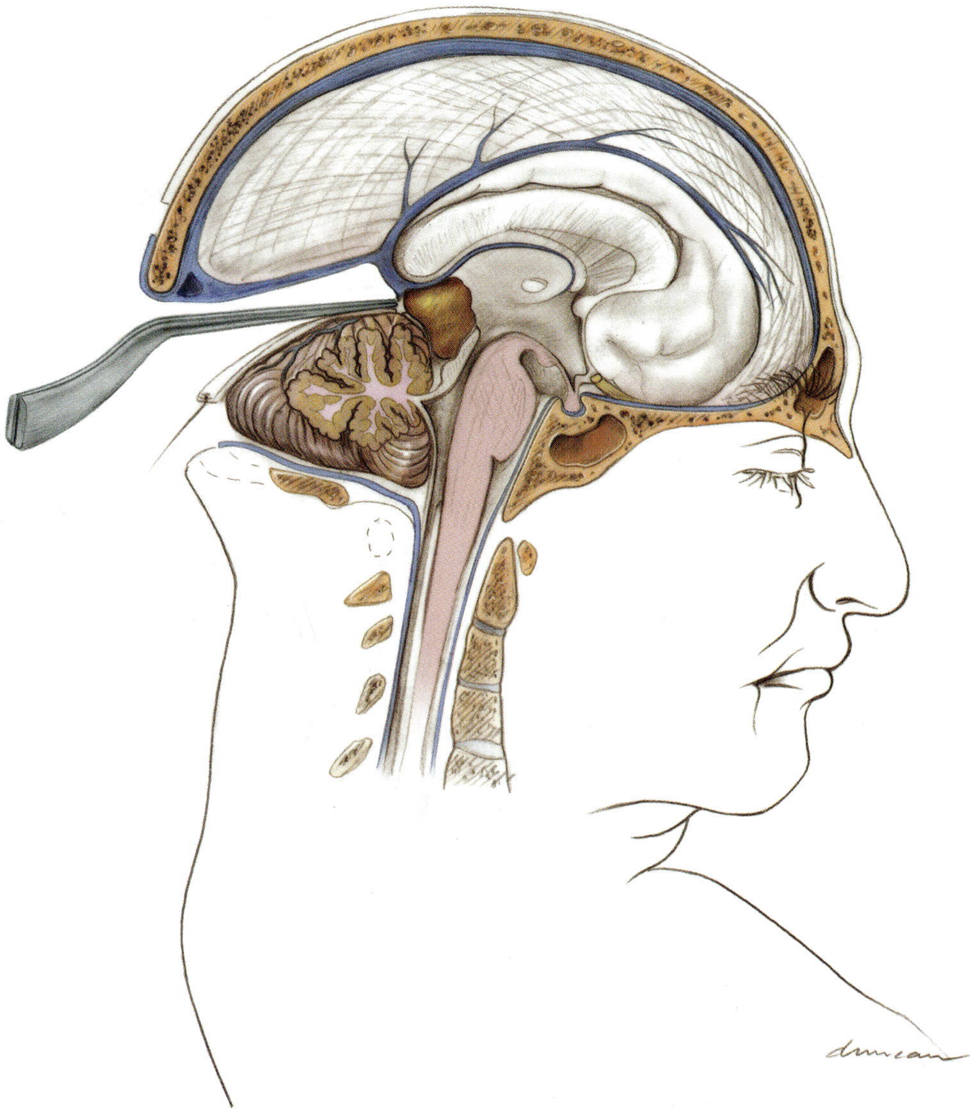

Figure 9–13.

Step 4. After the precentral vein has been divided, the caudal aspect of the tumor is usually encountered, covered in arachnoid. The arachnoid should be divided and peeled laterally to better define the posterior margin of the tumor capsule.

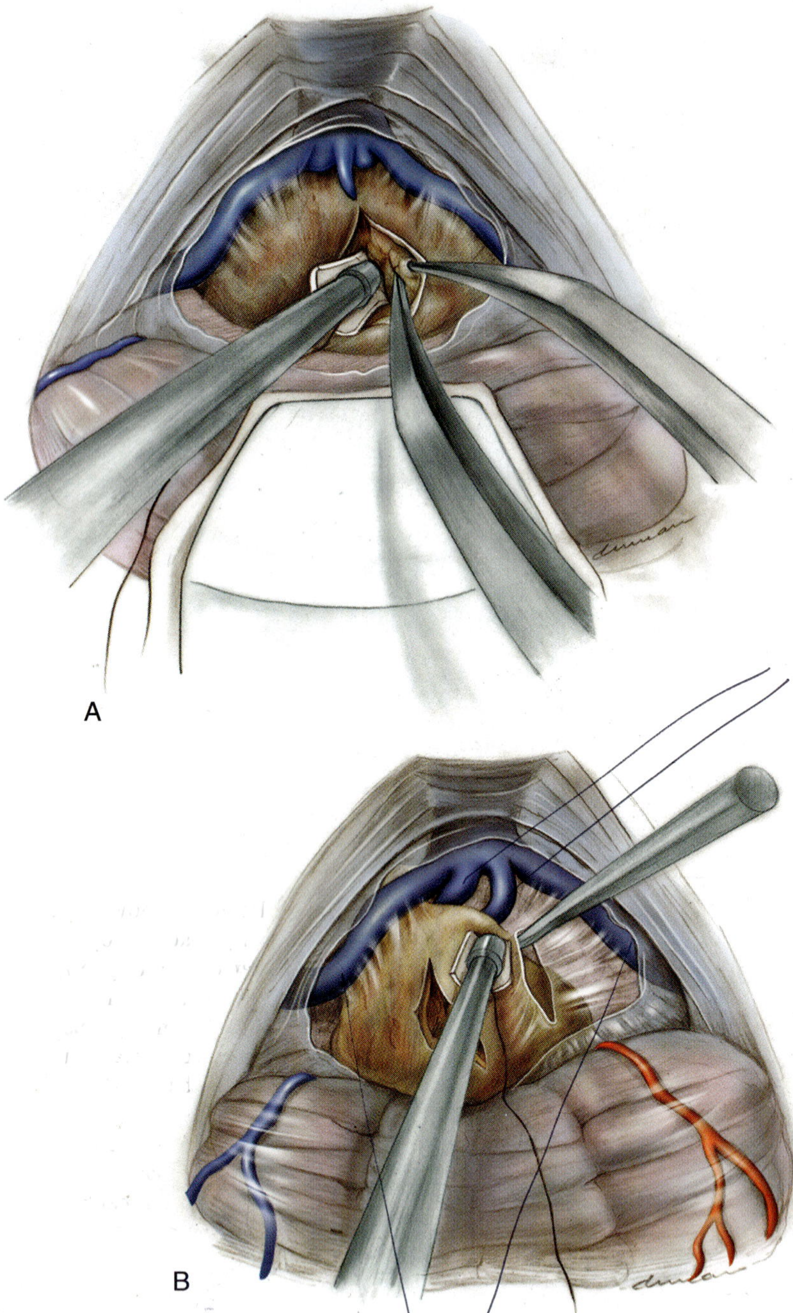

Figure 9–14.

Step 5. There are usually adhesions between the tumor capsule and the basal veins of Rosenthal and the internal cerebral veins. *A*, A dissecting spatula can be used to separate the tumor capsule from these venous structures. It is best to incise the tumor and perform internal debulking. Because of the complexity of tumors in this region, as much specimen as possible should be preserved for pathologic examination.

B, After internal debulking has been performed, the anterior margin of the tumor capsule is dissected off the internal cerebral veins, which lie rostrally and ventrally to the tumor. Depending on the type of tumor, complete removal may not be possible. If necessary, remnants of the tumor should be left intact instead of injuring the major deep draining veins.

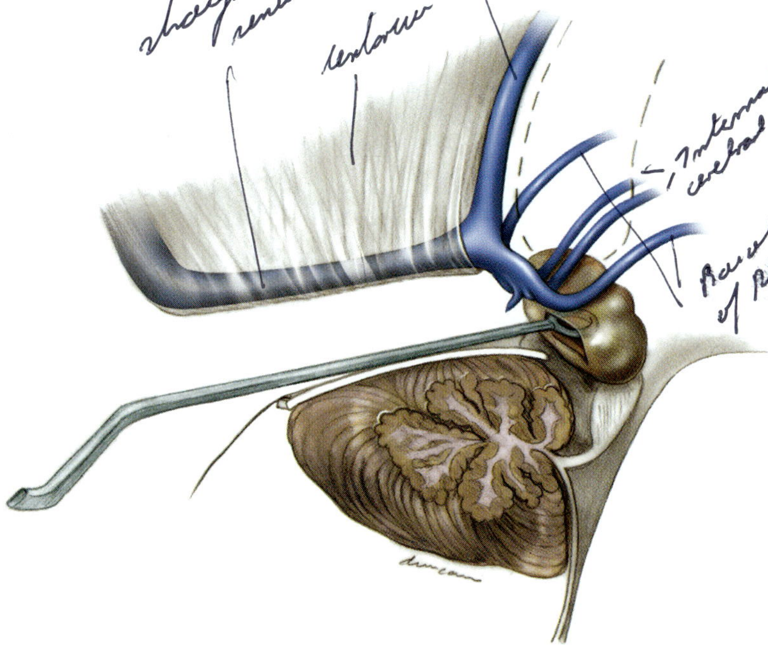

Figure 9–15.

Step 6. With the supracerebellar approach, access to tumors with a significant caudal extension may be difficult. It may be helpful to retract the cerebellum and to rotate the operating room table to alter the surgeon's line of sight. Usually, a spatula can be used to gently work the tumor capsule upward into the operative field. A malleable fiberoptic scope or mirror may be useful to inspect this deeper portion to better understand the dissecting plane if direct visualization is not optimum. For tumors with a very large caudal extension, a combined occipital transtentorial and supracerebellar approach can be used, as described in Chapter 5.

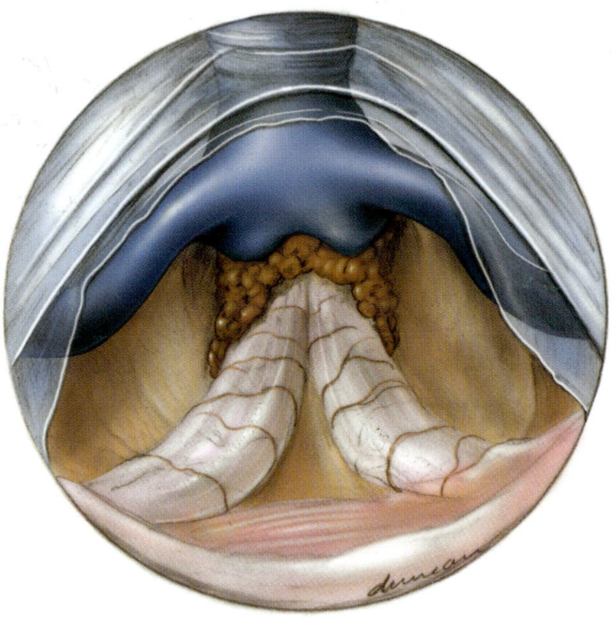

Figure 9–16.

Step 7. This is the typical view following removal of a pineal tumor. The third ventricle is framed laterally by the splenium and basal vein of Rosenthal, anteriorly by the internal cerebral vein, and inferiorly by the thalamus. It is important to irrigate the third ventricle thoroughly to flush out any debris. The veins should be inspected to make sure there is no thinning of the vascular wall. If the structural integrity of one of the veins is questioned, the vein should be buttressed with absorbable gelatin sponge. The cerebellum is inspected to make sure there are no hematomas or subpial hemorrhage. The author prefers to close the dura mater with a graft and not to replace the bone flap. This provides good decompression of the posterior fossa.

MEDULLOBLASTOMA

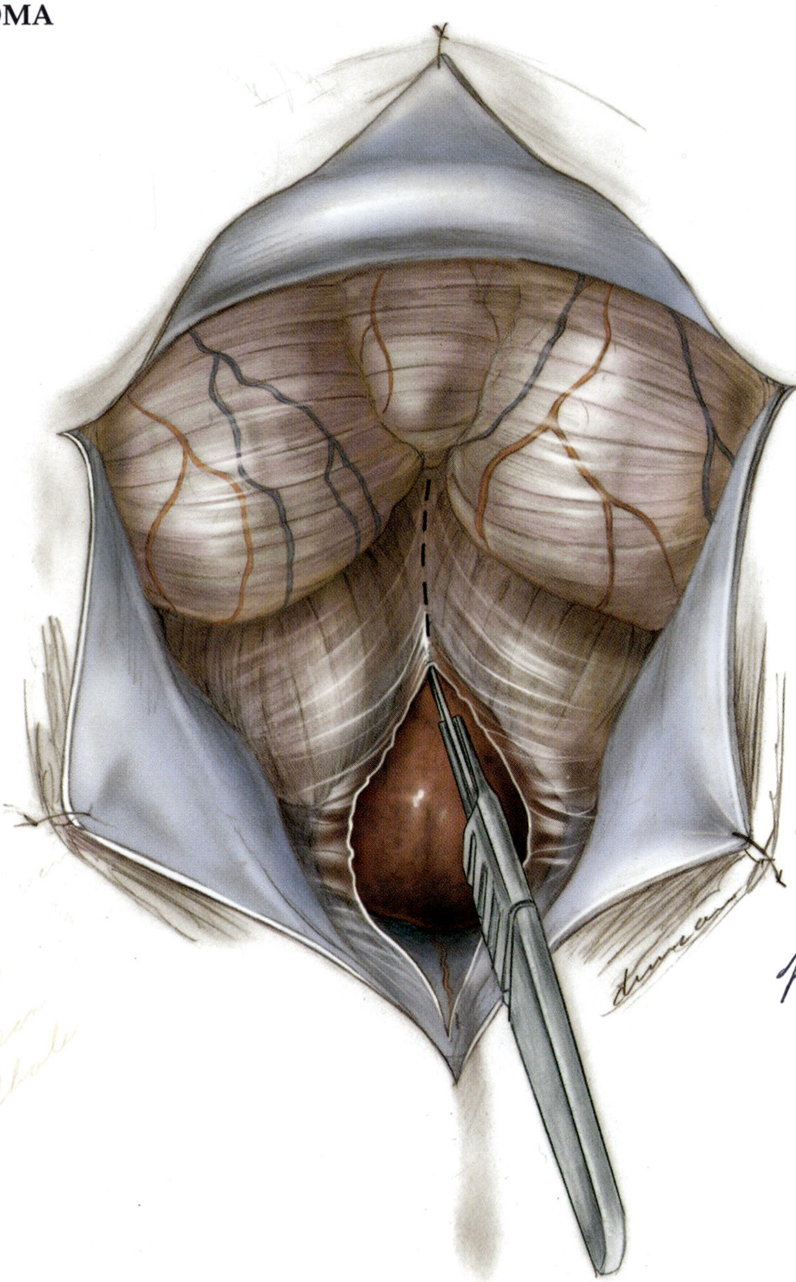

Figure 9–17.

Step 1. The approach to a medulloblastoma is similar to that for a Chiari malformation. The patient can be placed in either a sitting or prone position. The patient's head does not need to be flexed as much as for a supracerebellar approach to a tumor in the pineal region. Bony removal is similar to that for Chiari decompression. In addition to removing the posterior rim of the foramen magnum, a laminectomy of vertebra C-1 should also be performed. The dura mater is opened in a Y-shaped fashion and tacked to the margins of the muscle. Often, the tumor can be seen bulging out underneath the arachnoid, splaying the two cerebellar tonsils laterally. The arachnoid is incised first over the cisterna magna for drainage of cerebrospinal fluid. The arachnoid incision is then extended upward. The arachnoid can be held laterally by tacking it to the dura mater with either a suture or small hemostatic clips.

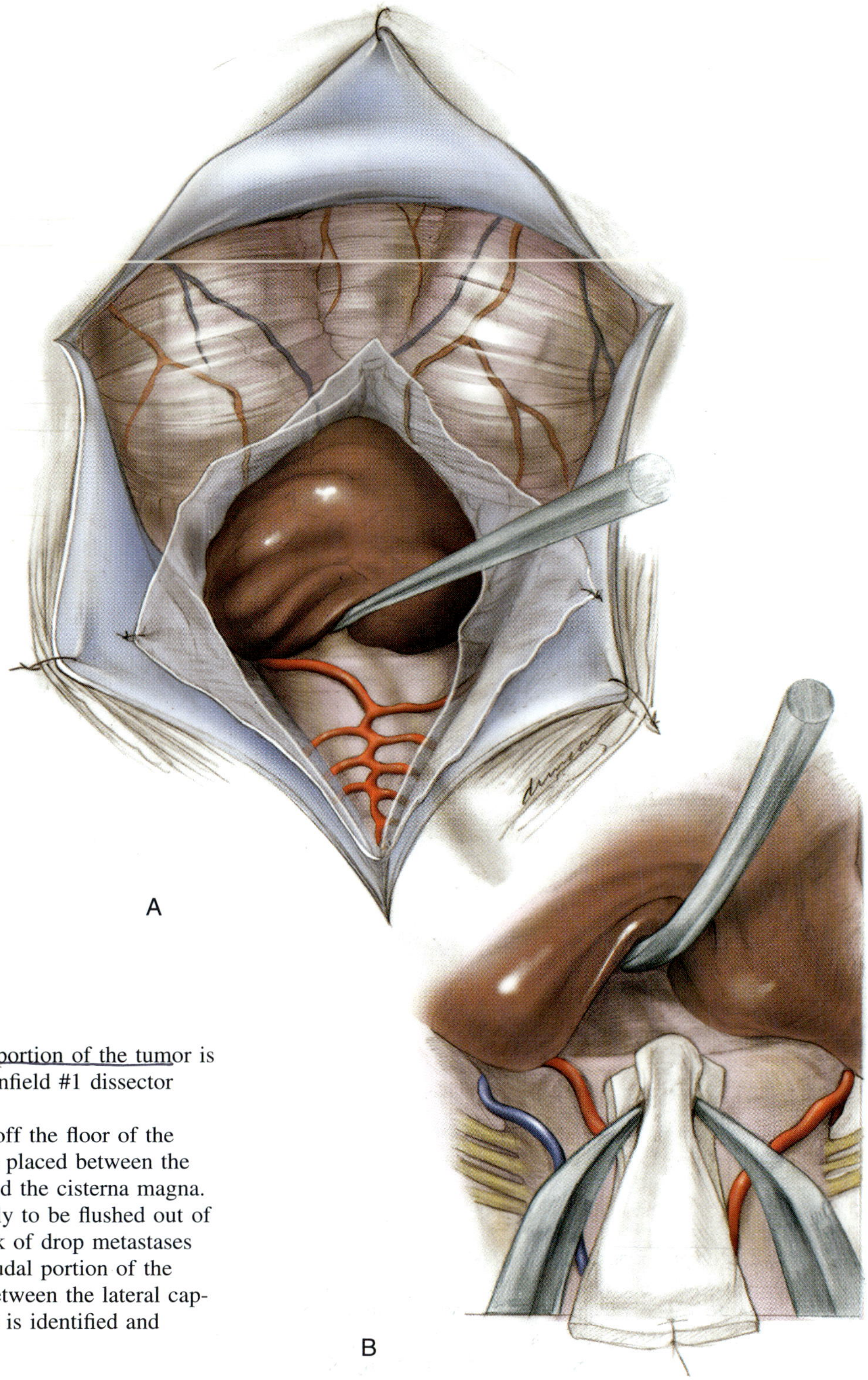

Figure 9–18.

Step 2. *A*, The caudal, or inferior, portion of the tumor is separated first from the medulla. A Penfield #1 dissector works well for this maneuver.

B, After the tumor has been lifted off the floor of the fourth ventricle, several cottonoids are placed between the tumor and the floor of the ventricle and the cisterna magna. In this way, tumor debris is more likely to be flushed out of the surgical wound, decreasing the risk of drop metastases entering the spinal canal. After the caudal portion of the tumor has been dissected, the plane between the lateral capsule of the tumor and cerebellar tissue is identified and defined by placement of cottonoids.

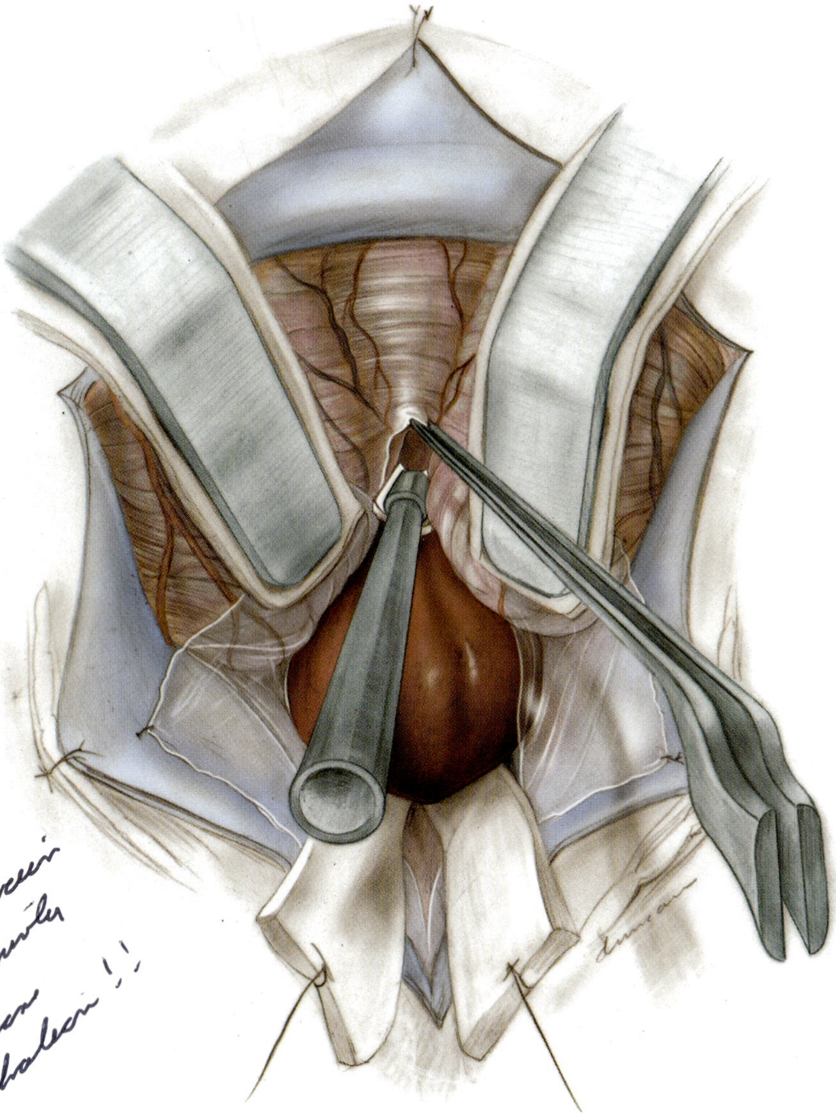

Figure 9–19.

Step 3. The attachment of the tumor is at the superior medullary velum. A #5 or #7 suction tip and bipolar cautery are used to develop the plane over the rostral and ventral portions of the tumor. It is important to ensure that the edge of the tumor is identified and that the dissection is approximately 5 to 10 mm above this edge to allow for a more aggressive resection of this infiltrative zone. At the depths of the rostral dissection, the surgeon will punch through into the fourth ventricle. It is important not to injure the floor of the ventricle. For small tumors, during the initial exposure of the tumor at the foramen magnum and before beginning the dissection, the surgeon can insert a cottonoid all the way up along the floor of the fourth ventricle underneath the tumor. This maneuver is more difficult to accomplish with large tumors.

With large tumors, it can be advantageous to retract both cerebellar tonsils with self-retaining retractors. Alternatively, the tonsil can be retracted with a suction tip and cottonoid. Using the suction tip as a retractor is faster because the surgeon can move it rapidly as the dissection is carried laterally and anteriorly.

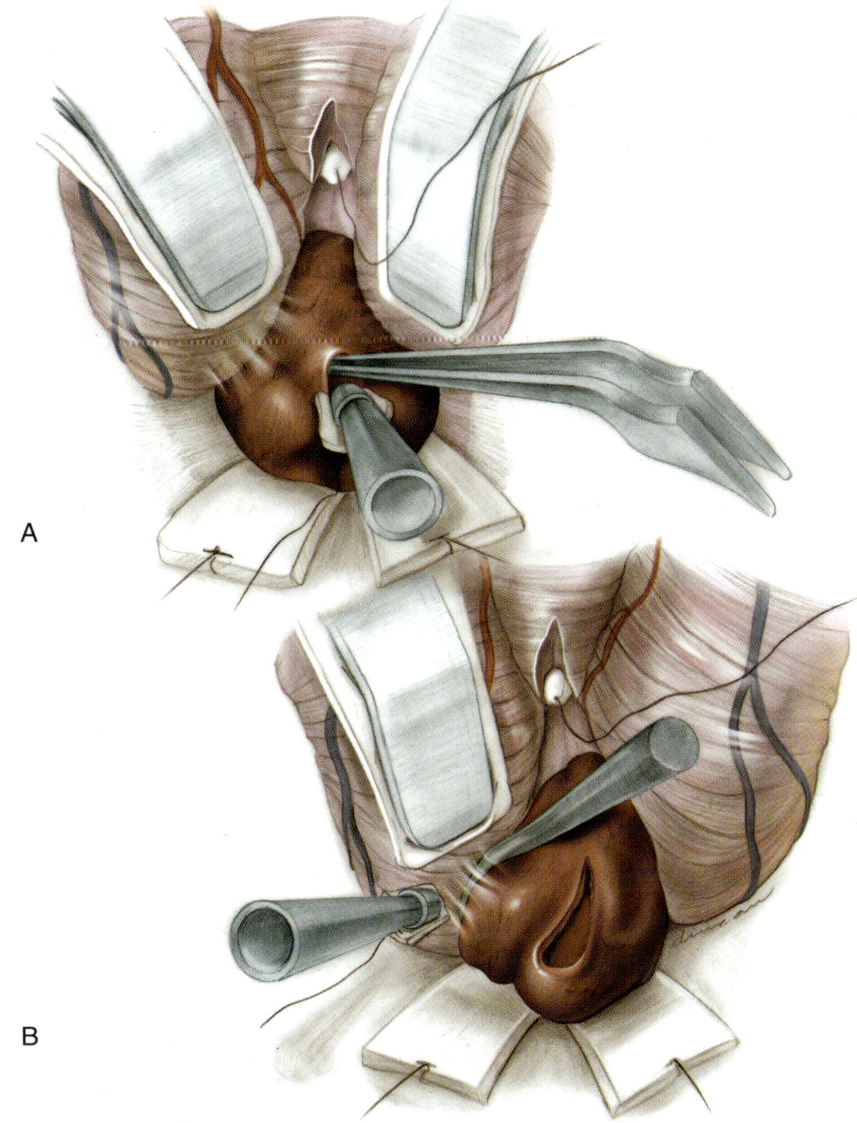

Figure 9–20.

Step 4. *A*, With large tumors, internal debulking is advantageous to collapse the tumor and to decrease the need for cerebellar retraction. Before the tumor is debulked, cottonoids should be placed over the cisterna magna to prevent tumor debris from entering the spinal canal.

B, After the tumor has been debulked, its lateral capsule is peeled off the overlying cerebellar tissue. In most circumstances, this plane is easy to establish and preserve. As tumor resection is carried deeper, the surgeon must follow this plane carefully to prevent inadvertent injury to the middle cerebellar peduncle.

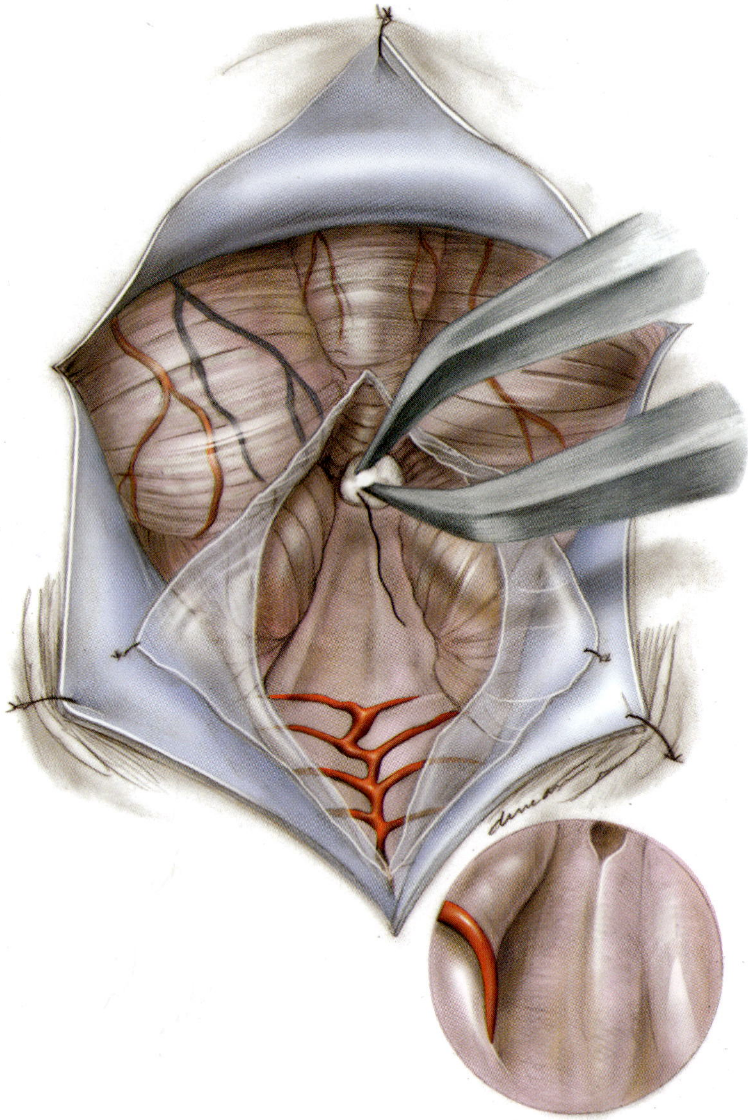

Figure 9–21.

Step 5. After the tumor has been resected, the underside of the cerebellar vermis and its extension into the superior medullary velum should be inspected thoroughly for any remnants of the tumor. Thereafter, it is meticulously cauterized. With most medulloblastomas, the floor of the fourth ventricle is not invaded. Any thickened or abnormal-appearing arachnoid along the cisterna magna should be harvested and examined pathologically for evidence of tumor dissemination.

EPENDYMOMA

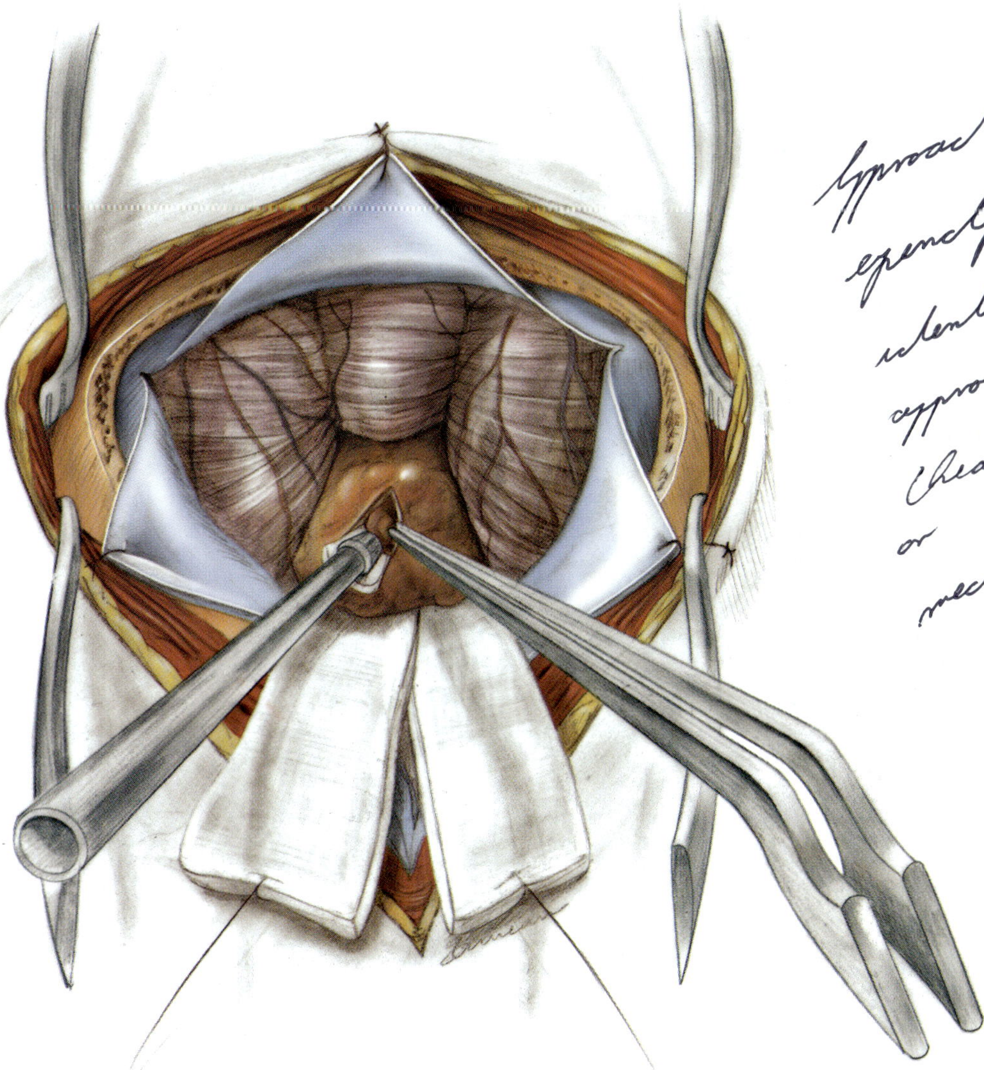

Figure 9–22.

Step 1. The position of the patient, the skin incision, and the bony exposure for resection of an ependymoma are identical to those used for medulloblastoma or Chiari malformation. After the dura mater has been opened, the arachnoid over the cisterna magna is opened to drain cerebrospinal fluid to decrease pressure within the posterior fossa. After the arachnoid has been opened, the caudal portion of the tumor closest to the surgeon is dissected or lifted off the cervicomedullary junction. For large tumors, there may be adhesions between the tumor capsule and the arachnoid and vascular structures in this region that require sharp dissection. After this posterior tongue of tumor has been dissected, cottonoids are placed between it and the medulla and the cisterna magna. In sequence, each cerebellar tonsil is retracted laterally so that the tumor capsule can be dissected off the overlying cerebellum. The tumor rarely invades the cerebral hemispheres; therefore, this plane usually is easy to identify and to maintain by placing cottonoids on the lateral side of the tumor capsule. The tumor is incised and internally debulked using suction, bipolar cautery, or an ultrasonic aspirator.

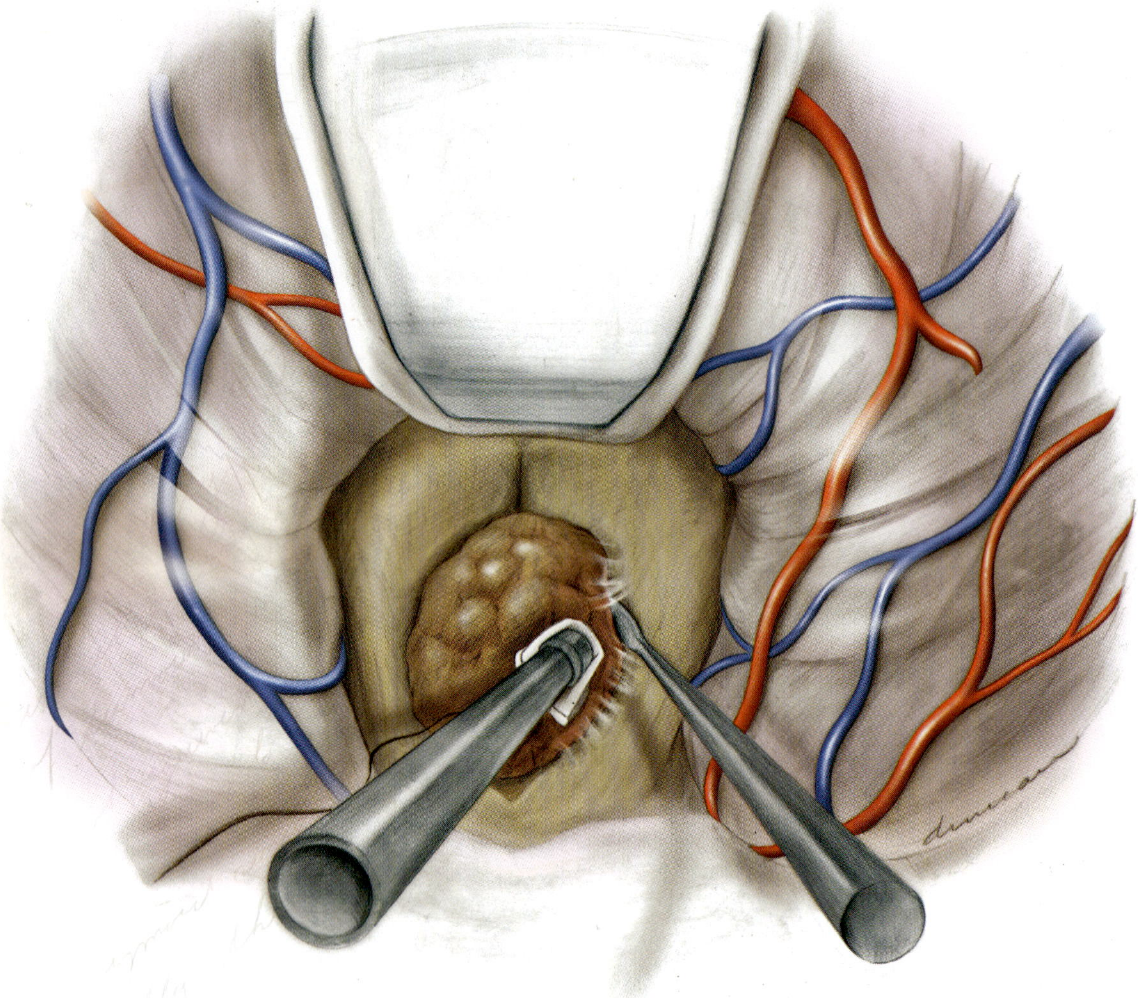

Figure 9–23.

Step 2. It is important to recognize that ependymomas originate from the floor of the fourth ventricle. Therefore, as debulking of the tumor proceeds into the fourth ventricle, the surgeon must exercise every caution to prevent inadvertent injury to the medulla. Furthermore, it may be difficult to separate the tumor from the lateral aspect of the ventricular floor, at its junction with the middle cerebellar peduncle. As the surgeon enters the fourth ventricle, a small cottonball can be placed rostral to the tumor at the opening of the aqueduct to prevent excessive drainage of cerebrospinal fluid from the lateral ventricles. This maneuver is especially helpful when the patient is in the sitting position and a mass in the fourth ventricle is being resected.

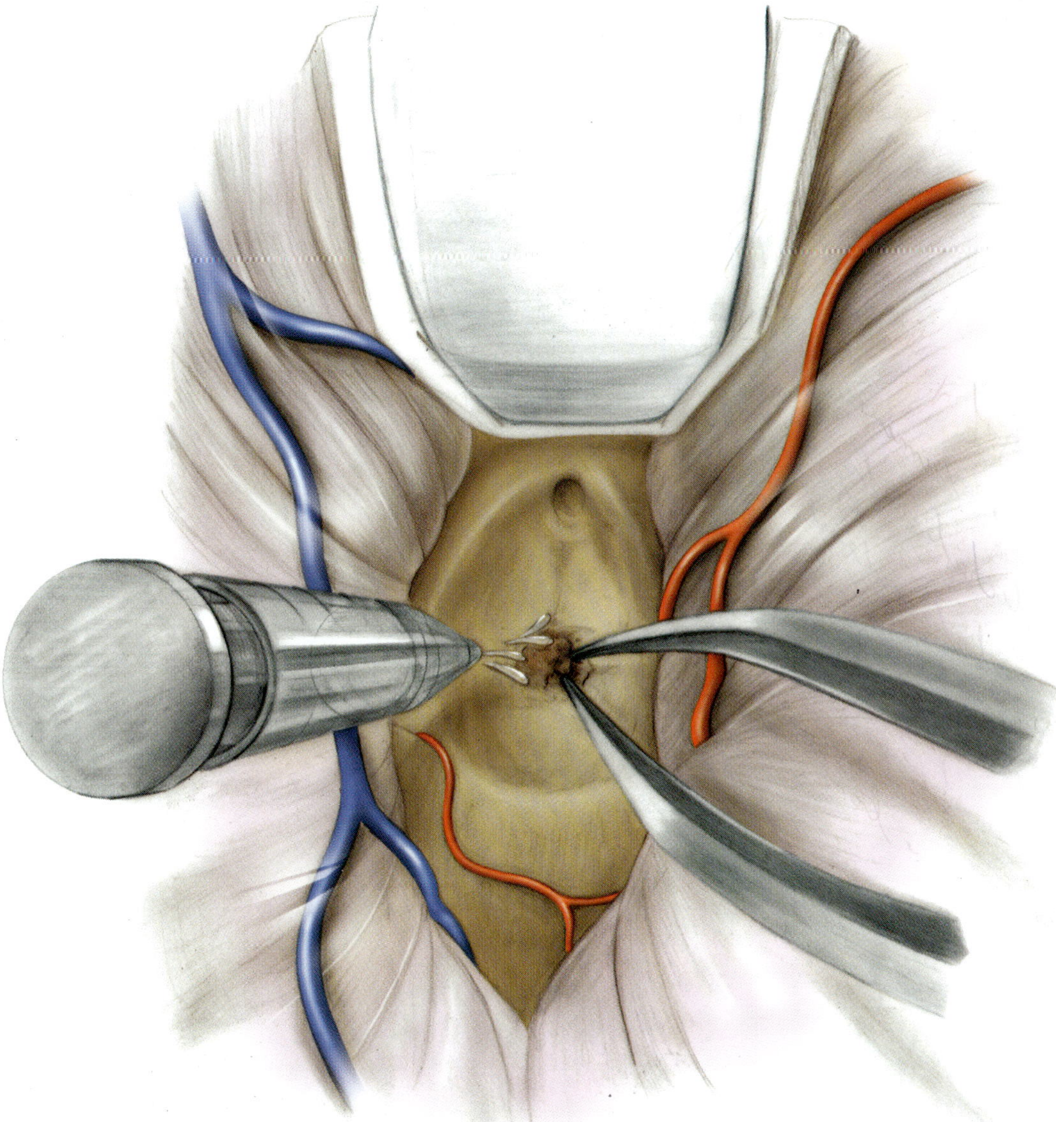

Figure 9–24.

Step 3. Under high magnification, the tumor is separated from the floor of the fourth ventricle, but small deposits of infiltrative tumor will remain. Creation of this plane is based on visual cues. Electromyographic monitoring of the lower cranial nerves can be useful when dissecting a tumor off the floor of the fourth ventricle, because it alerts the surgeon to the location of functional tissue along the facial and vagal trigones.

FORAMEN MAGNUM TUMOR

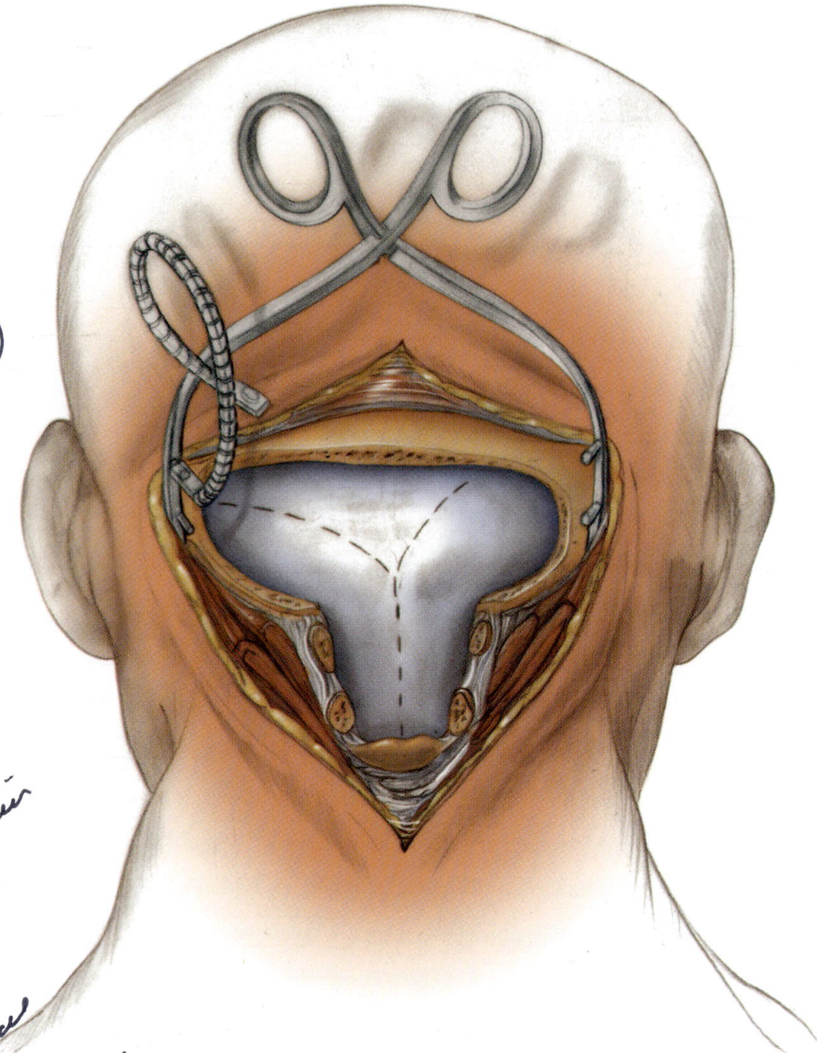

Figure 9–25.

Step 1. The position of the patient, the skin incision, and the bony removal for resection of a foramen magnum tumor are similar to those used for treating Chiari malformation. In a foramen magnum tumor, the extent of cervical laminectomy is determined by the caudal extension of tumor into the cervical spinal canal. It is not necessary to expose bone up to the torcular or lateral to the sigmoid sinus. However, at the foramen magnum, it is necessary that the bony removal extend to the occipital condyle on the side of the tumor. The medial one-third of the occipital condyle can be removed with a high-speed air drill and small diamond bur, which limits bleeding from the small bony venous channels.

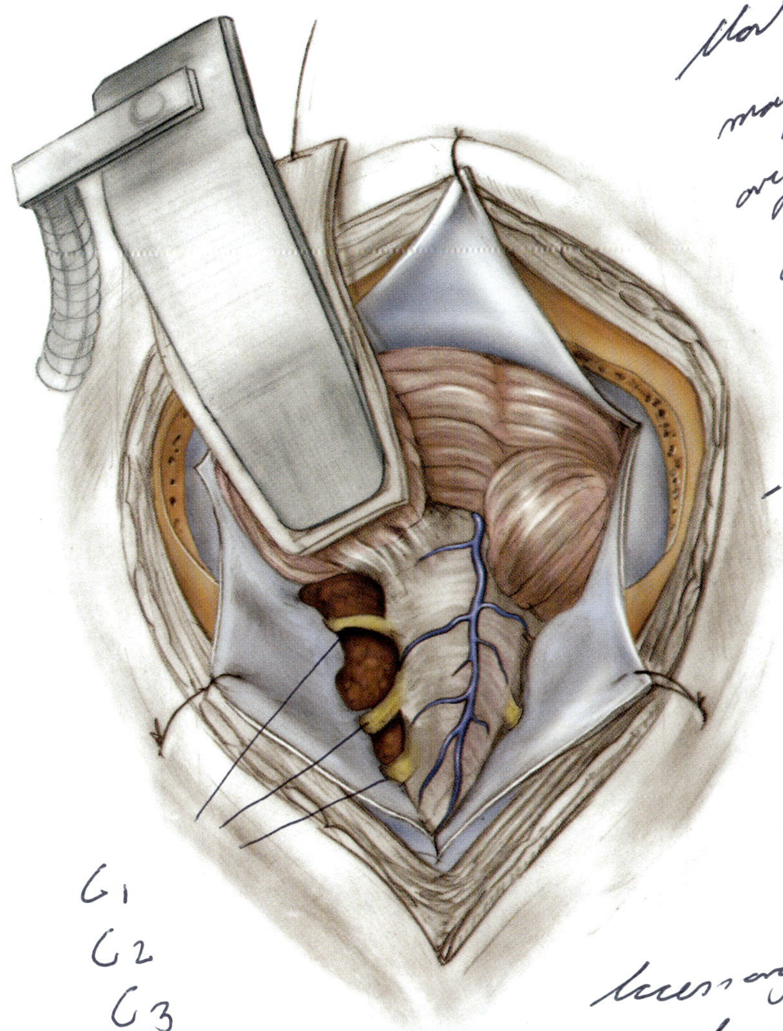

Figure 9–26.

Step 2. After the dura mater has been opened, the arachnoid over the cisterna magna is opened and tacked to the dura. Most foramen magnum tumors originate from the anterolateral foramen magnum. Thus, the cervicomedullary junction is typically displaced posteriorly and laterally by the tumor mass. This natural displacement assists the surgeon, and retraction of the spinal cord is not necessary. A single stitch can be placed in the dentate ligament to preserve this displacement until tumor resection has been completed. The rootlets of C-1 and C-2 usually overlie the tumor. If necessary, these posterior rootlets can be sectioned to provide additional exposure. The spinal accessory nerve is usually displaced laterally against the dura mater of the posterior fossa. The position of the vertebral artery varies, and the artery may be encased by tumor. This artery usually is anterior, especially when the tumor originates from the lateral aspect of the foramen magnum.

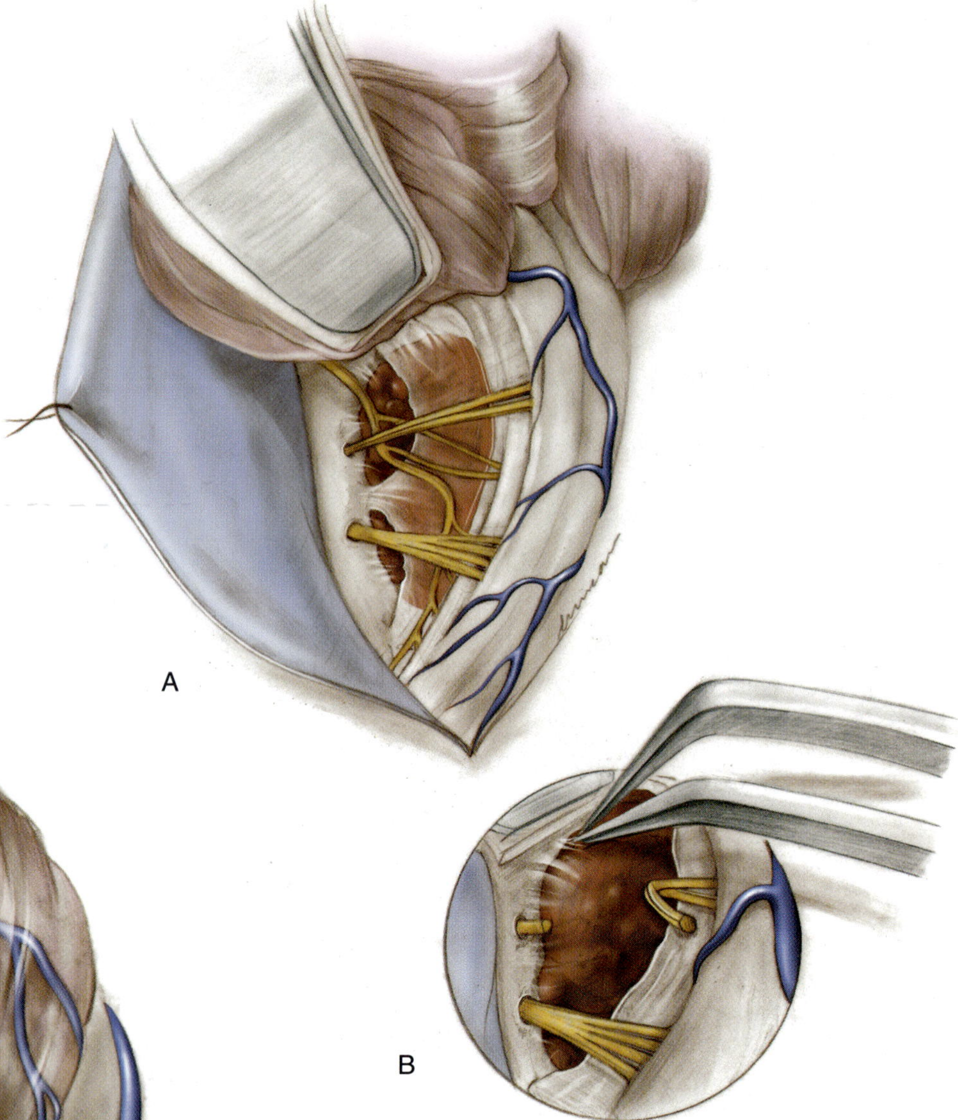

Figure 9–27.

Step 3. *A*, The arachnoid, which may partially overlie the tumor capsule, is peeled laterally. The plane between the medial aspect of the tumor and the lateral cervicomedullary junction is easily identified. It is advantageous to aggressively debulk the tumor internally, working above and below the rootlets of C-1 and C-2.

Step 4. *B*, After the tumor has been debulked, its attachment to the dura mater of the foramen magnum should be cauterized to decrease the vascular supply of the tumor.

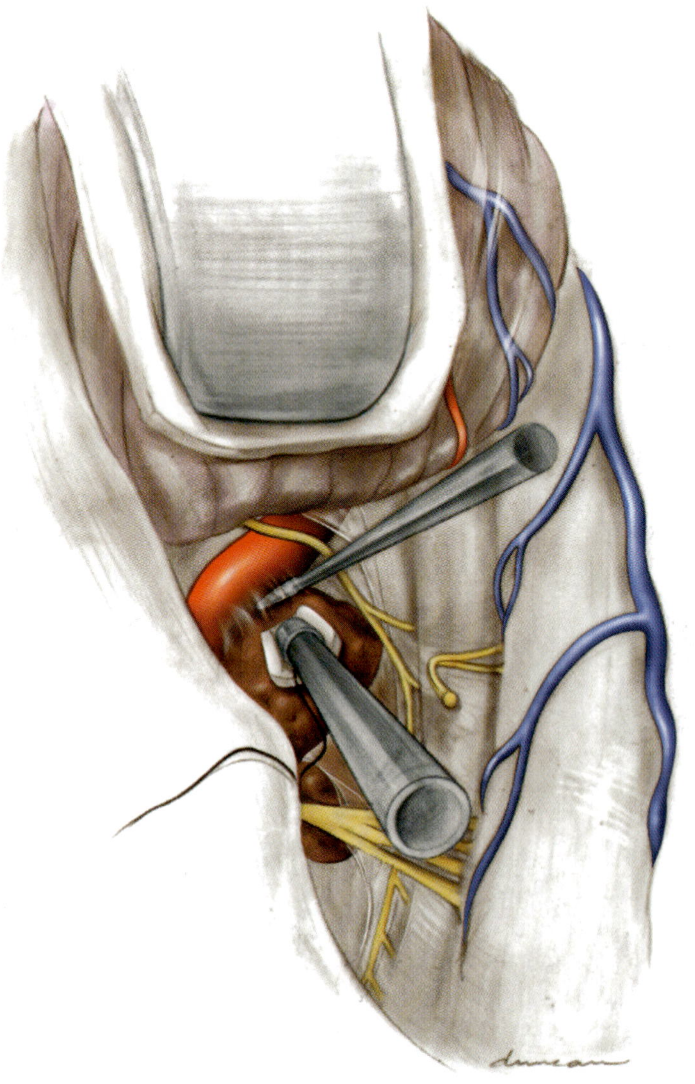

Figure 9–28.

Step 5. As the resection of the tumor extends deeper into the foramen magnum, it is important to identify the vertebral artery, which may be encased by tumor. A suction tip and small dissecting spatula work well for peeling tumor off the artery. If tumor is adhesive to either the vertebral or basilar artery or their perforating vessels, it may be necessary to leave small remnants of tumor. This may occur if a tumor of the foramen magnum has extended up to involve the lower two-thirds of the clivus.

10

Transsphenoidal Approach

Copyright © 1999 Mayo Foundation.

The transsphenoidal route is an excellent approach for resecting various sellar lesions, including pituitary adenomas, Rathke's cleft cysts, and intrasellar craniopharyngiomas. On preoperative radiographic imaging, the best clue that a transsphenoidal approach will work well for resecting a sellar/suprasellar lesion is enlargement of the sella turcica. Even pituitary macroadenomas with massive suprasellar extensions can be removed grossly through a transsphenoidal approach. However, an apparent extension or bulging of a tumor, with displacement of the diaphragma sellae inferiorly, without enlargement of the pituitary fossa (as often seen in a craniopharyngioma) indicates that the tumor needs to be removed through a transcranial approach. Cushing initially developed the translabial transseptal approach to the sella turcica but subsequently abandoned it for a transcranial route because of a high incidence of leakage of cerebrospinal fluid and meningitis. Transsphenoidal surgery was subsequently rejuvenated by Guiot, Thibaut, Hardy, and Wigser, with excellent surgical results.

Most transsphenoidal surgery is performed for resection of pituitary adenomas. These tumors may be either functional or nonfunctional. Approximately 75 percent of all pituitary adenomas are functional, and 40 to 50 percent are prolactinomas, 15 to 25 percent are growth hormone-secreting tumors, and 5 percent are adrenocorticotropic hormone (ACTH)–producing tumors. Of prolactinomas, approximately 70 to 75 percent of microadenomas and 30 percent of macroadenomas have long-term cure rates after transsphenoidal surgery, with normalization of serum levels of prolactin. One of the most significant prognostic indicators for successful prolactinoma surgery is the preoperative level of prolactin. Specifically, if the serum level of prolactin is less than 500 ng/mL preoperatively, the cure rate after transsphenoidal surgery is approximately 50 to 70 percent. However, if the preoperative serum level is greater than 1,000 ng/mL, the cure rate is less than 25 percent.

The surgical results are similar for growth hormone–producing tumors. Overall, the cure rate for somatotroph tumors is approximately 60 percent, with postoperative growth hormone levels less than 5 ng/mL. However, similar to prolactinomas, there is an inverse relationship between preoperative levels of growth hormone and long-term surgical cure. The success rate for surgical tumor control appears to decrease significantly when the preoperative level of growth hormone is greater than 50 ng/mL.

The surgical treatment of Cushing's disease is complicated. Reportedly, approximately 85 percent of patients with biochemical documentation of Cushing's disease have a pituitary adenoma even if the results of preoperative magnetic resonance imaging are unremarkable. Some experienced surgeons have reported a long-term cure rate of 80 to 90 percent with noninvasive microadenomas. With large ACTH-producing tumors, there often is an extension into the cavernous sinus and long-term surgical cure rates accordingly fall below 50 percent. At surgery, the presence of a microadenoma may be difficult to find because the tumor occasionally is located within the midportion of the pituitary gland and not lateralized. Also, in some patients with Cushing's disease, the source of excessive ACTH production is pituitary hyperplasia instead of a discrete pituitary adenoma. Cushing's disease is a life-threatening condition; therefore, the surgeon should strongly consider performing a complete hypophysectomy if a discrete adenoma is not found at surgery, because if transsphenoidal surgery for Cushing's disease fails, additional procedures and treatments will be required, for example, bilateral adrenalectomy. If there is residual pituitary adenoma, Nelson syndrome is a risk after adrenalectomy. Consequently, irradiation of the pituitary fossa is often recommended after adrenalectomy if the original biochemical data clearly support the presence of Cushing's disease instead of Cushing's syndrome. Because of the potential for the sequence of events, a strong argument can be made for performing a near-complete hypophysectomy if a discrete microadenoma is not found intraoperatively. A complete hypophysectomy can be performed with minimal traction on the infundibulum of the pituitary. Thus, the need for vasopressin postoperatively is often limited. The long-term endocrine implications for management of patients with Cushing's disease who undergo hypophysectomy instead of resection of a microadenoma are not dramatic in adult males. However, in children and in women who might desire to have children, the implications of a complete hypophysectomy are significant. It is debatable, but in children and in women desiring children, bilateral adrenalectomy instead of complete hypophysectomy might be best after a failed transsphenoidal exploration.

ANATOMY

The sella turcica is bounded by the sellar floor anteriorly and inferiorly, the dorsum sellae posteriorly, the diaphragma sellae superiorly, and the dura mater of the cavernous sinus laterally. The diaphragma sellae may be incompetent; therefore, a small pouch of arachnoid may be present within the sella turcica. Within the diaphragma sellae is the circular venous sinus, which has a variable anatomy and consists of the following venous structures. Typically, small venous channels connect the cavernous sinuses and run posteriorly to the dorsum sellae. Also, a venous sinus runs anteriorly at the junction of the tuberculum sellae and the anterior wall of the pituitary fossa. Collectively, these small venous sinuses are the "circular sinus" and usually are of no consequence during transsphenoidal surgery. However, in patients with Cushing's disease, the circular sinus often appears larger than normal and may be a source of nuisance bleeding during transsphenoidal surgery.

The pituitary gland is divided into an anterior lobe (the pars distalis and the pars intermedia) and a posterior lobe (the pars nervosa). The pars intermedia is a remnant of Rathke's pouch, which separates the anterior and posterior lobes and occasionally may be seen at surgery as a small cleft. The location of Rathke's cleft explains why, during transsphenoidal resection of a cyst of Rathke's cleft, the surgeon first encounters a thin but normal pituitary gland after removing the sellar floor. The posterior pituitary lobe is the end of the pituitary stalk, which consists of axons whose cell bodies are in the supraoptic and paraventricular nuclei of the hypothalamus. This explains why a minimally traumatic hypophysectomy often produces only transient diabetes insipidus. A thin layer of cells extends from the anterior lobe and encircles the pituitary stalk to form the pars tuberalis. Immunohistochemical data suggest that corticotropin cells (ACTH) are located in the midline in the anterior lobe, lactotrophs (prolactinomas) posterolaterally, somatotrophs (growth hormone) laterally, and thyrotrophs (rare thyroid secreting tumors) anteriorly.

The blood supply to the pituitary gland is derived primarily from the superior and inferior hypophysial arteries. The superior hypophysial artery originates from the paraclinoid internal carotid artery and perfuses the pituitary stalk and hypothalamus. The inferior hypophysial artery originates from the meningohypophysial trunk and supplies most of the pituitary gland. The venous drainage of the pituitary gland is a portal system that originates in the hypothalamus and drains into the cavernous sinus through the lateral hypophysial veins. The parasellar structures, including the cavernous sinus, optic chiasm, and carotid artery, are discussed in Chapter 1.

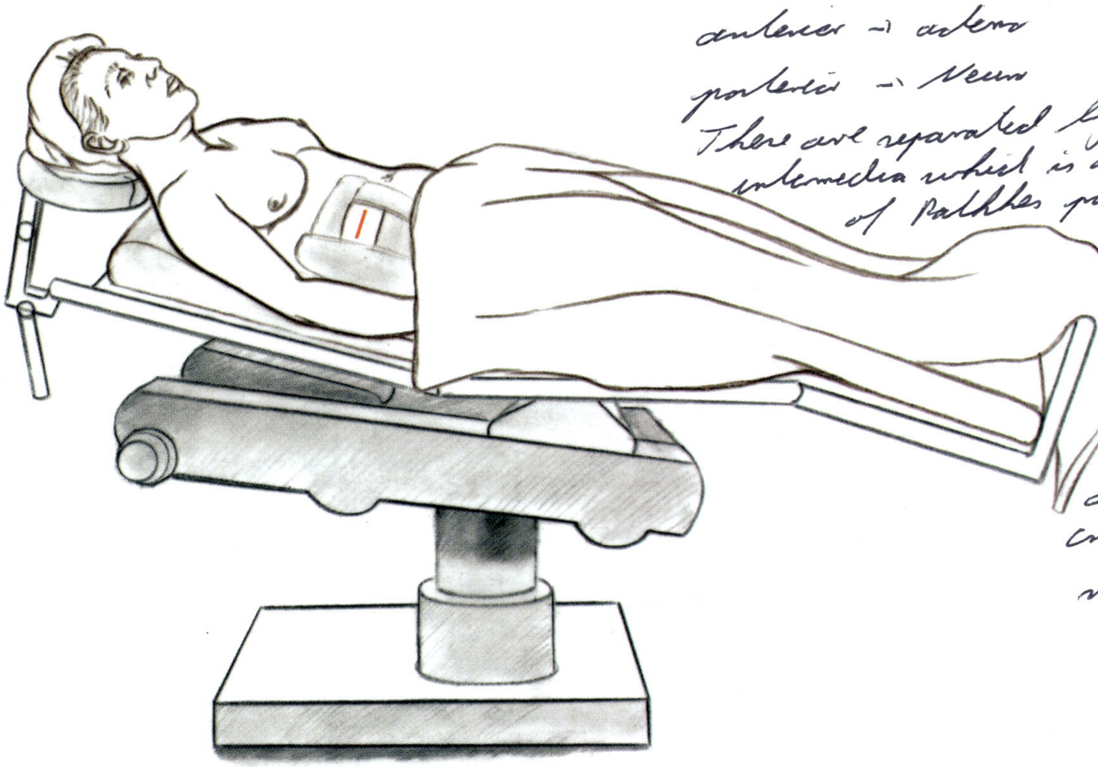

Figure 10–1.

For all transsphenoidal operations, the patient is positioned supine, with the operating table flexed and the patient's head supported in a horseshoe head rest. The horseshoe is advantageous over a rigid pinion system because it allows the head to be manipulated during the operation. The patient's nose should be parallel with the floor and angled approximately 30 to 45 degrees from the long axis of the body to allow the surgeon to stand comfortably and to rest his or her hands on the patient's chest. For large tumors with a suprasellar extension, a lumbar spinal drain can be placed for intraoperative injection of approximately 10 to 15 mL of air into the thecal sac. Because the patient's head is slightly elevated, the air ascends into the suprasellar cistern and helps displace the tumor downward into the operative field. The abdomen or right thigh is prepared for a possible fat or muscle graft.

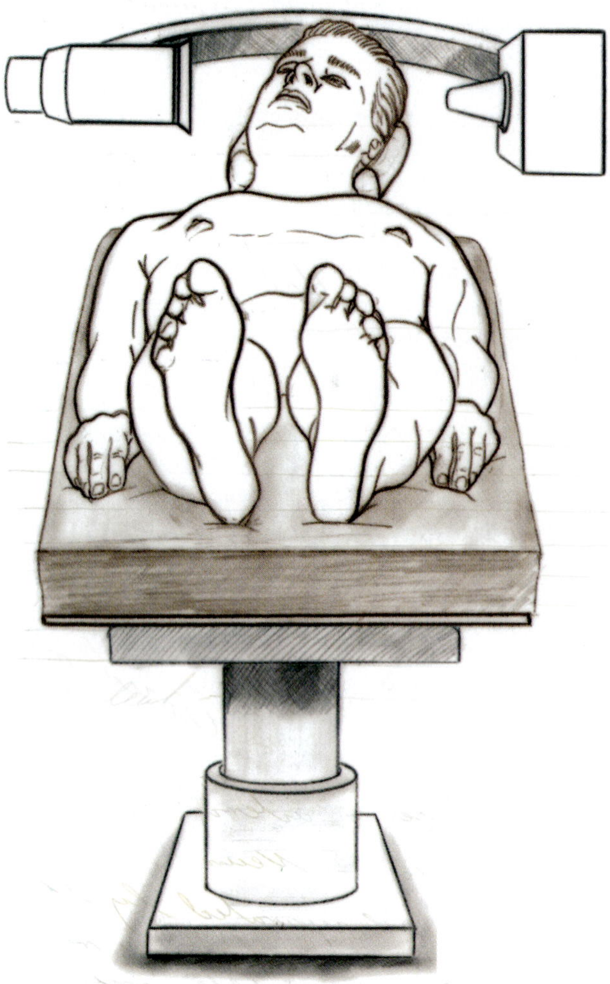

Figure 10–2.

It is important to use an image intensifier during the operation. It allows the neurosurgeon to confirm that the sella turcica has been reached through the transsphenoidal approach. With large tumors, the sella turcica is enlarged and thin and its identification is apparent; however, with microadenomas, it is less obvious. Radiographic confirmation of the pituitary floor is important before bone is removed. Inadvertent removal of the frontal fossa bone at the junction of the anterior sella turcica has the risk of cerebrospinal fluid leakage because the dura mater in that area is thin. Unplanned removal of the upper clivus carries a risk of neurovascular injury, bleeding from small venous sinuses, and cerebrospinal fluid leakage. The use of an intraoperative image intensifier also allows the surgeon to visualize the location of the ring curets during resection of the suprasellar component of the tumor.

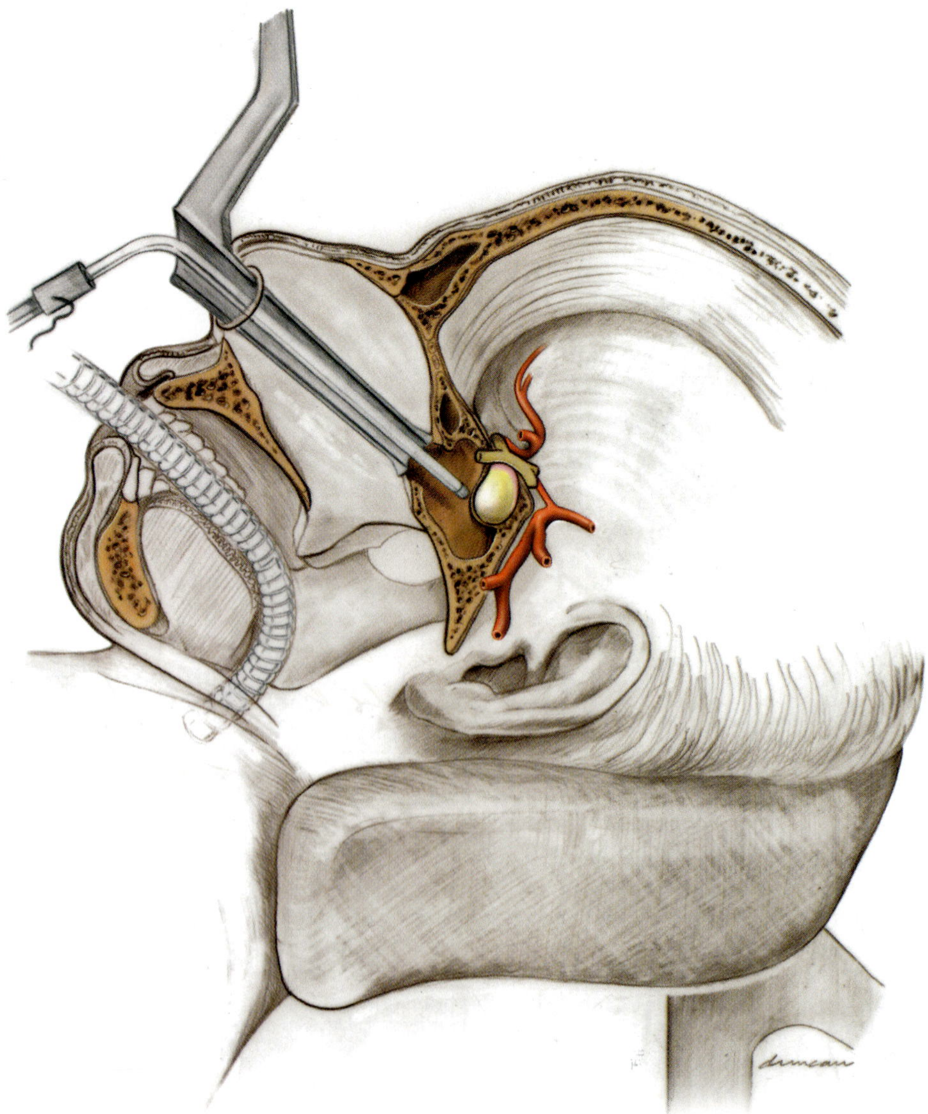

Figure 10–3.

This drawing illustrates the transnasal transsphenoidal approach to the sella turcica. The introduction of the endoscope has allowed resection through a transnasal approach instead of a sublabial approach. The transnasal approach has several advantages. There is no gingival incision or resection of the anterior nasal spine; therefore, there is less numbness of the upper teeth. Also, because the approach is less traumatic, the patient has less postoperative discomfort. A disadvantage of the transnasal route is that the approach is more angled and, thus, slightly crosscourt when working in the sella turcica. After the rostrum of the sphenoid sinus has been removed, a bivalved Hubbard or Hardy speculum is inserted. At this point, the operating microscope is brought into view. The rest of the lateral sphenoid sinus is removed to enhance exposure. Small bony septa and sinus mucosa are removed with a small bone punch. After this, the floor of the sella turcica is identified visually and confirmed on the image intensifier.

Figure 10–4.

There are several techniques for opening the floor of the sella turcica. If the floor is enlarged and thin, a microrongeur can be used to bite off the bone. Small angled Kerrison rongeurs can be used to enlarge the opening. If the sellar floor is not thin, a small chisel or high-speed air drill can be used to make the opening. In this illustration, a small chisel is used to make the initial cracks in the sellar floor. A bone forceps is used to crack off the initial body fragments, and an angled Kerrison is used to enlarge the bony removal. Regardless of the technique, it is mandatory to make sure that removal of the sellar floor is maximized. Specifically, it is important to remove the bone laterally as far as the junction of the sellar dura mater and the cavernous sinus and up to the junction with the floor of the frontal fossa. Similarly, it is important to remove bone down toward the clivus. Because most microadenomas are lateral, the lateral bony removal to the cavernous sinus is most important. Removal of the inferior floor down toward the clivus is necessary only for large macroadenomas or if hypophysectomy is planned.

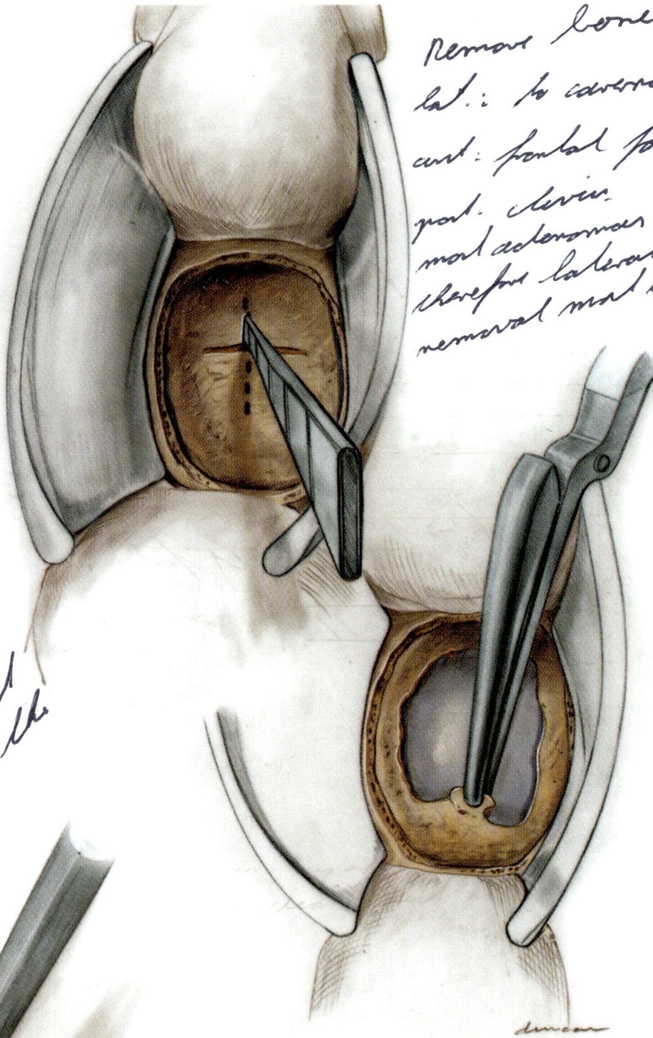

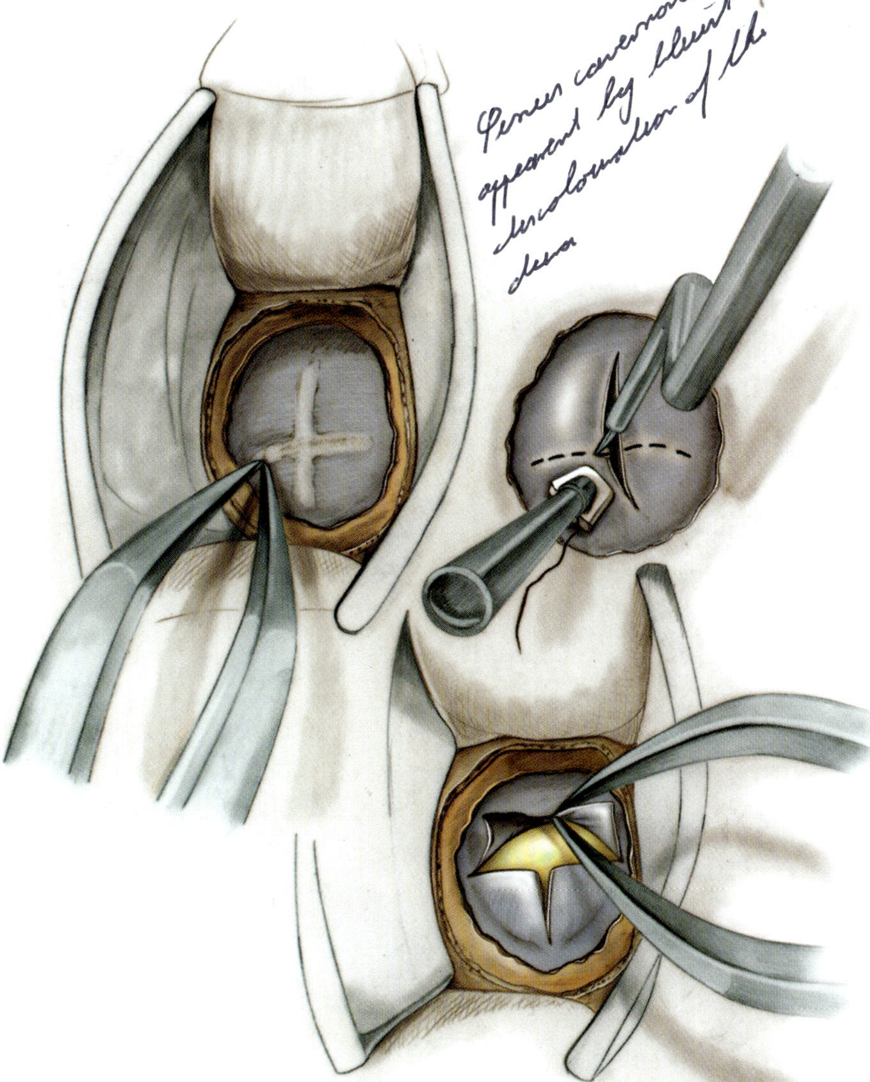

Figure 10–5.

After the floor of the sella turcica has been removed, the dura mater is cauterized with either a bipolar cautery or suction cautery. Occasionally, the tumor infiltrates or extends through the dura mater. It is important to cauterize up to the junction of the normal dura mater with the cavernous sinuses. Usually, the sinuses can be identified by a slight bluish discoloration of the dura mater. After the dura mater has been cauterized, an incision is made with a #11 blade knife and the dura mater is further cauterized. When incising the dura mater, it is important to stay 2 to 3 mm lateral to the apparent location of the cavernous sinuses. This safety margin will help decrease intraoperative venous bleeding. Sometimes bleeding occurs from venous sinuses at the junction of the dura mater and the bony removal. This bleeding usually can be controlled with small pieces of absorbable gelatin sponge (Gelfoam) placed under tamponade.

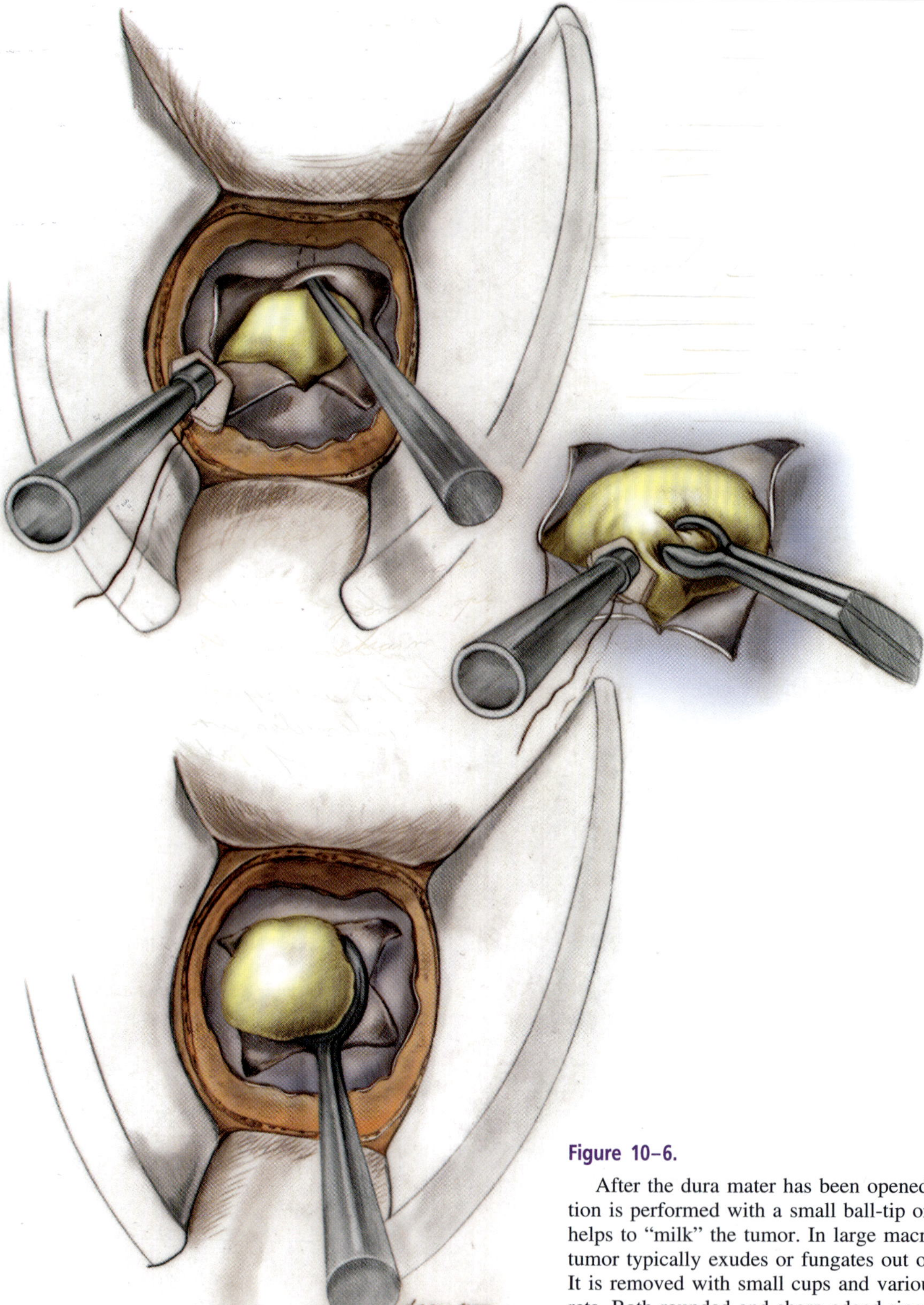

Figure 10–6.

After the dura mater has been opened, a subdural dissection is performed with a small ball-tip or flat dissector. This helps to "milk" the tumor. In large macroadenomas, the tumor typically exudes or fungates out of the dural opening. It is removed with small cups and various angled ring curets. Both rounded and sharp-edged ring curets can be used. Sharp-edged ring curets are good for cutting the tumor and scraping it off normal pituitary tissue.

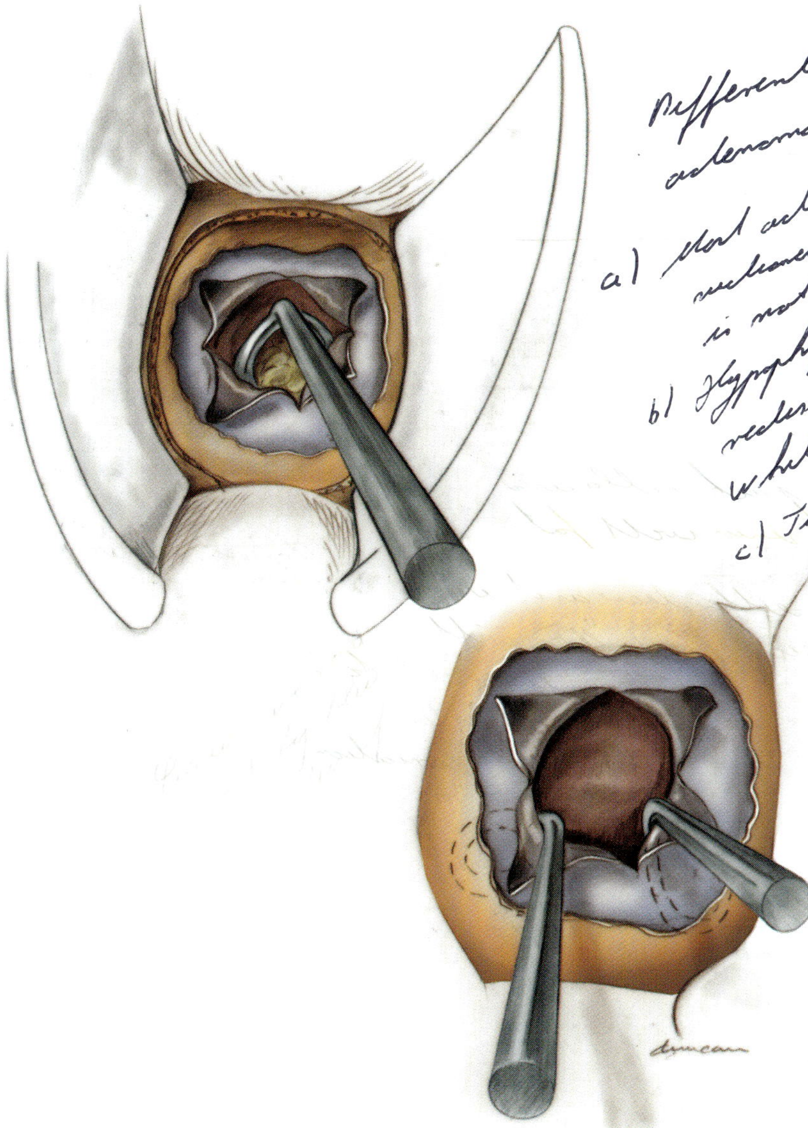

Figure 10–7.

As the tumor is removed, progressively larger ringed curets are used. It is important to explore methodically all recesses of the sella turcica. With large adenomas, large Vanderbilt ring curets can be used. The image intensifier is useful in confirming the location of the ringed curets, especially when the surgeon is above the clinoid process. Injection of 10 mL of air through the spinal needle helps to push the tumor down into the operative field. Most often, the tumor descends into the sella turcica without the injection of thecal air, because these tumors are usually under pressure and the dural opening creates an automatic route for decompression. When scraping tumor out of the lateral gutters, it is important to hold the ring curets gently between the thumb and index finger to avoid inadvertent entry into or injury to the cavernous sinus. Thickened, exposed dura mater should be cauterized. Because of the location of these macroadenomas, the pituitary gland is usually displaced rostrally. Therefore, as more tumor is removed, the pituitary gland descends into the pituitary fossa. Most macroadenomas are easily suctioned, but the normal gland is not. This can be an important technique for differentiating tumor from normal gland. Also, the normal gland has a more pinkish or reddish hue, whereas tumors are typically yellow-white. Furthermore, a thin layer of reactive tissue or fibrosis often occurs between the normal gland and the adenoma.

Figure 10–8.

After resection of large macroadenomas, it is prudent to reconstruct the floor of the sella turcica. If cerebrospinal fluid is leaking or oozing from the sella turcica, it is best to harvest an abdominal fat or thigh muscle graft and pack the sella. Importantly, the sella turcica should not be overly packed. Some surgeons advocate packing a large sella turcica even if there is no cerebrospinal fluid leak to prevent downward herniation of the optic chiasm. After the sella turcica has been packed, a piece of nasal cartilage is placed subdurally to reconstruct the sellar floor. With the transnasal approach, little cartilage is usually available for reconstruction. If there is a definite cerebrospinal fluid leak, it is best to pack the entire sphenoid sinus with abdominal fat.

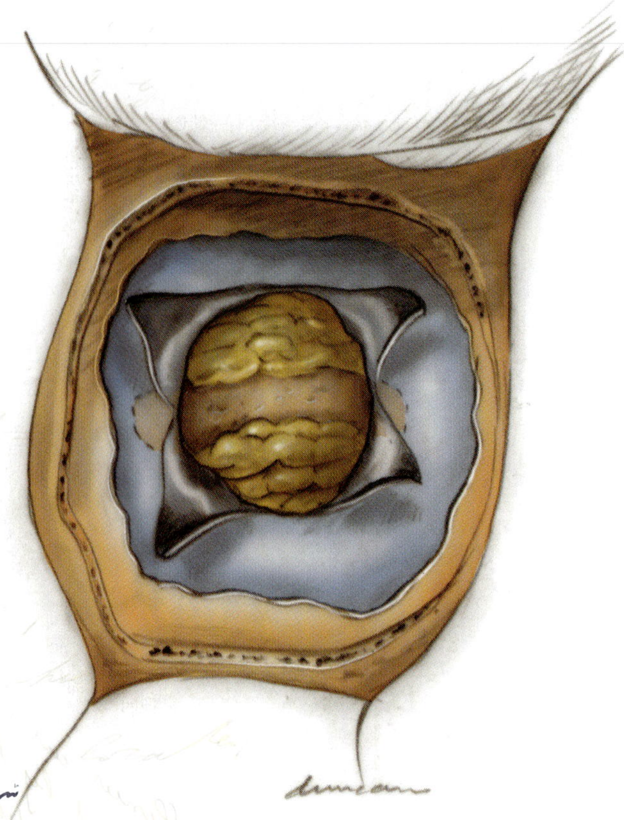

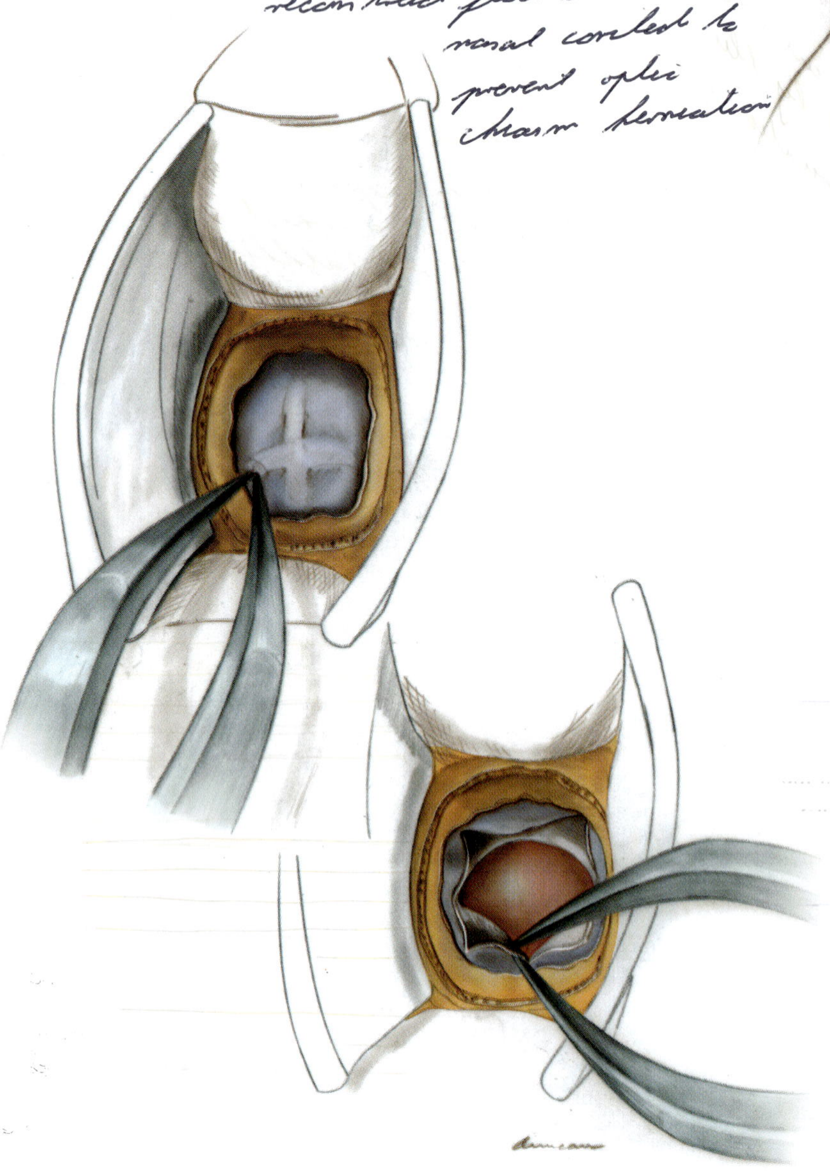

Figure 10–9.

Sequence for removal of a pituitary microadenoma. In contrast to macroadenomas, microadenomas usually do not cause enlargement of the sella turcica. Therefore, the surgeon has to work in a smaller space. Thorough study of the preoperative magnetic resonance images and biochemical data in Cushing's disease (if petrosal sinus sampling was performed) are helpful in developing an idea about where the tumor is located. After the bony floor has been removed, the dura mater is cauterized with a bipolar cautery and opened with a #11 blade knife and further cauterized. It is important to prevent heat injury to the normal pituitary gland when cauterizing the dura mater. Heat injury to the normal pituitary gland may make it more difficult to identify the adenoma. Some surgeons have reported the use of microultrasonography in locating microadenomas within the pituitary gland.

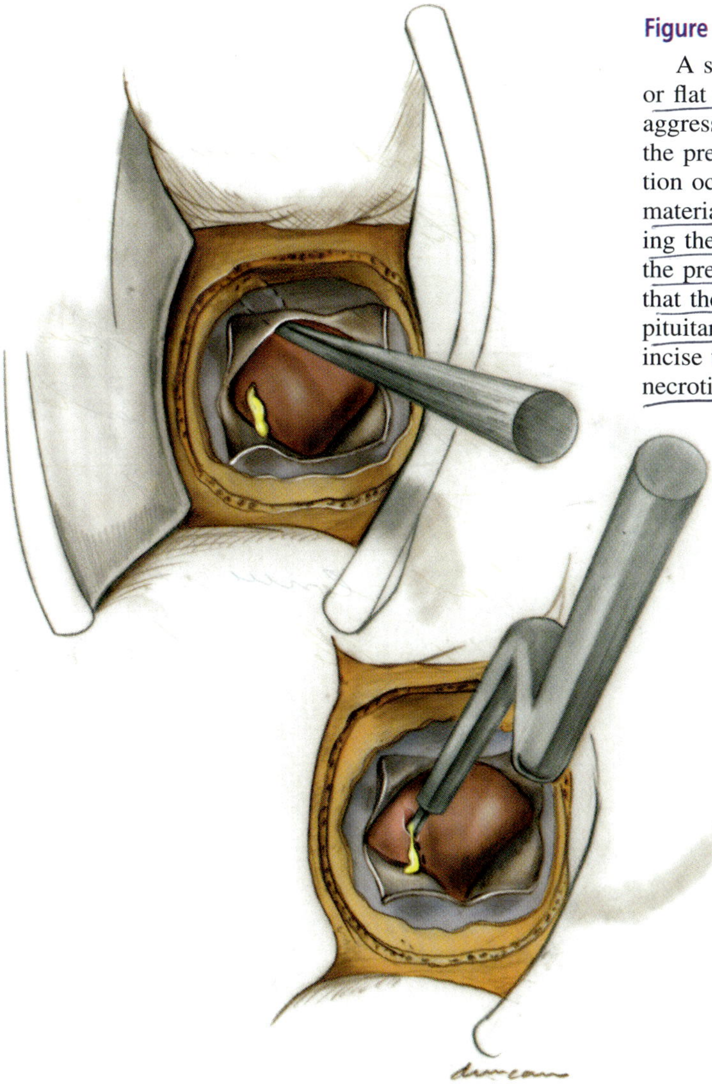

Figure 10–10.

A subdural dissection is performed with a small ball-tip or flat dissector. This helps to "milk out" the tumor. An aggressive subdural dissection can be useful in identifying the presence of a lateral microadenoma. The subdural dissection occasionally causes oozing of tumor exudate or necrotic material. This early visual identification is important in locating the site of the tumor. In the operation illustrated here, the preoperative magnetic resonance imaging study indicated that the tumor likely was located within the right side of the pituitary gland. Therefore, a #11 blade knife was used to incise the right lateral gland. This usually leads to oozing of necrotic tumor.

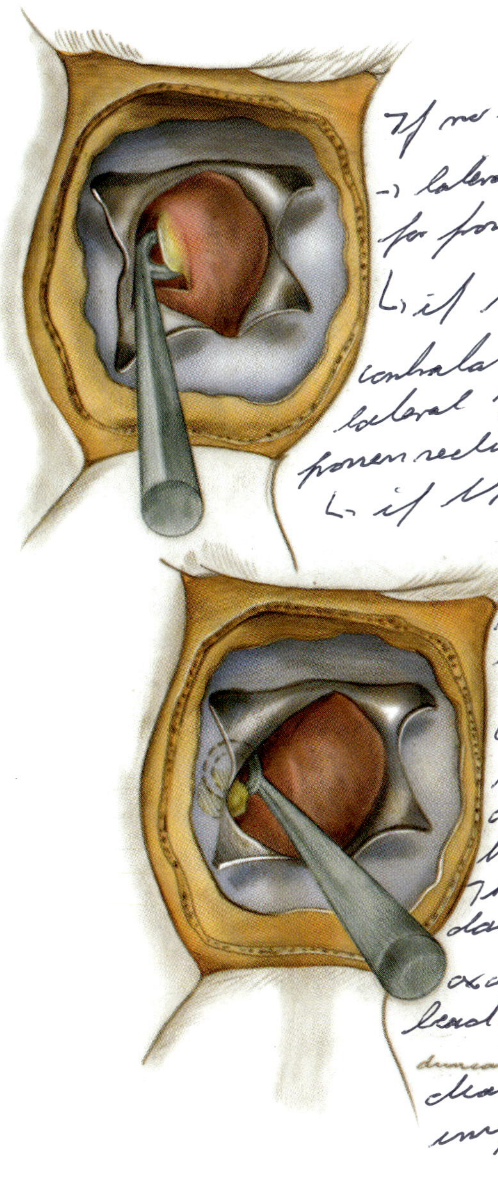

Figure 10–11.

After the tumor cavity has been identified, small curets are used to work within the tumor to debulk it. A sharp ring curet can be useful in peeling the tumor off its junction with normal pituitary tissue. For microadenomas that are located laterally, it is important to use ring curets to dissect the lateral gutter adjacent to the cavernous sinus. In patients with Cushing's disease, identification of the microadenoma may be a problem. However, an idea about where the tumor is located can be developed on the basis of preoperative imaging studies and petrosal sinus sampling. Therefore, the suspicious part of the pituitary gland should be incised first. If no obvious adenoma is identified, the lateral one-third of the pituitary should be removed en bloc and sent for pathologic examination of frozen sections. If no tumor is identified, an identical procedure should be performed with removal of the opposite lateral one-third of the pituitary. If neither side (one-third) of the pituitary contains tumor, an incision should be made in the midline to determine whether the adenoma is sitting in the midportion of the pituitary. If necessary, this remaining one-third of the pituitary can be removed to perform a hypophysectomy. When performing a hypophysectomy, it is important not to exert any downward traction on the middle third of the gland to prevent long-term injury to the infundibulum.

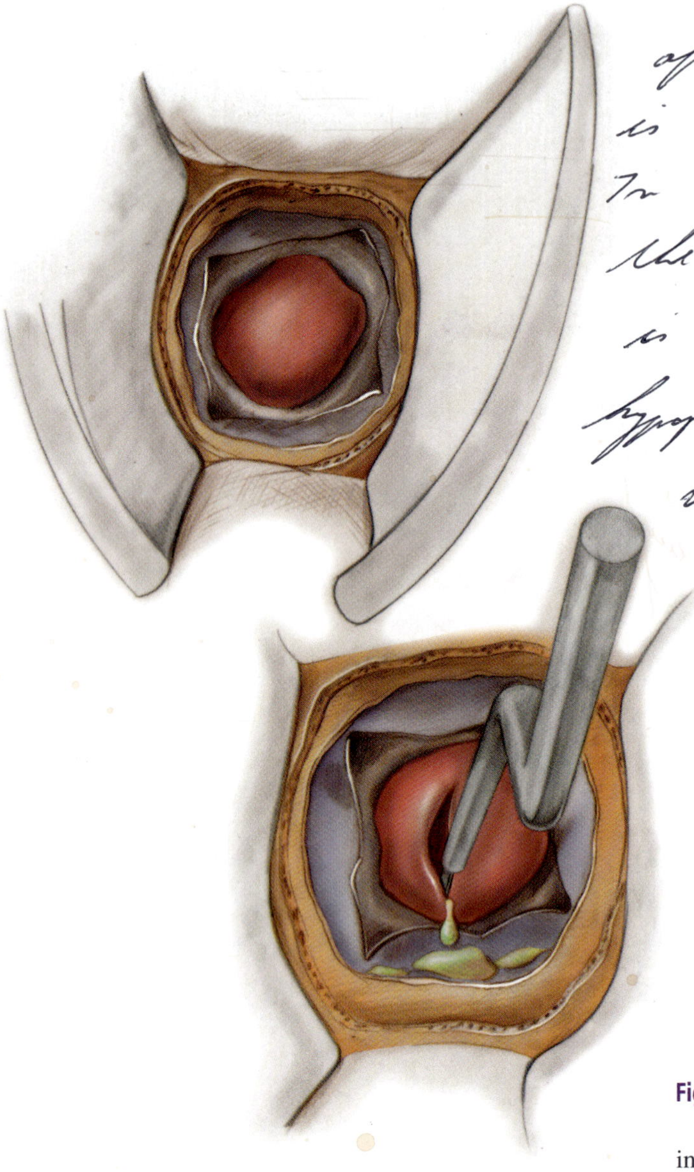

Figure 10–12.

Sequence for removal of a cyst of Rathke's cleft cyst or intrasellar craniopharyngioma. In both cases, the sella turcica is usually enlarged and the bony floor is thin. After the standard removal, the dura mater is cauterized and opened in a cruciate fashion. Whether a cyst or craniopharyngioma, the first tissue encountered is thin pituitary gland. Therefore, pituitary tissue sits between the surgeon and the lesion. The pituitary gland is incised vertically to encounter the cyst. The pituitary gland usually is no more than 2 to 3 mm thick. When the cyst is encountered, there is expression of xanthochromic fluid.

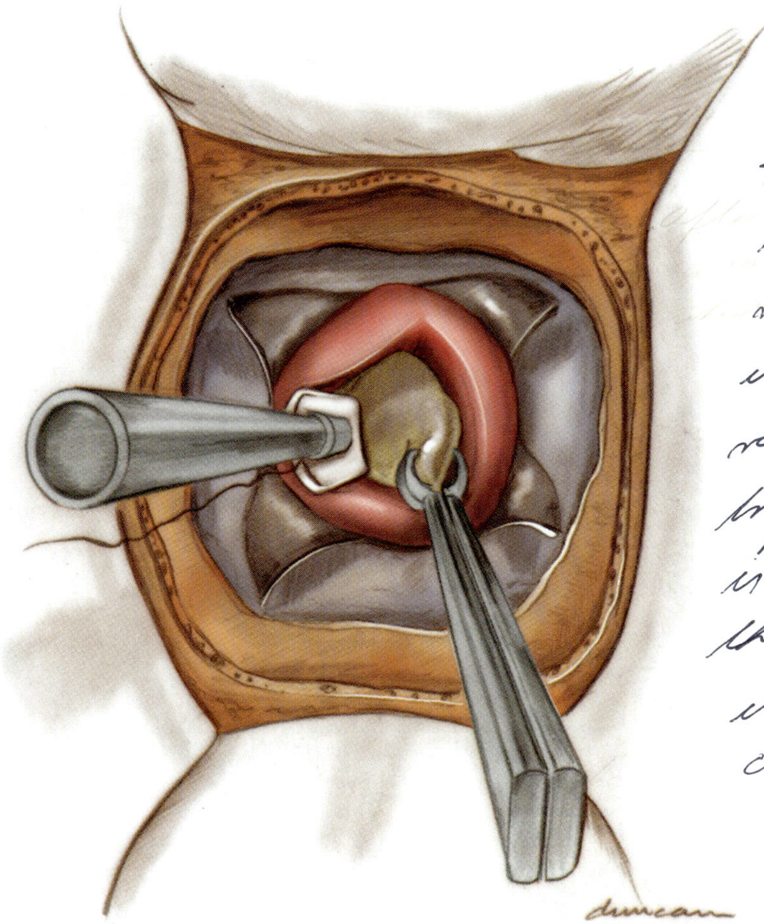

Figure 10–13.

After the cyst has been entered, the pituitary gland collapses into the operative field because of the decompression. Therefore, a suction tip and small cottonoid (Americot) are used to hold one wall open while the contents of the cyst are explored. The wall of a true cyst of Rathke's cleft is thicker than normal arachnoid. Parts of the cyst wall generally can be dissected off the normal pituitary gland with a long thin spatula or dissecting probe. Occasionally, the involved cyst is so thin that it cannot be removed without injuring the underlying pituitary gland. In this case, it is best to leave those small filament attachments alone. When exploring the interior of a cyst of Rathke's cleft, it is important to look for any grumous, yellowish firm material. The presence of this material suggests that the tumor is in fact a craniopharyngioma. Any solid tissue or tumor should be removed with small ring curets and punches.

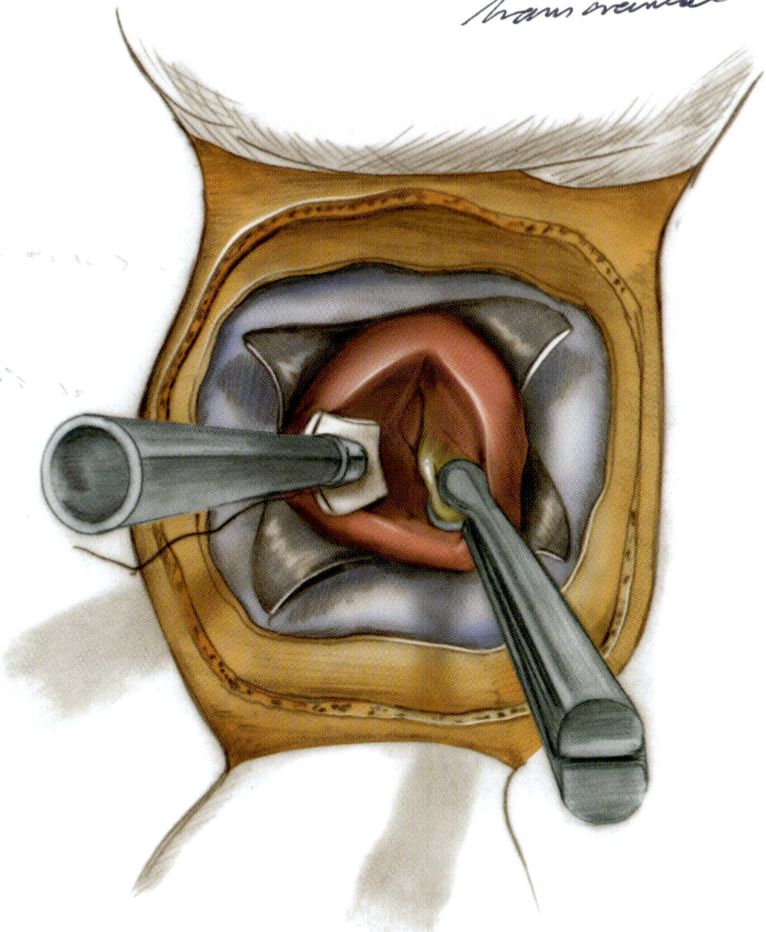

Figure 10–14.

The entire contents of the cyst should be examined to make sure there is no solid tissue. Small malleable endoscopes may be useful in this regard. With intrasellar craniopharyngiomas, the capsule is often adherent to the diaphragma sellae and pituitary stalk, requiring sharp dissection. With intrasellar craniopharyngiomas or a cyst of Rathke's cleft, there is often a cerebrospinal fluid leak. Therefore, it is necessary to pack the sella turcica with abdominal fat and to reconstruct the sellar floor. It also is necessary to pack the sphenoid sinus with abdominal fat, especially if a future transcranial resection of a craniopharyngioma is anticipated. It can be difficult to control postoperative rhinorrhea if a patient undergoes a cranial approach after a transsphenoidal procedure unless the pituitary fossa and the sphenoid sinus have been adequately packed.

11

Extracranial Vascular Approaches

Copyright © 1999 Mayo Foundation.

EXPOSURE OF THE CAROTID ARTERY

A curvilinear incision along the anterior border of the sternocleidomastoid muscle is used to expose the common carotid artery. The top of the incision curves posteriorly approximately 1.5 cm underneath the mastoid process. The lower end of the incision curves anteriorly 2 to 3 cm above the clavicle, usually along a fold of skin. The skin incision is made with a scalpel and extended through the platysma muscle. This skin incision usually severs the transverse cervical nerve, which can be relatively large in some patients. Sectioning of this nerve leads to numbness anterior to the skin incision underneath the mandible. Several small arteries tend to run through the platysma muscle. Hemostasis throughout this operation is achieved best with a bipolar cautery. Use of bipolar instead of monopolar current decreases the risk of injury to cranial nerves and blood vessels. Because heparin will be administered to the patient, it is best to spend several minutes using the bipolar cautery to cauterize small arteries along the platysma and the underside of the skin margin. It usually is not necessary to use skin clips or hemostats.

The surgeon and assistant retract the two edges of the skin incision with sponges. A scalpel is used to carry the incision deeper throughout its length to identify the anterior border of the sternocleidomastoid muscle. The upper end of the omohyoid muscle is also identified. The angle formed by the sternocleidomastoid muscle and the omohyoid muscle points to the common carotid artery. With dissecting scissors, the deeper relatively avascular fascia between the sternocleidomastoid muscle and the trachea is incised and spread to identify the artery. At this point, fishhook retractors are placed throughout the length of the incision, both medially and laterally. The fishhooks should be placed to grab the fascia that envelops both the trachea and the sternocleidomastoid muscle, thus retracting these structures medially and laterally, respectively. Here, the dissecting scissors are used to incise the deep cervical fascia on top of the common carotid artery up toward its bifurcation.

It is critical when exposing the common carotid artery to dissect on top of it. The surgeon should not dissect medially because of possible injury to the recurrent laryngeal nerve. At the level of the bifurcation of the common carotid artery, the surgeon should never work medial to the superior thyroid artery. When dissecting the proximal common carotid artery, it is important to clear the underside of the artery to facilitate placement of vascular loops. However, one should not dissect underneath the bifurcation of the common carotid artery because of the possibility of dislodging emboli or of injuring the superior laryngeal nerve. Leaving the underside of the bifurcation attached to the deep cervical fascia decreases the risk of these two complications.

At or just above the level of the bifurcation of the common carotid artery, the facial vein is identified. It should be dissected sharply free to make sure that the hypoglossal nerve is not hidden along its backside. Thereafter, the facial vein is doubly ligated and divided.

It can be useful to identify the descending hypoglossal nerve and to follow it proximally to the hypoglossal nerve. The descending hypoglossal nerve can be severed close to its junction with the hypoglossal nerve to allow better mobilization of the hypoglossal nerve distally. The superior thyroid artery is identified at the level of the bifurcation of the common carotid artery. A temporary hemostatic clip can be placed on this structure.

With sharp scissors, the external carotid artery is dissected free from the medial carotid sinus. Approximately 1 to 2 cm above the bifurcation of the common carotid artery, the external carotid artery gives off several branches, including the facial and occipital arteries. A vascular loop is placed around the proximal trunk of the external carotid artery. The surgeon then identifies the medial aspect of the internal carotid artery and frees it from the carotid sinus. Sharp scissors are used to dissect the distal internal carotid artery above the bifurcation of the common carotid artery by at least 3.0 cm. For a carotid endarterectomy, the surgeon can gently palpate the internal carotid artery and determine where the atherosclerotic plaque ends. Occasionally, the plaque can be visualized under magnification. In either case, it is best to have at least 1.0 cm of the internal carotid artery free above the presumed end of the plaque to facilitate placement of a shunt if one is needed. As the dissection is carried distally under the angle of the jaw, the fishhook retractors are placed under more tension. This tends to lift the carotid artery complex up out of the wound. The dissection usually is carried to the belly of the digastric muscle.

The tissue above the bifurcation of the common carotid artery between the external and internal carotid arteries contains the nerves that innervate the carotid body and the carotid sinus. Injecting approximately 1.0 mL of 1 percent lidocaine into this tissue helps to decrease the side effects of excessive stimulation of the carotid sinus, including fluctuations in blood pressure and cardiac rhythm. It is best to look between this neural sheath and the medial side of the external carotid artery to determine whether an ascending pharyngeal artery originates from the backside of the bifurcation of the common carotid artery. If this artery is present, a temporary hemostatic clip is used to occlude it.

At this point in the operation, two vascular loops are placed around the common carotid artery and one around the external carotid artery. The author prefers not to place any vascular loops around the distal internal carotid artery. After the loops have been placed, the surgeon must again determine whether the dissection has been extended far enough distally. Typically, increased exposure can be obtained by using blunt dissection with the finger and developing the plane between the anterior border of the sternocleidomastoid muscle and the parotid gland underneath the angle of the jaw. The fishhooks can be placed deeper into the belly of the sternocleidomastoid muscle close to its junction with the parotid gland. Occasionally, additional exposure is required.

EXPOSURE OF THE DISTAL INTERNAL CAROTID ARTERY

Exposure of the distal internal carotid artery is an important ancillary technique that can be useful in performing a complex carotid endarterectomy, in which the bifurcation of the common carotid artery is high or the atherosclerotic plaque has a distal extension. It also is important to expose the distal internal carotid artery close to the base of the skull when operating on extracranial aneurysms of the internal carotid artery or large tumors of the carotid body. During high exposures, the cranial nerves at risk include the facial, glossopharyngeal, vagus, and hypoglossal nerves. Careful anatomic dissection of the distal internal carotid artery minimizes injury to these functionally important cranial nerves.

In exposing the distal internal carotid artery, the following three points are important. One, it is useful to have the patient intubated nasally. This allows the mouth to be closed, which increases exposure under the angle of the jaw by approximately 1.0 to 1.5 cm. Although some surgeons report planned dislocation of the mandible during high exposures, this has not been necessary in the author's experience. Two, it is important to have the anesthesiologist prepared to use induced hypertension during cross-clamping of the internal carotid artery. With very high exposures, as for large aneurysms, placing the shunt beyond the lesion at the base of the skull may not be technically feasible. Induced hypertension can be a valuable technique in providing cerebral protection during cross-clamping by increasing collateral blood flow. Three, use of the operating microscope is important during high dissections. Both illumination and magnification are essential in minimizing injury to the cranial nerves. Because the operative field can become cluttered, self-retaining retractors will compromise the exposure. Accordingly, fishhooks are useful not only for optimizing exposure but for preventing injury to the lower cranial nerves from excessive retraction.

The lower part of the skin incision parallels the anterior border of the sternocleidomastoid muscle and curves posteriorly just underneath the earlobe. The superior portion of the incision sits in the postauricular sulcus around the earlobe and ascends in a pretragal skin crease in front of the ear. In rare cases, the incision extends up to the zygoma, which allows complete mobilization of the parotid gland and the facial nerve. This incision results in a triangular bend underneath the ear and allows for better alignment of the incision at closure.

The initial exposure is described in the preceding section. The descending hypoglossal nerve is followed rostrally to identify the hypoglossal nerve. Because the hypoglossal nerve will be retracted upward and medially under the mandible, the descending hypoglossal nerve must be severed. It is best to leave a good stump of this nerve branch because a suture can be placed through it into the submandibular fascia to retract the hypoglossal nerve. Occasionally, a muscular branch of the occipital artery that supplies the sternocleidomastoid muscle can be identified. Because this muscular branch can tether the hypoglossal nerve, it may be beneficial to doubly ligate and divide this artery as it sweeps over the superior margin of the hypoglossal nerve, thus facilitating displacement of the nerve.

Next, the sternocleidomastoid muscle is dissected rostrally, often bluntly, with the surgeon's finger. This better defines the border between the anterior edge of the sternocleidomastoid muscle and the caudal edge of the parotid gland. There is some loose fascia that is relatively avascular; it can easily be divided with dissecting scissors. At this point, the digastric muscle usually is seen along the upper margins of the operative exposure. Depending on the degree of exposure required, the digastric muscle can be retracted upward with either an Army-Navy type retractor or a self-retaining Henley retractor. If a higher exposure is required, the digastric muscle must be divided. The digastric muscle should be followed to its insertion in the mastoid groove and divided there. However, before this muscle is ligated, it is important to make sure that the main trunk of the facial nerve is not compromised. The stylohyoid muscle, which lies superior and parallel to the digastric muscle, can also be divided, which exposes the deeper stylomandibular ligament. This deeper stylomandibular ligament also can be resected to increase exposure of the internal carotid artery at the base of the skull.

Before the digastric and stylohyoid muscles are ligated, it is useful to identify the facial nerve. Accordingly, the incision at the lower end in front of the ear is made and extended caudally to connect with the incision in front of the sternocleidomastoid muscle. Deep to this incision, the parotid gland is identified in its enveloping fascia. Several hemostats or an Army-Navy retractor can be placed on the parotid gland and used as retraction by the surgeon's assistant. The posterior border of the parotid gland is exposed further and elevated. The anteroinferior surface of the tragus is followed deep to the medial triangular projection of cartilage. This deep cartilaginous projection "points" to the facial nerve. The parotid fascia is incised further between the mastoid process and the posterior margin of the parotid gland. Placement of the surgeon's finger on the mastoid tip directed anteriorly and forward points to and overlies the main trunk of the facial nerve. After the main trunk of the facial nerve has been identified, the lower division and the marginal mandibular nerve, which form the upper limit of the deep dissection, can be traced forward by sharp dissection and safely elevated by using the mobilized parotid tissue. At this point, the digastric and stylohyoid muscles can be ligated safely. Sectioning of the stylomandibular ligaments facilitates displacement of the mandible medially. Additional distal exposure of the internal carotid artery can be achieved by removing the styloid process with a small rongeur.

The Facial Nerve

The facial nerve exits the base of the skull through the stylomastoid foramen and travels forward and laterally into the parotid gland. It lies superior to the digastric muscle and, thus, can easily be damaged. Before the digastric muscle is ligated, it is necessary to identify the main trunk of the facial nerve. This is why it is essential to dissect the fascia between the parotid gland and the sternocleidomastoid muscle adjacent to the mastoid process. Placing fishhooks in the submandibular fascia and the parotid gland during prolonged operations helps limit injury to the marginal mandibular branch of the facial nerve.

The Glossopharyngeal Nerve

The glossopharyngeal nerve contains important sensory fibers of the soft palate and the oropharynx. Damage to the branches of this nerve may result in the patient having difficulty initiating swallowing. Small filaments from the glossopharyngeal and the vagus nerves to the pharynx are sometimes anterior and lateral to the internal carotid artery.

The Vagus Nerve

The pharyngeal branch of the vagus nerve exits from the trunk of the nerve at the level of the first cervical vertebra. It enters the superior constrictor muscle of the pharynx and supplies all the muscles of the pharynx and the soft palate except the stylopharyngeus and the tensor palati muscles. These motor branches leave the vagus nerve and course laterally and deep to the external carotid artery, well above the bifurcation of the common carotid artery. Therefore, during a typical carotid endarterectomy, they are never visualized. However, they are at risk during an operation for a large aneurysm of the cervical internal carotid artery or a carotid body tumor. The branches of these nerves are quite small, and they may be either anterior or posterior to the internal carotid artery.

The superior laryngeal nerve leaves the vagus nerve at the lower margin of the first cervical vertebra and descends. It is medial to both the internal and the external carotid arteries. The superior laryngeal nerve divides into an internal and an external branch. The internal branch is sensory and innervates the mucus membrane covering the epiglottis and the portion of the larynx above the vocal cords. The external branch is motor and innervates the cricothyroid muscle and the inferior constrictor muscle of the pharynx. Damage to the superior laryngeal nerve results in marked difficulty with swallowing because the patient is unaware of food particles lodged in and around the area of the epiglottis and because there is partial weakness of the inferior constrictor muscle of the pharynx and unilateral paralysis of the cricopharyngeus muscle (which allows the opposite cricopharyngeus muscle to distort the normal position of the cricoid cartilage). The superior laryngeal nerve can be injured during a routine carotid endarterectomy when the surgeon dissects underneath the bifurcation of the common carotid artery. Therefore, it is best not to mobilize underneath this bifurcation, not only to help prevent injury to the superior laryngeal nerve but also to decrease the risk of emboli from excessive mobilization. The superior laryngeal nerve also can be injured if the surgeon dissects medial to the superior thyroid artery.

Superiorly, the primary trunk of the vagus nerve descends between the internal carotid artery and the internal jugular vein, and inferiorly, between the common carotid artery and the internal jugular vein. In most patients, the vagus nerve is posterior to the artery and vein and, thus, is rarely injured. Occasionally, the vagus nerve can have a wandering course and be anterior to the carotid artery. It also can originate from the hypoglossal nerve and be confused with the descending hypoglossal nerve. Accordingly, any large nerve on top of the common carotid artery should be preserved and protected.

The recurrent branch of the vagus nerve is never visualized during a routine exposure of the internal carotid artery. It ascends between the trachea and the esophagus. On the right side, the recurrent branch arises from the vagus at the base of the neck in front of the right subclavian artery. It then loops around this artery (passing below and behind the artery) and runs superiorly and medially, crossing obliquely behind the common carotid artery to gain access to the groove between the trachea and the esophagus, where it ascends to the lower border of the cricoid cartilage. At this point, the recurrent branch of the vagus nerve becomes the inferior laryngeal nerve and innervates many of the intrinsic muscles of the larynx. Damage to the recurrent laryngeal nerve leads to unilateral paralysis of the vocal cords and hoarseness.

The Spinal Accessory Nerve

The spinal accessory nerve is identified adjacent to the jugular vein as it descends over the transverse process of the first cervical vertebra and disappears into the deep surface of the sternocleidomastoid muscle. Thus, this nerve has a medial to lateral course. While the sternocleidomastoid muscle is dissected off the mastoid process during a high internal carotid artery exposure, the spinal accessory nerve can be injured. Damage to this nerve leads to paralysis of the sternocleidomastoid and the trapezius muscles. Injury to the trapezius muscle leads to a partial shoulder drop and painful bursitis.

The Hypoglossal Nerve

As indicated above, the hypoglossal nerve can be mobilized rostrally after the descending hypoglossal nerve has been severed. This stump can be used to manipulate the hypoglossal nerve; it even can be tacked to the fascia underneath the mandible for improved exposure. Occasionally, the artery to the sternocleidomastoid muscle must be severed to allow the hypoglossal nerve to be displaced distally.

The Great Auricular Nerve

The cervical plexus has three major sensory nerves: the occipital nerve, the great auricular nerve, and the transverse cervical nerve. The great auricular nerve and the transverse cervical nerve enter the subcutaneous tissue by piercing the external cervical fascia along the posterior border of the sternocleidomastoid muscle. The transverse cervical nerve usually is cut during the skin incision, and this may result in patchy numbness along the incision. The great auricular nerve is encountered during the distal exposure when the parotid gland is mobilized. Severing the great auricular nerve leads to numbness of the earlobe. Depending on the location of this nerve in relation to the incision, it often can be dissected and mobilized. However, necessary exposure of the distal internal carotid artery should not be compromised by the anatomic preservation of the great auricular nerve. The cervical plexus contributes to the ansa cervicalis. The ansa hypoglossi supplies the motor innervation to the deep muscles of the neck. These branches usually are severed during exposure of the carotid artery without any resulting sequelae.

Carotid Endarterectomy

Approximately 3 minutes before the common carotid artery is cross-clamped, 5,000 units of heparin are administered intravenously. Also, the anesthesiologist is asked to use induced hypertension to increase the patient's systolic blood pressure to approximately 170 to 180 mm Hg. This induced hypertension facilitates collateral blood flow and significantly decreases the risk of cross-clamp ischemia and the need for a shunt. After time has been allowed for the heparin to circulate, the common carotid artery is occluded as low as the dissection permits with one "click" of a soft-shoe Fogarty clamp. Before the common carotid artery is occluded, it is important for the surgeon to palpate this vessel with the thumb and index finger to try to determine whether the clamp can be placed below any obvious atherosclerotic plaque in the common carotid artery. The external carotid artery is occluded by placing tension on the vascular loop or by using a temporary aneurysm clip. A small temporary aneurysm clip is placed across the distal internal carotid artery as far as the exposure will allow. These temporary aneurysm clips have a closing pressure of approximately 75 to 100 g. Use of a higher pressure closing clip has the risk of injuring the intima of the distal internal carotid artery.

The common carotid artery is opened with a stab wound made with a #11 blade knife. A Potts scissors is used to carry the incision distally through the bifurcation of the common carotid artery into the internal carotid artery above the level of the atherosclerotic plaque. It is important to extend the arteriotomy in the middle of the vessel instead of veering off to one side, which makes closure of the arteriotomy more difficult. After the initial arteriotomy, a small suction tip is used to remove blood in the lumen. The atherosclerotic plaque is inspected under magnification. It usually is necessary to extend the arteriotomy further, both distally and proximally, to expose completely the upper and lower ends of the lesion. In many patients, the plaque extends well down toward the aortic arch; therefore, clinical judgment must be used to determine how low the plaque is removed from the common carotid artery.

The atherosclerotic plaque is removed with a small spatula. Typically, the plane between the atherosclerotic plaque and the underlying intima can be identified along the medial or lateral side adjacent to the bifurcation of the common carotid artery. By using the spatula in a gentle back and forth motion along the long axis of the artery, the plaque is freed from the underlying intima. Usually, the plaque feathers free or breaks cleanly from the intima of the distal internal carotid artery. In some cases, the plaque blends imperceptibly with the intima distally. In these situations, a small incision with a microscissors is used to start the break. The break then can be continued by a peeling action of the plaque, with countertraction applied against the wall of the vessel. In most cases, the best separation of the plaque from the intima involves a tearing instead of a cutting motion. After a good separation of the plaque from the distal internal carotid artery has been achieved, the dissection is carried down along the common carotid artery.

After the atherosclerotic plaque has been removed from the internal carotid artery, the dissection is carried proximally along the lateral wall of the common carotid artery to the point that the surgeon thinks it is best to end plaque resection, at which place the plaque is incised with a Potts scissors. This is carried circumferentially around to the medial side of the common carotid artery. The spatula is used to dissect the plaque off the medial wall of the common carotid artery up to its bifurcation.

It is important to obtain good removal of the atherosclerotic plaque up the external carotid artery to prevent retrograde stump emboli. This is achieved best by using the spatula to work up the external carotid artery circumferentially around the plaque. The vascular loop is loosened gently and a hemostat is placed up in the external carotid artery as far as possible to grasp the plaque. In a simultaneous motion, the external carotid artery is everted and the hemostat is used to pull the plaque down, ideally obtaining a clean break in the distal external carotid artery. After the plaque has been removed, the entire endarterectomy bed is inspected meticulously for small flaps. Irrigation with a heparin solution usually will cause these small filaments to float upward, allowing better visualization and removal. It is important to use magnification to ensure that the endarterectomy bed is as smooth as possible. Again, the distal endarterectomy bed and its junction with the internal carotid artery are inspected to make sure there are no flaps or loose filamentous attachments, which can be the source of thrombus formation and emboli.

It should be emphasized that the complete atherosclerotic plaque up the distal internal carotid artery must be removed during the endarterectomy. It is common to find a subintimal extension of the plaque along the posterior wall of the artery. Strict attention to the plane between the plaque and the intima facilitates removal of the plaque from its subendothelial layer and the distal internal carotid artery. If after the plaque has been removed there is a ledge or concern about possible future flap formation, 6-0 double-arm monofilament sutures are used as tack sutures. They are placed from the interior of the vessel to the exterior. Use of double-arm instead of single sutures allows better placement of these tacking sutures, without stenosing the distal internal carotid artery.

Shunt Placement

Currently, the role of monitoring and the use of shunts are a matter of controversy. The author believes that continuous monitoring with intraoperative electroencephalography and selective shunting significantly decrease the risk of intraoperative ischemic complications. The criterion used for placement of a shunt is a significant electroencephalographic change, which occurs in approximately 10 percent of patients who undergo carotid endarterectomy. It is safe to place the shunt, if needed, after the plaque has been removed. This allows for better plaque removal and easier shunt placement. The shunt is placed by inserting it into the common carotid artery and securing it with two vascular loops. The Fogarty clamp is removed temporarily, allowing the shunt to be flushed. The common carotid artery is reoccluded, and the shunt is inserted into the internal carotid artery. After the shunt has been inserted into the internal carotid artery, it is secured with a Sundt-Kees clip graft. Thereafter, flow is restored up the shunt. Typically, within 1 to 2 minutes after the shunt has been placed, the electroencephalogram should normalize. If a significant electroencephalographic change persists, strong consideration should be given to performing intraoperative angiography through the shunt to determine whether there is an embolus in the middle cerebral artery.

Arteriotomy Closure

If the surgeon prefers, the vessel can be closed primarily with a running 6-0 monofilament suture. Clearly, the primary closure should be performed with magnification to avoid stenosis of the vessel because of incorporation of too much vessel wall in the suturing.

If the surgeon prefers to close with either a fabric or saphenous vein patch graft, it is sewn in place with a double-arm running 5-0 monofilament suture. The first stitch is placed through the distal end of the graft and arteriotomy up the internal carotid artery. This stitch is tied together with three overhand knots. One end of the monofilament suture is tagged to provide some countertraction. The other stitch is used to carefully anastomose the graft to the internal carotid artery. The first five or so stitches should be placed accurately to allow good taper of the graft to the internal carotid artery. These sutures should be approximately 1 mm deep and 1 mm apart. Each suture should purchase a full thickness of the intima and the vessel wall. Also, the suture should also go from inside the vessel to the outside to allow eversion of the suture line to the luminal surface. Accordingly, one suture line is performed largely with a backhand stitch. After the anastomosis is down into the common carotid artery, the backhand stitch can be rotated to allow a forehand suture from the abluminal to the luminal surface if desired. All sutures should be parallel, with an equal purchase of artery and graft, to prevent any irregularities along the suture line, which possibly could serve as a source of thrombus formation. As the graft approaches the proximal arteriotomy along the common carotid artery, it is tailored to provide a better fit. When sewing the graft to the artery, it is important to use these graft sutures as tacking sutures to secure the proximal plaque along the common carotid artery to the wall of the vessel. If a saphenous vein is used as a patch, it is best to reinforce it with a thin sheet of polytef (Teflon) to prevent formation of a pseudoaneurysm. Alternatively, if a synthetic expanded polytetrafluoroethylene (Gore-Tex) graft is used, a reinforcing polytef graft is not required.

Restoring Flow

Just before the closure of the arteriotomy is completed, the common carotid artery must be occluded if a shunt has been placed. The distal securing clip is loosened, and the shunt is removed. A temporary clip is placed again on the internal carotid artery, and then the final sutures in the arteriotomy are placed.

The last suture is kept loose to allow for back bleeding. The sequence of back bleeding and restoring flow is critical in preventing emboli. First, the clip is removed temporarily from the internal carotid artery to allow back bleeding from this vessel. After several seconds of back bleeding, the clip is reapplied. Second, the Fogarty clamp is loosened gently to allow bleeding up through the site of the last few stitches of the arteriotomy closure. After several seconds of bleeding up the common carotid artery, the Fogarty clamp is reapplied. Third, the clip on the internal carotid artery is again removed temporarily to allow for a final back bleeding. After this clip has been reapplied, the monofilament suture is tied. In tying the suture, a gentle force is used to tighten the entire suture line. Before flow is restored, the anesthesiologist is directed to reduce systolic blood pressure to 150 mm Hg to decrease the risk of hyperperfusion. Flow is restored, first, by removing the Fogarty clamp and, second, by loosening the vascular loop on the external carotid artery. During this time, the internal carotid artery is occluded. Accordingly, any loose fragments or emboli in the common carotid artery are flushed up the external carotid artery. After blood flow has been restored up the external carotid artery for 1 or 2 minutes, the clip is removed from the internal carotid artery. During this reperfusion period, the anesthesiologist is requested to palpate the pulse of the temporal artery by the ear. A good pulse means that the external carotid artery is patent. However, the absence of a pulse suggests there is an intimal flap in the distal external carotid artery. In this case, it is best to explore the external carotid artery by temporarily occluding it at its takeoff from the common carotid bifurcation and as far distally as the exposure will allow. An arteriotomy is made with a #11 blade knife and extended with Potts scissors up the external carotid artery. The surgeon usually will find a poor breakage of the atherosclerotic plaque. This generally can be dissected off the intima of the external carotid artery. Thereafter, the arteriotomy is closed primarily with a running 6-0 monofilament suture.

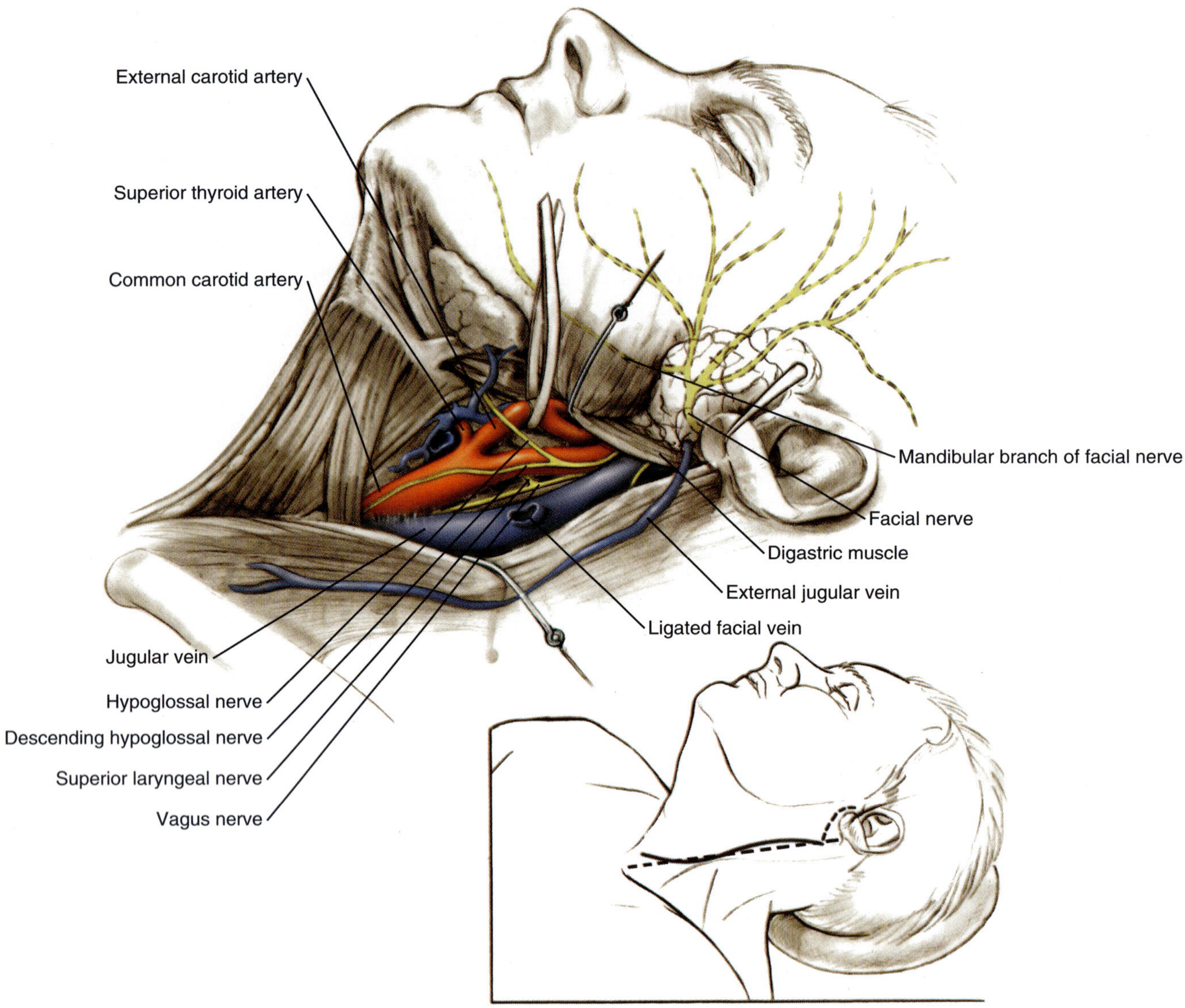

Figure 11–1.

This drawing shows the pertinent neurovascular anatomy and typical incision for carotid endarterectomy. If a high exposure is required for partial mobilization of the parotid gland, the incision is carried anterior to the ear.

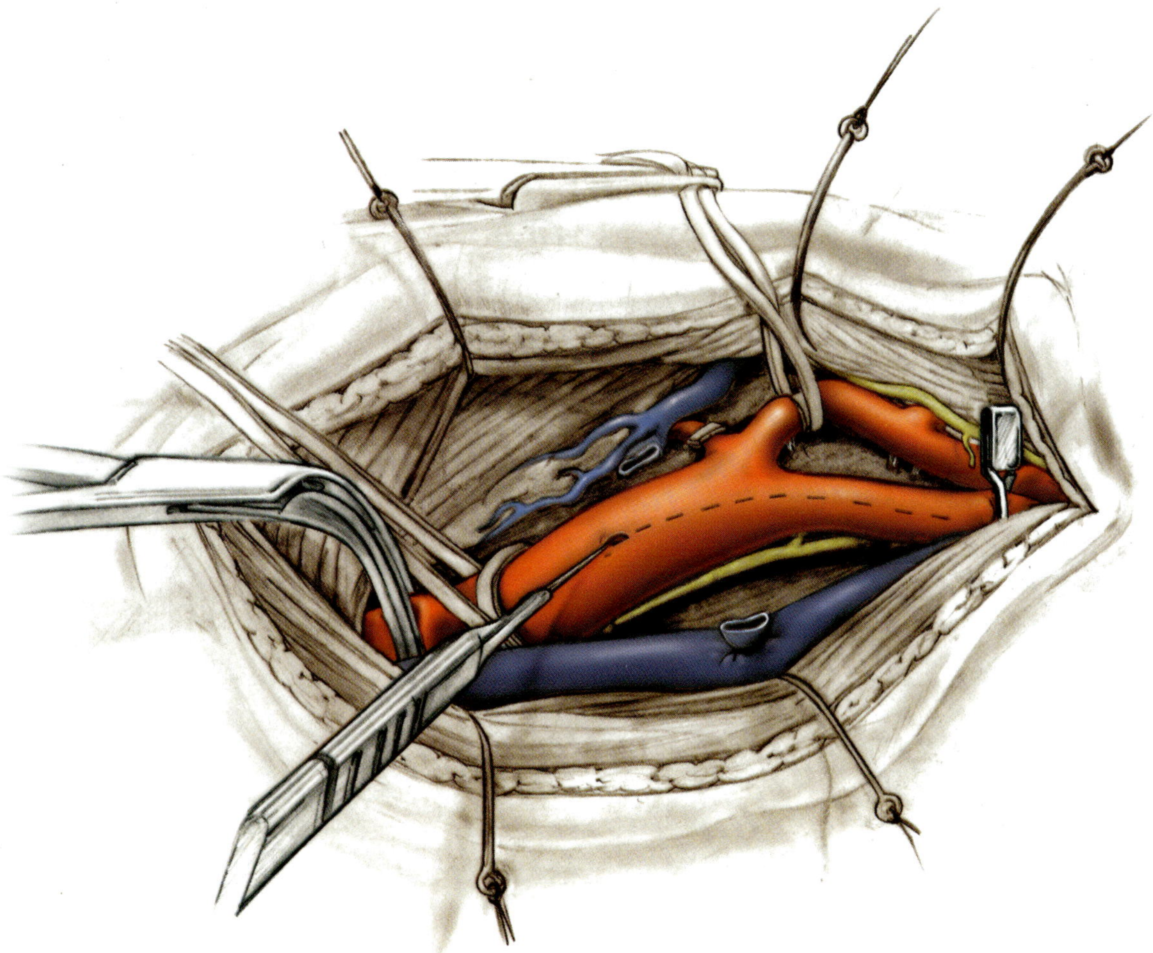

Figure 11–2.

Step 1. After 5,000 units of heparin have been given intravenously, the common carotid artery is occluded with a soft-shoe Fogarty clamp, the internal carotid artery with a temporary aneurysm clip, and the external carotid artery with a vascular loop. An arteriotomy is made in the common carotid artery with a #11 blade knife.

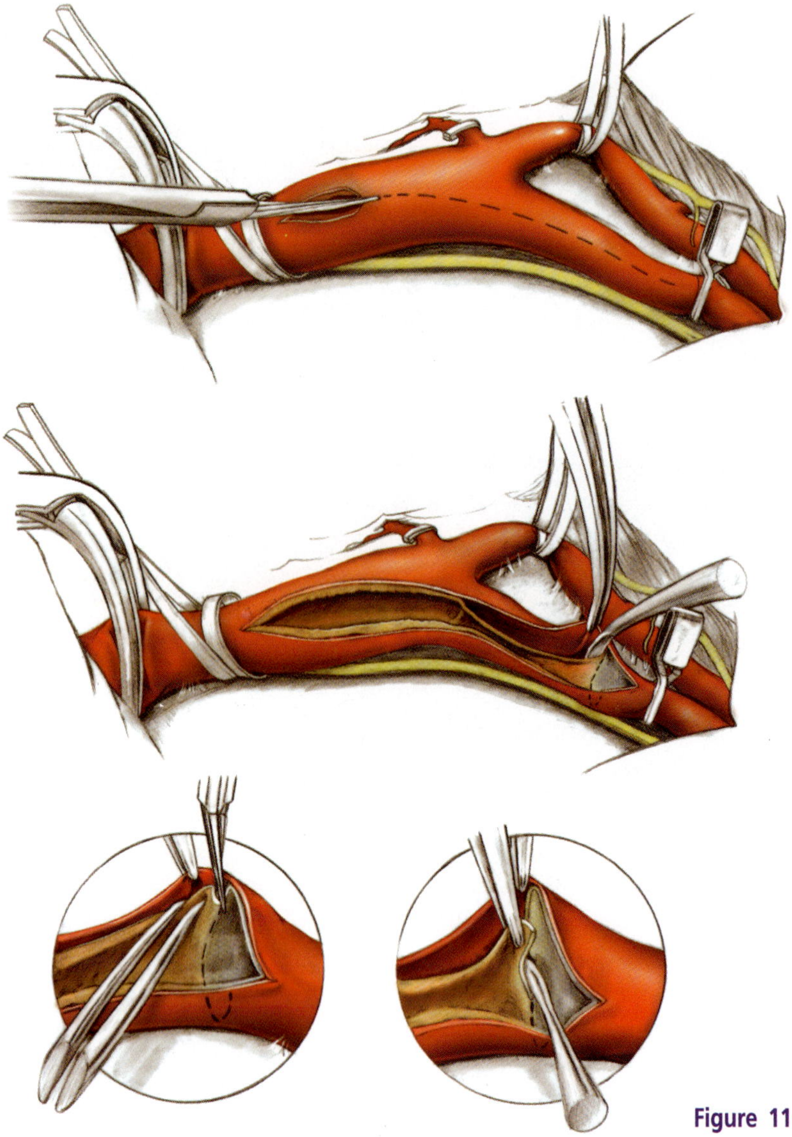

Figure 11–3.

Step 2. The arteriotomy is extended with Potts scissors up through and beyond the atherosclerotic plaque in the internal carotid artery. A plane of cleavage between the atherosclerotic plaque and intima at the bifurcation of the common carotid artery is identified with a spatula. The plaque first is removed up the internal carotid artery. The plaque generally breaks free and feathers out of the internal carotid artery. Occasionally, it is necessary to use microscissors to make a small cut in the plaque. After the starting cut has been made, the plaque is torn with a combination of countertraction and use of the spatula. Only atraumatic vascular forceps are used to grasp the vessel wall. Furthermore, to avoid traumatic injury, the intima of the internal carotid artery beyond the endarterectomy is never held directly with the forceps.

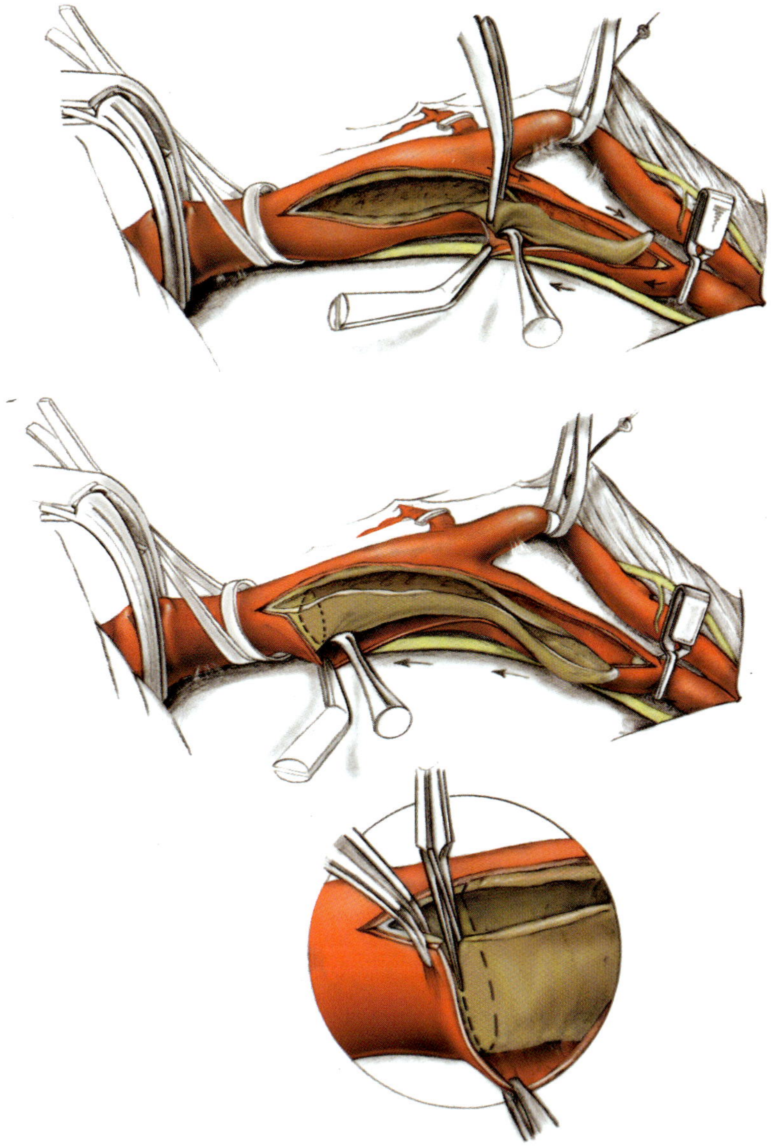

Figure 11–4.

Step 3. After the distal plaque in the internal carotid artery has been removed, the dissection is carried proximally down the common carotid artery with the use of the spatula and countertraction between the plaque and the vessel wall. The Potts scissors is used to cut the plaque in the common carotid artery in a circumferential pattern.

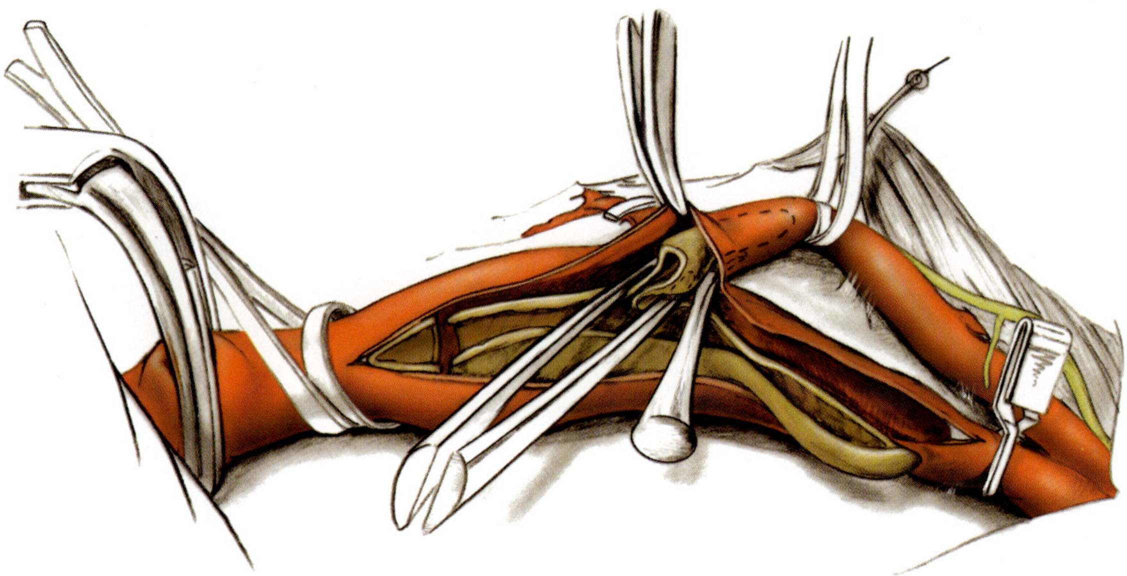

Figure 11–5.

Step 4. The spatula is used to dissect the plaque in a blind fashion circumferentially in the external carotid artery. The plaque is grasped with a hemostat, and an eversion technique is used to pull it out of the external carotid artery. After the plaque has been removed, the entire endarterectomy site is irrigated with heparin solution. Loose filaments are removed with microforceps. The internal carotid artery is inspected to make sure there are no flaps or ledges.

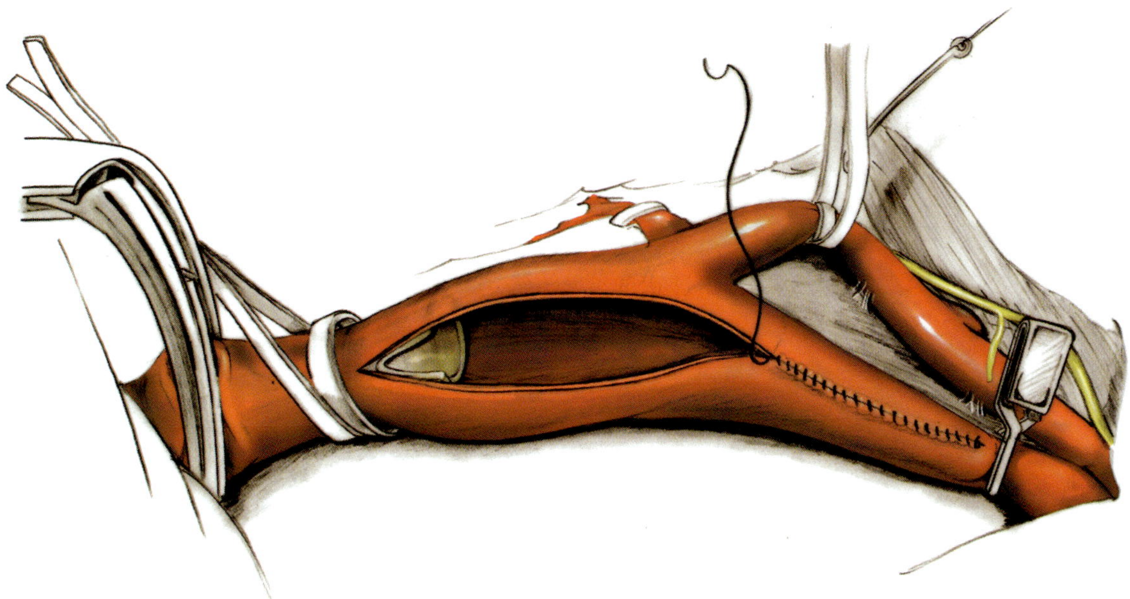

Figure 11–6.

Step 5. In large caliber vessels, the arteriotomy can be closed, under magnification, with a running 6-0 monofilament suture. Each suture should be full thickness, including the adventitia, to ensure that the closure has normal tensile strength. Just before the suture is tied, the aneurysm clip on the internal carotid artery is removed temporarily to allow back bleeding down this vessel. The artery is then reoccluded. The Fogarty clamp is removed temporarily from the common carotid artery to flush air and any grumous material out through the arteriotomy opening. The final suture is then tied. Blood flow is restored by removing the Fogarty clamp and loosening the loop around the external carotid artery. After 10 to 20 seconds, the clip on the internal carotid artery is removed. Accordingly, any thrombus or grumous material is flushed up the external carotid artery. This decreases the risk of an embolic event occurring during the restoration of blood flow after the carotid endarterectomy.

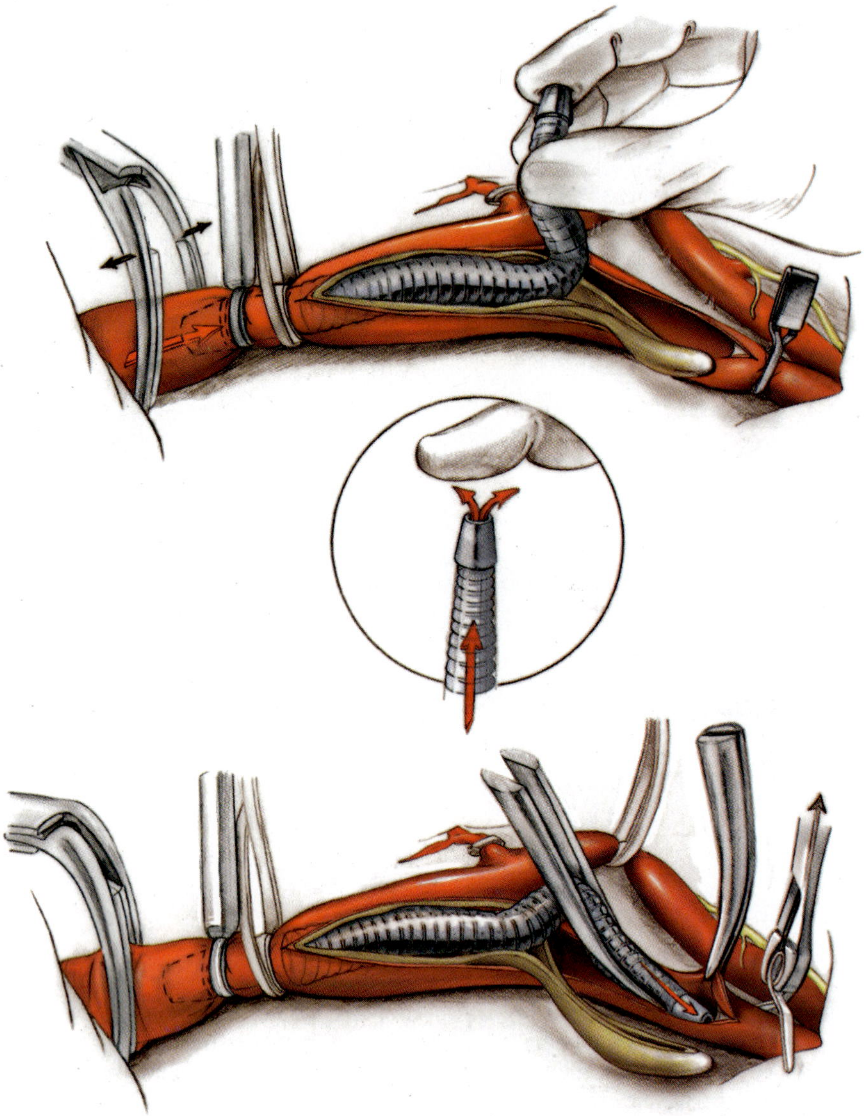

Figure 11–7.

In some cases, intraoperative monitoring, such as electroencephalography, indicates a significant change with cross-clamping of the common carotid artery. In such case, it is best to place a shunt. Before the shunt is placed, it is best to remove at least the plaque up the internal carotid artery. Often, the entire endarterectomy can be performed before a shunt is placed, thereby ensuring good plaque removal. First, the shunt is placed down the common carotid artery. The Fogarty clamp is released temporarily, and the shunt is flushed to dislodge any air. Second, the shunt is inserted into the internal carotid artery. The temporary clip is removed from the internal carotid artery to flush out this vessel. After the shunt has been inserted up the internal carotid artery, it is secured with a clip graft. The Fogarty clamp is then removed and blood flow is restored up the shunt. If the electroencephalogram does not normalize after several minutes, intraoperative angiography through the shunt should be considered to look for a possible embolus in the middle cerebral artery.

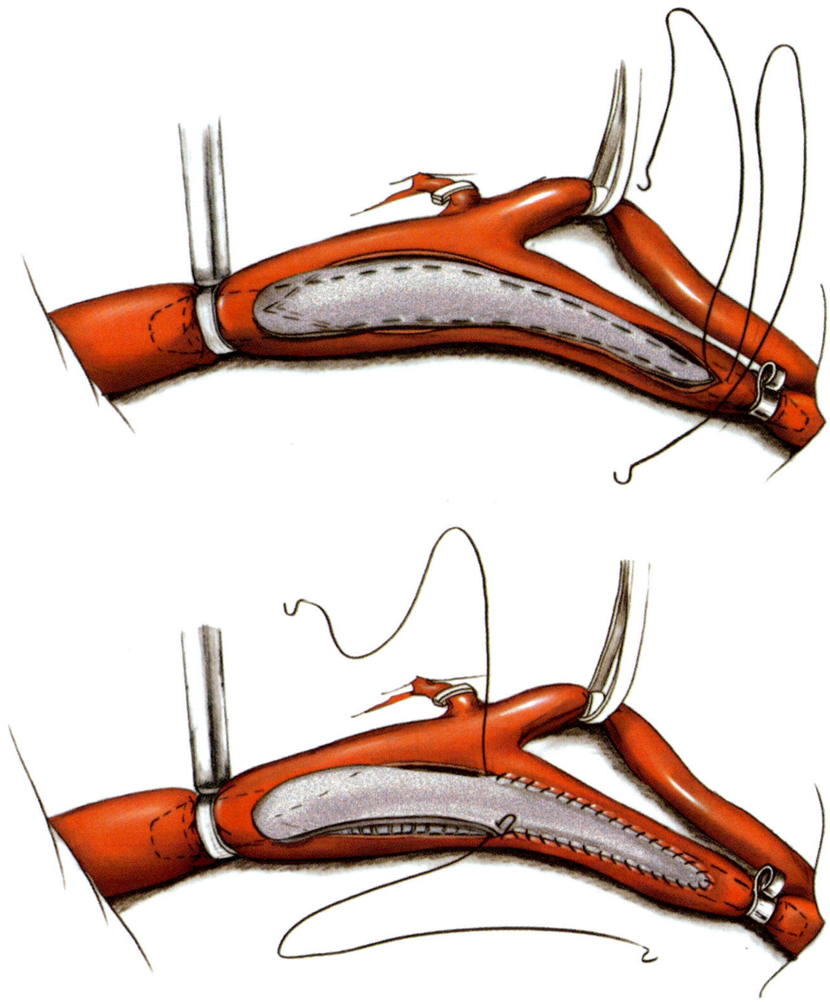

Figure 11–8.

The internal carotid artery often has a small caliber. In this case, it is best to close the arteriotomy secondarily with a patch graft. A saphenous vein or synthetic graft can be used. Illustrated here is repair of the arteriotomy with a graft and an indwelling shunt. A double-arm 24-inch 5-0 monofilament suture works best. It is optimum to sew from the graft to the vessel, thereby leading to eversion of the suture line. The first five or so stitches in the internal carotid artery should be approximately 1 mm wide and 1 mm deep. Thereafter, the stitches should be 2 mm wide and 2 mm deep. Exact placement of the sutures will lead to a smooth suture line, which will decrease turbulence and the risk of thromboembolic complications.

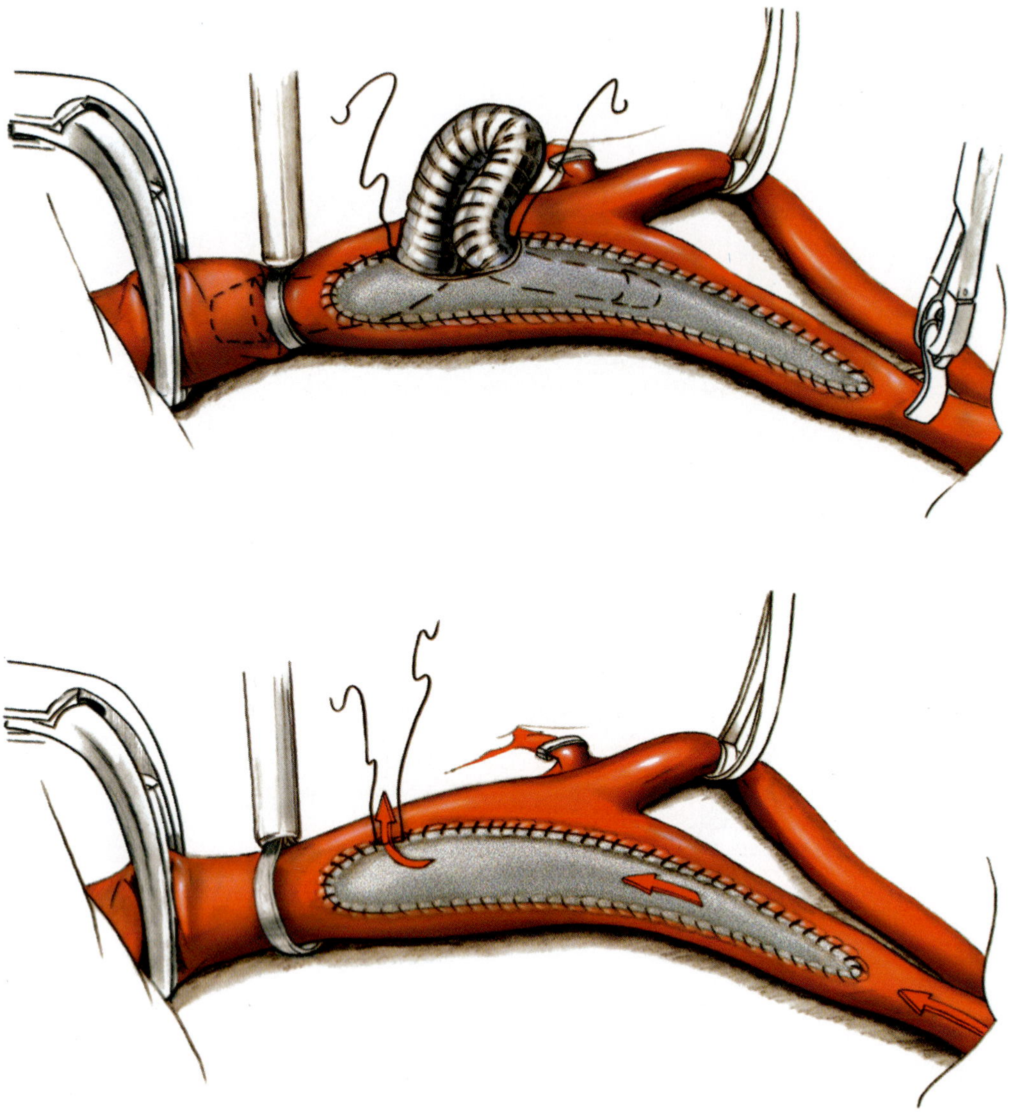

Figure 11–9.

Just before the suture line is closed, the common carotid artery is occluded again with a Fogarty clamp. The securing clip on the internal carotid artery is removed, and the shunt is extracted. This will also allow back bleeding down the internal carotid artery.

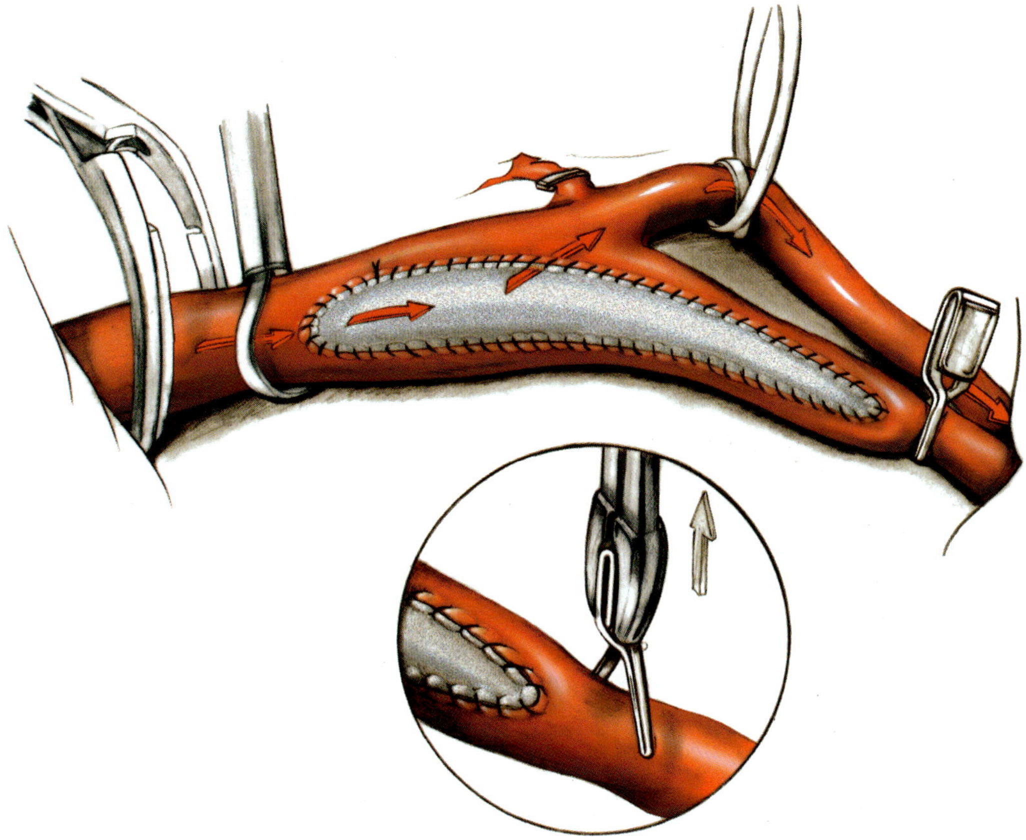

Figure 11–10.

After several seconds of back bleeding, the internal carotid artery is occluded again with a temporary aneurysm clip. The arteriotomy is then closed. The Fogarty clamp is removed, after which the vascular loop on the external carotid artery is loosened. This allows any potential embolic material to be flushed up the external carotid artery. After approximately 10 to 20 seconds, the clip on the internal carotid artery is removed.

CAROTID BODY TUMOR

Surgical Technique

It is useful to consider several general principles when resecting large tumors of the carotid body. First, it is important to perform the operation with intraoperative monitoring such as electroencephalography. If the common carotid artery must be occluded temporarily for hemostasis, it is important to know the status of the collateral blood flow to the ipsilateral cerebral hemisphere. Second, distal exposure of large tumors is obtained by mobilization of the parotid gland, as discussed above. This approach facilitates identification of the lower cranial nerves cephalad to the tumor and aids in their preservation. Third, these tumors are dissected in the capsular-adventitial plane instead of the subadventitial plane advocated by some surgeons. The capsular-adventitial plane is developed with bipolar coagulation techniques and magnification with either surgical loops or an operating microscope. Use of this plane minimizes the risk of injury to the arterial wall and, ultimately, hemorrhage. Fourth, great effort is taken to maintain the integrity of the external carotid artery. Fifth, although some authors recommend routine use of a shunt in patients with large tumors, shunts are used only when the electroencephalogram demonstrates insufficient perfusion if carotid occlusion is required. This procedure minimizes the risks associated with the use of a shunt. In most cases, meticulous dissection eliminates the need for either temporary occlusion of the carotid artery or placement of a shunt.

In all patients, the ipsilateral lower leg is prepared and draped in case a saphenous vein graft is required. The proximal common carotid artery is exposed, as described above, by dissection of the deep fascia anterior to the sternocleidomastoid muscle. This dissection is extended upward to the bifurcation of the common carotid artery, at which point the caudal limit of the tumor is encountered.

The common facial vein is often incorporated in the tumor capsule and must be ligated together with several draining veins surrounding the tissue. The tumor is isolated along its medial and lateral borders. The proper plane of dissection is identified, using the bipolar forceps under visual magnification between the lower pole of the tumor and the common carotid artery. Because the main blood supply of the tumor is from the bifurcation of the common carotid artery and the external carotid artery, the dissection delineates these attachments first. There usually is an areolar plane between the tumor and the artery, except for the subadventitial attachment of the tumor at the posterior wall of the bifurcation of the common carotid artery. With the use of a bipolar cautery, the many perforating arteries arising from the vasa vasorum are coagulated and divided. The tumor is often fed by large proximal branches of the external carotid artery, which should be ligated individually, as should the large feeding arteries from the vertebral and thyrocervical trunk that develop in very large tumors. The tumor is grasped with forceps and rotated superolaterally to expose the interface between the tumor and the carotid artery. By dissecting in the periadventitial layer close to the arteries, the risk of injuring the superior and recurrent laryngeal nerves is minimized.

Rarely, the vagus nerve is incorporated in the tumor bed; if it is, it must be carefully dissected free. The identification of the vagus nerve in relation to the tumor is facilitated by mobilization of the parotid gland. The other cranial nerve that can be injured at this point in the dissection is the hypoglossal nerve. The tumor usually displaces the hypoglossal nerve posteriorly and superiorly. It is important to identify this nerve in the submandibular region to preserve it. The mandibular branch of the facial nerve can be injured by excessive retraction under the angle of the jaw; however, mobilization of the parotid gland usually provides sufficient room for the dissection. In tumors that have a large lateral extension, the surgeon must be alert for the accessory spinal nerve.

After the feeding branches from the common and external carotid arteries have been dissected and ligated, the lateral and superior poles of the tumor are further mobilized. Laterally and somewhat posteriorly, it is common for the tumor to derive a major share of its blood supply from the carotid sheath. These vessels often are quite large, but they can be well controlled with bipolar coagulation techniques. As the exposure is extended higher, the parotid gland is mobilized so that the most cephalic portion of the tumor can be identified. The digastric muscle generally is severed at its connection with the mastoid process to aid in dissecting the upper limits of large tumors. The last portion of the tumor that is dissected free is the medioposterior attachment between the internal and external carotid arteries. In this manner, most of the tumor can be rotated to visualize better the vagus nerve and its extremely important superior laryngeal branch. As the tumor is elevated from its bed, the superior laryngeal nerve is worked away from the tumor capsule. After the tumor has been excised, the arteries are inspected carefully for any injury to the arterial wall. If a segment of artery appears to be injured, the artery is occluded and a local arteriotomy is made. The appropriate arterial repair and, if necessary, endarterectomy are performed.

Rarely, a massive tumor of the carotid body may extend up to and erode the foramen lacerum and the petrous bone. Tumors that extend into the posterior fossa require suboccipital craniectomy. Tumors that invade the foramen lacerum can be approached through a petrosectomy, but often these tumors are not completely resectable.

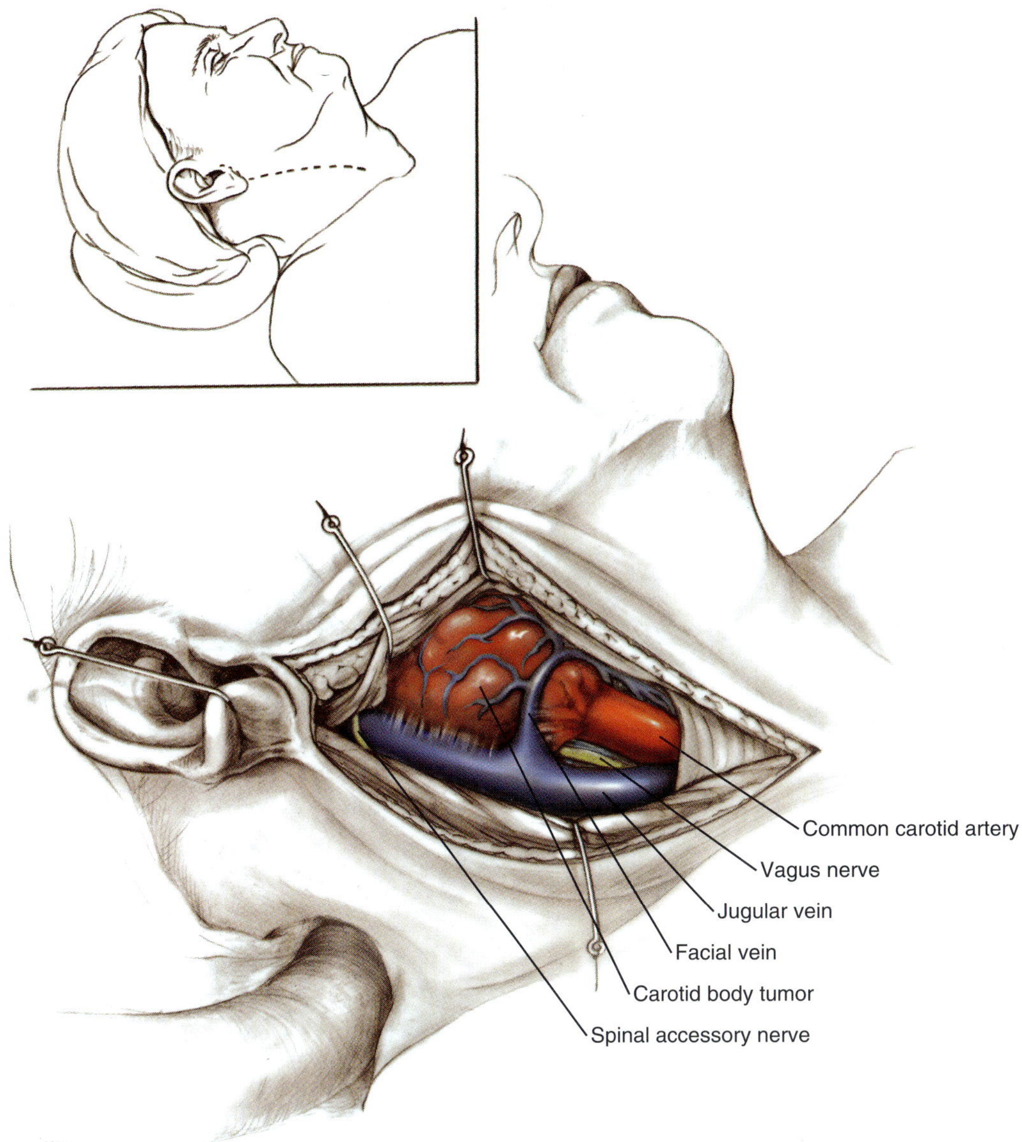

Figure 11–11.

Step 1. The typical exposure of a carotid body tumor requires some mobilization under the parotid gland. The digastric muscle must be either retracted or sectioned at its attachment to the mastoid process. The facial vein usually is incorporated in the capsule of the tumor.

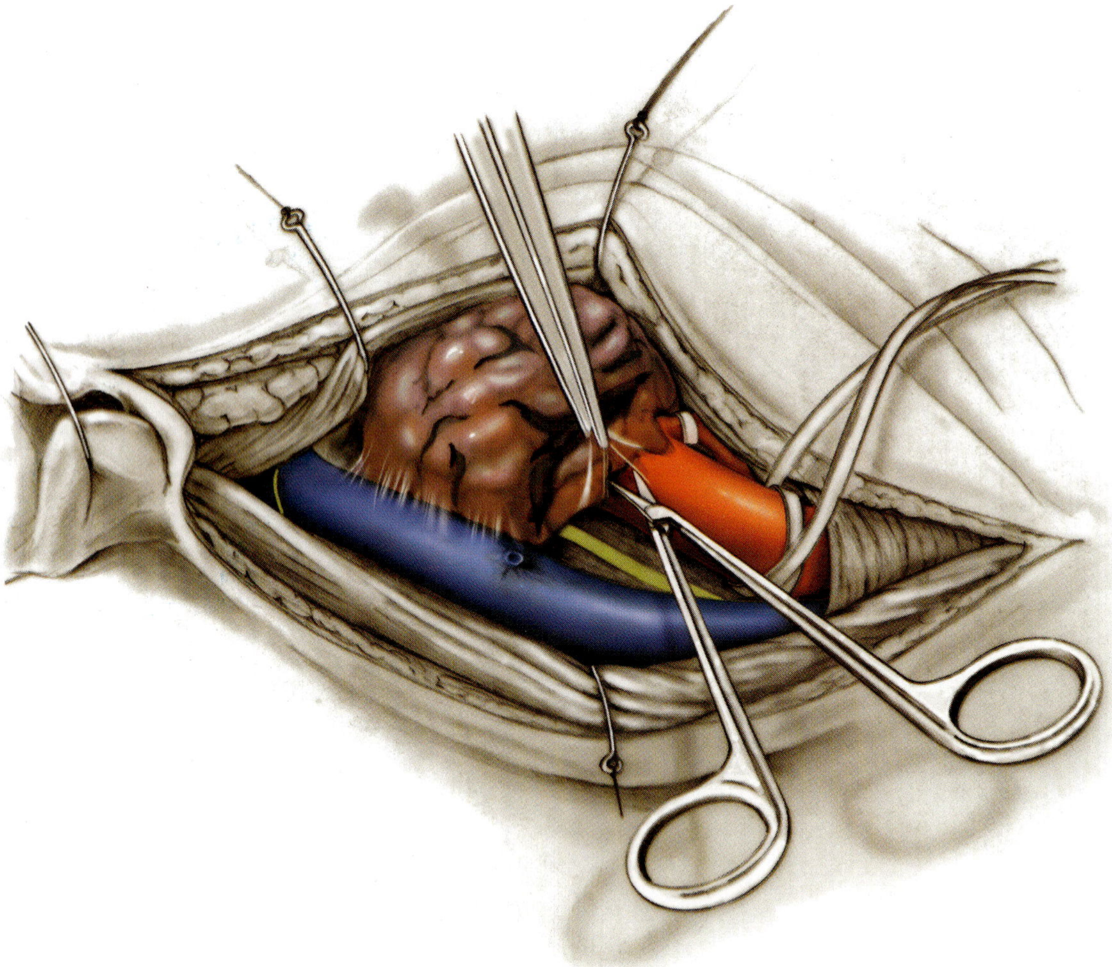

Figure 11–12.

Step 2. The dissection starts at the origin of the carotid body tumor at the bifurcation of the common carotid artery. The proximal internal and external carotid arteries are identified and dissected sharply free. There typically are numerous vascular feeding vessels from the bifurcation of the common carotid artery and the external carotid artery that are obliterated with the bipolar cautery.

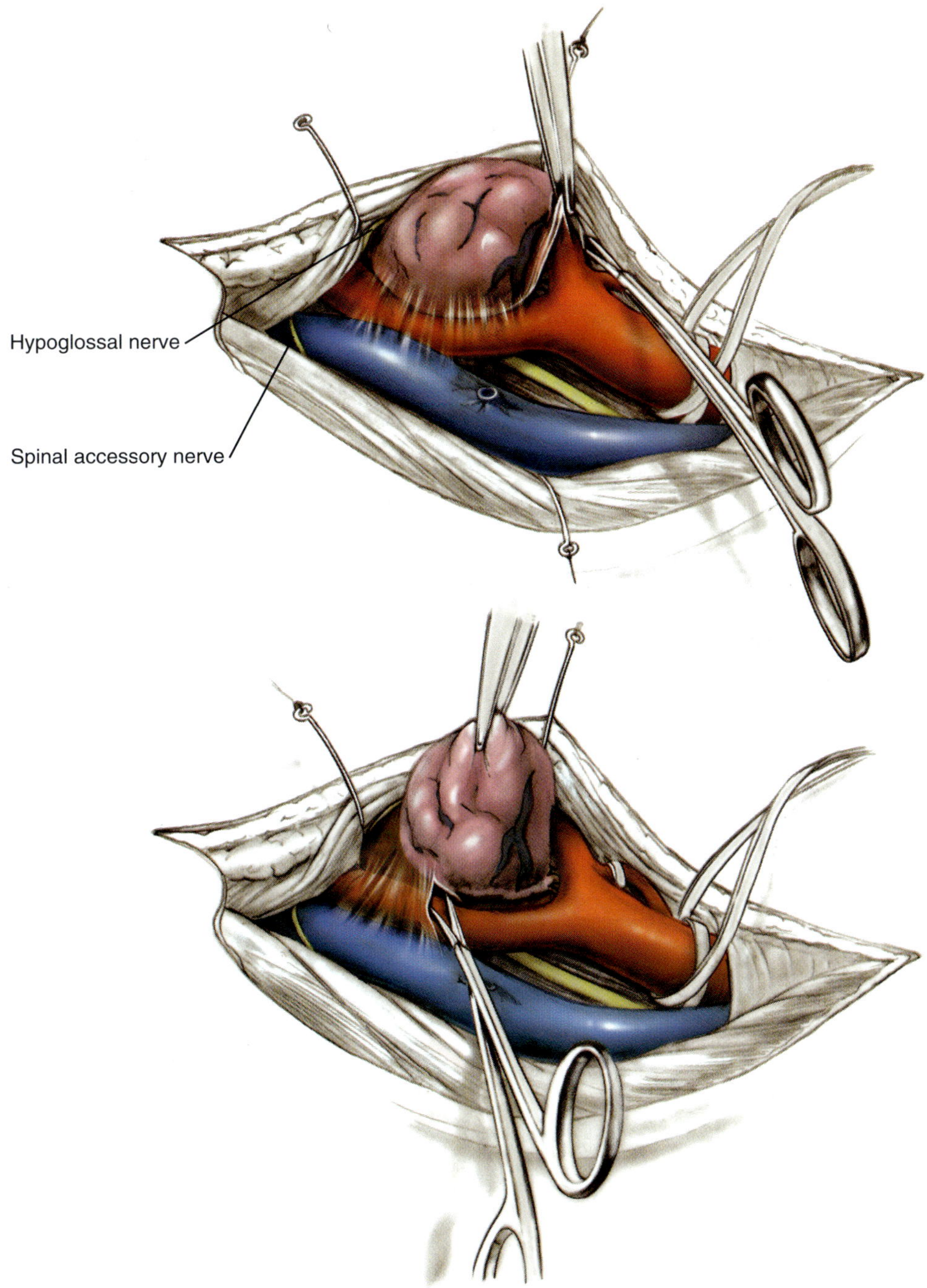

Figure 11–13.

Step 3. The dissection proceeds up the external carotid artery, where major arterial feeding vessels can be identified. Some of these vessels need to be ligated individually. The tumor capsule is somewhat fibrous; therefore, with greater mobilization, the tumor can be rotated to facilitate the dissection. After the tumor has been freed from the external carotid artery, the surgeon identifies the proximal internal carotid artery and dissects it off the tumor capsule.

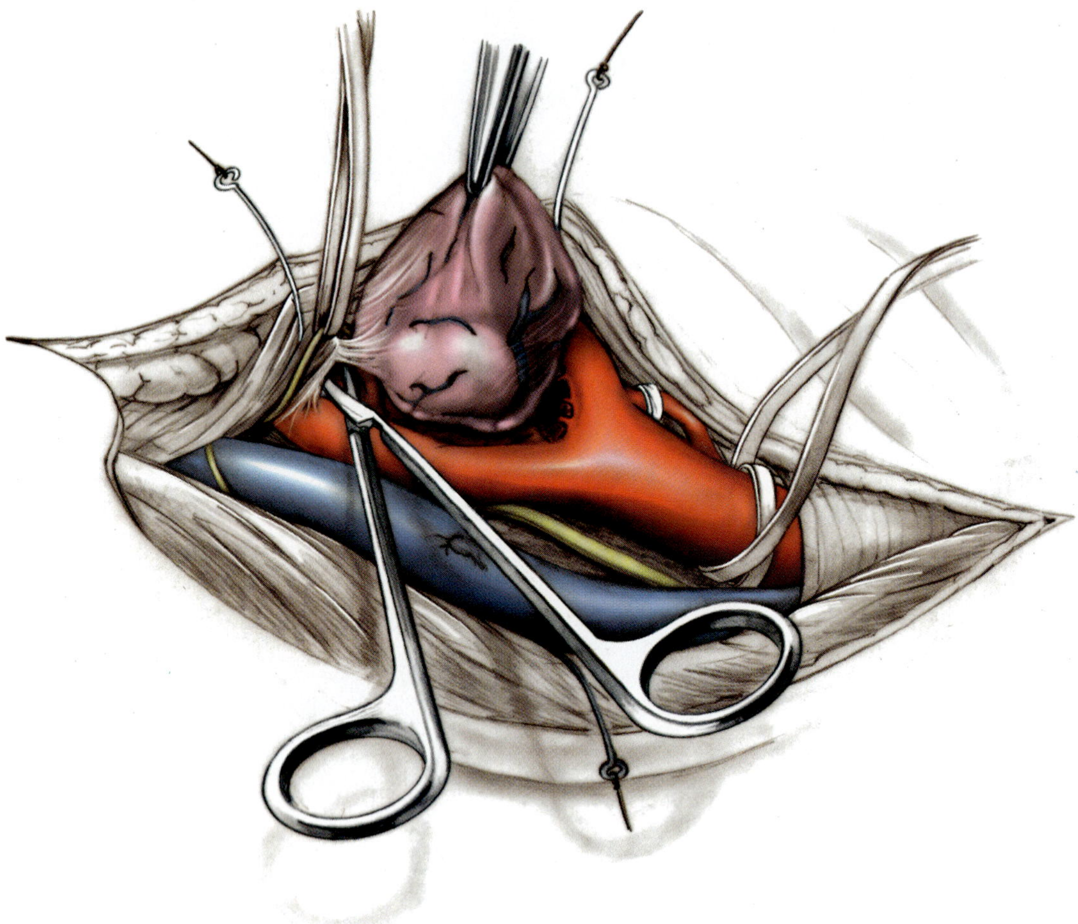

Figure 11–14.

Step 4. At the upper limit of the tumor, the hypoglossal nerve is usually identified under the belly of the digastric muscle. It is dissected sharply free from the tumor capsule. The tumor is displaced or retracted downward to facilitate identification of this plane.

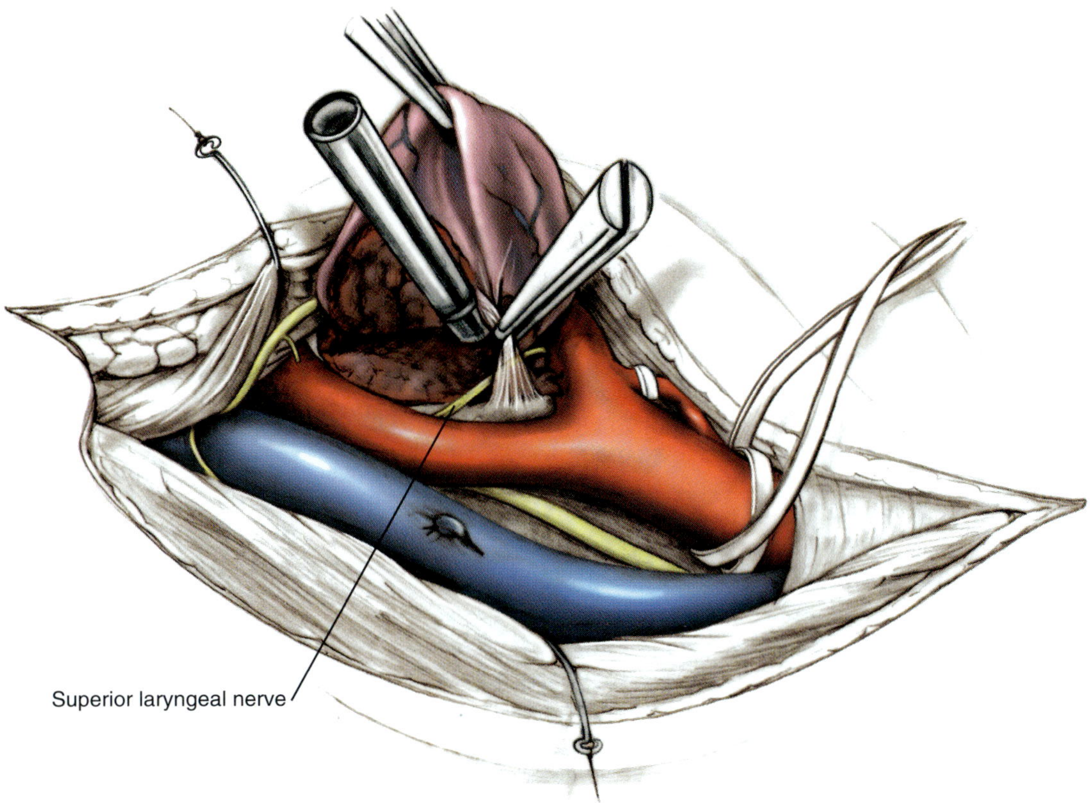

Figure 11–15.

Step 5. The attachment of the tumor to the deep fascia between the internal and external carotid arteries is dissected sharply free. It is important to recognize that branches of the superior laryngeal nerve that run in this fascia need to be protected, otherwise the patient will have difficulty swallowing.

CAROTID ARTERY ANEURYSM

Surgical resection of an aneurysm of the cervical internal carotid artery uses many of the techniques described above for carotid endarterectomy and high exposures. It is important to emphasize that it is mandatory to obtain adequate exposure distal to the aneurysm. Often, this requires partially mobilizing the parotid gland and sectioning the digastric and stylohyoid muscles. It is beneficial to have a neuroradiologist perform a trial balloon occlusion of the internal carotid artery proximal to the aneurysm during preoperative transfemoral cerebral angiography. This trial balloon occlusion in combination with blood flow studies can provide valuable information about the degree of collateral blood flow. Thus, before the operation, the surgeon knows whether a shunt will be necessary when the carotid artery is occluded and the aneurysm is resected.

If a trial balloon occlusion cannot be performed, the following intraoperative assessment with electroencephalography should be performed. After the common carotid artery and its bifurcation have been exposed, it is best to do a test clamping of the carotid artery to assess the potential for collateral blood flow when the arteries are occluded for resection of the aneurysm. During this test occlusion, the common carotid artery and the external carotid artery are occluded. Alternatively, the internal carotid artery is occluded just beyond the bifurcation of the common carotid artery if this exposure has already been achieved. During this cross-clamping trial, the intraoperative electroencephalogram is observed for 3 to 5 minutes to determine whether there is sufficient collateral blood flow. If this trial occlusion produces a change in the electroencephalogram, blood flow is restored immediately and the patient is made hypertensive. Next, a second trial occlusion is performed to determine whether this induced hypertension has significantly increased collateral blood flow. These measures are necessary because it is considerably easier to perform an interposition graft without having to use a shunt.

After the degree of collateral flow and the potential need for a shunt have been determined, the aneurysm is dissected free to identify the distal internal carotid artery. During this distal dissection, care is taken to identify and to protect the hypoglossal nerve and possibly filaments coming from the vagus nerve. After the distal and the proximal ends of the aneurysm have been identified, the arteries are occluded with temporary aneurysm clips and the aneurysm is resected.

The interposition graft between the stump of the internal carotid artery and the distal internal carotid artery can be performed with either a dilated saphenous vein or a synthetic vascular graft. Several anastomoses are illustrated to provide a smooth transition between vessels and grafts of different caliber. The distal anastomosis is performed first, using an operating microscope and interrupted 6-0 monofilament sutures. The anastomosis commences with the back wall. It is best to use interrupted instead of running sutures to avoid stenosis of the anastomosis site. Typically, the angle-spatulated anastomosis works best. After the distal anastomosis has been performed, the graft is irrigated with a solution of heparin and then sewn to the proximal internal carotid artery using several different types of anastomoses, depending on the difference in caliber between the graft and the proximal internal carotid artery. Although interrupted sutures are more time-consuming, they tend to work best. Just before the last several sutures are tied, it is best to back bleed both down the distal and the proximal internal carotid arteries to prevent emboli from going up through the graft.

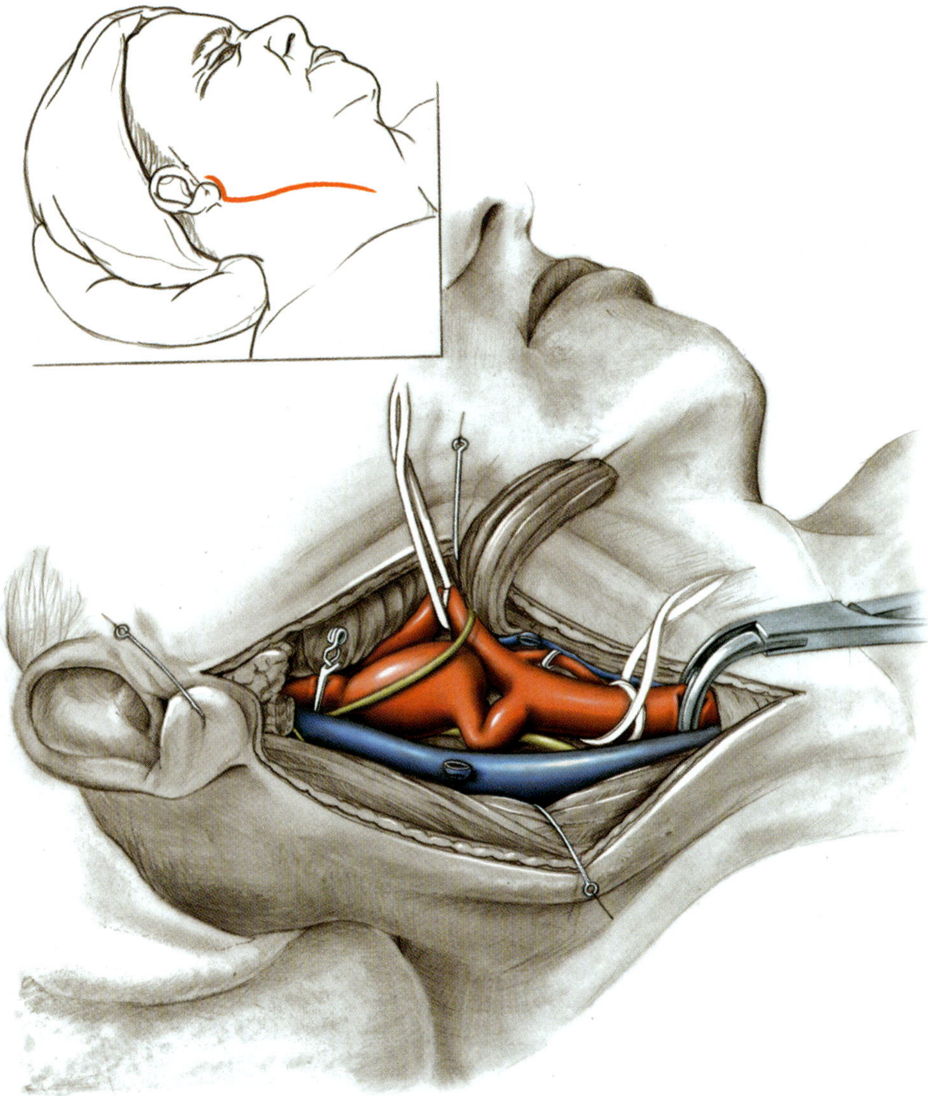

Figure 11–16.

The primary treatment of an aneurysm of the cervical internal carotid artery is resection of the aneurysm and reconstruction of the internal carotid artery. Reconstruction of the internal carotid artery can be performed by direct reanastomosis of the proximal and distal internal carotid artery if there is sufficient redundancy in the vessel. Otherwise, an interposition graft will be necessary. It often is necessary to work underneath the angle of the jaw and to partially mobilize the parotid gland to expose the distal internal carotid artery beyond the aneurysm. As illustrated here, the digastric muscle and the stylohyoid muscle have been severed and reflected medially.

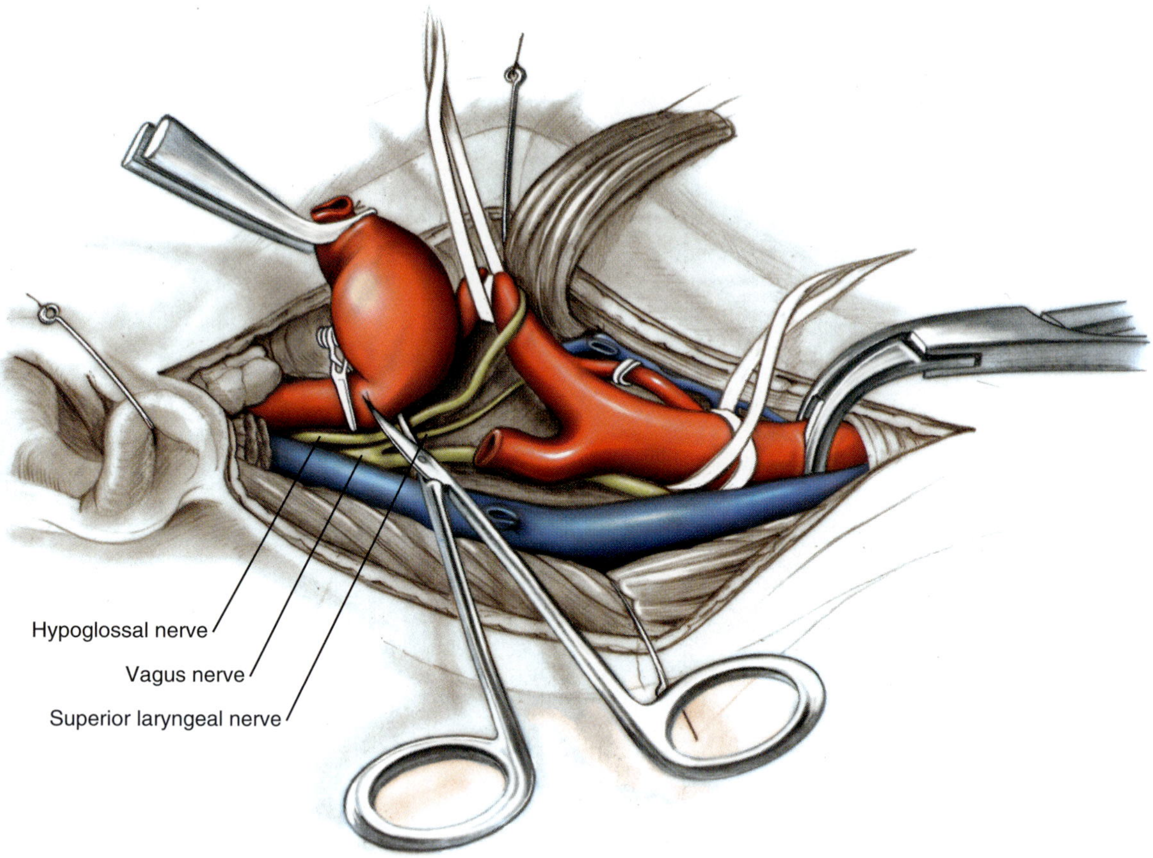

Figure 11–17.

After 5,000 units of heparin have been administered, the arteries are occluded. A soft-shoe Fogarty clamp is used to occlude the common carotid artery, and a temporary aneurysm clip is used to occlude the distal internal carotid artery beyond the aneurysm. The external carotid artery can be secured with either an aneurysm clip or a vascular loop. Next, the aneurysm is dissected from the surrounding tissue. The nerves at risk for injury include the hypoglossal nerve, the vagus nerve, and the superior laryngeal nerve.

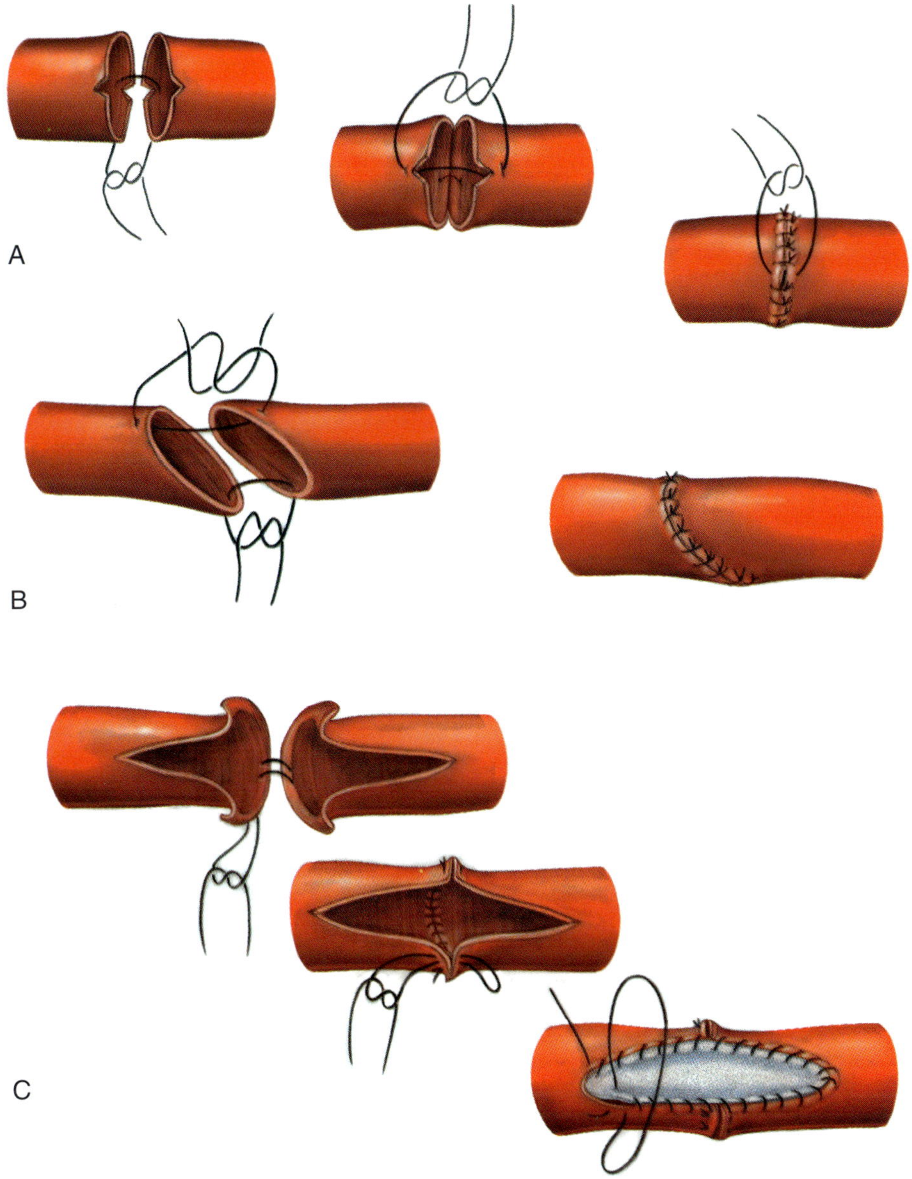

Figure 11–18.

Various anastomoses are useful for sewing interposition grafts. The goal of these anastomoses is to prevent stenosis at the site of the anastomosis. *A*, The first anastomosis is a fish mouth maneuver. It is important to use double-arm monofilament sutures and to sew from inside to outside to allow eversion of the vessel and, therefore, proximation of the intima with either the intima of the saphenous vein graft or the inner lining of the fabric graft.

B, The second anastomosis is a spatulated anastomosis. Again, it is important to make sure that the anastomosis line is everted. Although a running suture can be used, it has a higher risk of stenosis. Therefore, interrupted sutures are often preferable for reconstructing smaller vessels, although these sutures take more time.

C, The third anastomosis is a back wall–roofpatch reconstruction. This anastomosis is useful in providing the best taper between two vessels of significantly different diameters. The back wall is sewn with interrupted 6-0 monofilament sutures. If a saphenous vein is used as the interposition graft, a segment of the vein can be used for the patch graft. If a synthetic graft is used, either the graft itself or a small vein can be used as the patch.

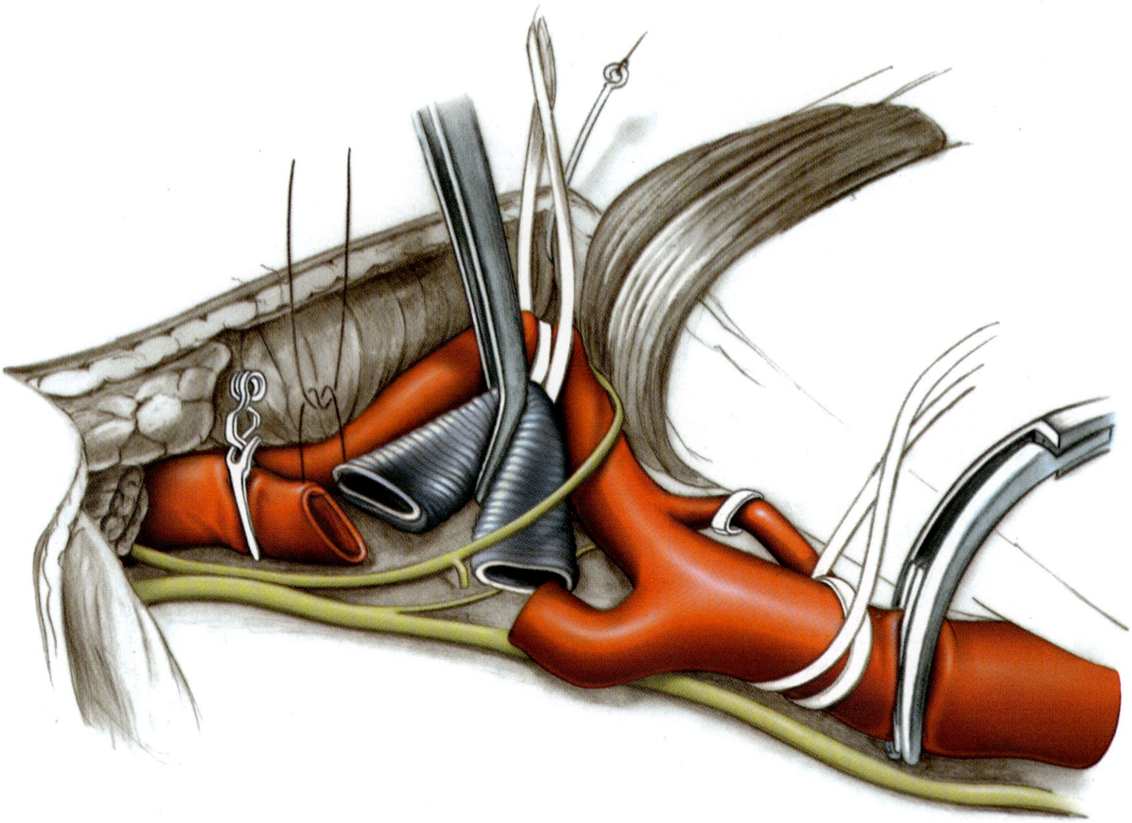

Figure 11–19.

In this illustration, an interposition graft is being constructed with a polyethylene terephthalate (Dacron) fabric ribbed graft. The distal hookup is a spatulated anastomosis.

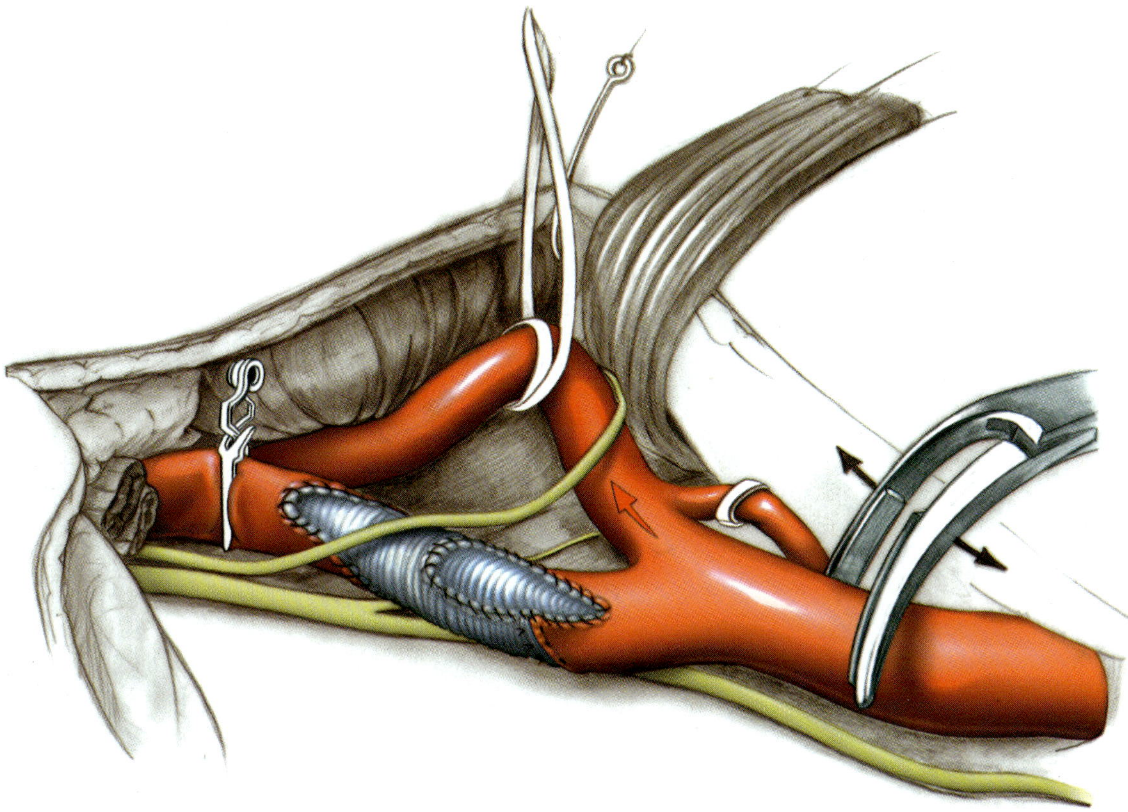

Figure 11–20.

A proximal anastomosis using a back wall–roofpatch graft reconstruction. As in any interposition graft, it is important to make sure that the interposition vessel is of sufficient length that neither anastomosis is under excessive tension. After the reconstruction has been performed, the Fogarty clamp is removed from the common carotid artery, and the external carotid artery is reopened. This allows any thrombus or grumous material to be flushed up the external carotid artery. Thereafter, blood flow is restored through the internal carotid artery.

RECURRENT CAROTID STENOSIS

Reoperation for recurrent carotid stenosis is becoming a more frequent surgical procedure. The most common causes of recurrent stenosis are recurrent atherosclerosis and myointimal hyperplasia. Operating on a recurrent carotid stenosis is more difficult than performing the original operation because of the dense scar tissue that forms in the neck after the initial procedure. Dissecting the carotid artery can be hazardous not only because of injury to the arteries but also to the cranial nerves. Also, in approximately one-half of the patients with recurrent atherosclerosis, endarterectomy cannot be performed because the plaque is tightly adherent to the underlying intima by scar tissue. It quickly becomes apparent to the surgeon whether the recurrent plaque can be removed. If a plane cannot be identified easily, in all likelihood an interposition graft from the common carotid artery to the internal carotid artery above the recurrent stenosis will be required.

The interposition graft can be fashioned from either a dilated saphenous vein or a synthetic expanded polytetrafluoroethylene graft. The techniques and anastomoses for this graft are identical to those described above for surgical resection of aneurysms of the cervical internal carotid artery. It is important to emphasize that induced hypertension before cross-clamping the carotid artery can significantly reduce the need for placement of a shunt. Performing an interposition graft without an indwelling shunt is technically easier. It also is important to administer 5,000 units of heparin before cross-clamping the carotid artery. Although this leads to temporary leaking at the two sites of anastomosis, it decreases the incidence of thromboembolic complications.

The treatment of recurrent stenosis due to myointimal hyperplasia is enlargement of the artery with a roofpatch graft. In myointimal hyperplasia, the lesion consists of a thickening of the entire arterial wall in the region of the previous endarterectomy. Because there is no plane in which an endarterectomy can be performed, angioplasty with a patch graft works best.

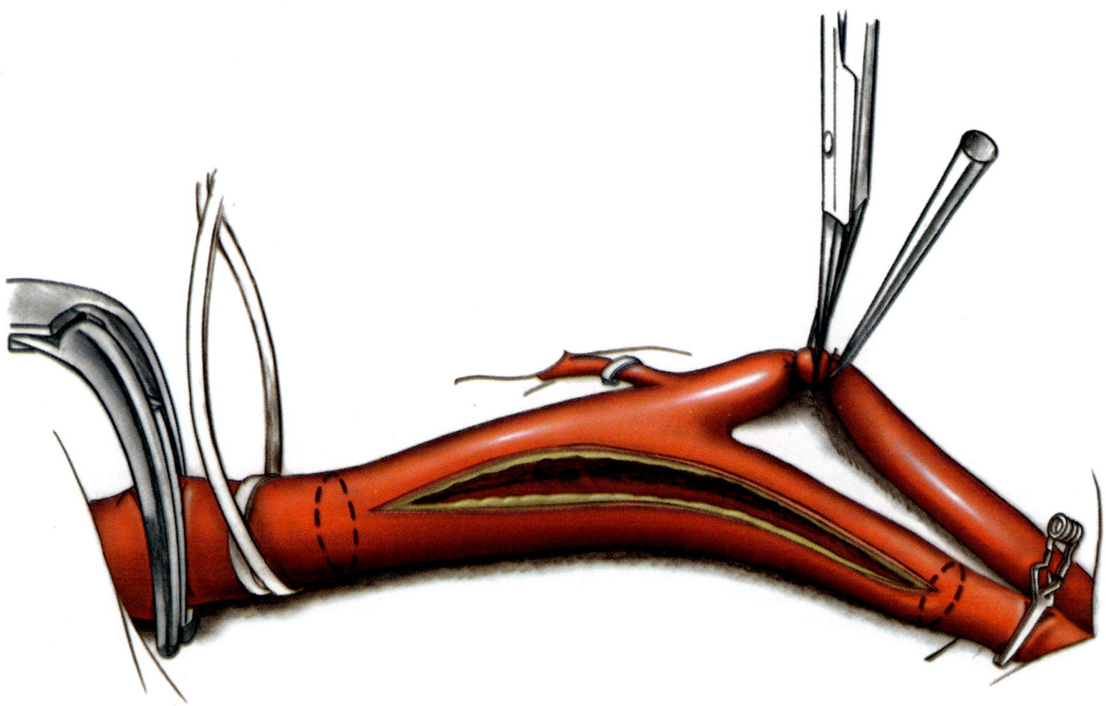

Figure 11–21.

An arteriotomy is made in a standard fashion extending from the common carotid artery up through the internal carotid artery. In approximately 50 percent of patients, no plane separates the recurrent atherosclerotic plaque from the underlying intima; thus, an interposition graft must be performed. The external carotid artery is doubly ligated and divided. The superior thyroid artery is also ligated. The common carotid artery below the arteriotomy and the internal carotid artery distal to the arteriotomy are cut, leaving stumps of each vessel. It is unnecessary—and in fact dangerous—to remove the bifurcation of the common carotid artery because it will be scarred to its underlying fascia, and the superior laryngeal nerve will be exposed to injury during attempted removal. Thus, it is best just to lay the interposition graft within the opening vessel and to leave the bifurcation of the common carotid artery in situ.

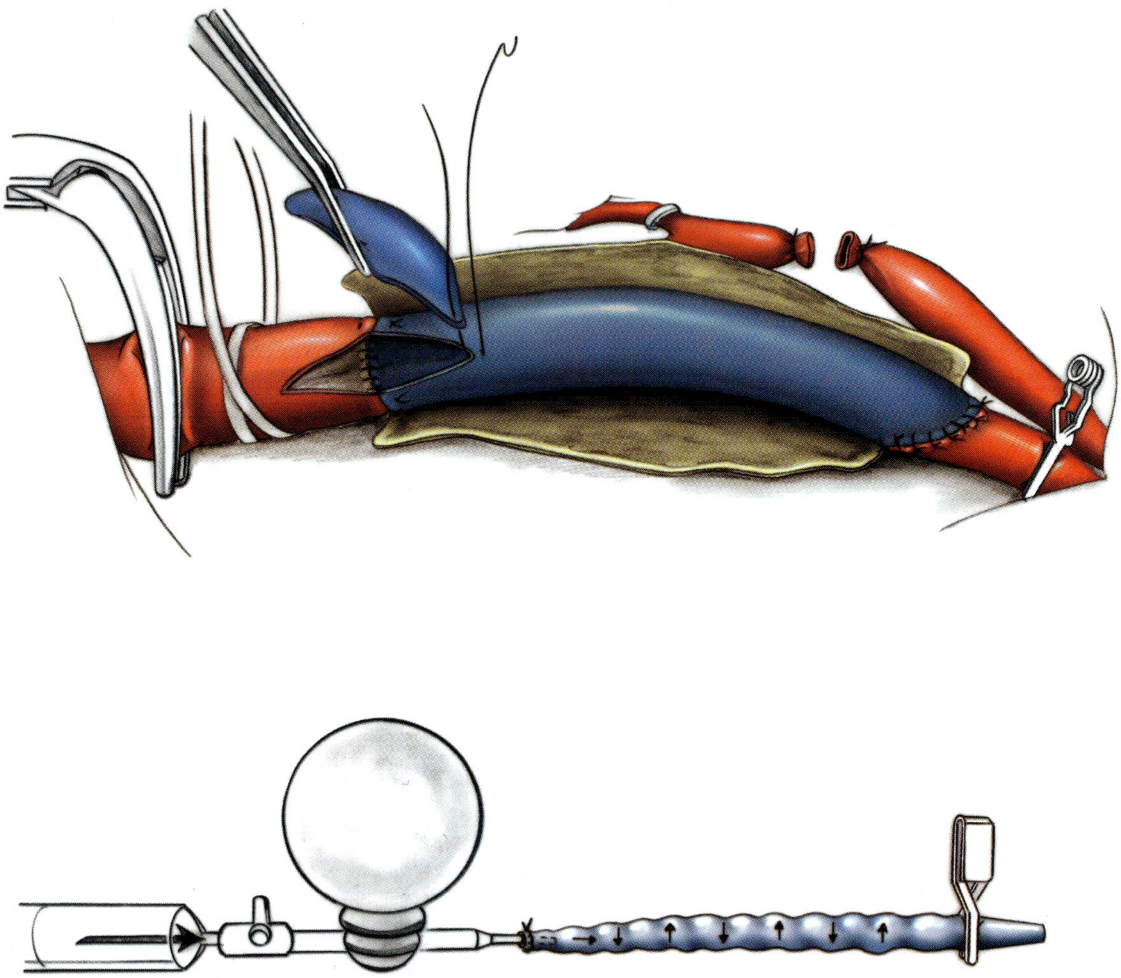

Figure 11–22.

In the case illustrated here, a saphenous vein has been harvested from the leg. It is being dilated with cold papaverine-heparin solution. Use of this balloon vein dilatation kit prevents overdilatation and injury to the intima of the vein. The saphenous vein is sewn in place, anastomosing it from the common carotid artery to the internal carotid artery. The distal anastomosis is performed first, usually with a fish mouth anastomosis. Next, the proximal anastomosis is completed. Just before the last few sutures of the proximal anastomosis are tied, both antegrade and retrograde back bleeding are performed from the internal and the common carotid arteries to prevent an embolus from traveling up the internal carotid artery.

MOYAMOYA DISEASE

Several surgical techniques have been used in the treatment of moyamoya disease. The operation advocated here always uses an encephalomyosynangiosis, with grafting of the temporalis muscle to the cortical surface. This is combined with either an encephaloarteriosynangiosis or a direct superficial temporal artery-to-middle cerebral artery anastomosis, depending on the caliber of the temporal artery and the cortical vessels. Specifically, if the temporal artery or cortical branches of the middle cerebral artery are small, an arteriosynangiosis is performed by dissecting the temporal artery free but leaving it in continuity with the scalp. This temporal artery graft is placed onto the cortical surface and held in place by two bands of dura mater. The surrounding bony defect is covered with the temporalis muscle. Alternatively, if the temporal artery and recipient branches of the middle cerebral artery are of sufficient caliber, a direct superficial temporal artery-to-middle cerebral artery anastomosis is performed. The remaining craniotomy defect is repaired with a temporalis muscle graft.

It is important to emphasize that cerebral blood flow in patients with moyamoya disease is tenuous. Several rules need to be followed. First, the patient's $PaCO_2$ should be kept normal and hyperventilation should be avoided. Hyperventilation can lead to an intraoperative steal phenomenon, resulting in strokes both in and out of the circulation that is being treated surgically. Second, the patient should be kept euvolemic, with close attention paid to blood loss throughout the surgical procedure. Third, the bone flap should be reattached to the skull with sutures to avoid rigid fixation. Because the temporalis muscle sits underneath the bone, close approximation of the bone flap to the cranium can result in a significant mass effect and a stroke. Fourth, because the temporal artery is harvested from the skin flap, it is important to design a flap that has a broad pedicle. Furthermore, the topical application of nitroglycerin paste to the skin flap can be beneficial in decreasing ischemic necrosis of the scalp.

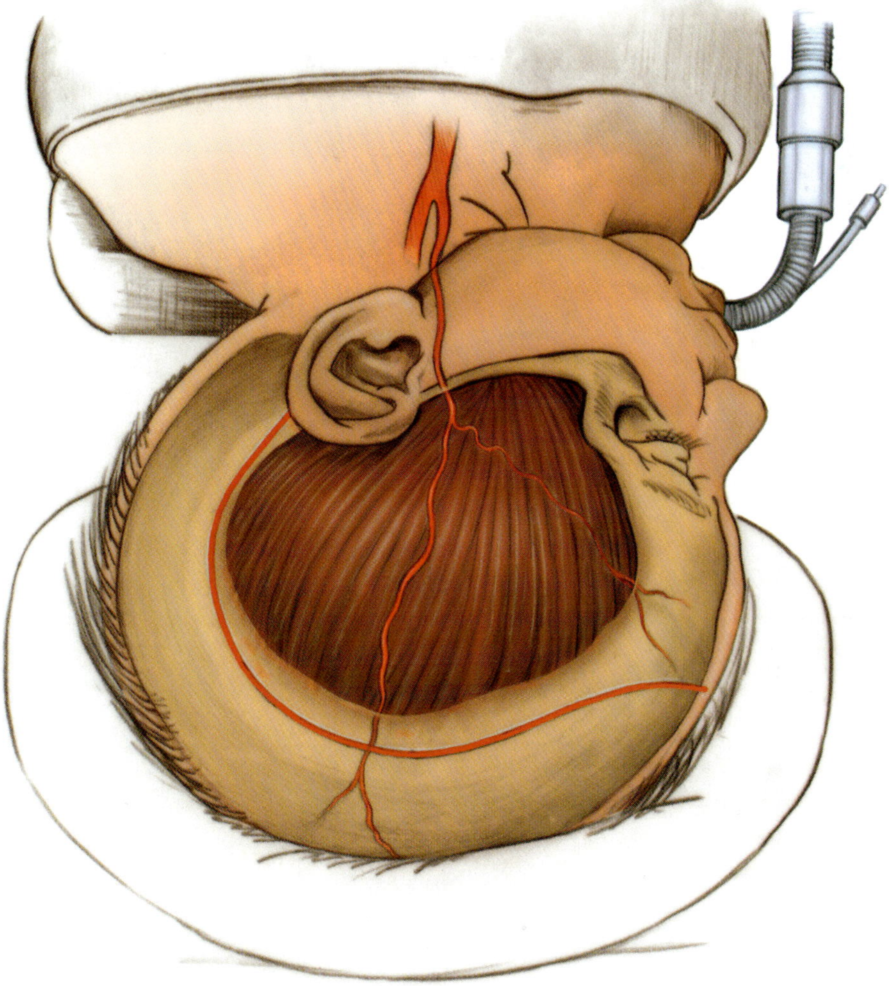

Figure 11–23.

Step 1. The skin flap is designed so that the temporal artery can be harvested from the scalp and dissected free of the temporalis muscle but preserved in continuity in case an encephalomyoarteriosynangiosis will be performed. This type of skin flap works better than a horseshoe type because there is less risk of ischemic necrosis of the scalp flap.

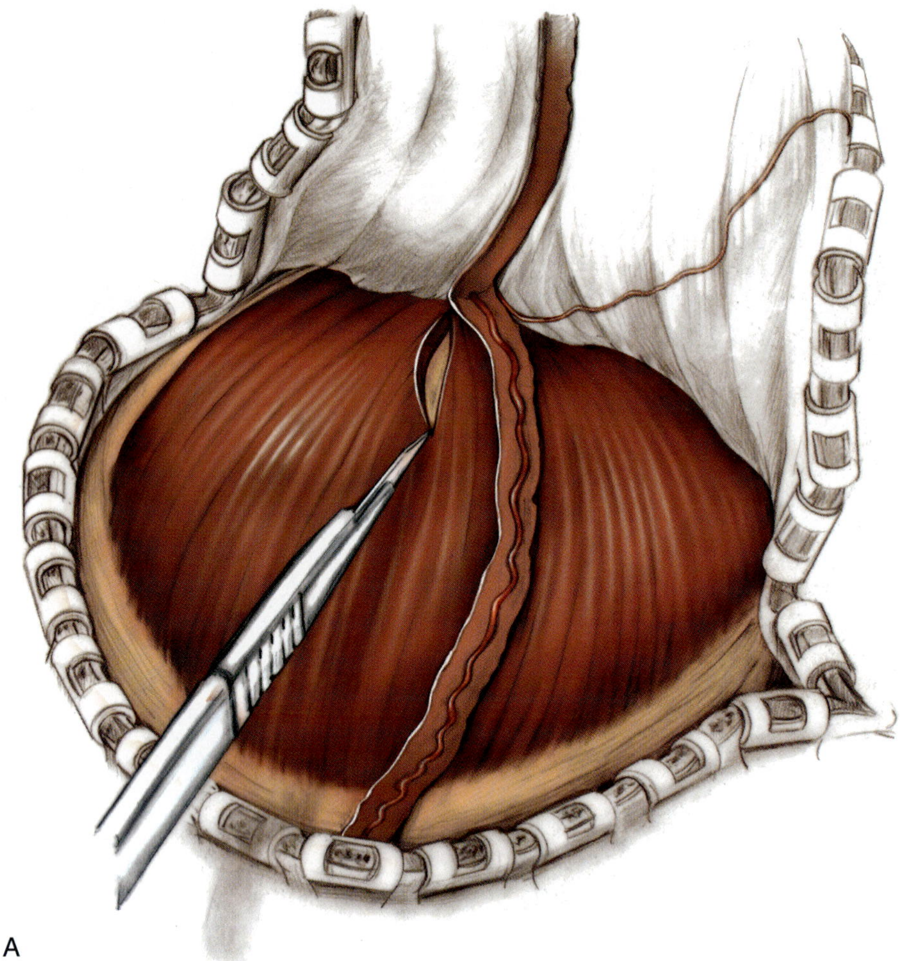

A

Figure 11–24.

Step 2. *A* and *B,* The temporal artery is dissected free from the galea aponeurotica but preserved in continuity. The temporalis muscle is dissected off the calvarium and split to allow passage of the temporal artery in preparation for an encephalomyoarteriosynangiosis.

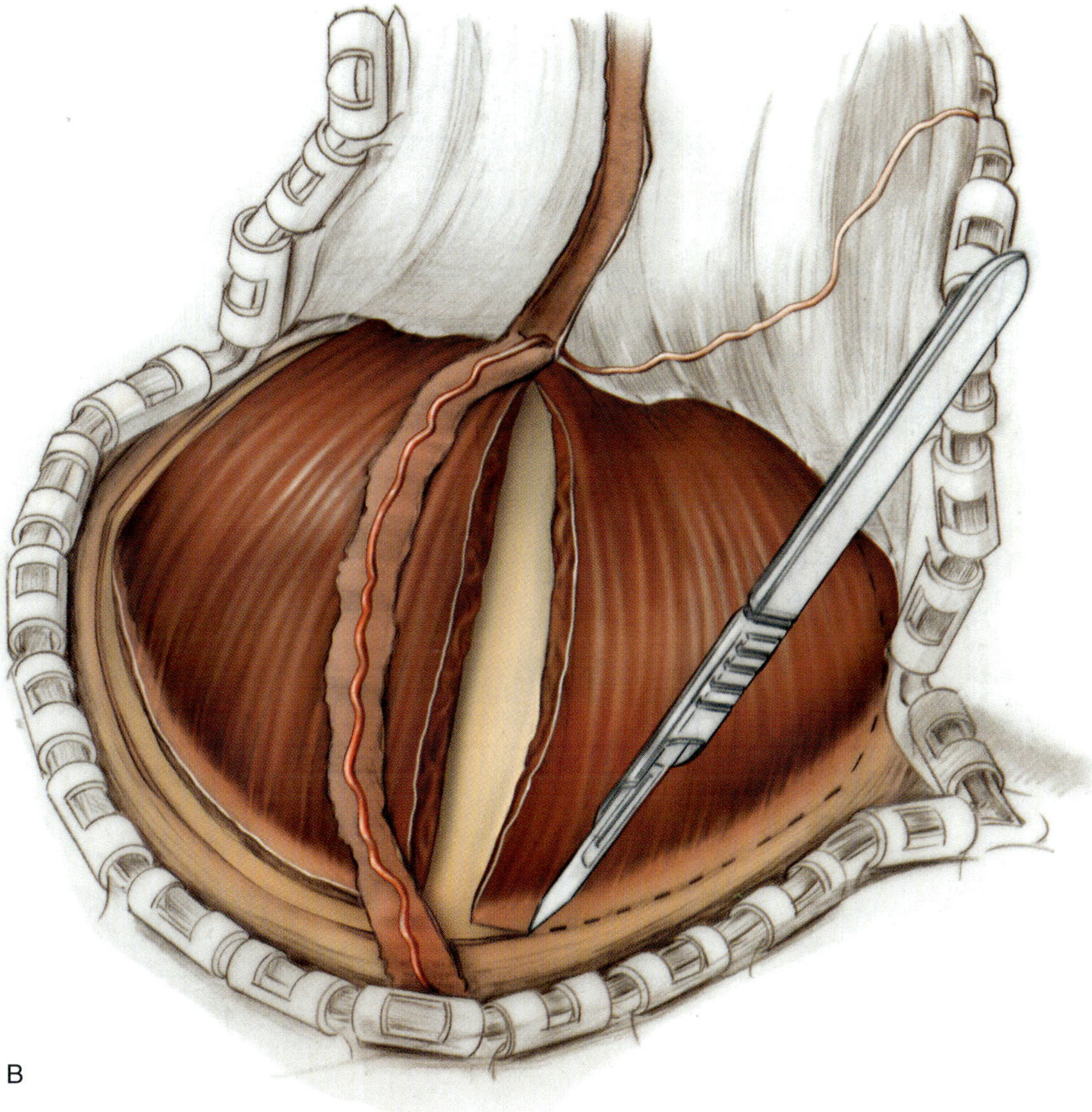

B

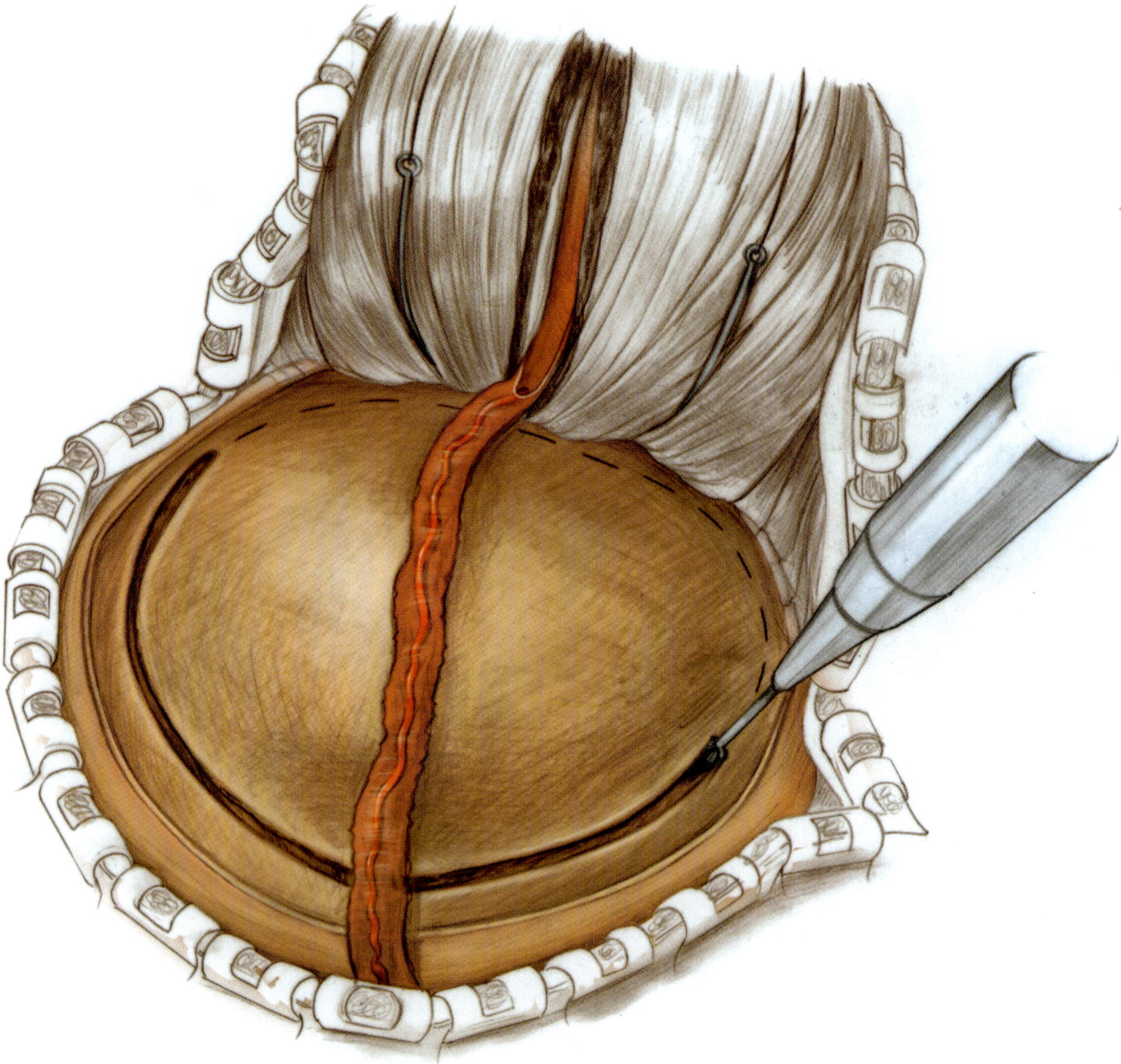

Figure 11–25.

Step 3. The temporalis muscle is retracted with fishhooks. A large frontotemporoparietal craniotomy is performed with a high-speed air drill and diamond bur or craniotome. During this process, the temporal artery pedicle is protected.

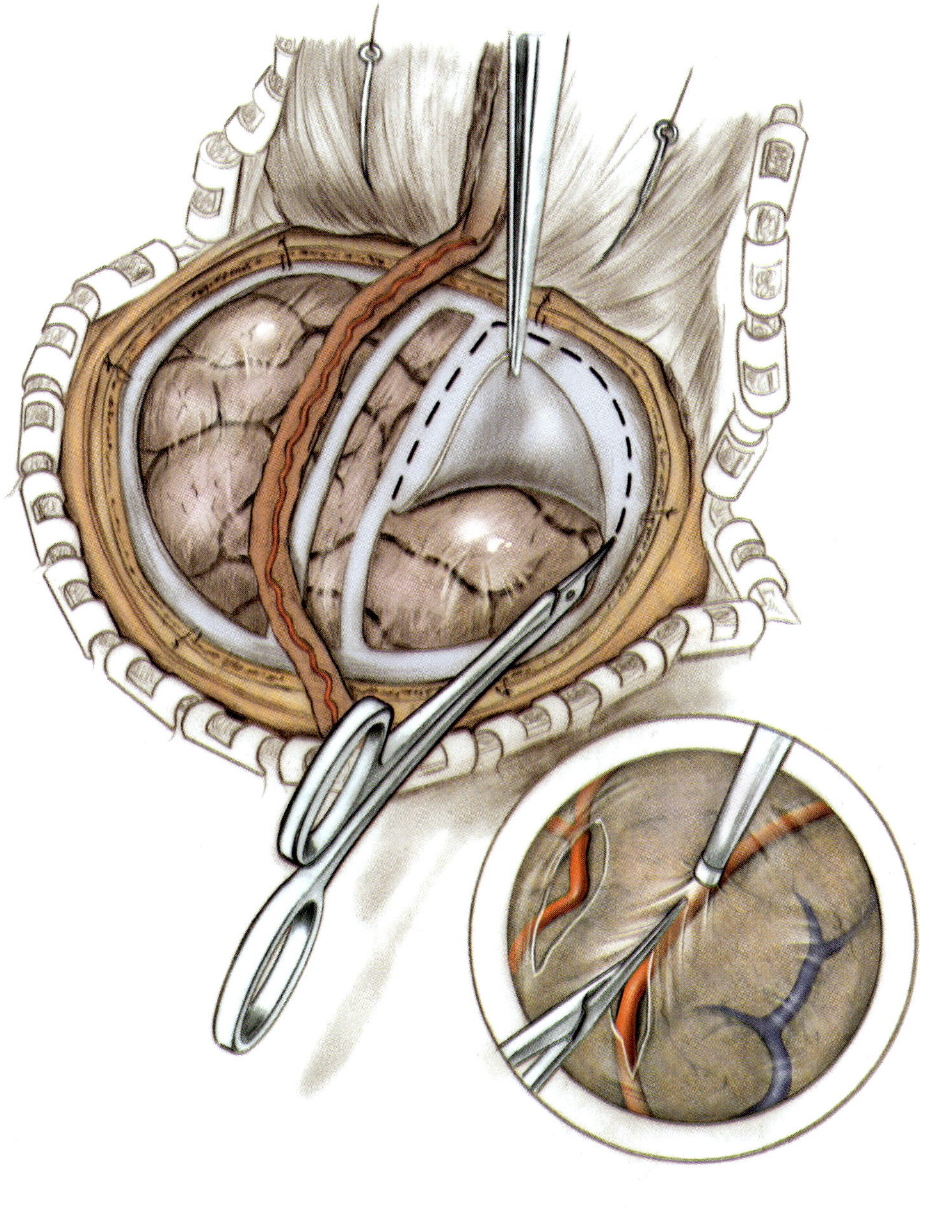

Figure 11–26.

Step 4. The dura mater is opened widely and tacked to the margins of the bone. If an encephalomyoarteriosynangiosis is to be performed, two bands of dura mater are left intact. The temporal artery pedicle is sewn to these dural bands to approximate the graft to the cortical surface. After the dura mater has been opened and tacked to the margins of the bone, numerous incisions are made in the arachnoid with use of the operating microscope. Usually, a sharp #11 blade knife is used to make the initial incision in the arachnoid over a cortical vessel, and then a straight microscissors is used to lift up the arachnoid and to cut it over the length of the vessel as far as the subarachnoid space permits.

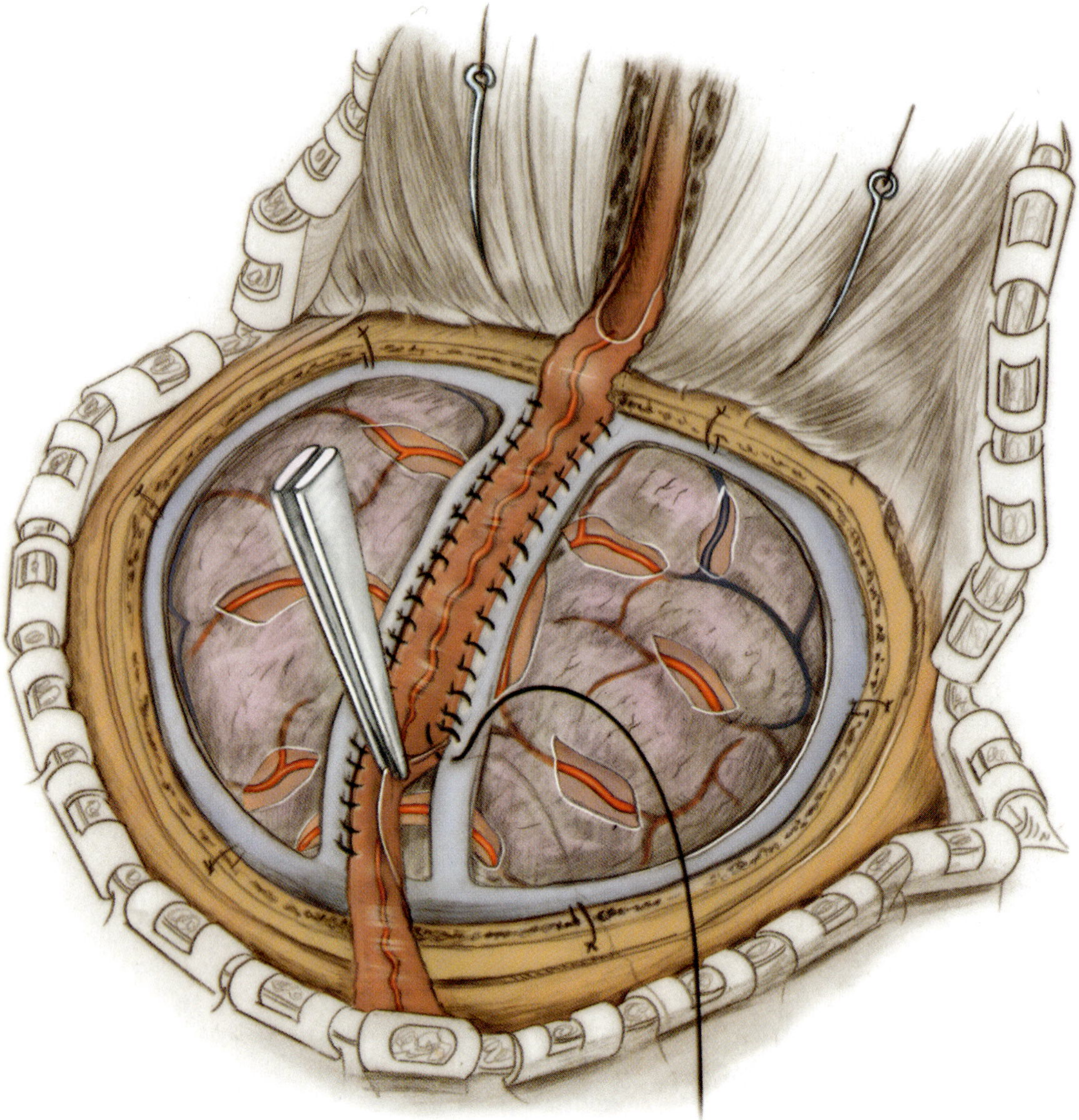

Figure 11–27.

Step 5. After the arachnoid has been incised, the temporal artery pedicle is approximated to the two dural bands with either interrupted or running sutures. With each successive incision in the arachnoid, there will be some drainage of cerebrospinal fluid, which makes the next incision more difficult. Accordingly, the surgeon should start by incising the arachnoid over the largest vessels closer to the ear and work toward the midline. The collection of cerebrospinal fluid tends to be gravity-dependent; therefore, despite the incisions in the arachnoid over the temporal lobe and Sylvian fissure, there usually are some large subarachnoid spaces along the parietal lobe close to the inferior edge of the bone that can be incised.

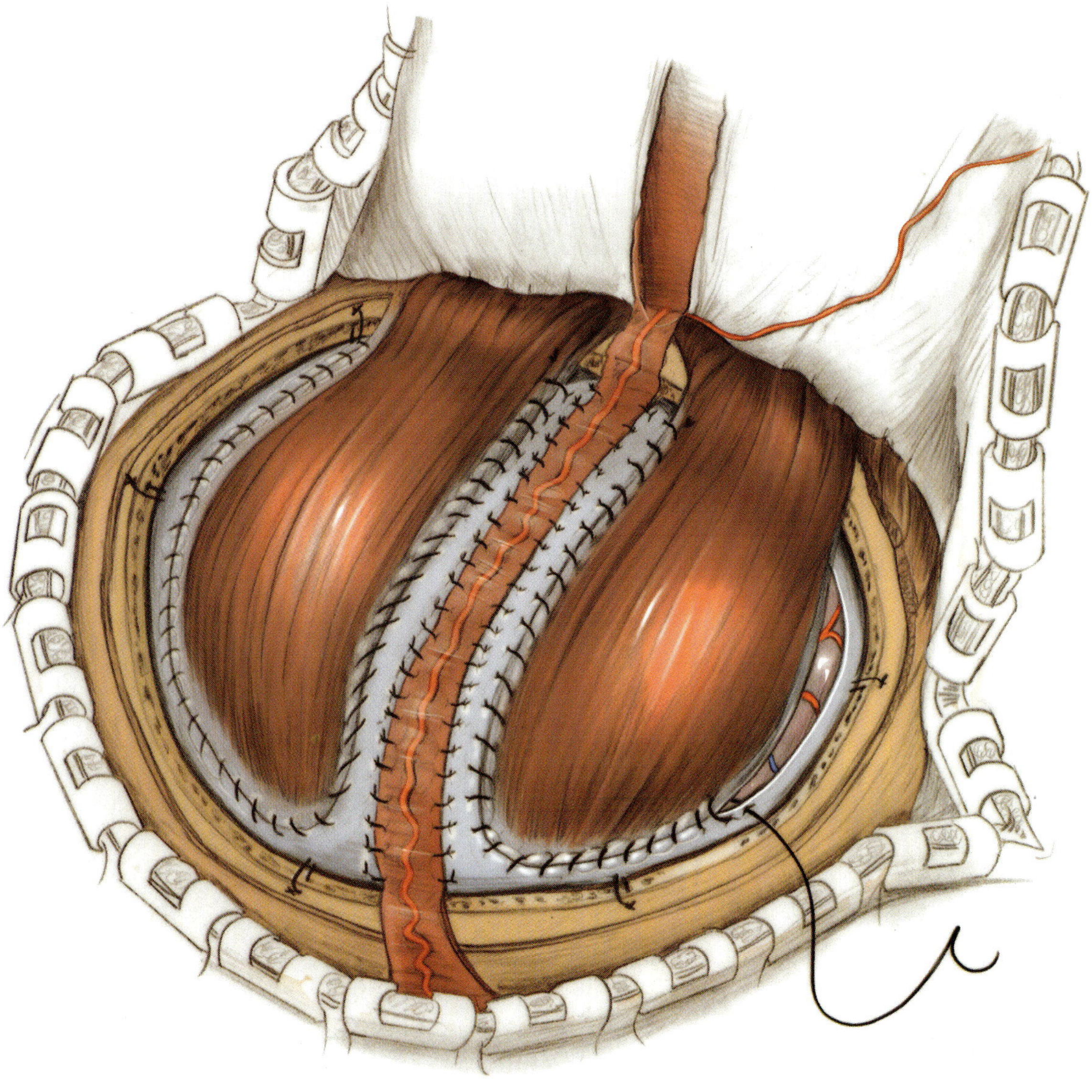

Figure 11–28.

Step 6. The myosynangiosis is performed by sewing the temporalis muscle and its fascia to the cut edge of the dura mater covering all the exposed cerebral cortex. After the encephalomyoarteriosynangiosis has been performed, the bone flap is applied loosely with monofilament sutures. The skin flap is closed in two layers. Nitroglycerin paste is applied to the scalp, and a loose head dressing is applied.

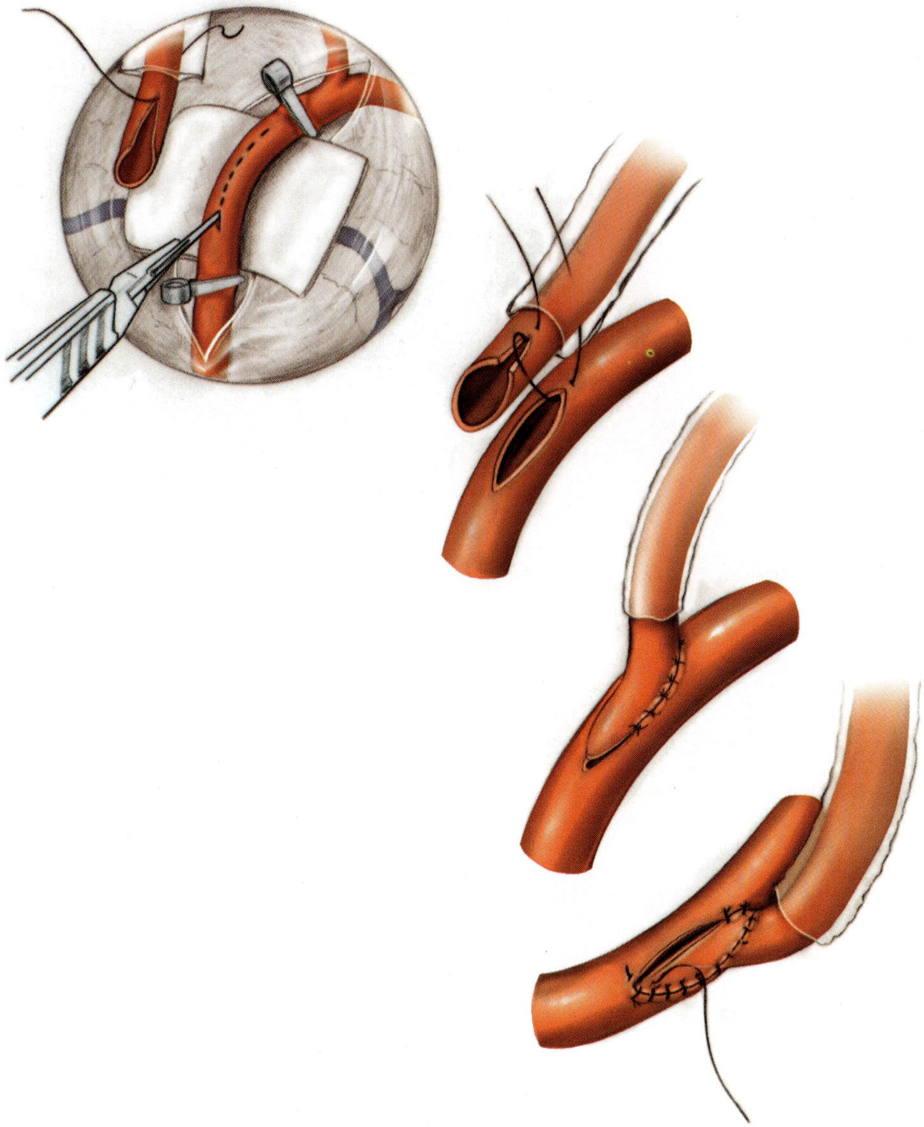

Figure 11–29.

If the temporal artery and cortical vessels are of sufficient size, a direct superficial temporal artery-to-middle cerebral artery anastomosis should be performed. The recipient cortical vessel is dissected free from its arachnoid over a distance of approximately 1.5 cm. A rubber dam is placed under the vessel to prop it up. Before the artery is occluded temporarily, thiopental (2 to 3 mg/kg) is administered to provide some cerebral protection. The artery is occluded temporarily with two microwire clips. An arteriotomy is made with a broken razor blade or a sharp #11 blade knife and extended with straight microscissors. Depending on the surgeon's preference, the anastomosis can be performed either with running or interrupted 10-0 or 9-0 monofilament sutures. During preparation of the cortical vessel, the temporal artery is irrigated with a papaverine-heparin solution and then occluded at its base to prevent thrombus formation within the vessel. After the anastomosis has been performed, some oozing may occur from the suture line. This usually can be stopped by applying an absorbable gelatin sponge (Gelfoam).

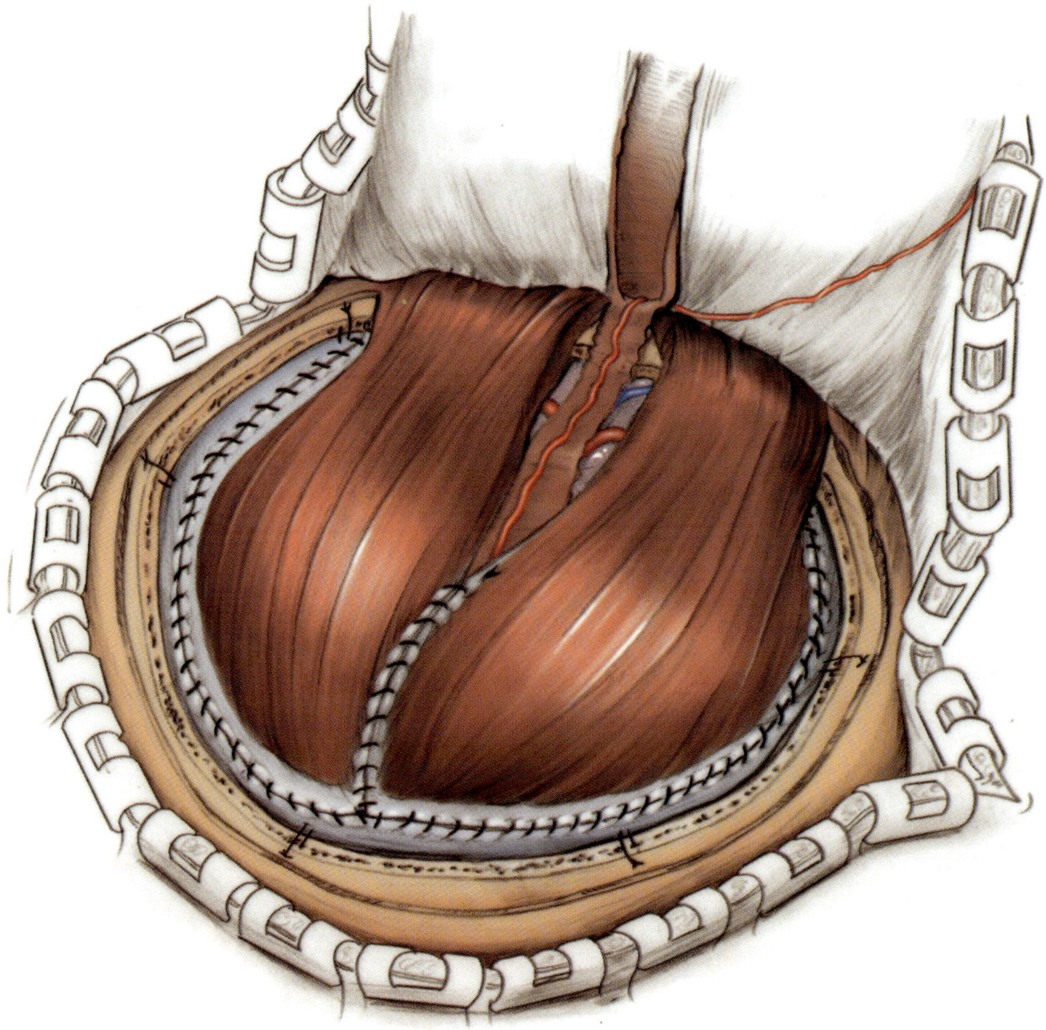

Figure 11–30.

After the superficial temporal artery-to-middle cerebral artery bypass has been completed, the myosynangiosis is performed by anastomosing the temporalis muscle and its fascia to the cut edge of the dura mater. The wound is closed as described above.

VERTEBRAL ARTERY TRANSPOSITION

The incision is placed approximately one fingerbreadth above the clavicle. It extends for 7 to 8 cm laterally from the suprasternal notch. The platysma, sternocleidomastoid, sternohyoid, and sternothyroid muscles are divided. This exposes the common carotid artery, the internal jugular vein, and the vagus nerve. The artery and vein are separated free from their loose fascial tissue. The vertebral artery can be exposed by two routes. First, the jugular vein and the vagus nerve can be retracted laterally and the vertebral artery identified in the deep cervical fascia. Exposure in this way does not require sectioning the anterior scalene muscle or displacing the phrenic nerve. On the right side, the surgeon should be alert for the recurrent laryngeal nerve, which needs to be protected if visualized. On the left side, the thoracic duct may be visualized; if it is, it should be ligated. The second type of exposure requires displacement of the jugular vein medially. The phrenic nerve is identified on top of the scalene muscle, running from lateral to medial. This nerve is retracted laterally by using a small vascular loop. The anterior scalene muscle is incised horizontally to allow the proximal vertebral artery to be identified. The vertebral artery is dissected free from its surrounding tissue and its submergence behind the longest colli muscle. Occasionally, sympathetic fibers cross the vertebral artery; they are divided.

After the vertebral artery has been mobilized, it is ligated proximally and divided. The common carotid artery is occluded temporarily with two soft-shoe Fogarty clamps. A Goosen punch is used to create an opening in the common carotid artery. The anastomosis of the vertebral artery to the common carotid artery is performed under the operating microscope using interrupted 8-0 monofilament sutures. It is best to use interrupted sutures because a running suture may lead to stenosis of the anastomosis. The back wall is sewn in place first. Before the opening is made in the common carotid artery, it is important to determine the best angle and course of the vertebral artery that will allow a gentle curve without causing kinking or tension along the suture line. Occasionally, if there is significant atherosclerotic plaque in the common carotid artery, it may be necessary to perform an endarterectomy before the vertebral artery transposition. To increase collateral blood flow, induced hypertension should be used during the operation, as should intraoperative encephalography.

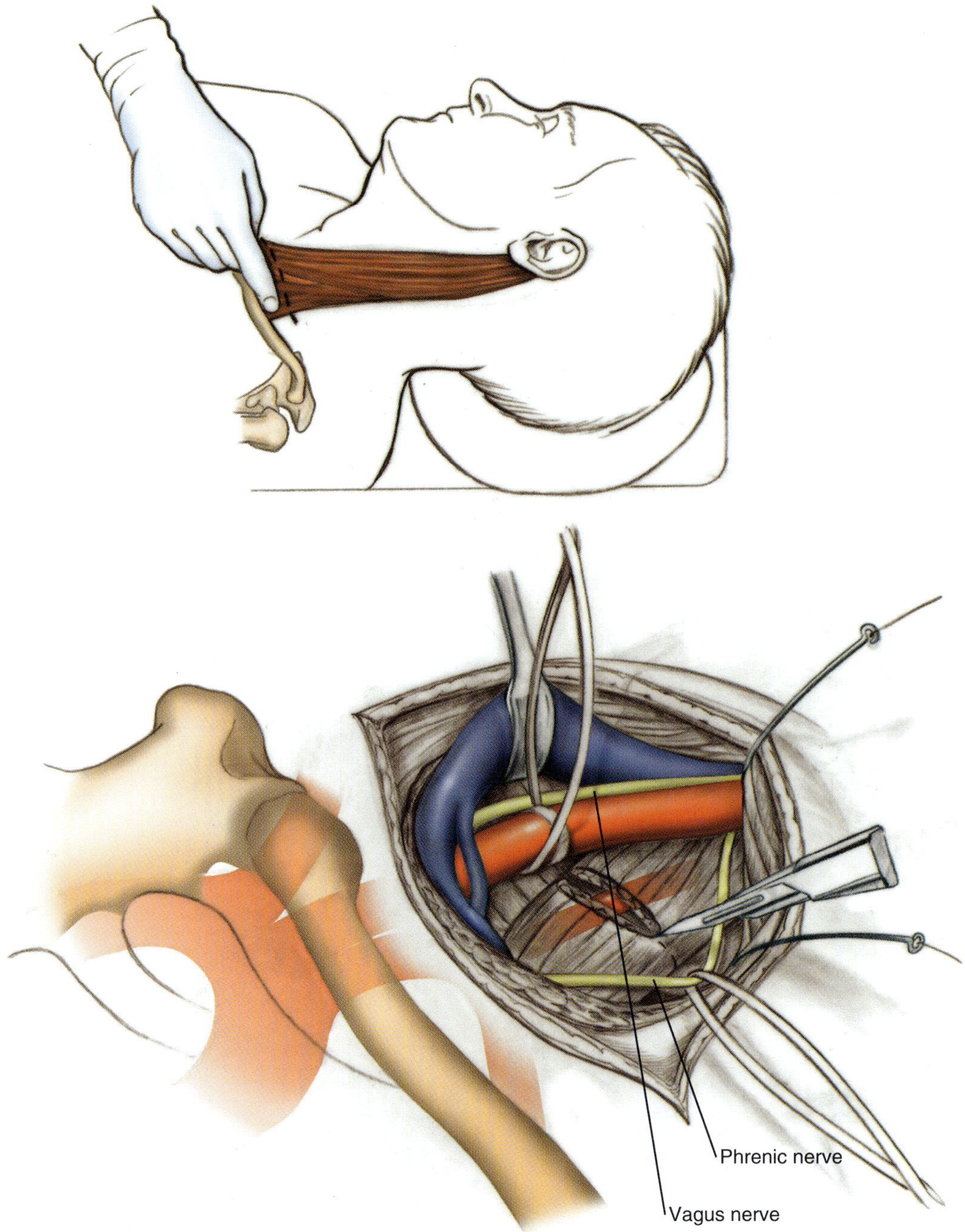

Figure 11–31.

The incision is made approximately one fingerbreadth above the clavicle. It extends for 7 to 8 cm laterally from the suprasternal notch. As illustrated here, the jugular vein and the vagus nerve are retracted medially and the phrenic nerve is retracted laterally. This allows exposure of the anterior scalene muscle, which is divided to expose the vertebral artery. The thoracic duct may be visualized on the left side; it should be ligated. A sufficient length of the vertebral artery needs to be mobilized.

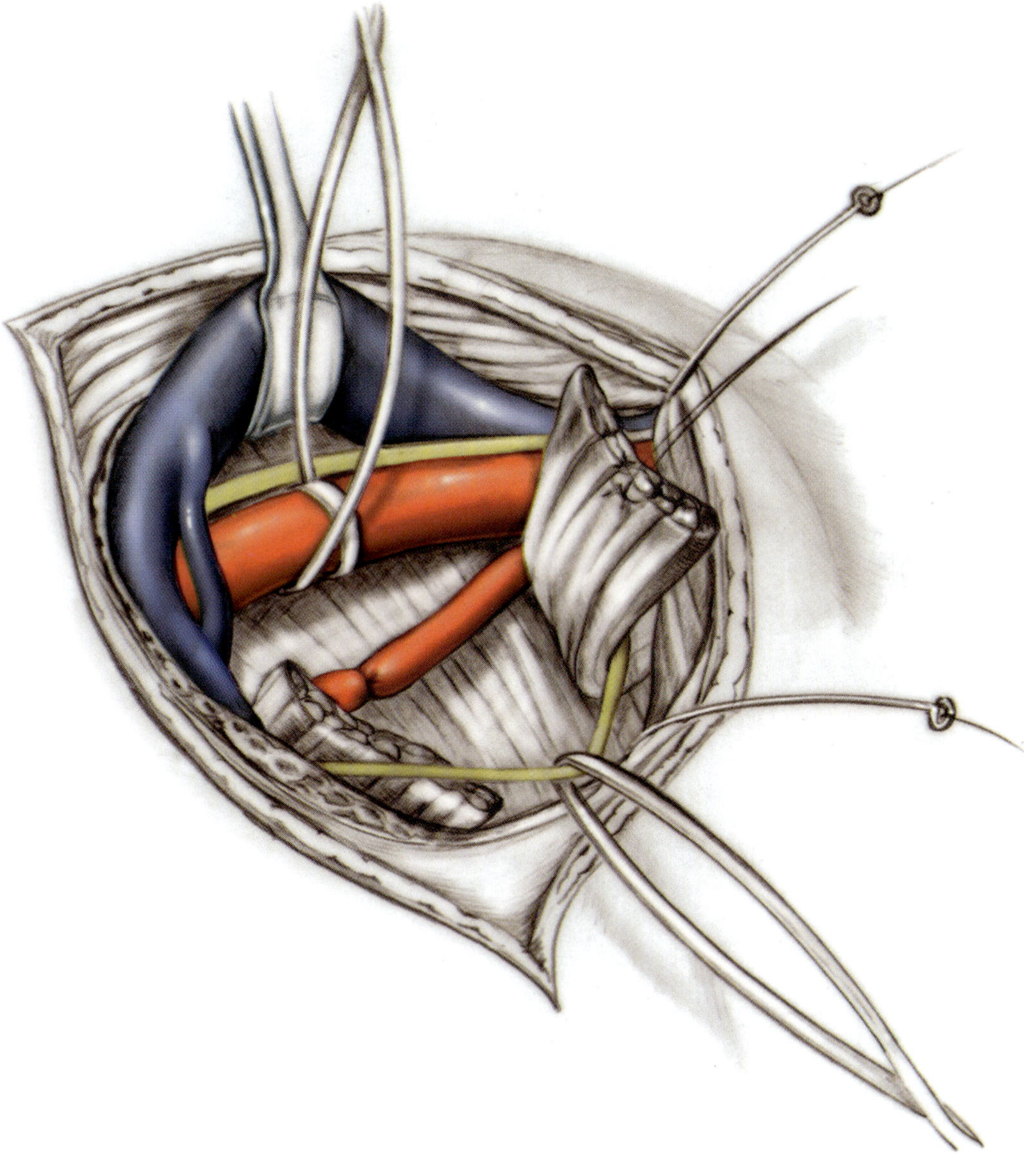

Figure 11–32.

A small vascular loop can be placed around the phrenic nerve and gently retracted laterally to keep this nerve out of harm's way. After the anterior scalene muscle has been sectioned, the vertebral artery is dissected free from the surrounding soft tissue and ligated as low as possible in the operative field. The more the vertebral artery is mobilized, the easier the anastomosis.

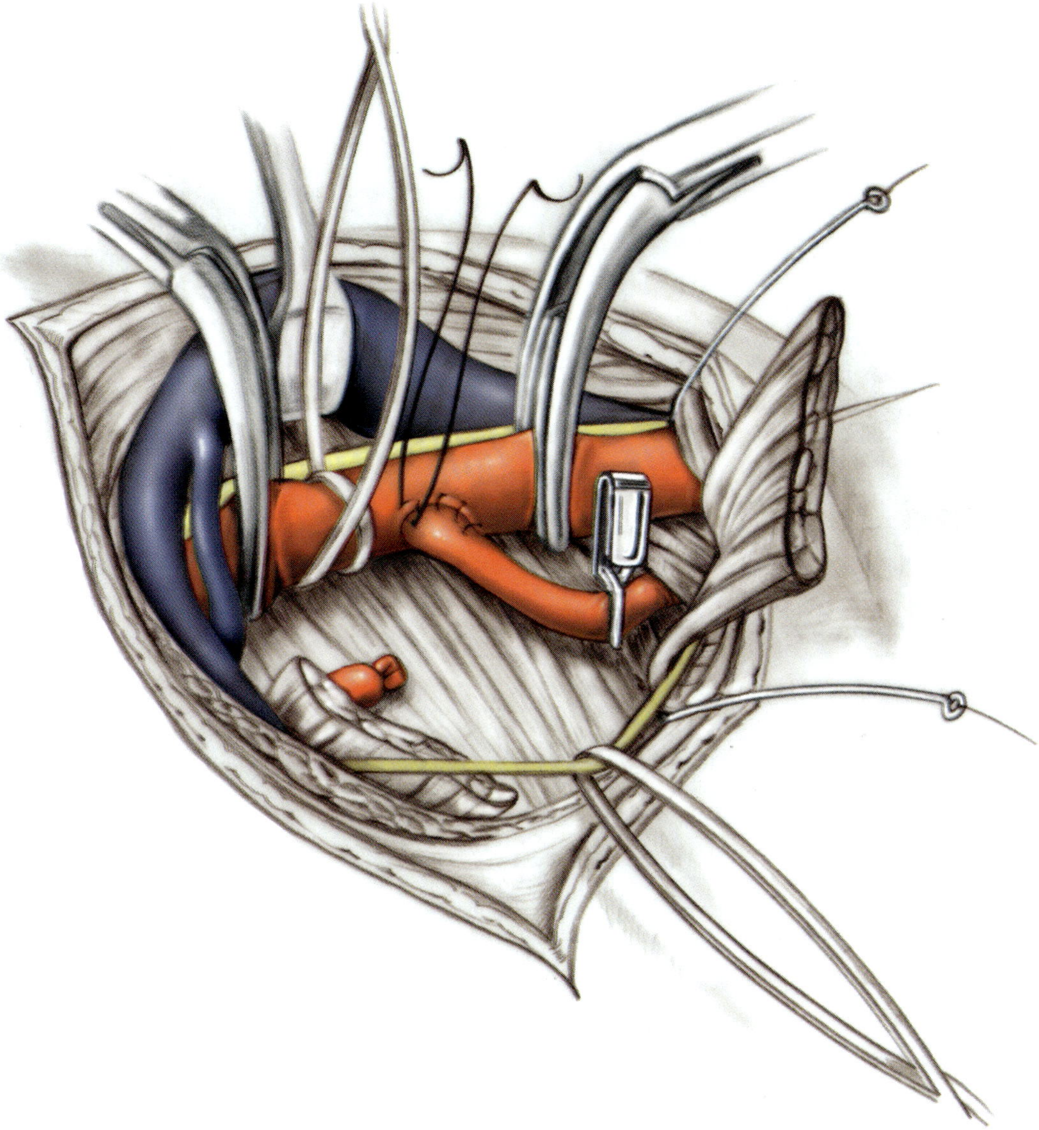

Figure 11–33.

The common carotid artery is occluded with two soft-shoe Fogarty clamps. A Goosen punch is used to create the opening in the common carotid artery. It is important to place this opening in such a location that the vertebral artery makes a gentle curve without kinking. Under the operating microscope, the vertebral artery is sewn in place to the common carotid artery with interrupted 8-0 monofilament sutures. During the carotid occlusion, induced hypertension is used to increase collateral blood flow.

SAPHENOUS VEIN BYPASS

Saphenous vein bypass procedures can be beneficial in treating both ischemic disease and large broad-based fusiform type giant intracranial aneurysms. For example, a saphenous vein bypass graft from the cervical carotid artery to the posterior cerebral artery may be useful in treating medically refractory high-grade stenosis of the basilar artery. Giant aneurysms of the internal carotid or middle cerebral artery can sometimes be treated by the combination of proximal ligation or trapping and a distal bypass.

An extremely important component of this operation is correct harvesting of the saphenous vein. First, it should not be overly manipulated during the dissection, and the adventitia surrounding the vessel should be preserved. The small branches and tributaries are ligated with 5-0 or 6-0 monofilament sutures instead of bipolar cautery. Before the saphenous vein is removed, a 6-0 monofilament suture is sewn loosely into the adventitia from proximal to distal to allow for the correct orientation of the vein (Garrett line). This prevents the vein from twisting during its placement through the subcutaneous tunnel from the craniotomy to the neck. After the vein has been harvested, it is irrigated with a cold solution of papaverine-heparin. A vein dilatation kit is used to prevent overdistention of the vein.

For procedures on the anterior circulation, either the supraclinoid internal carotid artery or the middle cerebral artery is exposed through a standard pterional craniotomy. For anastomosing into the middle cerebral artery, an M_2 segment is best. Sewing into the middle cerebral artery is technically easier than performing a direct end-to-end or end-to-side anastomosis to the supraclinoid internal carotid artery. The anastomosis is performed with interrupted 9-0 or 8-0 monofilament sutures. Although a running suture requires less time, there is a small risk of stenosis at the site of the anastomosis. The length of the anastomosis is approximately 1.0 cm. Before the middle cerebral artery or the internal carotid artery is occluded, thiopental (3 to 5 mg/kg) or etomidate is administered intravenously. Induced hypertension is used to increase collateral blood flow.

For procedures on the posterior circulation, the subtemporal approach is used to expose the posterior cerebral artery. The craniotomy is carried low to the floor of the middle cranial fossa. Also, cerebrospinal fluid is drained through a lumbar needle and mannitol is injected to achieve brain relaxation. In the subtemporal approach, it is important to protect the vein of Labbé with absorbable gelatin sponges and cottonoids (Americot). The entire temporal lobe is protected with hemostatic fabric (Surgicel) and cottonoids before it is retracted. This is an important point because before the posterior cerebral artery is occluded, 5,000 units of heparin are administered. As the posterior cerebral artery courses around the peduncle, it is dissected free from the arachnoid. Typically, the anterior half of the P_2 segment is chosen for the anastomosis posterior to the oculomotor nerve. This segment of the posterior cerebral artery usually has no perforating vessels. Specifically, the thalamoperforating arteries arise along the P_1 segment and the posterior choroidal and posterior temporal arteries arise from the distal P_2 segment. The distal anastomosis in a posterior circulation bypass is an extremely exacting and technically difficult procedure. The anastomosis is approximately 1.0 cm long. It is performed with running 9-0 monofilament sutures. A running suture is preferable to interrupted sutures because limited space at the depth of the wound makes tying the suture difficult; therefore, the use of running sutures saves time.

Before the distal anastomosis is performed, a #20-French Argyle trocar catheter is inserted into the temporalis muscle and passed over the zygoma, through the deep layers of the subcutaneous tissue in front of the ear, superficial to the parotid gland, and down into the neck wound. A #2 silk suture is then brought through this catheter with a trocar. The saphenous vein is tied to the silk suture and brought through the Argyle catheter. The previously placed Garrett line is used to make sure that the vein is not rotated in the Argyle catheter.

The importance of the proximal anastomosis needs to be emphasized. A poorly constructed proximal anastomosis will lead to occlusion of the vein graft. Various proximal anastomoses can be used. For a posterior circulation bypass, the saphenous vein should be sewn to the stump of the external carotid artery with either a fish mouth or spatulated anastomosis. For giant aneurysms of the anterior circulation in which trapping is performed, it still is useful to sew to the external carotid artery. In this way, a saphenous vein can be constructed completely before the internal carotid artery is occluded, thereby decreasing the risk of ischemic injury. If the external carotid artery is small, an end-to-side anastomosis to the common carotid artery can be performed using a Goosen punch. If a preoperative trial balloon occlusion suggests that temporary occlusion of the internal carotid artery can be tolerated, the saphenous vein can be sewn directly end-to-end to the internal carotid artery.

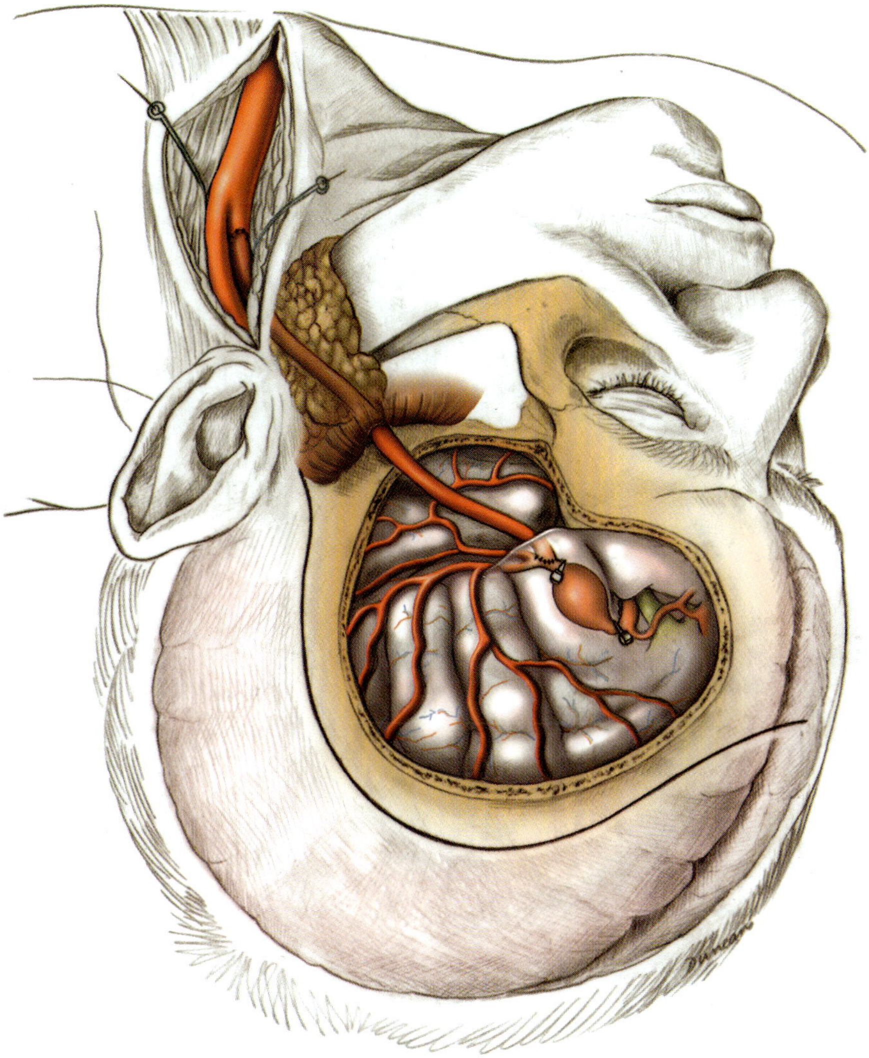

Figure 11–34.

This is the general scheme for intracranial-to-extracranial bypass using a long-vein saphenous vein bypass. In this illustration, a giant fusiform aneurysm of the middle cerebral artery is being trapped. Blood flow to the distal middle cerebral artery is preserved through a saphenous vein graft from the external carotid artery to the middle cerebral artery beyond the aneurysm.

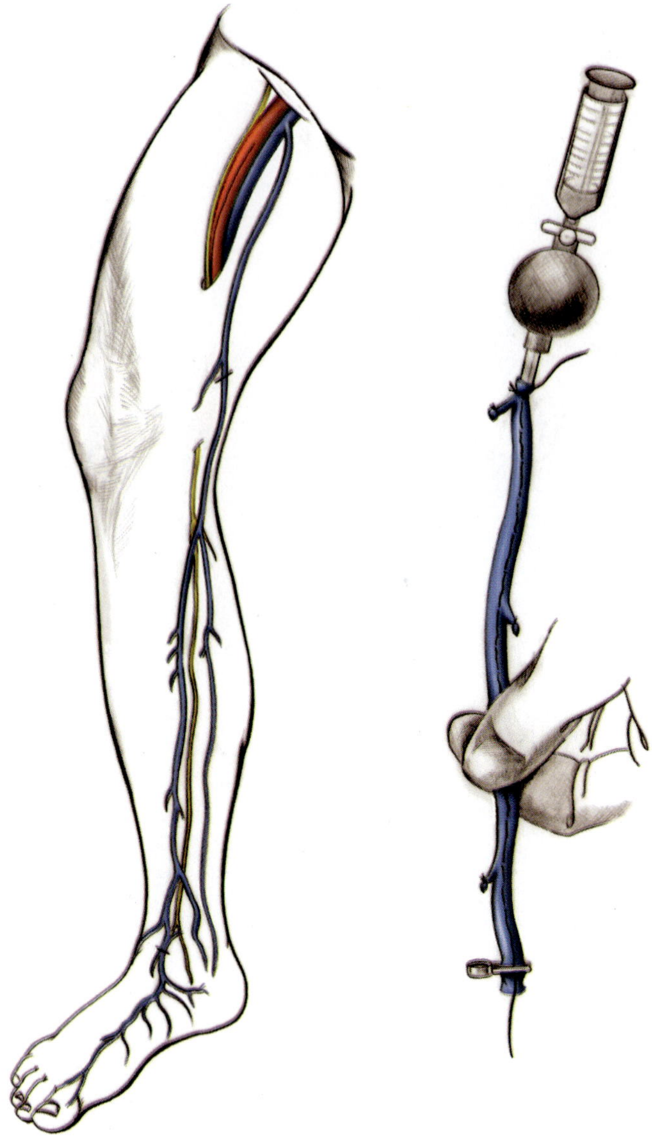

Figure 11–35.

A critical step in the preparation for this type of bypass is harvesting the saphenous vein from the leg. The saphenous vein is identified adjacent to the medial malleolus and dissected upward just beyond the popliteal fossa. During this dissection, the various branches of the saphenous vein are ligated with a 6-0 monofilament suture instead of bipolar cautery. The adventitia of the vein should be preserved. Before the vein is removed from the leg, a Garrett line is sewn in place with a 6-0 monofilament suture. This Garrett line is important in maintaining the correct orientation of the vein as it is passed through the subcutaneous tunnel from the craniotomy to the neck. After the vein is removed, a mechanical spasm usually occurs. This spasm can be broken with gentle massage. Dilatation of the vein is achieved with a standard vein dilatation kit, using a cold papaverine solution. After the vein has been expanded, it is irrigated with a heparin solution.

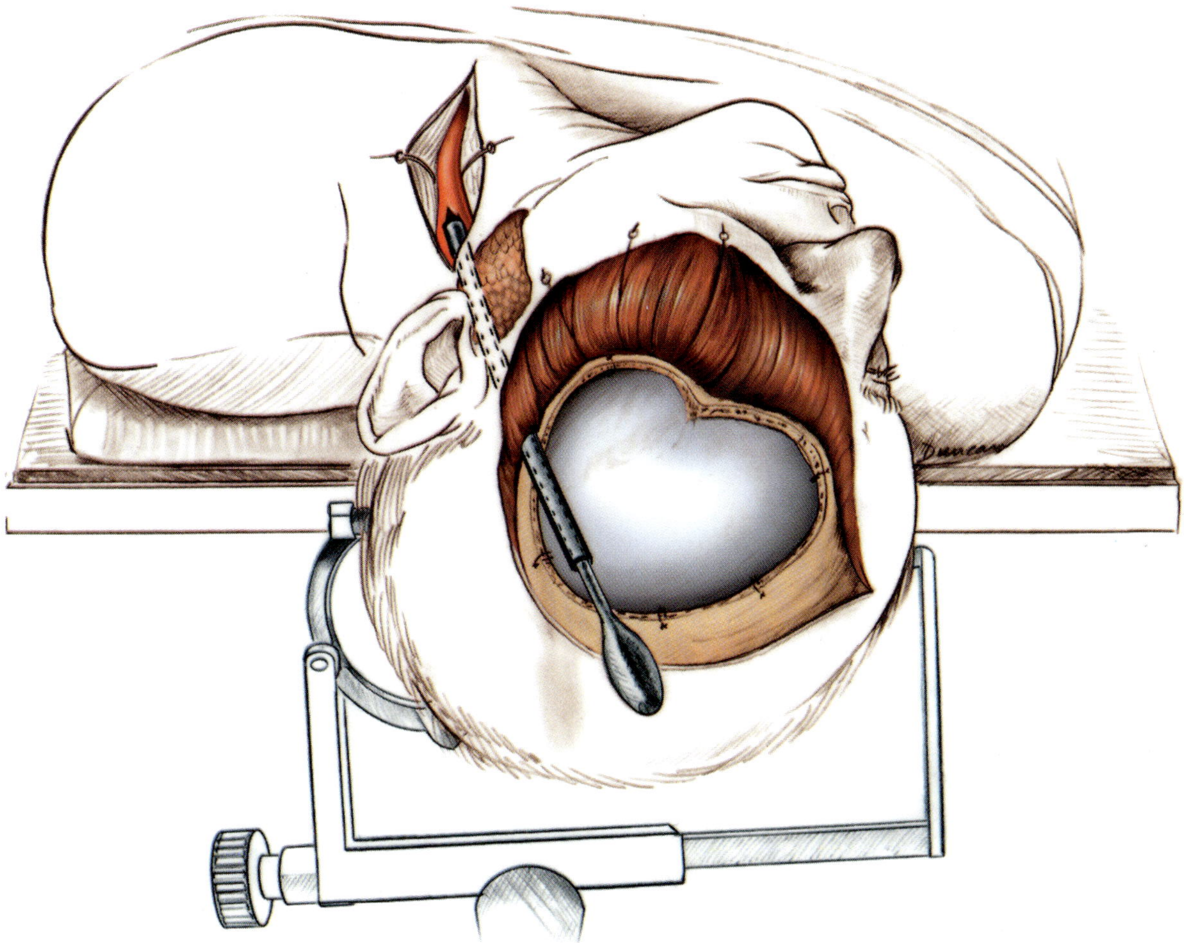

Figure 11–36.

The subcutaneous tunnel from the craniotomy to the cervical carotid artery is achieved with a #20-French Argyle trocar catheter. The trajectory of this catheter is in front of the ear and superficial to the parotid gland. After the Argyle tube has been placed, a #2 silk suture is brought through it. This is attached to the vein, which then is also brought through the catheter using the Garrett line to preserve the correct orientation.

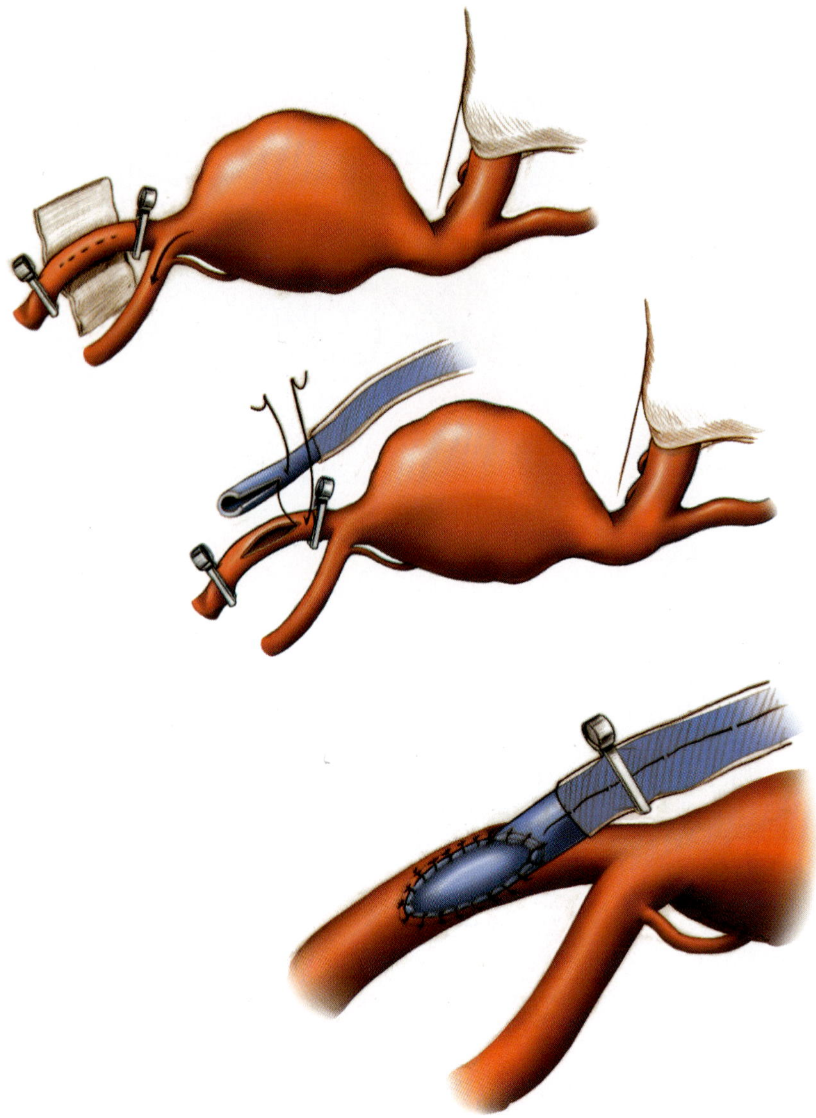

Figure 11–37.

In this illustration, a branch of the M_2 segment has been chosen for the site of the anastomosis so that blood will still flow through most of the middle cerebral artery complex during the temporary occlusion required for the anastomosis. A rubber dam is useful in propping up the middle cerebral artery. The length of the anastomosis is approximately 1.0 cm. Although running sutures work well, there is a small risk of stenosis at the site of the anastomosis; thus, interrupted sutures are preferable. After the distal anastomosis has been achieved, the temporary clips on the middle cerebral artery are removed. The saphenous vein is irrigated again with heparin, and a temporary clip is applied close to the distal anastomosis to prevent blood from running down the saphenous vein and possibly causing thrombus formation because of stagnation. When performing an extracranial-to-intracranial saphenous vein bypass for ischemic disease, 5,000 units of heparin should be administered systemically before the initial anastomosis is performed. However, whether heparin should be used during bypass surgery for intracranial aneurysms is a matter of controversy.

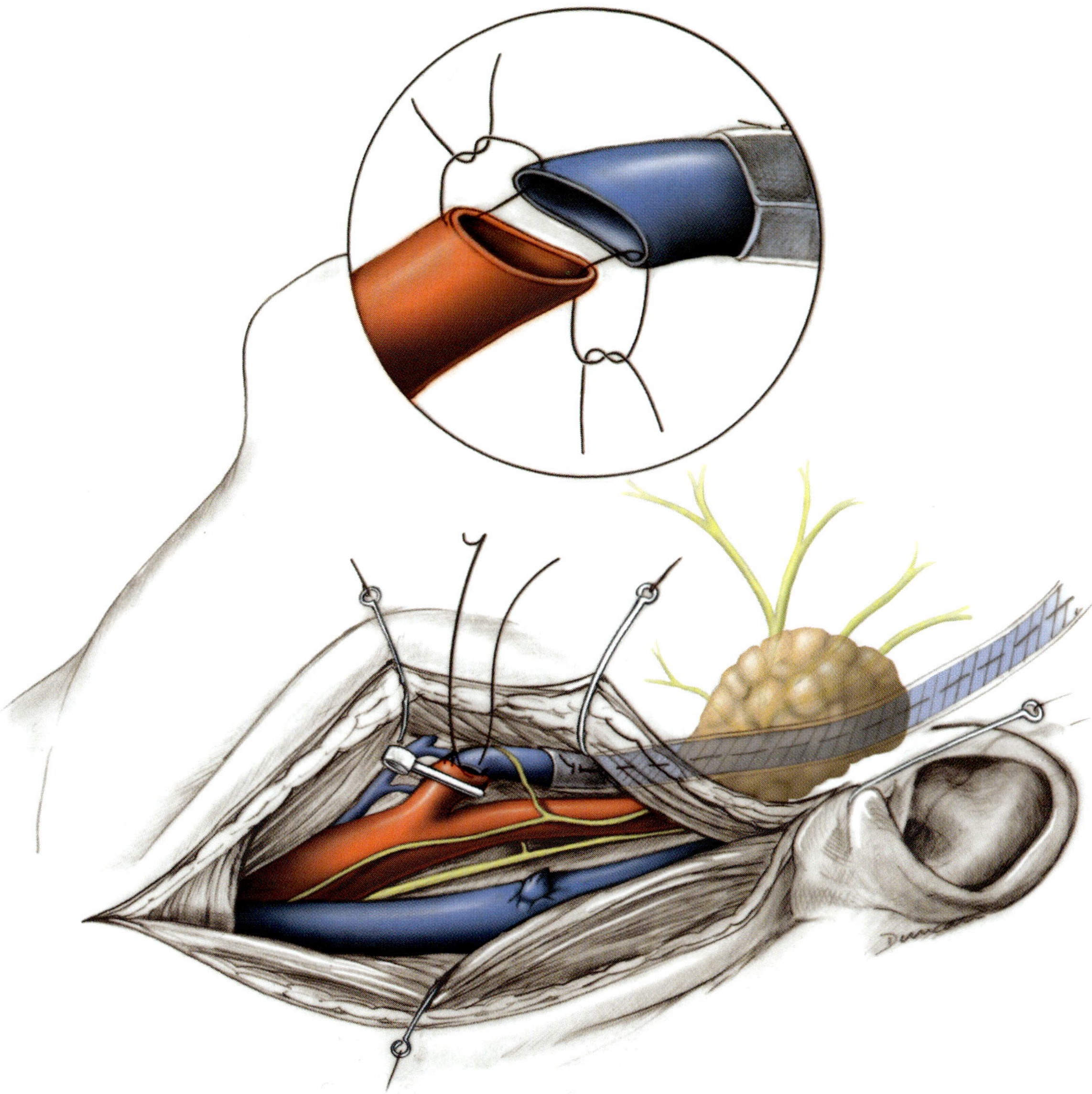

Figure 11–38.

As illustrated here, the saphenous vein is being sewn to the external carotid artery just beyond the bifurcation of the common carotid artery. With this procedure, blood flow is maintained through the internal carotid artery throughout the operation. Furthermore, after the aneurysm of the middle cerebral artery has been trapped, the internal carotid artery will continue to perfuse the anterior cerebral, the posterior communicating, and the anterior choroidal arteries. Often, the best proximal anastomosis is a spatulated type, using interrupted 6-0 monofilament sutures. Just before the last few sutures are tied, it is best to use back bleeding down the saphenous vein and up the external carotid artery to flush out any residual air in the graft. In the example shown here, the aneurysm is trapped with aneurysm clips after flow is restored. For ischemic disease procedures, the heparin is not reversed. It is important to give aspirin to all these patients after the operation.

12

Cerebrospinal Fluid Drainage Procedures

Copyright © 1999 Mayo Foundation.

EXTERNAL VENTRICULAR DRAIN

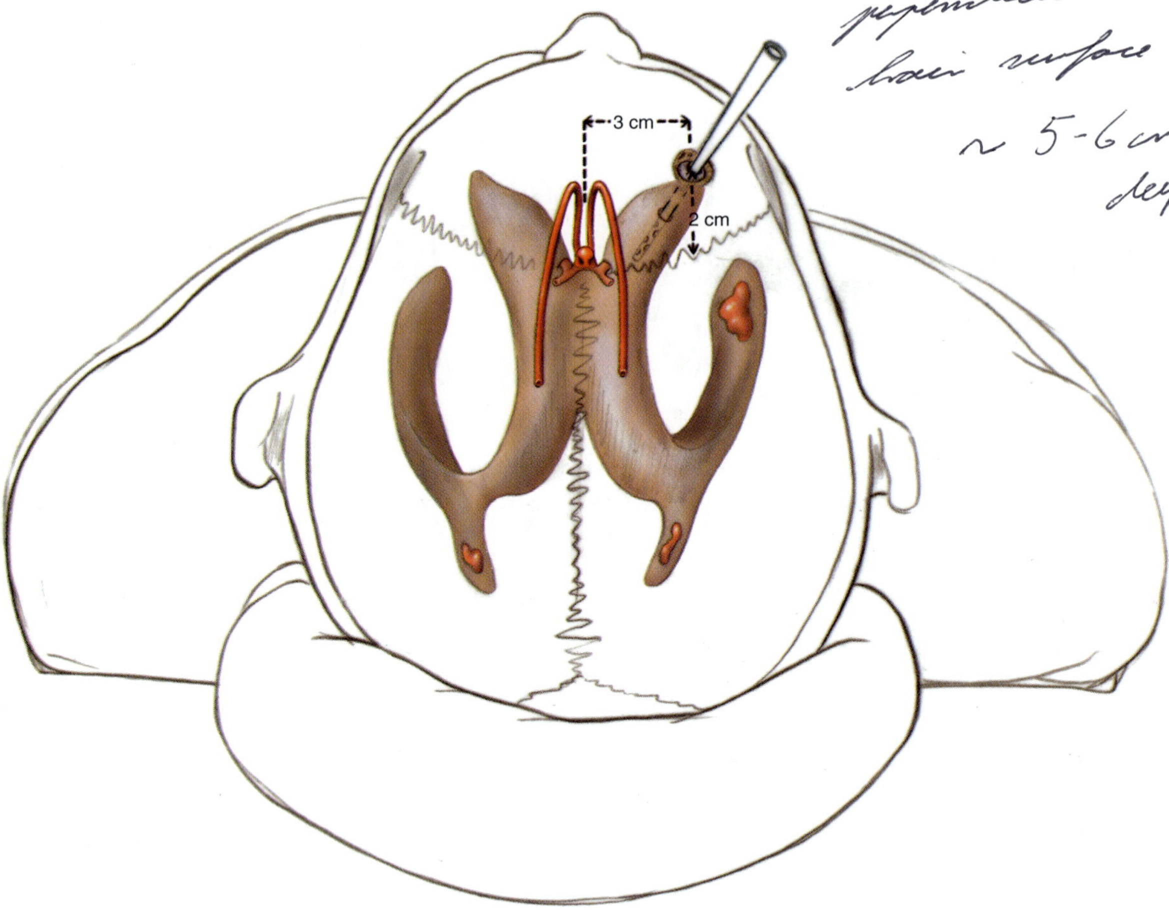

Figure 12–1.

Placement of an external ventricular drain can be performed at the bedside, in the emergency room, or in the operating room. The ease of placement depends on the size of the ventricles and the presence or absence of a midline shift. If the ventricle is very small, the use of stereotaxis or external scalp support devices should be considered. The patient's head is held in a donut or round wash basin in a straight up, slightly flexed position, with 0 degrees of rotation. It is useful to have the nurse or assistant hold the patient's chin underneath the drapes to prevent movement. The twist drill or bur hole should be placed 3 cm lateral to the midline and 1 to 2 cm anterior to the coronal suture. The ventricular catheter is passed perpendicular to the brain. Therefore, the trajectory will point to an imaginary line extending back from the inner canthus of the ipsilateral eye. In most cases, the surgeon will enter the lateral ventricle at 5 to 6 cm from the calvarium. Typically, there is a feeling of resistance and then popping as the lateral ependymal surface is punctured. After the ventricle has been cannulated, the catheter should be inserted an additional 2 cm. The metal stylus within the catheter is removed to ensure that there is good flow of cerebrospinal fluid. The catheter is reoccluded to prevent excessive drainage of cerebrospinal fluid. Most ventricular catheters have 5.0-cm markings.

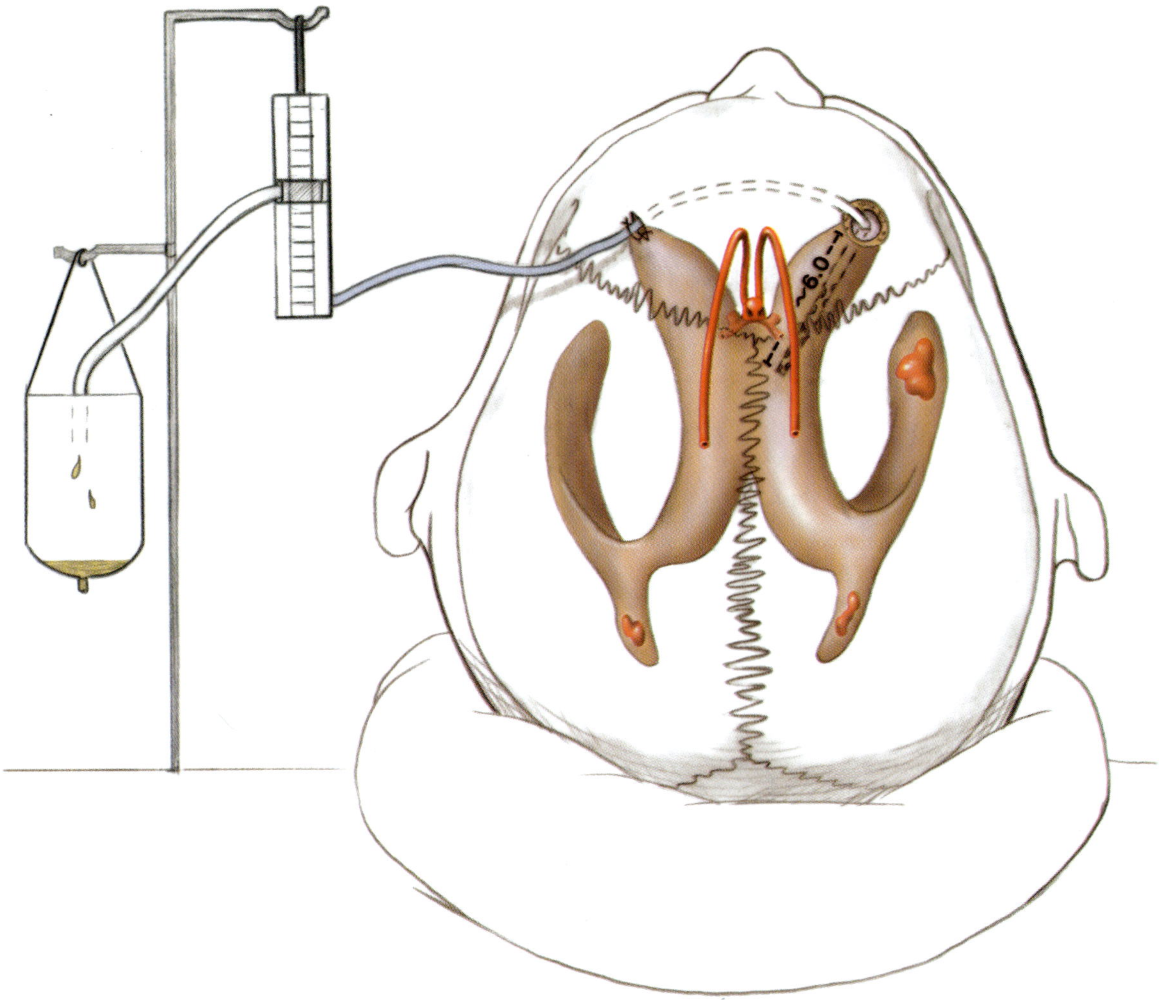

Figure 12–2.

It is optimum to have the catheter run underneath the galea for approximately 5 to 6 cm before it is brought out through the skin. Some evidence suggests that placing the catheter in a funnel decreases the risk of contamination and infection. The wounds are closed with a monofilament suture. Collodion can also be applied to the incision overlying the twist drill. A full head dressing is applied. Various draining systems can be used to regulate the amount of cerebrospinal fluid drainage and intracranial pressure.

VENTRICULOPERITONEAL SHUNT

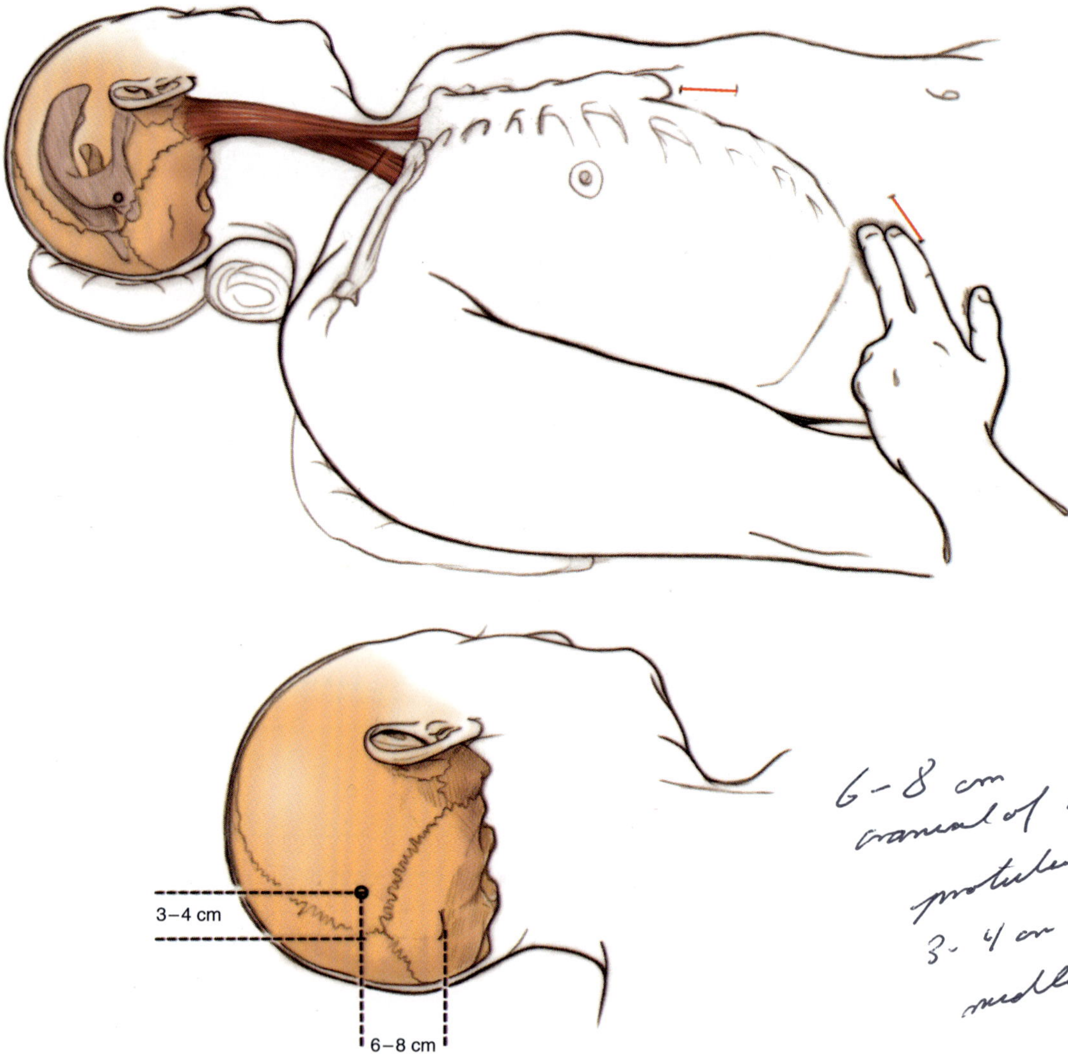

Figure 12–3.

Step 1. Illustrated here is the general body position for placement of a ventriculoperitoneal shunt. Under ideal circumstances, the head should be rotated laterally, parallel to the floor. Placement of a towel underneath the shoulder helps with head rotation. In older patients with cervical spondylosis, head rotation may be difficult. In fact, placement of a ventricular shunt through a frontal bur hole may be technically easier. For parietooccipital shunt placement, the bur hole should be made 6 cm up from the external occipital protuberance and 3 cm lateral from the midline. This will approximate the bur hole over the lambdoid suture. Placing the bur hole on top of the lambdoid suture is advantageous because frequently the dura mater is stuck to the underlying calvarium, which means there often is less epidural bleeding. Either a midline or a right subcostal incision can be used to expose the peritoneum.

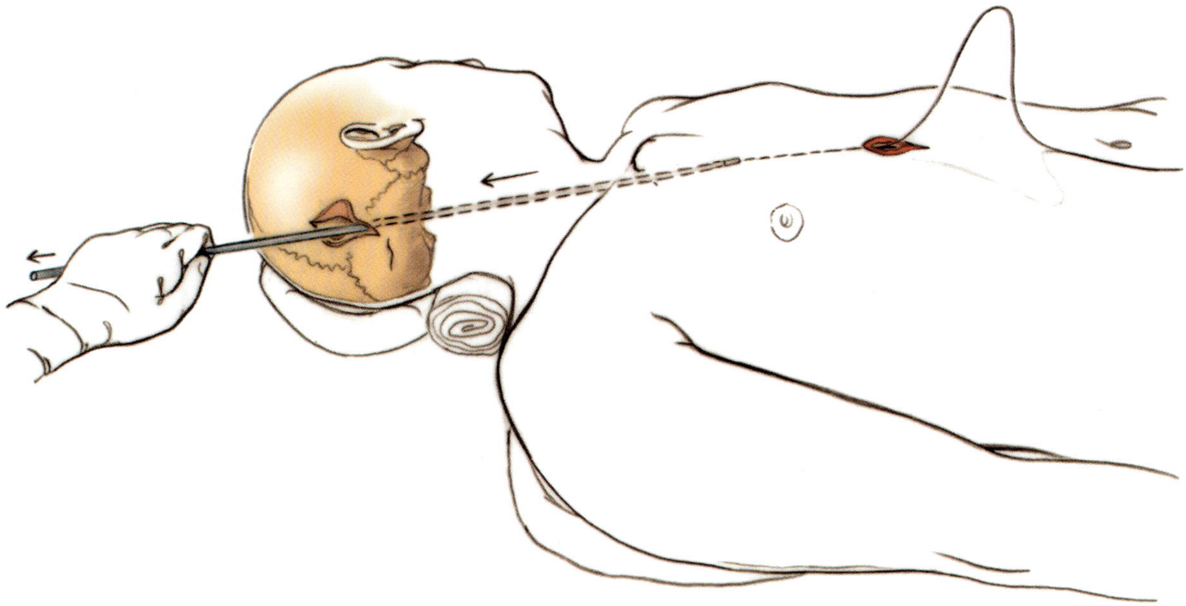

Figure 12–4.

Step 2. After the bur hole has been placed and the peritoneum exposed, a trocar is used to create a tunnel between the two incisions. A 2-0 suture is tied to the trocar and passed through the subcutaneous tunnel. Often, it is necessary to make a third incision near the clavicle. The subcutaneous tunnel adjacent to the occipital incision is spread with hemostats to create a subcutaneous pocket to contain the shunt valve.

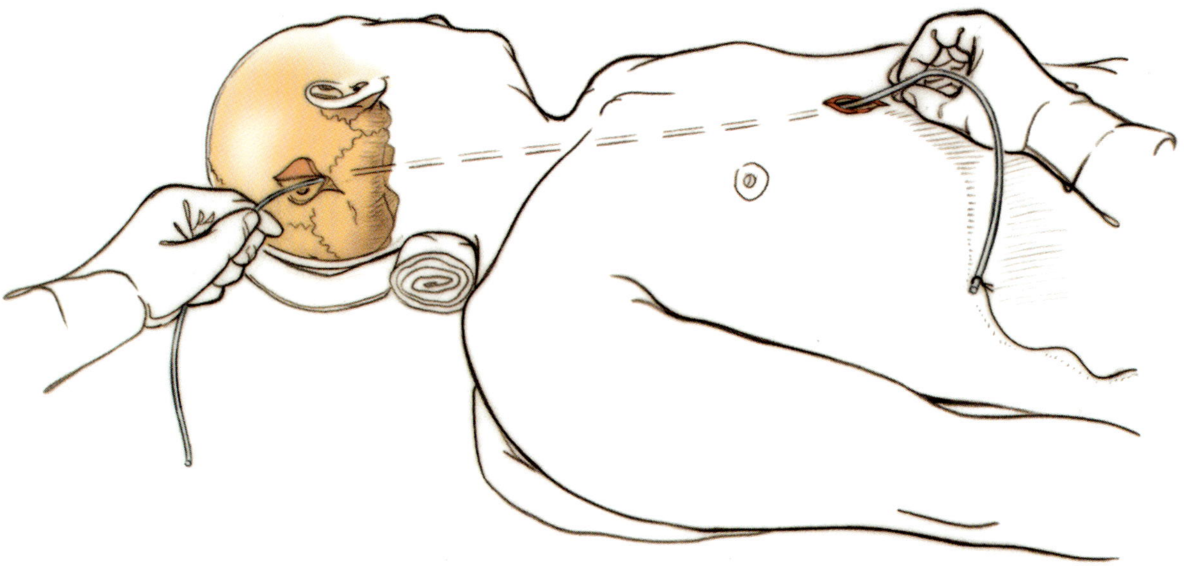

Figure 12–5.

Step 3. The shunt tube is passed between the two incisions. It is important not to let the shunt tube touch the skin. Because of this, the patient is draped with iodine-impregnated sterile (Steri) drapes to cover the skin overlying the surgical sites. After the shunt tube has been brought through the tunnel, the longer abdominal end is wrapped in a towel.

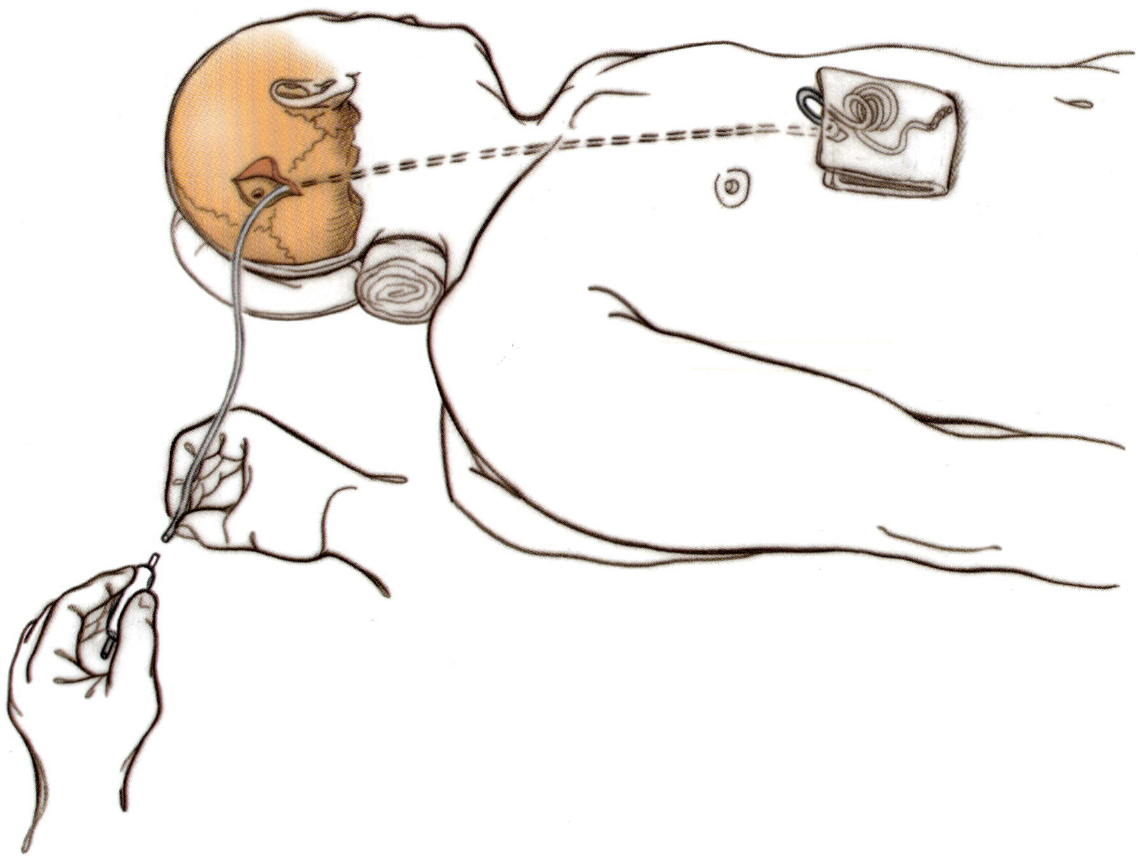

Figure 12–6.

Step 4. Many different shunt systems are available, and many of them have a peritoneal catheter already attached to the valve. If this is not the case, the chosen shunt valve is attached to the peritoneal catheter.

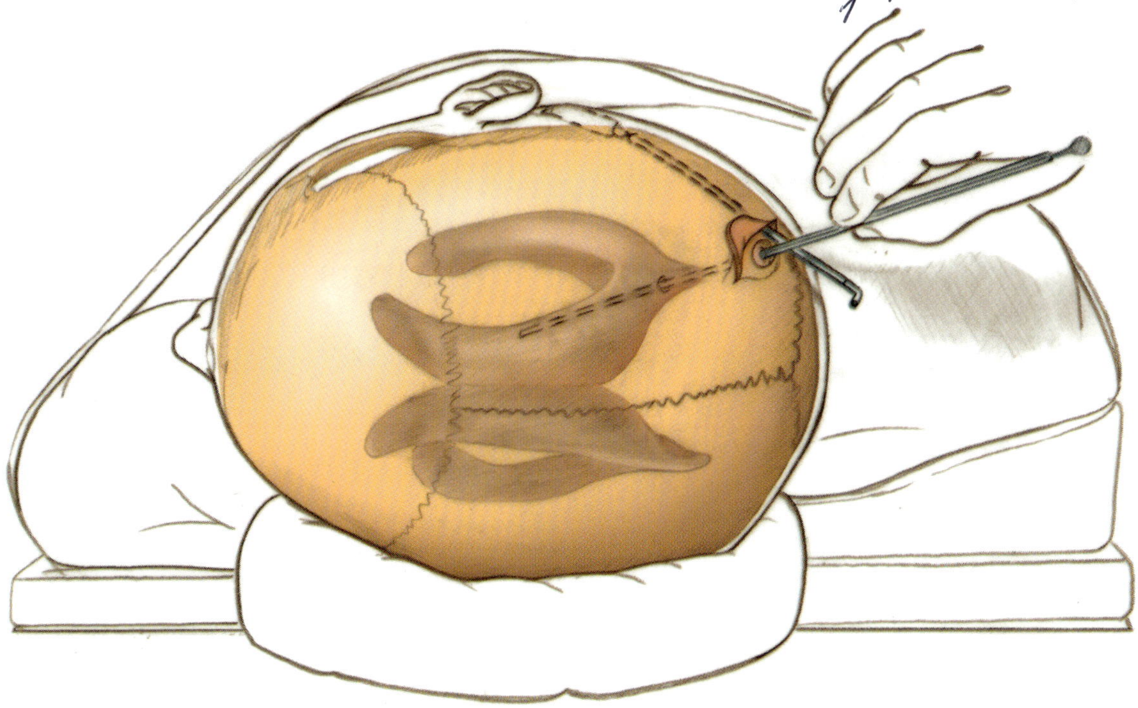

Figure 12–7.

Step 5. The dura mater is cauterized and opened in a cross fashion. It is important to not cut the dura mater back to the bone edge, otherwise nuisance bleeding may occur along the dural edge, which cannot be cauterized because of the overlying bone. The pia mater is cauterized and incised with a #11 blade knife, avoiding any major vessels in the area. Next, the ventricular catheter is passed into the ventricle using a trajectory that points the catheter toward a line extending posteriorly from the inner canthus of the ipsilateral eye. Because of this trajectory, the ventricular catheter will be perpendicular to the brain at its entry. It is important to recognize that a more lateral trajectory has the risk of injury to the posterior limb of the internal capsule. Alternatively, if the trajectory is too medial, the catheter will miss the ventricle and hit the falx cerebri. At approximately 5 to 6 cm, the catheter should have punctured the ependyma and be sitting within the atrium of the lateral ventricle. If the ventricle has not been cannulated by 7 cm, it is best for the surgeon to withdraw the catheter and try a slightly more medial instead of lateral trajectory.

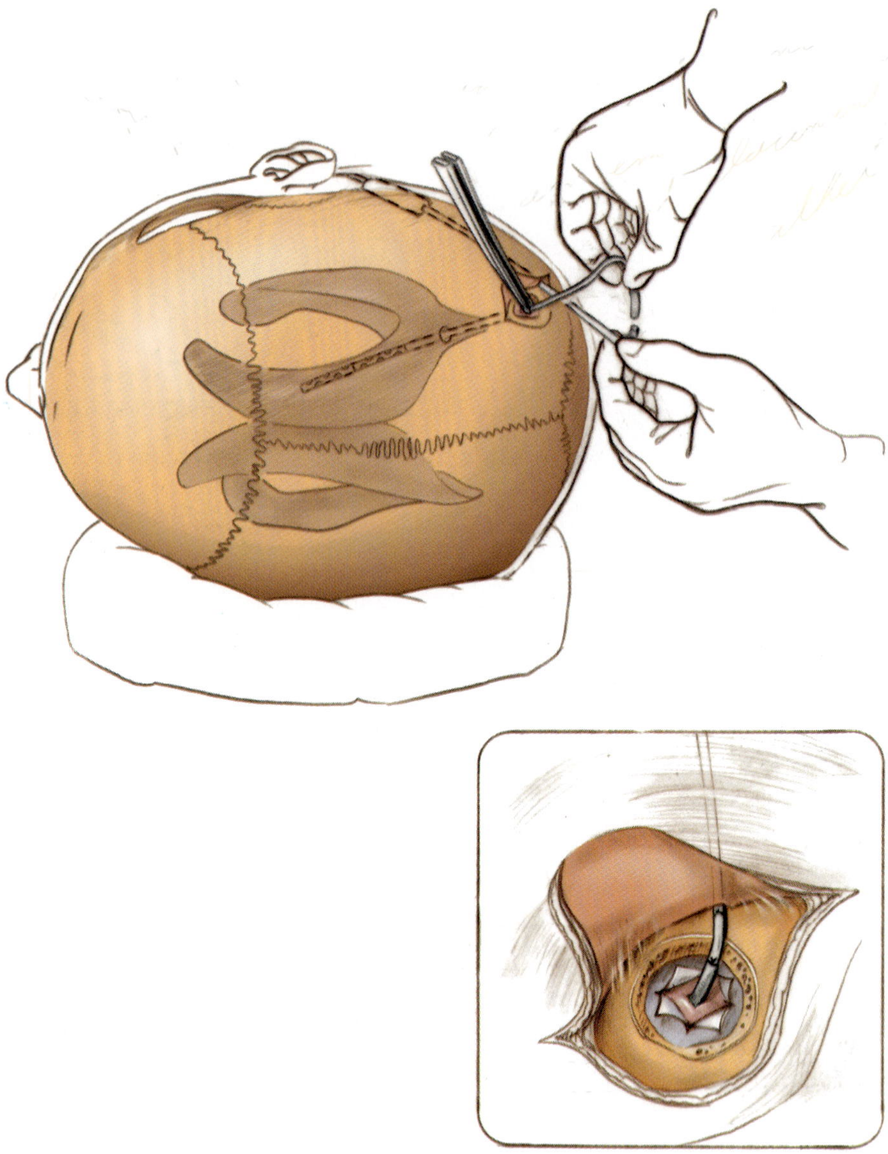

Figure 12–8.

Step 6. After the ventricle has been cannulated, the stylet is removed; the surgeon's assistant should immediately pinch the catheter with atraumatic forceps to prevent cerebrospinal fluid drainage. One cause of subdural hygroma in patients with normal pressure hydrocephalus is ventricular collapse due to excessive removal of cerebrospinal fluid at the time of shunt placement. There are several preferences for the length of the catheter that should be inserted into the ventricle. Some surgeons advocate placement of 10 cm of catheter, which places the tip in the frontal horn of the ipsilateral ventricle away from the choroid plexus. Other surgeons advocate a 7- to 8-cm placement, which places the catheter adjacent to the foramen of Monro. Whatever the choice, it is important to advance the catheter without a stylet to make sure that the catheter remains within the ventricle.

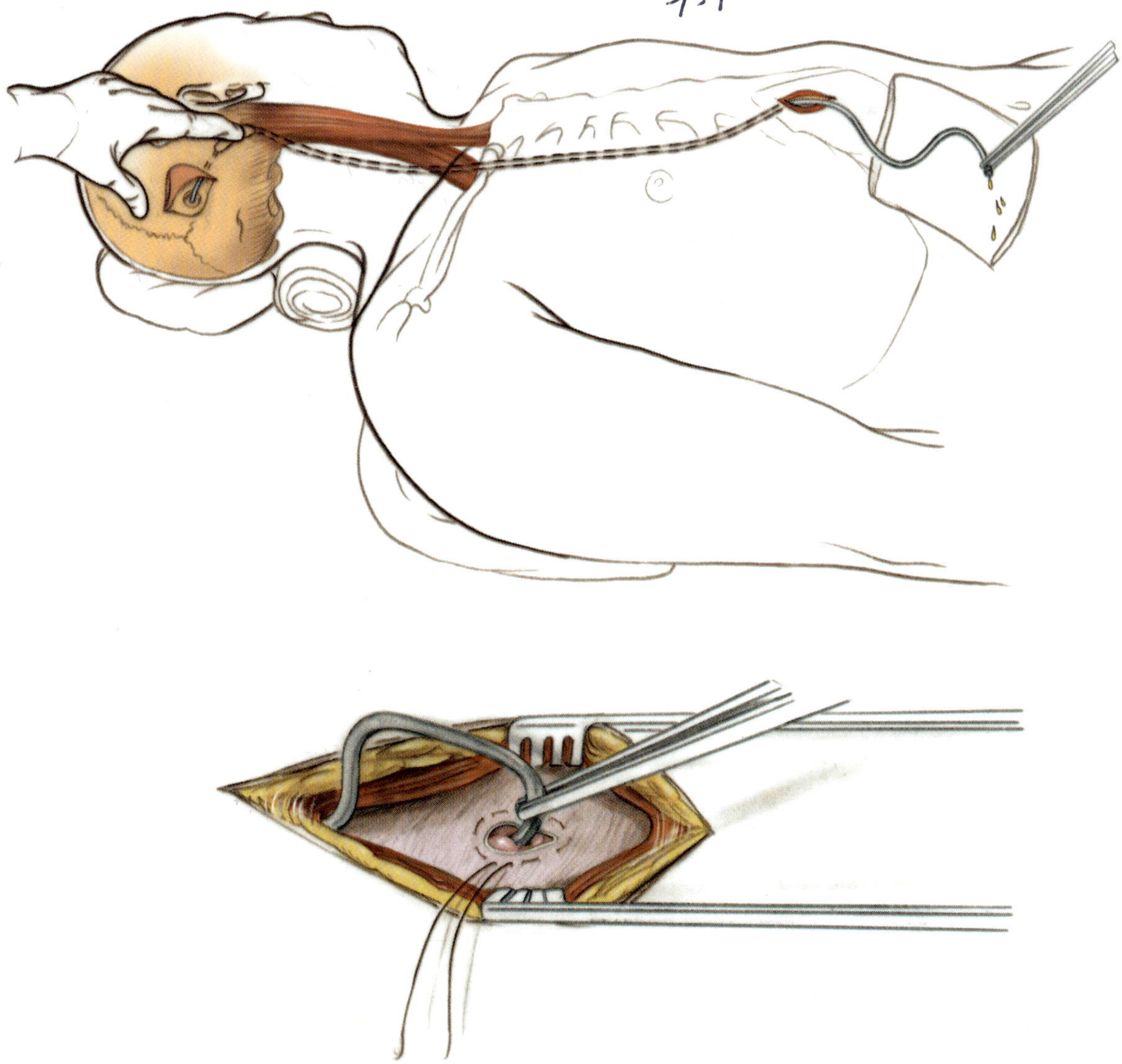

Figure 12–9.

Step 7. Often, the valve is connected to the shunt with an L-shaped connector. It is best to tack the valve to the adjacent pericranium with a small monofilament suture. The valve is pumped while the distal end is observed to make sure that there is expression of cerebrospinal fluid. Thereafter, approximately 25 cm of catheter is placed into the peritoneal cavity. All wounds should be closed in multiple layers. The use of absorbable monofilament instead of braided sutures may decrease the risk of shunt infection.

VENTRICULOATRIAL SHUNT

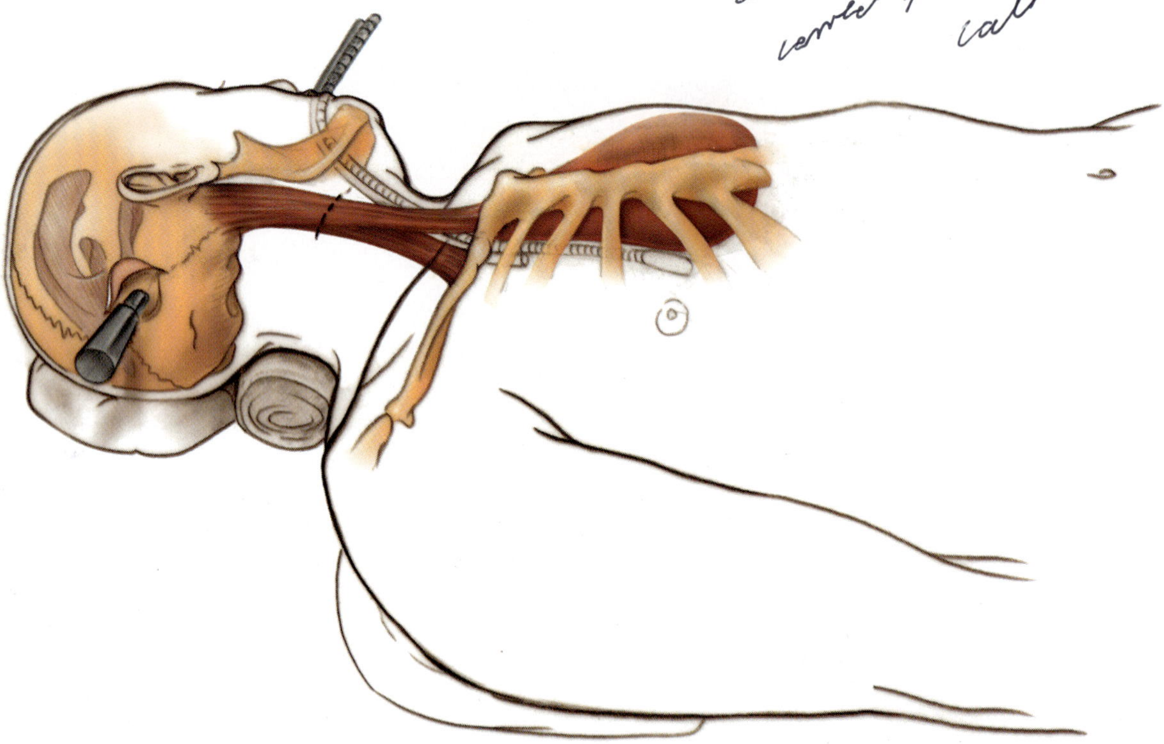

Figure 12–10.

Step 1. Illustrated here is the position for placement of a ventriculoatrial shunt. After induction, the anesthesiologist should insert a transesophageal echocardiography probe. This instrument can be quite useful in confirming the correct location of the atrial catheter within the right atrium. If transesophageal echocardiography is not available, other techniques are available to confirm correct catheter placement, including intraoperative radiography and electrocardiography. For the latter technique, an electrocardiographic clip is attached to the ventricular catheter, which is filled with saline. As the catheter is inserted from the superior vena cava into the right atrium, the P waves become progressively larger. As the catheter progresses into the right ventricle, the P waves become biphasic. At this point, the catheter is withdrawn back into the right atrium. It is important to fill the catheter with saline, because otherwise a current will not be conducted and the electrocardiogram will be useless. Overall, intraoperative transesophageal echocardiography is more accurate and easier to use. An additional advantage is that after the shunt has been placed, pumping of the valve causes an efflux of cerebrospinal fluid and air bubbles into the right atrium, which can be visualized on the echocardiogram, confirming shunt patency. The parietooccipital bur hole is placed 6 cm above the external occipital protuberance and 3 cm lateral from the midline. One of the more difficult aspects of a ventriculoatrial shunt procedure is identification of the facial vein. A horizontal incision two fingerbreadths below the angle of the jaw is used. The surgeon can usually palpate the notch created by the facial artery in the mandible, just anterior to the angle of the jaw. Running along with this artery is the facial vein. A horizontal incision should be placed below this notch.

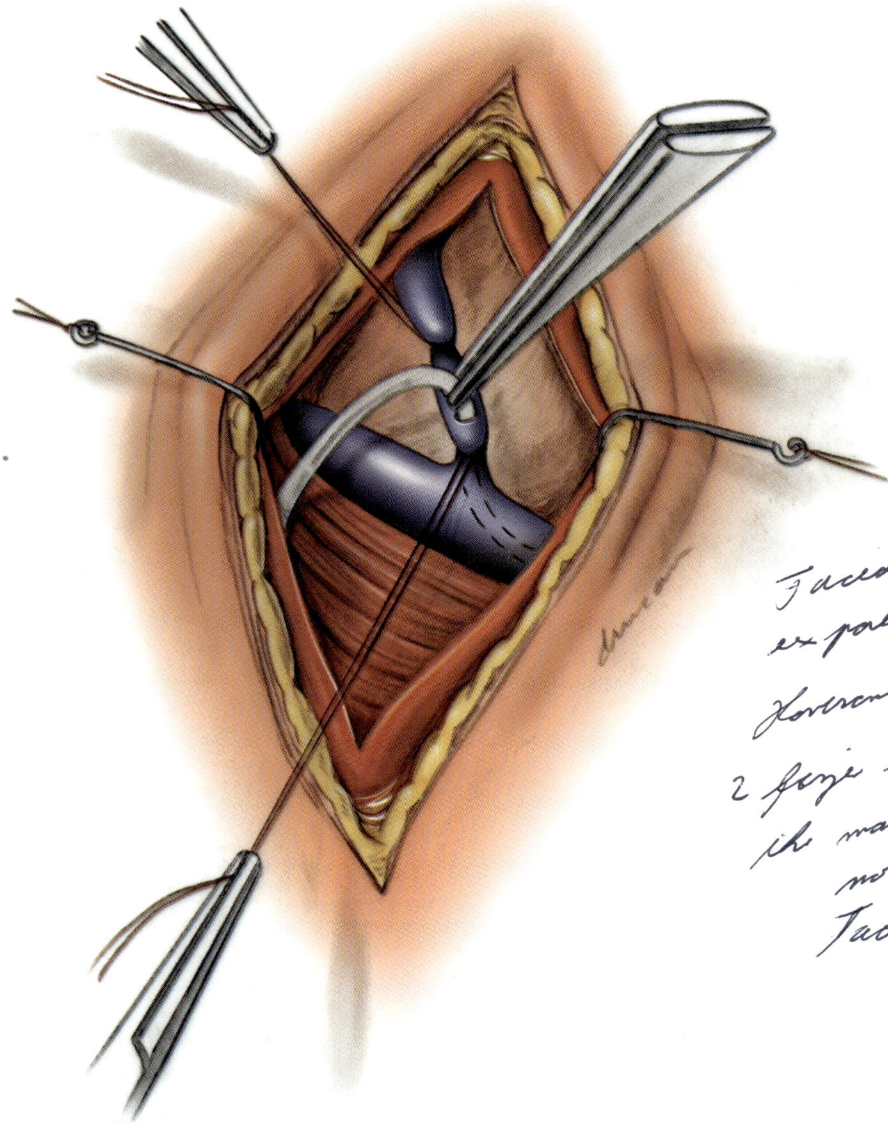

Figure 12–11.

Step 2. After the occipital bur hole has been placed, the facial vein is identified through a horizontal incision two fingerbreadths below the facial artery notch in the mandible. It is useful but not mandatory to isolate the facial vein down to its junction with the internal jugular vein. One suture is placed distally around the facial vein and held with some tension using a hemostat. A second loose suture is placed around the proximal facial vein under tension to prevent back bleeding. Thereafter, a linear incision is made, and the atrial catheter is inserted down into the jugular vein toward the superior vena cava. Before insertion, it is important to make sure that the atrial catheter has been flushed with saline and attached to a syringe. If significant resistance is met when passing the catheter, it is likely that the catheter is either in the external jugular vein or has turned laterally into the subclavian vein. The catheter should be withdrawn and reinserted. If resistance is met again, the cannulated vein should be dissected further to make sure that it is the facial vein that is entering the internal jugular vein.

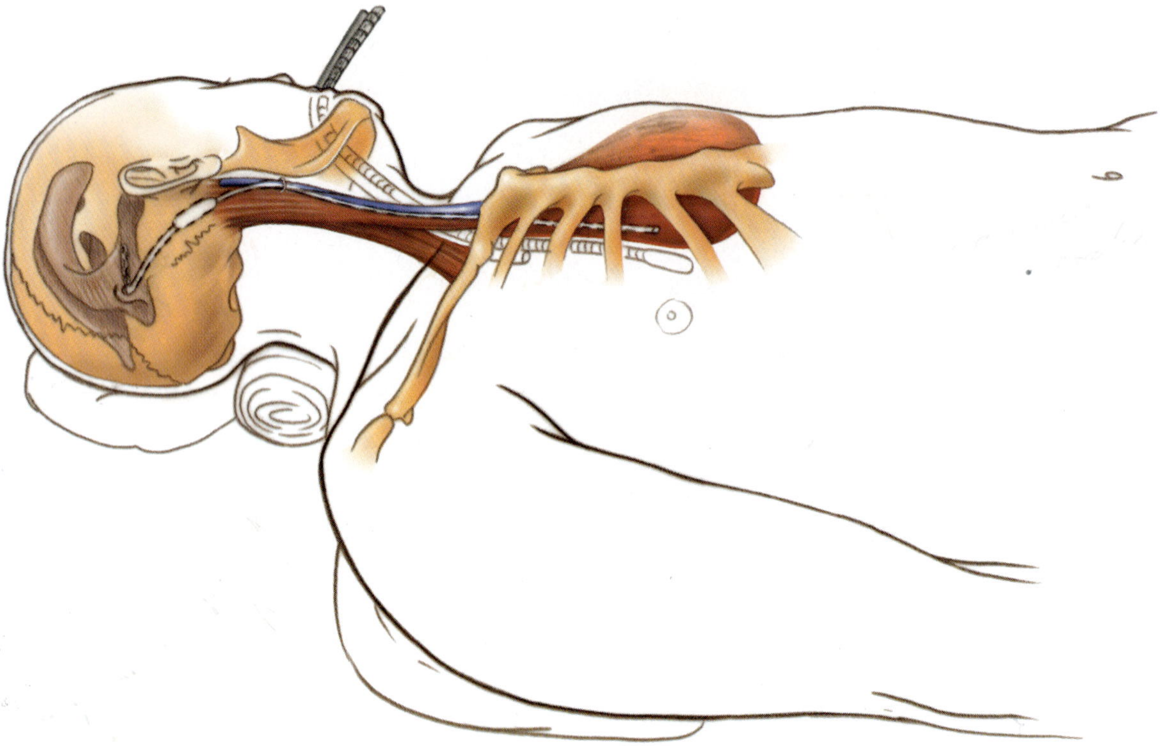

Figure 12–12.

Step 3. The atrial catheter is passed from the neck incision to the cranial incision through a subcutaneous tunnel previously made with a trocar. The valve is then attached. It is important during this time to make sure that the atrial catheter is filled with saline and occluded with a small atraumatic clamp to prevent blood from sitting in the atrial catheter and possibly forming thrombus. After the valve has been connected, it is useful to attach a manometer to ensure that the opening and closing pressures are correct. Next, the dura mater is cauterized and opened in a cross fashion. The pia mater is cauterized, and a ventricular catheter is inserted, similar to that described for placement of a ventriculoperitoneal shunt. This is hooked to the valve. The valve is then pumped to make sure there is normal compression and refilling. As mentioned above, echocardiography can be used to confirm shunt patency by visualizing air bubbles exiting from the atrial catheter.

THIRD VENTRICULOSTOMY

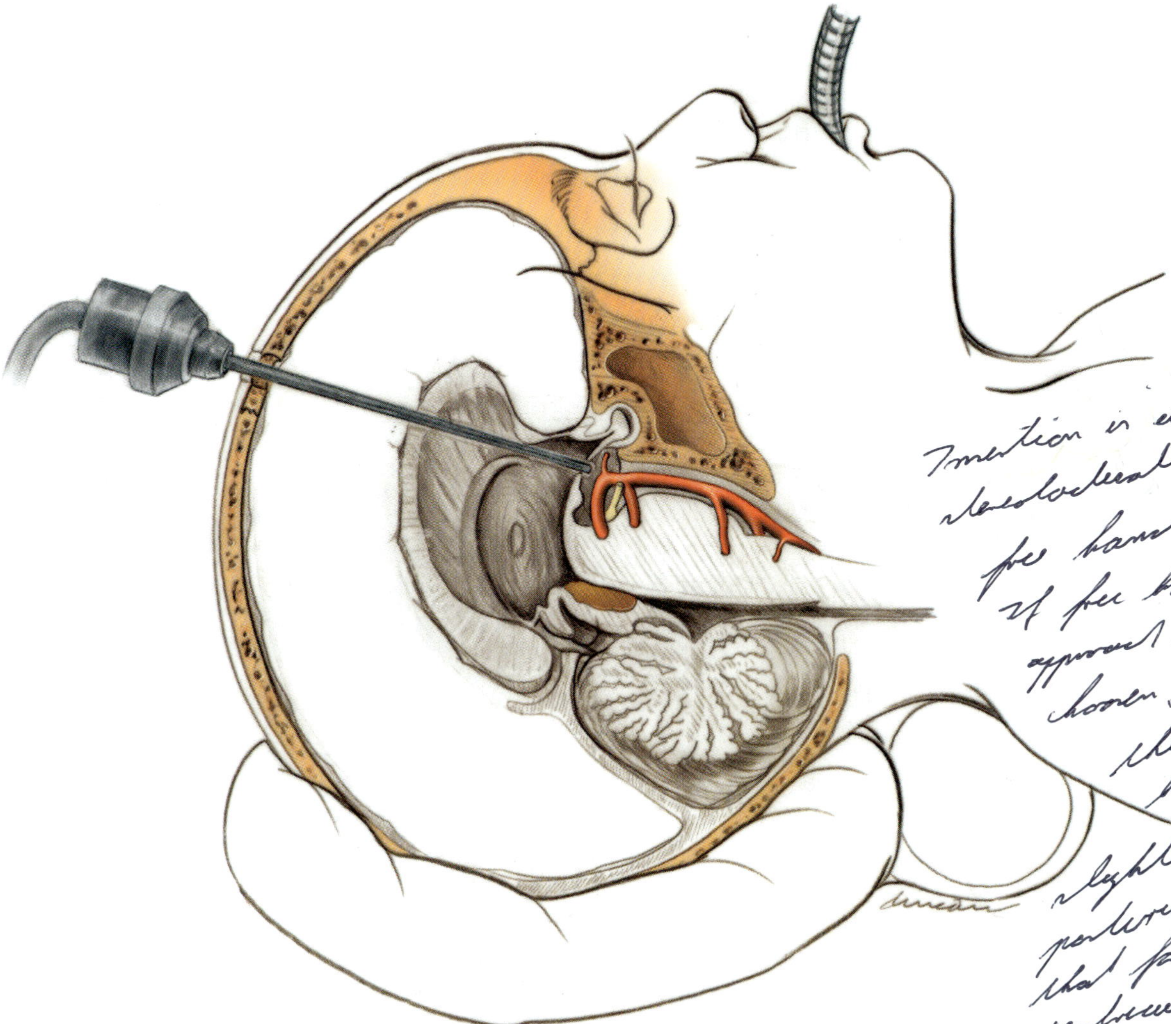

Figure 12–13.

Placement of a third ventriculostomy is an extremely useful procedure if the patient has obstructive hydrocephalus. In this illustration, the child has aqueductal stenosis due to a neoplastic process involving the tectal plate. **Step 1**. The patient is positioned supine with the head straight up, with 0 degrees of rotation, and slightly flexed. The use of stereotaxis increases the ease and success of a third ventriculostomy by permitting the surgeon to determine the best trajectory that allows the tuber cinereum to be punctured just anterior to the mammillary bodies by passing an instrument or scope through the foramen of Monro. Stereotaxis is especially useful when there is significant ventricular distortion caused by an inflammatory or neoplastic process. If a free hand approach is chosen, the bur hole is made 1 cm anterior to the coronal suture and 3 cm off the midline. This is slightly posterior to the bur hole used for placement of an external ventricular drain. A bur hole is used instead of a twist drill, because it is important to have some room to maneuver the scope in passing through the foramen of Monro.

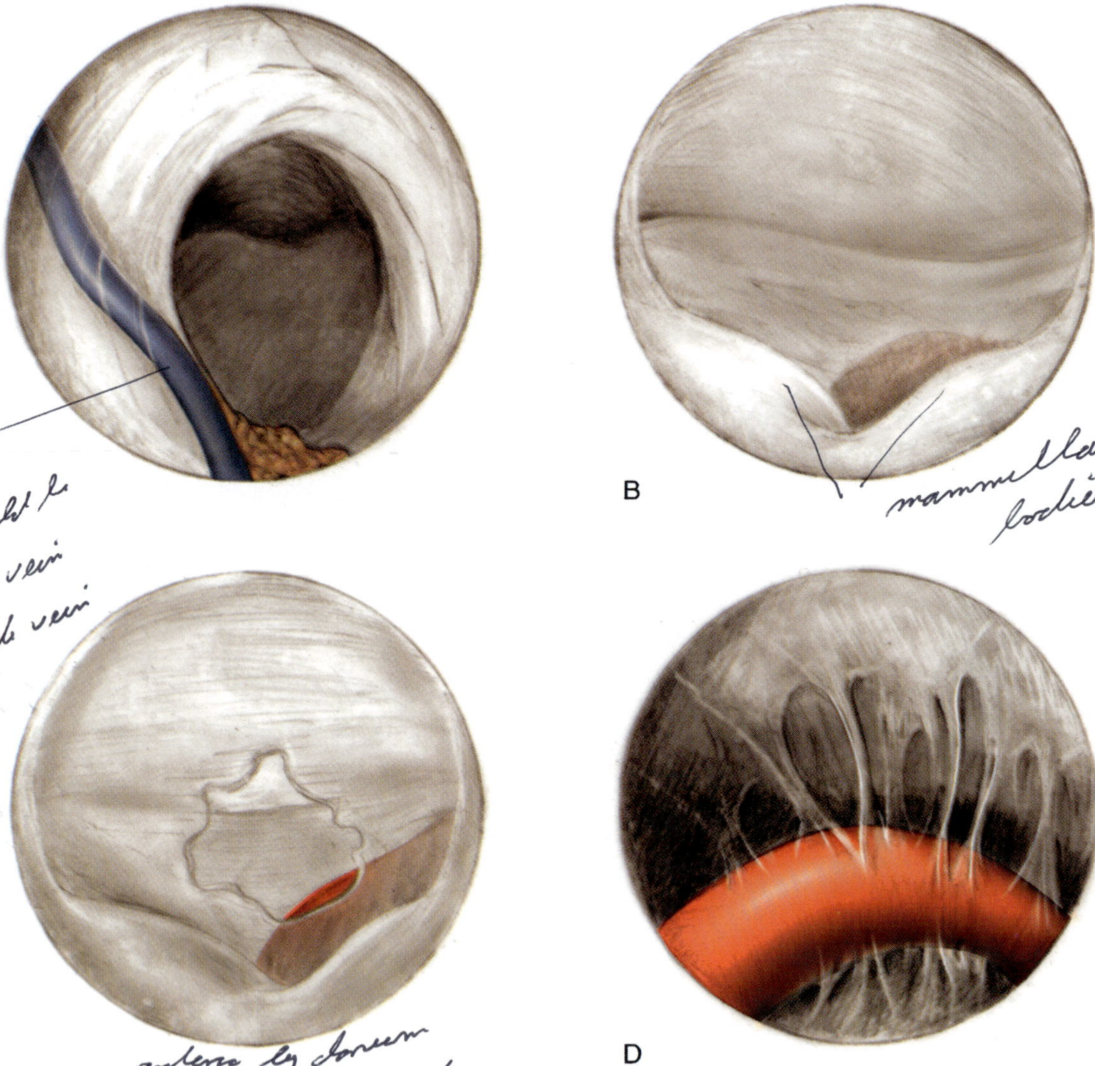

Figure 12–14.

Step 2. *A*, Illustrated here is the typical appearance of the right foramen of Monro as visualized through an endoscope. Usually, the foramen of Monro is enlarged because of the fornix being stretched. The typical intraventricular landmarks visualized include the medial septal vein, choroidal plexus, thalamostriate vein, and lateral anterior caudate vein. It is important not to traumatize the fornix as the endoscope passes through the foramen of Monro. Most endoscopes have a side port that can be used for irrigation. Irrigating through the scope as it is inserted through the foramen will gently push the fornix out of harm's way.

Step 3. *B*, As the scope is inserted through the foramen of Monro, the mammillary bodies become more visible. The point of puncture is anterior to the mammillary bodies in the tuber cinereum. Looking through the endoscope, anterior is the dorsum sellae and clivus. If the tuber cinereum is thin, the outline of either the basilar or the posterior cerebral artery may be seen.

Step 4. *C*, There are several techniques for puncturing the tuber cinereum. For example, the endoscope itself can be used. More sophisticated scopes have a side port that allows passage of a dilating balloon to enlarge the third ventriculostomy. Often, there is slight bleeding, which will stop with irrigation.

D, The endoscope can be inserted deeper to better visualize the basilar artery. Usually, there are strands of arachnoid between the clivus and the basilar artery. The surgeon should not attempt to cut or to lyse these arachnoid trabeculations. If the patient has a functioning shunt, it is important to ligate it to make sure that the flow of cerebrospinal fluid is directed through the third ventriculostomy to increase the likelihood of patency.

13

Percutaneous Procedures for Trigeminal Neuralgia

Copyright © 1999 Mayo Foundation.

Facial pain can be caused by many different disorders. It is essential that an accurate assessment of the pain be obtained before any treatment is initiated. The first step is a detailed history that includes a description of the onset, nature, location, and character of the pain and factors that either elicit or relieve the pain. On the basis of this information, it may be necessary to perform a computed tomographic or magnetic resonance imaging examination or to select laboratory studies to exclude neoplastic, infectious, or vascular causes of the pain. After this evaluation has been completed, neuralgic or non-neuralgic facial pain can be diagnosed in most patients.

Neuralgic facial pain is commonly classified as classic trigeminal neuralgia, trigeminal neuropathy, or atypical trigeminal neuralgia. Classic trigeminal neuralgia is characterized by intermittent, shock-like facial pains that can be exacerbated by various triggers. Patients with classic trigeminal neuralgia are pain-free between the episodes of facial pain. Patients with trigeminal neuropathy have a constant, unremitting pain that cannot be elicited with cutaneous triggering events. Atypical trigeminal neuralgia is defined as a combination of both episodic and constant facial pain.

Typical trigeminal neuralgia can be either idiopathic or secondary. Most authors believe that in idiopathic cases vascular compression of the dorsal root entry zone causes the trigeminal nerve to become hyperactive and dysfunctional. Secondary causes of trigeminal neuralgia include multiple sclerosis and tumors of the skull base that impinge on the trigeminal nerve or ganglion. For most patients with classic trigeminal neuralgia, medical management is successful in relieving pain for several years. However, if the patient becomes unresponsive to medical therapy or is unable to tolerate the side effects of the medications, surgical intervention may be required.

The goals of surgery for trigeminal neuralgia are twofold: one, to have the patient pain-free and not require medications after the procedure, and two, to minimize the chance of the tic pain converting into a differentiated pain syndrome such as anesthesia dolorosa. Microvascular decompression, as described in Chapter 8, is often recommended because it does not produce a destructive lesion in the trigeminal nerve or ganglion; thus, few patients have significant postoperative facial numbness. The incidence of anesthesia dolorosa is also quite low. However, many patients and some physicians are wary of the risks associated with a major intracranial procedure. Furthermore, many patients with trigeminal neuralgia are elderly and may be considered at increased risk for complications from general anesthesia. In these circumstances, less invasive techniques to treat the pain are desirable.

Several percutaneous techniques have been developed to treat pain by injuring the trigeminal ganglion. The modalities used to damage the ganglion include thermocoagulation by radio-frequency currents, chemical destruction with neurotoxic agents such as glycerol, and compression with a microballoon. Each procedure has its relative advantages and disadvantages. Of the percutaneous procedures, radio-frequency rhizotomy is associated with the lowest rate of pain recurrence. Studies have documented that pain-free outcomes are strongly associated with the degree of postoperative facial numbness after radio-frequency procedures. Thermal rhizotomy of the trigeminal nerve is associated with the highest incidence of anesthesia dolorosa. Glycerol rhizotomy is less likely to produce changes in facial sensation, and the incidence of postoperative differentiation pain is very low; however, the recurrence rate of pain has been estimated to range from 30 to 50 percent. Similar to thermal rhizotomy, the goal of balloon compression is facial numbness. Postoperative weakness of the masseter muscle occurs in approximately 25 percent of patients after ganglion compression.

Some physicians recommend injection into the peripheral facial nerves as a simple, effective means to treat facial pain. Although such procedures are generally considered palliative in nature, they offer many advantages, especially for an elderly patient with pain in a discrete region. The procedure is simple to perform, can be performed under local anesthesia, and has immediate results. The duration of pain relief is short, with a median duration of 6 to 12 months.

In contrast to the results of surgery for classic trigeminal neuralgia, in which approximately 90 percent of patients become pain-free, the results of peripheral procedures for patients with atypical facial neuralgias is poor. The mechanism of atypical facial neuralgia is thought to be located centrally in either the nucleus caudalis, the spinothalamic tract, or the ventral posteromedial nucleus of the thalamus. A few authors have reported good results after trigeminal tractotomy, mesencephalotomy, or thalamotomy for atypical facial neuralgias. In general, procedures aimed at either the trigeminal ganglion or nerve should not be performed on these patients.

ANATOMY

The successful completion of any peripheral trigeminal procedure depends on a thorough knowledge of the pertinent anatomy. The trigeminal nerve is the primary cutaneous sensory nerve of the head and face. The tactile and nociceptive fibers that compose the trigeminal nerve are axons of first-order sensory neurons with cell bodies in the trigeminal ganglion. The central processes of these sensory neurons synapse in either the main sensory nucleus or the spinal nucleus of the trigeminal nerve. The trigeminal (Gasserian) ganglion rests in a depression in the medial petrous temporal bone. A dural envelope surrounds the ganglion, producing a small cerebrospinal fluid cistern known as Meckel's cave. From the trigeminal ganglion emerge the three divisions of the trigeminal nerve. Each of these exits the cranium through foramina at the base of the skull: the ophthalmic division (V1) goes through the superior orbital fissure, the maxillary division (V2) goes through the foramen rotundum, and the mandibular division (V3) goes through the foramen ovale. After each division exits the skull, it divides further into the peripheral nerves that supply the skin of the head and face.

Percutaneous procedures aimed at the Gasserian ganglion require that the injurious agent (electrode, glycerol, or microballoon) be placed intracranially adjacent to the ganglion. Entrance into the intracranial space is achieved by passing a needle through the foramen ovale. If the tip of the needle is directed too medially, it will meet the lateral pterygoid plate and need to be repositioned. Fluoroscopic guidance facilitates the accurate and safe placement of the needle. Nearby foramina that can be penetrated inadvertently by the needle include the superior orbital fissure, carotid canal, and jugular fissure. Intraoperative fluoroscopy is also helpful in preventing the needle from penetrating too deep into the middle cranial fossa. Passage of the needle through the cheek and infratemporal fossa may injure branches of the external carotid artery. The usual consequence of such an injury is a hematoma of the cheek, but this resolves.

PERCUTANEOUS RETROGASSERIAN GLYCEROL RHIZOTOMY

Patients who are to have percutaneous retrogasserian glycerol rhizotomy are admitted to the hospital on the day of the operation. They are instructed to take their normal morning medications with a sip of water before coming to the hospital. However, aspirin or other nonsteroidal anti-inflammatory medications that may affect platelet function are not to be taken in the days preceding surgery. Preoperative studies are few. If the patient has no history of clotting difficulties, it is not necessary to perform coagulation studies or other blood tests.

Although general anesthesia is not required or desirable, intraoperative anesthetic management is crucial. An intravenous catheter is inserted while the patient is in the outpatient surgery area, and the patient is brought to the operating room or radiology suite. The patient's condition is monitored with intermittent cuff measurements of blood pressure, electrocardiography, and continuous pulse oximetry. Nasal oxygen is routinely given. To reduce anxiety, patients are often given a short-acting benzodiazepine (midazolam, 0.5-mg increments) upon arrival. Ideally, the patient will remain relaxed but awake and able to assist with positioning of the needle throughout the operation. Sometimes, it is also necessary to control pain with narcotics (fentanyl citrate, 25–50-μg increments). To reduce the chance of cardiac complications and hematoma formation, the patient's systolic blood pressure should be less than 150 mm Hg at the beginning of the procedure. Blood pressure greater than 150 mm Hg is generally associated with an anxious patient who will have difficulty with the procedure. In such cases, the operation is delayed until blood pressure can be brought under better control. Bradycardia and asystole can occur in response to placing the needle through the foramen ovale or to injecting the glycerol. Consequently, the anesthesiologist should be prepared to administer cholinergic blocking agents (atropine sulfate, 0.4 mg) if the patient has a significant vasovagal reaction. To minimize patient discomfort, either a short-acting barbiturate (methohexital sodium) or propofol (10–20 mg intravenous bolus) is given before the needle penetrates the foramen ovale. These measures are important to blunt cardiovascular responses during the procedure. Although rare, postoperative cardiac ischemia has been reported after percutaneous needle procedures for the treatment of trigeminal neuralgia.

PERCUTANEOUS GASSERIAN MICROCOMPRESSION

Percutaneous microcompression of the trigeminal ganglion developed by Mullan uses an approach to the foramen ovale similar to that for glycerol or radio-frequency rhizotomy. Under fluoroscopic control, an 18-gauge needle is initially used to locate the rim of the foramen ovale, then a blunt-tip 14-gauge needle is threaded over a wire stylet and inserted into the foramen ovale. Following radiographic confirmation, a #3 or #4 Fogarty catheter is passed through the 14-gauge needle into the foramen and inflated to 0.5 to 0.75 mL for 1 or 2 minutes. The pain relief following balloon compression is reported to be equal to that after glycerol rhizotomy. One disadvantage of this approach is the indiscriminate compression of the Gasserian ganglion, which may lead to hypesthesia (more apparent in V2 and V3 divisions of the trigeminal nerve).

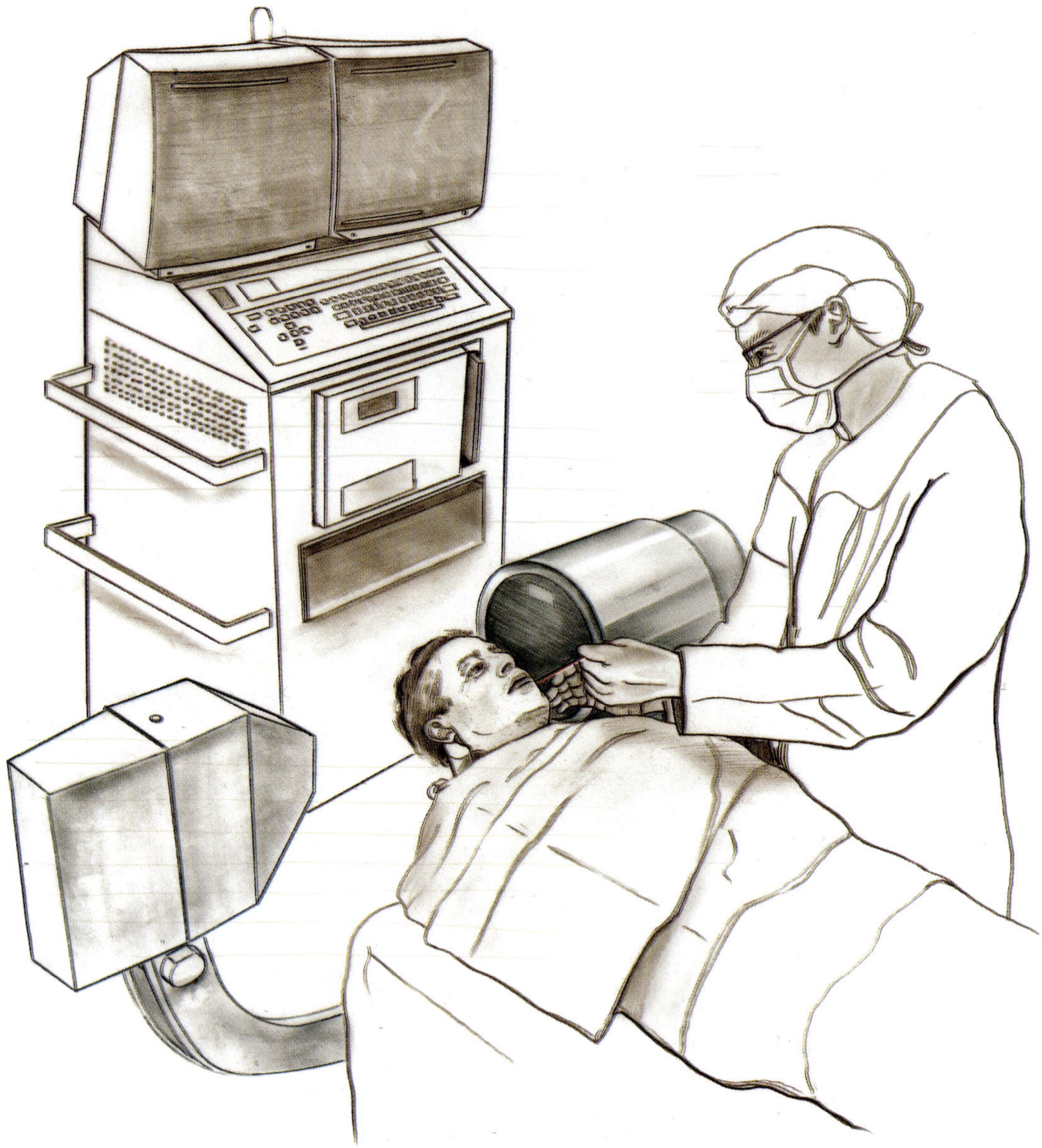

Figure 13–1.

The safe and effective completion of the procedure requires high-quality fluoroscopic guidance. Depending on the surgeon's preference, the procedure can be performed in either a radiology suite where multiplane fluoroscopy is available or in the operating room with C-arm fluoroscopy. All personnel in the operating room should be adequately protected with lead gowns from radiation exposure. The procedure begins with the patient supine on an operating room table. The patient's head is supported throughout the procedure by a standard cerebellar headholder.

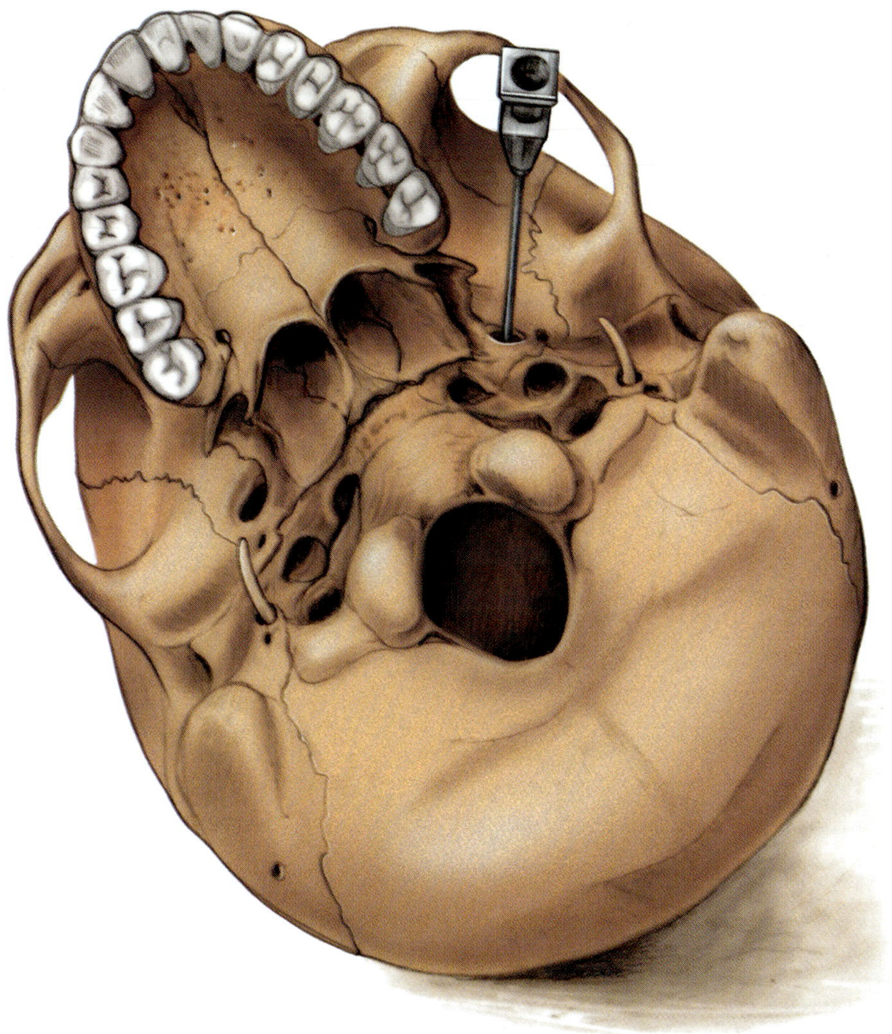

Figure 13–2.

Two primary methods are used to ensure accurate placement of the needle through the foramen ovale. The first, developed by Håkanson, uses a combination of anterior-posterior (AP) and lateral projections to guide needle placement. A true AP projection is obtained so that the petrous ridge appears at the level of the inferior orbital rim. The lateral projection should have the internal auditory canals superimposed on one another. The second method, advocated by Apfelbaum, depends on an oblique, submental projection to visualize the foramen ovale.

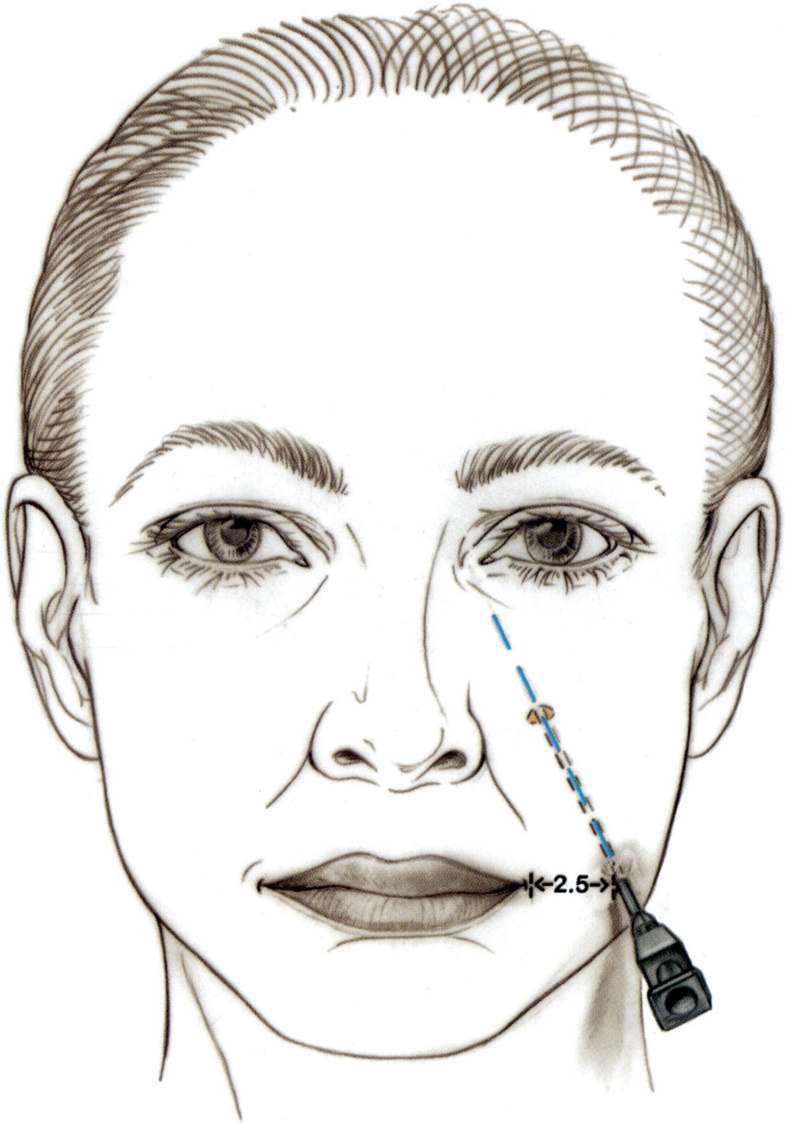

Figure 13–3.

After the patient has been properly positioned and the fluoroscopic equipment has been tested, the procedure can begin. Towels are placed on the chest and neck, and the face is cleansed with alcohol. The needle used for the procedure is a 20- or 22-gauge spinal needle, 90 mm long. The usual site of needle entry is 2.5 cm lateral to the angle of the mouth.

Figure 13–4.

From this point, two lines are drawn with a marking pen. They serve as the initial guide for needle placement. The first line directs needle placement in the AP and superior-inferior planes and extends along the zygoma to a point 25 mm in front of the ear. The second line directs needle placement in the left-right direction and extends to the ipsilateral medial canthus. The skin at the site of needle entry is infiltrated with lidocaine. As the needle is passed through the cheek, the surgeon places his or her finger in the patient's mouth to provide proprioceptive guidance and to ensure that the needle does not penetrate the oral cavity. If the needle enters the mouth, it is withdrawn and the procedure is started again with a new sterile needle. Fluoroscopy should be checked frequently to ensure the proper trajectory of the needle. Ideally, the needle can be placed on the first attempt, to minimize the chance of injury to a branch of the external carotid artery. If the trajectory needs to be corrected, it is best to withdraw the needle several centimeters before redirecting it in a new plane. When the needle is in the correct position at the base of the skull, the patient is given either a short-acting barbiturate or propofol to make penetration of the foramen ovale as painless as possible.

The needle is advanced in millimeter increments through the foramen ovale, using lateral fluoroscopy each time to guarantee that the needle is not advanced too far intracranially. The surgeon will feel the needle pass through the foramen, much like the passage of a spinal needle through the yellow ligament during a lumbar puncture. In a small percentage of patients (1 or 2 percent), it is impossible to advance the needle because of abnormalities at the base of the skull. In such cases, it may be helpful to switch to the oblique "needle" view to better visualize the foramen. After the position of the needle has been confirmed fluoroscopically, the stylet is removed to check for the flow of cerebrospinal fluid. The flow of cerebrospinal fluid does not confirm that the needle is in the cistern, because a lateral position can also result in brisk flow of this fluid from the subarachnoid space subtemporally. If cerebrospinal fluid flow is not observed, the needle can be advanced incrementally to the clival line. The absence of cerebrospinal fluid flow is generally due to scarring of the cistern caused by other previous procedures or placement of the needle into the nerve itself.

If the needle position is correct radiographically, with or without the flow of cerebrospinal fluid, the patient should be

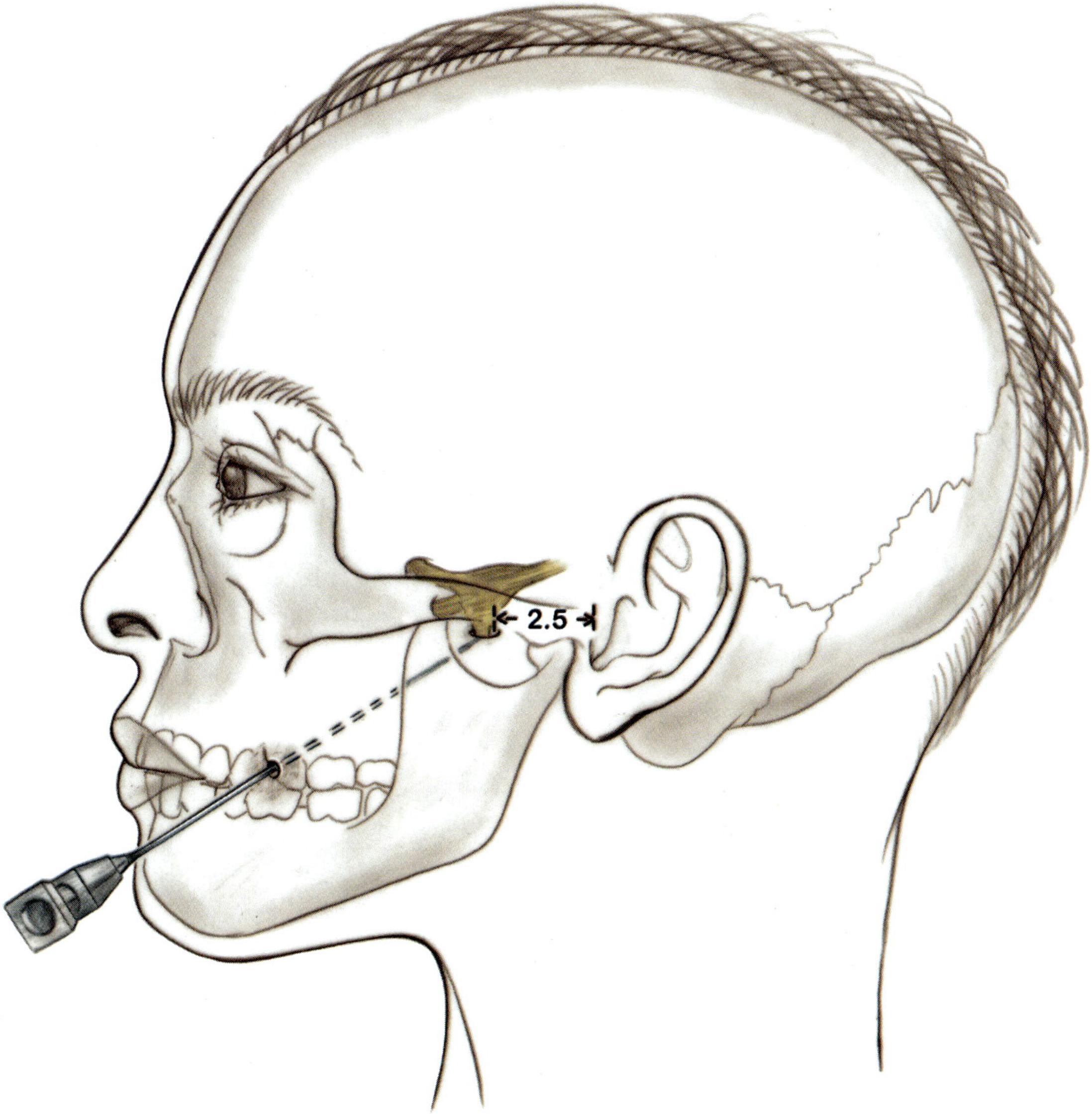

Figure 13–4 *Continued*

sat upright so contrast cisternography can be performed. Under lateral fluoroscopic guidance, a water soluble, nonionic contrast agent is injected with a 1-mL tuberculin syringe to confirm placement of the needle in the trigeminal cistern and to measure the volume of the cistern. The contrast agent is injected until it is seen to escape into the posterior fossa. The average volume of the cistern is approximately 0.25 mL (range, 0.1 to 0.5 mL). If injection of the contrast agent does not outline the cistern, the needle tip most likely lies subtemporally and needs to be repositioned more medially. After the position of the needle has been confirmed, the contrast agent is evacuated from the cistern by drainage through the needle or by returning the patient to a supine position, with the neck extended.

With the patient again in an upright position, the glycerol is mixed with sterile tantalum powder to provide a permanent marker of the trigeminal cistern. The glycerol-tantalum mixture is quite viscous, and a tight seal is necessary between the tuberculin needle and the syringe. The amount of glycerol injected is related to the location of the patient's pain. For patients with V3 pain, approximately one-half of the cistern is filled with glycerol; for V2 pain, approximately two-thirds; and for V1 pain, the cistern is filled completely. Tailoring the amount of glycerol injected to the patient's symptoms will decrease the incidence of postoperative facial numbness. After the glycerol has been injected, the needle and syringe are removed together and a small adhesive bandage is applied to the site of needle insertion. The patient is kept in the upright position with the neck slightly flexed for the first several hours after the operation to maximize the exposure of the ganglion and nerves to the glycerol. The patient is dismissed several hours later.

Patients often experience relief from pain in the first hours after the operation. Factors that predict a good result include easy penetration of the foramen ovale, free flow of cerebrospinal fluid, normal appearance of the trigeminal cistern, and ipsilateral V1 pain during the injection of glycerol. Patients are instructed to continue taking their preoperative medications until they notice a significant reduction in pain. At that point, the dosage of the medications is tapered slowly over the course of days to weeks. If the pain returns during the tapering, the patient is instructed to continue taking the medications at the lowest possible dosage that provides control of the symptoms.

PERIPHERAL NERVE INJECTIONS

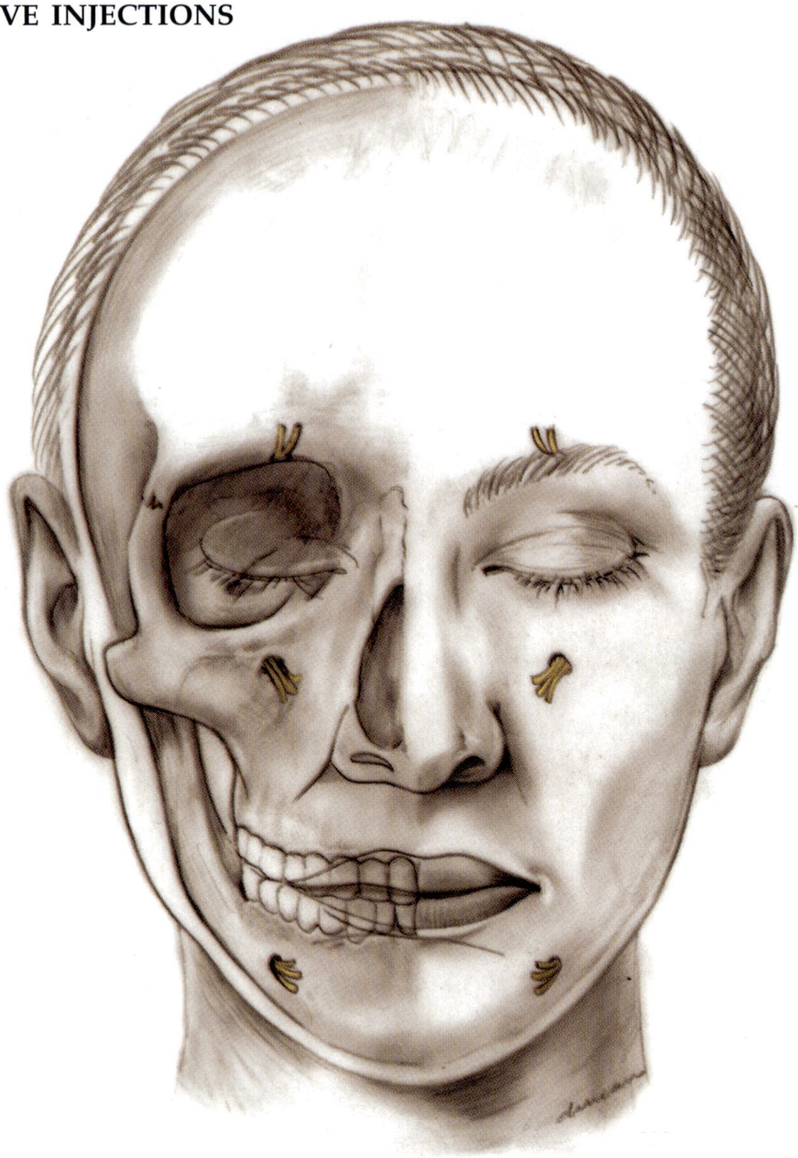

Figure 13–5.

Injection of absolute alcohol into one of the peripheral branches of the trigeminal nerve is often useful in elderly patients with pain localized to a discrete region. The procedure generally can be performed under local anesthesia in a physician's office. However, it often is more comfortable for the patient to have some anesthetic support to relieve anxiety and to minimize discomfort. Patients generally complain of paresthesias in the appropriate distribution whenever the needle is placed adjacent to the desired nerve. A test injection with a local anesthetic solution (lidocaine) is performed before the injection of alcohol. If the patient states that the pain relief is satisfactory, the injection is repeated with absolute alcohol (0.5 mL). No preoperative studies are needed.

The patient is placed in the supine position. The appropriate region is then cleansed with alcohol. For injection into the supraorbital and supratrochlear nerves, the medial one-third of the superior orbital rim is palpated for the supraorbital notch. After the overlying skin has been anesthetized, the needle is advanced into the supraorbital foramen in an inferior-superior direction and absolute alcohol is injected. The infraorbital nerve can be injected with alcohol at the infraorbital foramen. The foramen can be palpated at a point 1.5 cm lateral to the nasolabial fold and 1 cm below the inferior rim of the orbit. The needle should be advanced in an inferior-superior and slightly medial to lateral direction. For lower jaw pain, the mental nerve can be injected with alcohol where it exits the mental foramen. The mental foramen is often difficult to palpate. To estimate its position, a line is drawn through the supraorbital and infraorbital foramina onto the mandible. The needle is advanced in a superior-inferior and slightly lateral to medial direction. Again, to ensure a satisfactory clinical result, it is important that the patient report paresthesias in the expected distribution during needle placement before alcohol is injected. Injections into peripheral nerve can be repeated as required, although pain relief often is not as good after subsequent procedures.

Index

Page numbers in *italics* refer to figures.

C

D

E

F

M

N

O

P

R

S

T